# Anesthesia Oral Board Review

# Anesthesia Oral Board Review

## Knocking Out the Boards

*Second Edition*

Edited by
**Jessica A. Lovich-Sapola**
Cleveland Clinic, Cleveland, Ohio

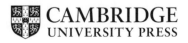

CAMBRIDGE
UNIVERSITY PRESS

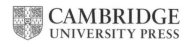

Shaftesbury Road, Cambridge CB2 8EA, United Kingdom

One Liberty Plaza, 20th Floor, New York, NY 10006, USA

477 Williamstown Road, Port Melbourne, VIC 3207, Australia

314–321, 3rd Floor, Plot 3, Splendor Forum, Jasola District Centre, New Delhi – 110025, India

103 Penang Road, #05–06/07, Visioncrest Commercial, Singapore 238467

Cambridge University Press is part of Cambridge University Press & Assessment, a department of the University of Cambridge.

We share the University's mission to contribute to society through the pursuit of education, learning and research at the highest international levels of excellence.

www.cambridge.org
Information on this title: www.cambridge.org/9781107498310

DOI: 10.1017/9781316181492

First Edition published 2010

Second Edition published 2023

Printed in the United Kingdom by TJ Books Limited, Padstow Cornwall

*A catalogue record for this publication is available from the British Library.*

*A Catologing-in-Publication data record for this book is available from the Library of Congress.*

*Library of Congress Cataloging-in-Publication Data*

ISBN 978-1-107-49831-0 Paperback

# Contents

Contents

## Section 7 Pediatric Anesthesia

## Section 8 Endocrine

## Section 9 Trauma Anesthesia

## Section 10 Emergency Events

## Section 11 Organ Transplant

## Section 12 Post-Anesthesia Care Unit

# Contributors

## Contributing Editors

### Editor

**Jessica A. Lovich-Sapola, MD, MBA, FASA**
Professor of Anesthesiology, Cleveland Clinic Lerner College
of Medicine at Case Western Reserve University School
of Medicine
Anesthesiology Institute at Cleveland Clinic, Cleveland, Ohio

### Associate Editor

**Brian M. Sapola, BS, MA**
Associate Lecturer, Graduate Nursing, Nurse Anesthesia
Associate Lecturer, Allied Health, University of Akron, Akron,
Ohio
Part-Time Faculty, Graduate Nursing, Nurse Anesthesia,
Youngstown State University, Youngstown, Ohio
Adjunct Instructor of Biology, Cuyahoga Community College,
Cleveland, Ohio

## Contributors

**Konstantinos Alfaras-Melainis, MD, MSc**
Assistant Professor, University of Pittsburgh Medical Center,
Pittsburgh, PA

**Ali G. Ali, DO**
Assistant Professor of Anesthesiology, Case Western Reserve
University, Cleveland, OH
Metrohealth System, Cleveland, OH

**Jonathan A. Alter, MD**
Assistant Professor, Case Western Reserve University School
of Medicine, Cleveland, OH
Metrohealth Medical Center, Cleveland, OH

**Brendan J. Astley, MD**
Assistant Professor, Case Western University, Cleveland, OH
MetroHealth Medical Center, Cleveland, OH

**Sennaraj Balasubramanian, MBBS, MD, FCARCSI, EDRA**
Assistant Professor of Anesthesiology,
Washington University School of Medicine in St. Louis, St.
Louis, Missouri

**Kara M. Barnett, MD, FASA**
Associate Clinical Member, Memorial Sloan Kettering Cancer
Center, New York, NY

**Elvera L. Baron, MD, PhD, FASA, FASE**
FASE Associate Professor, Case Western Reserve University
School of Medicine, Cleveland, OH
Cardiothoracic Anesthesiologist, Louis Stokes Cleveland VA
Medical Center, Cleveland, VA

**Michael Dale Bassett, MD**
Assistant Professor, Case Western Reserve University,
Cleveland, OH
MetroHealth Hospital Systems, Cleveland, OH

**Nicholas Bigler, DO**
Resident, South Pointe Hospital Cleveland Clinic Foundation,
Cleveland, OH
Anesthesia Institute Cleveland Clinic, Cleveland, OH

**Vera V. Borzova, MD, FASA**
Assistant Professor, Cleveland Clinic Lerner College of
Medicine
Pediatric Anesthesiologist, Cleveland Clinic Foundation,
Cleveland, OH

**Chris P. Boutton, MSN, CRNA**
MetroHealth Medical Center, Cleveland, OH

**Taylor Bowman, DO**
Anesthesia Resident CA-2, Cleveland Clinic South Pointe
Hospital, Cleveland, OH

**Cory Rene Brune, DO**
Staff Anesthesiologist, Jefferson City Medical Group, Jefferson
City, MO

**Monica Cheriyan, MD, MPH**
Program Director, Obstetric Anesthesiology Fellowship
Clinical Assistant Professor of Anesthesiology, Anesthesiology
Institute – Regional & Obstetric Anesthesia, Cleveland Clinic,
Cleveland, OH

**Elliott Chiartas, DO**
Anesthesiology Resident, Cleveland Clinic-South Pointe
Hospital, Cleveland, OH

Anesthesiology Institute at the Cleveland Clinic, Cleveland, OH

**Melvyn J. Y. Chin, MD**
Anesthesiologist, Anesthesia Associates of Rochester, P.C., Rochester, NY

**Samuel DeJoy, DMD, MD, FASA**
Assistant Professor, Case Western Reserve University School of Medicine, Cleveland, OH
Director, Neuro-Anesthesiology, MetroHealth Medical Center, Cleveland, OH

**Jagan Devarajan, MD, MBA, FASA**
Associate Professor of Anesthesiology, Cleveland Clinic Lerner College of Medicine at Case Western Reserve University School of Medicine, Cleveland, OH
Department of Regional Practice Anesthesiology, Cleveland Clinic, OH

**Varun Dixit, MD**
Cardiac Anesthesiologist, Chippenham Hospital, Richmond Virginia

**Wesley G. Dougall, MD**
Anesthesiology Resident, Case Western Reserve University, Cleveland, OH
Metrohealth Medical Center, Cleveland, OH

**Jennifer Eismon, MD**
Assistant Professor of Anesthesiology, Cleveland Clinic Lerner College of Medicine at Case Western Reserve University School of Medicine, Cleveland, OH
Anesthesiologist at the Anesthesiology Institute at Cleveland Clinic, Cleveland, OH

**Dylan Elder, DO**
Anesthesia Resident, Cleveland Clinic, Cleveland, OH

**Erica Fagelman, MD**
Assistant Professor, Department of Anesthesiology, Perioperative and Pain Medicine, The Icahn School of Medicine at Mount Sinai at Mount Sinai Hospital, New York, NY

**Garietta Falls, MD**
Assistant Professor, Case Western Reserve School of Medicine, Cleveland, OH
Metrohealth System, Cleveland, OH

**Emma Fu, MD**
Anesthesiology Resident, Case Western Reserve University, Cleveland, OH
MetroHealth System, Cleveland, OH

**Meaghan Fuhrmann, MD, MA**
Pediatric Anesthesiology Fellow, Cincinnati Children's Hospital Medical Center

**John George, MD, MS, FASA**
Assistant Professor of Anesthesiology, Cleveland Clinic Lerner College of Medicine, Cleveland Clinic, Cleveland, OH

**Adrienne Gomez, MD**
Chief Resident, Case Western Reserve University, Cleveland, OH
MetroHealth Medical Center, Cleveland, OH

**Rushi Gottimukkala, MD**
Anesthesia Resident, MetroHealth Medical Center, Cleveland, Ohio

**Daniel Guay, MD**
Anesthesia Resident, MetroHealth Medical Center, Cleveland, OH

**Ryan J. Gunselman, MD**
Education Director, Department of Anesthesiology, HCA Healthcare|Mission Health, North Carolina Division

**Maureen S. Harders, MD**
Assistant Professor, Case Western Reserve University School of Medicine, Cleveland, OH
Director of Anesthesia Operations, Anesthesiologist, at MetroHealth Medical Center, Cleveland, OH

**Cassandra Hoffman, MD**
Pediatric Anesthesiologist, Akron Children's Hospital, Akron, Ohio

**Mariam Naeem Ibrahim, MD, MBBS**
Anesthesiology Resident, MetroHealth Medical Centre, MetroHealth Medical Centre, Cleveland, OH

**Marcos A. Izquierdo, MD**
Assistant Professor, Case Western Reserve University, Cleveland, OH
MetroHealth Medical Center, Cleveland, OH

**Kaitlyn Jakubec, MSN, CRNA**
Certified Registered Nurse Anesthetist at Cleveland Clinic, Avon Hospital at Richard E. Jacobs Campus, Cleveland, OH

**Mathew A. Joy, MD**
Assistant Professor of Anesthesiology, Case Western Reserve University School of Medicine, Cleveland, OH
Anesthesiologist, MetroHealth Medical Center, Cleveland, OH

**Robert St. Jules, MD**
Assistant Professor, Division of Liver Transplantation, Department of Anesthesiology, Perioperative and Pain Medicine, The Icahn School of Medicine at Mount Sinai Hospital, New York, NY

**Zaid H. Jumaily, MD, MSc**
Adult Cardiothoracic Anesthesia Fellow, New York University, New York, NY
Langone Health, New York, NY

**Saima Karim, DO, FACC, FHRS**
Associate Professor of Medicine, Case Western Reserve University, Cleveland, OH
MetroHealth Medical Center, Cleveland, OH

**Maureen Keshock, MD MHSA, FASA**
Assistant Professor, Cleveland Clinic Lerner College Medicine, Cleveland, OH
Medina Hospital, Medina, OH,
Cleveland Clinic Foundation, Cleveland, OH

**Casey L. Kohler, MD**
Assistant Professor, Case Western Reserve University, Cleveland, OH
MetroHealth Medical Center, Cleveland, OH

**Hoaky Lam, DO**
Anesthesia Resident, Cleveland Clinic South Pointe Hospital, Warrensville Heights, OH

**Michael Leeds, MD**
Anesthesiology Resident, Case Western Reserve University School of Medicine, Cleveland, OH
MetroHealth Medical Center, Cleveland, OH

**Serle Levin, MD**
Chairman, Regional Practice Anesthesiology, Anesthesiology Institute, Cleveland Clinic, Cleveland, OH

**Jessica A. Lovich-Sapola, MD, MBA, FASA**
Professor of Anesthesiology Cleveland Clinic Lerner College of Medicine at Case Western Reserve University School of Medicine
Anesthesiology Institute at Cleveland Clinic, Cleveland, Ohio

**Jocelyn Loy, MD**
Assistant Professor of Anesthesiology, Case Western Reserve University School of Medicine, Cleveland, OH
Anesthesiologist, MetroHealth Medical Center, Cleveland, OH

**Vijay R. Mohan, DO**
Anesthesia Resident, Cleveland Clinic – South Pointe Hospital, Cleveland, Ohio

**Jeffrey Neurock, DO**
Medical Director of Anesthesiology, Anesthesiology Associate Program Director, Cleveland Clinic – South Pointe Hospital, Warrensville Heights, OH

**Jodi-Ann Oliver, MD**
Associate Professor, Department of Anesthesiology and Perioperative Medicine, Division of Anesthesiology, Critical Care and Pain Medicine, The University of Texas MD Anderson Cancer Center, Houston, Texas

**Lori-Ann Oliver, MD**
Assistant Professor, Cleveland Clinic Lerner College of Medicine, Cleveland, OH
Anesthesiology Institute at Cleveland Clinic, Cleveland, OH

**Brian M. Osman, MD**
Associate Professor of Anesthesiology, Department of Anesthesiology, Perioperative, Medicine, and Pain Management, University of Miami Miller School of Medicine, Miami, FL

UHealth Tower, University of Miami Health System, Miami, FL

**Kristen Oswald, MSN, CRNA**
Nurse Anesthetist, Cleveland Clinic, Cleveland, Ohio

**Neel Pandya, MD**
Anesthesiologist, Buena Vista Anesthesia Medical Group, Pasadena, CA

**John L. Parker, DO**
Resident, Department of Anesthesiology, Case Western Reserve University, Cleveland, OH
MetroHealth Medical Center, Cleveland, OH

**Fouseena Pazheri, MD**
Assistant Professor, School of Medicine, Case Western Reserve University, Cleveland, OH
Metro Health Medical Center, Cleveland, OH

**Cristian M. Prada, MD**
Assistant Professor, Case Western Reserve University School of Medicine, Cleveland, OH
MetroHealth Medical Center, Cleveland, OH

**Michael Prokopius, MD, MBA, FACS, CPPS**
Associate Professor of Ophthalmology, University of Cincinnati College of Medicine, Cincinnati, OH
UC Health and the Cincinnati VA Medical Center, Cincinnati, OH

**Aditya Reddy, MD**
Cardiac Anesthesiologist, St. Francis-Emory Healthcare, Columbus, Georgia

**Quratulain Samoon, MD, MRCS**
Assistant Professor, University of Pittsburg School of Medicine, Pittsburg, PA
Associate Director, Division of Cardiac Anesthesia, UPMC Altoona, Altoona, PA

**Brian M. Sapola, BS, MA**
Associate Lecturer, Graduate Nursing, Nurse Anesthesia
Associate Lecturer, Allied Health, University of Akron, Akron, OH
Part-Time Faculty, Graduate Nursing, Nurse Anesthesia Youngstown State University, Youngstown, OH
Adjunct Instructor of Biology, Cuyahoga Community College, Cleveland, OH

**Kamaljit K. Sidhu, MD**
Assistant Professor, Department of Physical Medicine and Rehabilitation, University of Rochester, Rochester, NY

**Maninder Singh, MBBS, MD, MSc, FRCPC**
Assistant Professor, Metrohealth Medical Center, Cleveland, OH

**Winston Singleton, MD, MHI**
Fellow, Pain Medicine, The Ohio State University, Columbus, OH

**Augusto Torres, MD**
Assistant Professor, Case Western Reserve University School of Medicine, Cleveland, OH

**Luis A. Vargas-Patron, MD**
Fellow in Pediatric Anesthesiology, Boston Children's Hospital, Boston, MA
Clinical Fellow in Anesthesia, Harvard Medical School, Boston, MA

**Karl Wagner, MD, FASA**
Associate Professor, Case Western Reserve University School of Medicine, Cleveland, OH
Bel-Park Anesthesia Associates, Youngstown, OH

**Brian Wheatley, CAA**
Certified Anesthesiologist Assistant, MetroHealth System, Cleveland, OH

Simulation Instructor, Case Western Reserve University, Cleveland, OH

**Andrew Yurkonis, MD**
Resident Physician, Case Western Reserve University, Cleveland, OH
Metrohealth Medical Center, Cleveland, OH

**Sarah Zach, MSN, APRN-CRNA**
Metrohealth Medical Center, Cleveland, OH

**Sierra Ziska, DO**
Resident, South Pointe Hospital, Cleveland Clinic Foundation, Cleveland, OH

# Acknowledgments

I want to especially thank my wonderful husband, Brian, and my two great kids, Rachel and Jeremy, for allowing me the time to work on this project. They understand how important it is for me to help my colleagues to not only pass this exam and become board certified, but also become amazing anesthesiologists.

To all of the authors and consulting editors, I appreciate all of your time and hard work, more than you could imagine. This book would not have been possible without all of your help. Thank you!

I want to send a special thanks to my father, James Lovich, and son, Jeremy Sapola, who put in hours of their time to draw many of the book's illustrations.

I also want to thank the anesthesia department at MetroHealth Medical Center in Cleveland, Ohio, for helping me to become the anesthesiologist I am today. Also, I want to thank my new department at the Cleveland Clinic for supporting me on the continued journey of my career.

# Letter from the Associate Editor

I would like to make a few comments about Dr. Lovich-Sapola – about the person, the physician, and the professional – to give you, the reader, some insight into how this book has come about, my role as assistant editor, and our intended purpose for this book.

First, let me introduce you to "Jessica," as I call her. Of course, I could tell you about how we met, got married, had two beautiful children, and so on, but what is important to you is this: I have never met a more ambitious learner than Jessica. That is how this book came about. She was so intent on mastering the ABA oral examination that when she was studying she took meticulous notes on every possible question the examiners could ask. She became infatuated with that test. Of course, she passed and became board certified. But then she had a bunch of notes, and she formulated these into case studies and reviews that she shared with her residents and candidates for the test. The residents said, "This could be a book, Dr. Lovich." And that's how this book happened.

If you have read the list of editors and contributors, you might be wondering why I'm the associate editor for the book. You might be saying, "This guy is not a board-certified anesthesiologist. He's not even a doctor!" I do teach physiology to nurse anesthesia students, but I've only been in an operating room as a patient. So, why did she ask me, other than for the sake of convenience?

Well, I have something in common with you. We're both *not* board-certified anesthesiologists! I have edited this book to make each chapter have the same format and have them be independently readable and understandable. I wanted this book to introduce the science, the physiology, the acronyms, and the materials and methods in a way that makes sense. Therefore, not only is this book intended to be the must-have anesthesia oral board review book for the ABA candidate, but it should be an invaluable reference for the anesthesia resident as well as preparation for medical students or anesthetist students on an anesthesiology rotation at a hospital. I was the medical knowledge litmus test for my wife. I made sure that this book didn't intimidate you or confuse you by assuming you know all of the anesthesia acronyms. She made sure that it didn't insult your anesthesia knowledge. Both of us want you to become a competent, board-certified anesthesiologist.

If you are a medical student and you are going into an anesthesia rotation, you can look up cases and read the clinical issues so that you know what's going on in the operating room. If you are a PGY-1 intern, this book will give you some background knowledge that you can use for CA-1 anesthesia residency day one. If you are an anesthesia resident, you can read the Knockout Treatment Plan to be knowledgeable for when the attending starts grilling you. And, of course, to the ABA candidates, you want to read this entire book, including the TKO sections that tell you how to approach the answer on the day of your oral exam in order to satisfy the examiners and pass. In fact, you're going to do more than pass – you're going to KNOCK IT OUT!

**Brian M. Sapola**

# How to Use This Book

This book is an anesthesia oral board review book. I have tried to cover all of the essential topics required to pass the anesthesia applied exams. It does not have every question that you could be asked, nor is it exhaustively complete. This book should be used as a guide to understand and memorize facts so that you can easily discuss the topics as an anesthesia consultant. For a more in-depth understanding of the topics, the major textbooks or journals should be referenced. However, you should know all of the information presented in this book like the back of your hand. The more prepared you are, the easier it will be for you to think on your feet during the actual exam. Memorizing this book will not guarantee a passing score. You must take this knowledge and practice, practice, practice. The key to passing the oral boards is oral preparation. You must take this basic knowledge and then practice answering questions out loud. Study hard. Good luck!

# Format

Each chapter starts with a sample case. This is an example of how the topic may be presented on the real exam. The clinical issues section covers specific details that require your time to understand, learn, and memorize. The final section is the KO treatment plan. This section usually references the sample case. It gives you a written dialogue demonstrating how you could answer the sample case questions on the actual exam. Prior to reading this section, try to talk out loud about what you would say and do in the sample scenario. Then read this section. At times, there will be TKO sections that stress the points that you need to memorize in order to pass the exam.

# Applied Exam Tips for Success

## Criteria for Becoming a Board-Certified Anesthesiologist

1. Complete an approved anesthesia residency accredited by the ACGME.
2. Pass the ABA Basic and Advanced Written Board Exams.
3. Pass the ABA Applied Exams: Standardized Oral Exam (SOE) and the Objective Structured Clinical Exam (OSCE).
4. Have adequate physical and sensory faculties.
5. Be free from the influence of or dependency on chemical substances.
6. Have no felony on record.

## Standardized Oral Exam

1. Two 35-minute sessions
2. Assessment of your judgment, adaptability, and organization

## Starting Note

1. You walk in the door **passing**.
2. You have 70 minutes to **not** prove otherwise to the examiners.
3. Statistically, your best chance for passing the exam is the first time you take it.
4. The ABA's general recommendations are:
   a. Study, especially the topics you are the least comfortable with.
   b. Practice out loud daily.
   c. Use your daily cases as a chance to talk though your plan.
   d. Read journal articles.

## Objective Structured Clinical Exam

1. Seven eight-minute stations
2. Four minutes between each session
3. Four stations assess professional communication.
4. Three stations evaluate technical competency.

## Dress Code

1. Men: coat and tie
2. Women: office attire
3. I recommend a suit for men.
4. Most women also wear a dark pants suit.

## Behavior

1. Maintain good eye contact.
2. Speak up.
3. Maintain good posture.
4. Act professionally.
5. Do not argue with the examiners.
6. Give the examiners a firm handshake at the beginning and the end of the exam, even if you feel that you did poorly.
7. Avoid slang and informality.
8. Don't play with your pen or jewelry.
9. Talk with the examiners like you are a colleague.
10. Do not talk down to the examiners or be overly cocky or smug.

## What to Bring to the Exam

1. Basically nothing
2. You can't bring anything into the room except a pen and your identification.

## Exam Rooms

1. Every room is adjusted for equal lighting and temperature.
2. In each room you are given water, a pen, and a piece of paper.
3. The examiners will verify the case with you.
4. They will check your wrist band.
5. The examiners will introduce themselves to you.
   a. At this time you can switch rooms if you feel that you know an examiner.
   b. There may be an observer in the room who does not grade you.

## Exam

1. The exam is based on general knowledge of all anesthesia-related fields.
2. The examiners follow a strict script.

## Who Writes the Exams?

1. Practicing anesthesiologists who serve as examiners submit the cases.
2. The ABA takes care to ensure reasonable content sampling.

## What Facts Do They Expect the Examinee to Know?

1. In-depth knowledge of all drugs used and their effects on normal and abnormal body functions
2. Pathogenesis
3. Alternate methods of management
4. Mechanism of drug action
5. Methods of measurement including routine lab studies and normal measurements
6. Ability to anticipate, diagnose, and provide rational therapy for any complications that are likely to arise

## Format for SOE

1. Briefing session
2. Two parts, 35 minutes each

## Part A

1. 10 minutes to look at the information. Take notes.
2. Intra-operative: 10 minutes (senior examiner)
3. Post-operative/critical care: 15 minutes (junior examiner)
4. Three extra cases: 10 minutes (senior examiner)

## Part B

1. 10 minutes outside the exam room to look at the case. Take notes.
2. Pre-operative: 10 minutes (senior examiner)
3. Intra-operative: 15 minutes (junior examiner)
4. Three extra cases: 10 minutes (senior examiner)

## Audits of the Exam

1. The actual exam questions are graded by the examiner for content and difficulty prior to giving the exam.
   a. Content: excellent, good, acceptable, marginal
   b. Difficulty: too difficult, appropriate level of difficulty, or too easy

2. This score is also used in the final grading.

## Examiners Are Briefed on Their Roles

1. They get the exam the night before.
2. They are able to look up the general topics.
3. They are told to limit their preparatory research.

## What the Examiners Know About You

1. Your name
2. That's it!

## Audits of the Examiners

1. The examiners are audited a few times during the week.
2. The ABA maintains strict quality control.

3. If the ABA has a problem with an examiner, he or she is not asked to serve as an examiner again.
4. Each examiner is ranked yearly as being an easy, moderate, or hard examiner.

## What Are Examiners Audited For?

1. Questioning
   a. Asking vague questions
   b. Asking confusing questions
   c. Asking for facts instead of judgment (giving a superficial exam)
   d. Being unprepared to ask another question
   e. Giving inappropriate positive or negative reinforcement
   f. Asking rhetorical questions
   g. Acting in an aggressive or threatening manner
   h. Asking multiple questions without waiting for a response
   i. Pursuing factual minutiae
   j. Staying on schedule
   k. Covering all of the script
   l. Knowing when to change topics
   m. Being well prepared and informed
   n. Asking too many yes/no questions. They should ask more open-ended questions.
   o. Examiners should be unemotional and give no feedback.

2. Evaluating
   a. Not taking into account the difficulty of the question
   b. Not recognizing nongradable questions/answers
   c. Trying to guess the co-examiner's rating and matching those ratings
   d. Fretting over a split with a co-examiner leading to failure to concentrate on the next examination

## Diplomate Attributes

1. Application of knowledge
   a. Be able to apply the factual knowledge to a clinical scenario. The primary goal is not the recall of cognitive information.
   b. Show the ability to assimilate and analyze data so as to arrive at a rational treatment plan.

2. Judgment
   a. Use sound judgment in making and applying decisions.

3. Adaptability
   a. Be able to respond to a change in the patient's clinical condition.
   b. Be willing to change your plan in response to a change in the situation or patient's condition.

4. Organization and presentation

a. Do you communicate well with peers, patients, family, and community?

b. Are you an anesthesia consultant?

c. Can you be a leader of an anesthesia care team?

d. Can you prioritize and organize your presentation?

e. Can you structure your answers?

f. Are you able to define the priorities in the care of the patient?

## Scoring

1. You are not scored on one question. You are scored overall.

2. In the past, a person may have failed over one missed critical question. This is not true of the current exam.

3. The score is related to the difficulty of the test.

4. The score is also related to the difficulty of the examiner.

5. The score is scaled.

6. The score is based on the exam and the examiner.

7. The analysis is multifaceted.

8. One examiner can't fail you!

## Be Able to Answer

1. Why?

2. Why not?

3. Why not something else?

## Tips for Answering the Question

1. At times, there is **no** right or wrong answer!

2. Don't be too regimented.

3. It is okay to say you are not comfortable with a certain technique, but you must know that it is possible.

## Questions?

1. Just answer the question.

2. Do not ask questions. Examiners don't have any more information than they have told you.

3. You can ask for a clarification if you really don't know what they are asking.

4. Always assume that your patient is healthy. The examiner will let you know if this is not the case.

## You Are Asked a Question . . .

1. Listen to the question and answer it.

2. Immediately justify why that was your answer.

3. Say: I am doing "X" and this is why.

4. Examiners don't want to hear all the things you could do. Pick one!

5. Say "I would," not "I could . . . "

6. They expect you to be able to defend your selected plan of management.

7. They will interrupt when you have said enough.

8. Explain things to the examiners assuming they do not understand anesthesia.

9. The explanation is more important than the answer.

## More Tips

1. Imagine yourself in the operating room. Only do things that you would normally do.

2. Don't be afraid to "consult" another service or physician. This shows that you know when to ask for help as opposed to compromising the patient's safety.

3. Write down any numbers or labs the examiners give you.

4. If you do not know the answer, say "I don't remember at this time." Don't ever make up answers.

5. Don't quote a book or article unless you are prepared to have a detailed discussion.

6. Always keep the patient safe!

## Bad Things Happen

1. Bad things are going to happen, no matter how good you are.

2. They are written into the script.

3. Treat the problem and don't stress over whether it was your fault.

## So, You Realize You Made a Mistake . . .

1. They don't want you to be wishy-washy, so stick to your guns.

2. But don't go down with the sinking ship.

3. If you realize that you made a big, killing mistake, say, "I am sorry, but I . . . "

## Problem Candidates . . .

1. Have superficial knowledge

2. Have good knowledge, but . . .

a. They can't apply it or adapt to clinical conditions.

b. They can't express or defend why they do something.

c. They don't realize that "we do it every day at my hospital" does not count.

3. Try to control the exam by

a. Asking too many questions

b. Giving deliberately slow responses

4. Talk a lot, but say little

5. Can't express ideas or defend a point of view in a convincing manner

6. Are indecisive

7. Show faulty judgment

8. Do not take the test seriously and are not prepared

## Failure

1. In case you have to retake the exam

   a. You will never be re-examined by the same people.

   b. The examiners have no way of knowing if this is your first or twentieth time taking the exam.

## Bibliography

American Board of Anesthesiology. 2008 ABA non-examiner workshop. Fort Lauderdale, FL April 14–15, 2008.

American Society of Anesthesiologists. www.asahq.org /education-and-career/asa -resident-component/study -resources-and-education/aba-applied- exam-oral-and-clinical-assessment- resources

# Standard ASA Monitors

Karl Wagner

## Sample Case

A 30-year-old male comes to the radiology suite for an MRI of his lower spine for cauda equina syndrome. He has lower extremity weakness, morbid obesity, and obstructive sleep apnea. He is too afraid to enter the scanner and would rather be paralyzed than get into the machine. The only way an MRI will be obtained is if the patient has general anesthesia as per the radiologist. He is fasted and ready to go in the scanner when you get the call.

## Clinical Issues

"Standard ASA monitors" is a buzz phrase that we use every day in practice.[1] We will also use the term when we sit for the boards. Do not forget what these monitors are.

1.  Standard I: A person who is qualified to monitor, evaluate, and care for the patient must be present in the room.
2.  Standard II: During all anesthetics, the patient's oxygenation, ventilation, circulation, and temperature should be continuously evaluated.

    a.  Oxygenation

        i.   Oxygen analyzer: used to measure the oxygenation of the inspired gas
        ii.  Pulse oximeter: used to measure the oxygenation of the blood

    b.  Ventilation

        i.   The adequacy of ventilation should be monitored at all times.
        ii.  Monitor expired carbon dioxide ($EtCO_2$)
        iii. Respiratory volumes (if on a ventilator) should be measured.

        iv.  Disconnect-alarms on the ventilators should be used.
        v.   It is important to have audible alarms when practical and available.

    c.  Circulation

        i.   EKG, blood pressure, and heart rate must be measured and evaluated at least every five minutes.
        ii.  We also must be able to palpate pulses, auscultate heart sounds, and/or visualize a continuous arterial wave form or pulse using plethysmography.

    d.  Body temperature

        i.   Temperature should be continuously monitored in all patients receiving anesthesia.
        ii.  This is especially important if clinically significant changes in body temperature are anticipated.

## KO Treatment Plan

This patient may become paralyzed, secondary to the cauda equine syndrome, if he does not get the MRI scan. The surgeons cannot operate without the scan. No matter what technique you choose (laryngeal mask airway or endotracheal tube), you must monitor all of his vital signs. Do not let the radiology technicians tell you it is only a short scan and that you do not need monitors. Every anesthetic gets the standard ASA monitors. You should always have access to MRI-compatible monitors.

---

[1] These standards were approved by the House of Delegates on October 21, 1986, and last amended on December 13, 2020. They can be viewed at the ASA website www.asahq.org/standards-and-guidelines/standards-for-basic-anesthetic-monitoring

# Pulse Oximetry

Jessica A. Lovich-Sapola, Brian M. Sapola, and Jonathan A. Alter

## Sample Case

You are called to the emergency room to evaluate the airway of a patient found unconscious after a failed suicide attempt. He was found in his garage with his car running. His pulse oximetry reading is 97%. He is very somnolent. You determine that the patient needs to be intubated. The medical student standing nearby wants to know why you would intubate him if his "oxygenation" is normal.

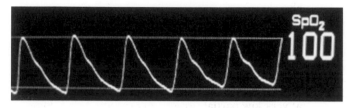

**Figure 2.1** Pulse oximetry reading. Photo credit: J. Lovich-Sapola, MD, MBA, FASA.

## Clinical Issues

### Mechanism of Function

1. The color of the blood is a function of oxygen saturation.
2. The change in color results from the optical properties of hemoglobin and its interaction with oxygen.
3. The ratio of oxyhemoglobin and reduced hemoglobin can be determined by absorption spectrophotometry.
4. Light-absorbance measurements of pulsatile blood are used to determine the concentration of various species of hemoglobin.
5. Adult blood contains four species of hemoglobin: oxyhemoglobin, reduced hemoglobin, methemoglobin, and carboxyhemoglobin.
6. Each of these species of hemoglobin has a different light-absorption profile.
7. The oxygen saturation is determined by using the Beer–Lambert law.
8. Two wavelengths of light are used to distinguish oxyhemoglobin from reduced hemoglobin.
9. Light-emitting diodes (LEDs) in the pulse sensor emit red (660 nm) and infrared (940 nm) light.
10. Reduced hemoglobin absorbs more red (660 nm) light, while oxyhemoglobin absorbs more infrared (940 nm) light.
11. Carboxyhemoglobin has near-identical absorbance as oxyhemoglobin at 660 nm.
12. The percentage of oxygenated and reduced hemoglobin is determined by using a ratio of infrared to red light sensed by the photodetector.
13. The pulse oximeter then determines the difference in the amount of oxygenated hemoglobin in the pulsatile arterial blood from the nonpulsatile venous blood.

### Indications

1. Standard ASA monitor
2. Measurement of the pulse rate
3. Measurement of the oxygen saturation of hemoglobin (Fig. 2.1)
4. Tool for early warning of hypoxemia

### Contraindications and Limitations

1. No clinical contraindications
2. Does not ensure oxygen delivery
3. Does not ensure oxygen utilization by the tissues
4. Poor indicator of adequate ventilation
5. Rare reports of pressure necrosis and burns

### Benefits

1. Noninvasive
2. Continuous monitor
3. Can be used on patients of all age groups
4. Simple
5. Autocalibrating
6. Reliable

### Causes of Inaccuracy

1. Dyshemoglobins
2. Vital dyes
3. Nail polish (greatest effect with blue)
4. Ambient light
5. LED variability
6. Motion artifact
7. Background noise
8. Electrocautery
9. Loss of signal with hypoperfusion

10. Black henna
11. Surgical stereotactic positioning systems

## Errors in Pulse Oximetry

1. Carboxyhemoglobin: overestimates the fraction of hemoglobin available for oxygen transport because of the identical absorbance profile for these species at 660 nm.

   a. Carboxyhemoglobin is assumed by the pulse oximeter to be an $SpO_2$ of 90% oxyhemoglobin since although absorbance is identical at 660 nm, absorbance for carboxyhemoglobin is zero at 940 nm.

   b. Although the $SpO_2$ estimate would be 90%, this is still enough to alter the reading a great deal if $SaO_2$ is significantly less than 90% (with carboxyhemoglobin saturation greater than 10%), which is achievable even at very low partial pressures of carbon monoxide.

2. Methemoglobin: at high levels, the $SpO_2$ approaches 85%, independent of the actual oxygen arterial saturation ($SaO_2$).

3. Hemoglobin Köln: reduction of 8–10%

4. Transient decrease with indigo carmine, indocyanine green, high-dose isosulfan blue, and methylene blue

## Co-oximeter

1. The $SpO_2$ measured by pulse oximetry is not the same as the arterial saturation ($SaO_2$) measured by a laboratory co-oximeter.

2. The pulse oximeter measures "functional" saturation.

3. The co-oximeter uses multiple wavelengths to distinguish other types of hemoglobin by their characteristic absorption profile, which will remove the carboxyhemoglobin error artifacts of absorbance in the red range and methemoglobin at longer wavelengths.

4. The co-oximeter measures the "fractional" saturation.

5. If other hemoglobin moieties are present, the $SpO_2$ measurement will be higher than the $SaO_2$ reported by the laboratory.

6. Methemoglobin and carboxyhemoglobin are usually at such low concentrations in a normal patient that the functional saturation of hemoglobin approximates the fractional value.

## KO Treatment Plan

The sample patient is at high risk for carbon monoxide poisoning. Despite a "normal" pulse oximetry reading, one must assume that his true arterial oxygen saturation is likely low. An arterial blood gas should be sent immediately for a co-oximetry reading. This will give you the true levels of oxyhemoglobin and carboxyhemoglobin. Not only is the falsely high pulse oximetry reading deceiving, but also the characteristic cherry red appearance of the patient with high carbon monoxide levels can be deceiving as to the actual extent of the hypoxia. Carboxyhemoglobin is treated with oxygen therapy. The patient should be receiving 100% oxygen. Since this patient is somnolent and likely not able to protect his airway, intubation may be necessary.

## Bibliography

Barash PG, Cullen BF, Stoelting RK, et al. *Clinical Anesthesia*, 8th ed. Philadelphia: Lippincott Williams & Wilkins, 2017, pp. 709–10.

Ehrenwerth J, Eisenkraft J, Berry J. *Anesthesia Equipment Principles and Applications* 3rd ed. Philadelphia: Elsevier, 2020, pp. 253–70.

Gropper MA. *Miller's Anesthesia*, 9th ed. Philadelphia: Elsevier, 2020, pp. 1301–5.

# Capnography

Zaid H. Jumaily and Jessica A. Lovich-Sapola

## Sample Case

The patient is an 85-year-old female undergoing an anterior cervical fusion. One hour into the case her end-tidal carbon dioxide ($EtCO_2$) begins to drop from 35 to 15 mm Hg. What is your differential diagnosis? What are the appropriate steps to manage this change?

## Clinical Issues

### Terminology

1.  Capnography: the numerical measurement and graphic waveform display of the $CO_2$ concentration versus time or expired volume. Capnography provides three sources of information: numerical $CO_2$ values, the capnogram shape, and the arterial and end-tidal $PCO_2$ difference.
2.  Capnograph: the machine that generates the waveform.
3.  Capnogram: the continuous graphic waveform representation of the $CO_2$ concentration over time (Fig. 3.1). Characteristic waveforms can help in the diagnosis of underlying clinical or technical abnormalities such as partial airway obstruction, accidental extubations, circuit disconnects, and hypermetabolic states. This early recognition of a life-threatening problem allows for early intervention before irreversible damage occurs.
4.  Capnometry: the measurement and numerical display of maximum inspiratory and expiratory $CO_2$ concentrations during a respiratory cycle.
5.  Capnometer: the device that performs the measurement and displays the readings.

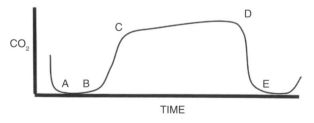

**Figure 3.1** Illustration of a normal capnogram of a patient undergoing mechanical ventilation. Drawing credit: Jeremy B. Sapola

A, B: Expiration begins, but the sampling line does not detect $CO_2$-containing gas secondary to the anatomic dead space.

B, C: $CO_2$-containing gas is detected and a sharp rise in the waveform is demonstrated.

C, D: Plateau phase, surrogate for alveolar gas sampling. Normally flat, but can slope upwards when there is a V–Q mismatch. Point D reflects $EtCO_2$.

D, E: Inspiration, and capnograph returns to zero. If the waveform does not return to zero, could indicate rebreathing.

6.  $EtCO_2$: end-tidal carbon dioxide; the measurement of the concentration of $CO_2$ at the end of exhalation. Normal value of partial pressure ranges between 35 and 45 mm Hg.
7.  $PaCO_2$: the partial pressure of $CO_2$ in the arterial blood.

## Indications

1.  Standard of care for anesthetic monitoring
2.  Used to monitor the accuracy of ventilation

## Contraindications

1.  There are no contraindications

## Clinical Application

1.  Causes of decreased $EtCO_2$
    a.  Decrease in metabolic rate
        i.   Hypothermia
        ii.  Hypothyroidism
    b.  Change in elimination
        i.    Increased dead space/COPD
        ii.   Hyperventilation
        iii.  Decreased cardiac output/cardiac arrest
        iv.   Decreased $CO_2$ production
        v.    Circuit leak or occlusion
        vi.   Pulmonary embolism (air, thrombus, gas, fat, marrow, or amniotic)
    c.  Other
        i.    Increased muscle relaxation
        ii.   Increased depth of anesthesia
        iii.  Surgical manipulation of the heart or thoracic vessels
        iv.   Wedging of the pulmonary artery catheter
2.  Causes of increased $EtCO_2$
    a.  Increased metabolic rate
        i.    Increased $CO_2$ production (malignant hyperthermia, thyrotoxicosis, and hyperthyroidism)
        ii.   Hyperthermia
        iii.  Shivering or convulsions
        iv.   Sepsis

b. Change in elimination

   i. Rebreathing (valve prolapse, failed $CO_2$ absorber)
   ii. Hypoventilation
   iii. Depression of the respiratory center with a decrease in tidal volume
   iv. Reduction of ventilation (partial paralysis, neurologic disease, high spinal anesthesia, weakened respiratory muscles, or acute respiratory distress)
   v. Increased or improving cardiac output
   vi. Right to left intracardiac shunt

c. Other

   i. Excessive catecholamine production
   ii. Administration of blood or bicarbonate
   iii. Release of an aortic/arterial clamp or tourniquet with reperfusion to ischemic areas
   iv. Glucose in the IV fluid
   v. Parenteral hyperalimentation
   vi. $CO_2$ used to inflate the peritoneal cavity during laparoscopy, pleural cavity during thoracoscopy, or a joint during arthroscopy
   vii. Subcutaneous epinephrine injection

3. Causes of minimal to zero $EtCO_2$ or a sudden drop to near-zero

a. Equipment malfunction
b. Endotracheal tube (ETT) disconnect, obstruction, or total occlusion
c. Bronchospasm
d. No cardiac output/cardiac arrest
e. Bilateral pneumothorax
f. Massive pulmonary embolism
g. Esophageal intubation
h. Application of positive end expiratory pressure (PEEP)
i. Cricoid pressure occluding the tip of the ETT
j. Sudden, severe hypotension

4. Errors in capnography

a. Water vapor
b. Disconnection

## KO Treatment Plan

### Intra-operative

1. Capnography is useful for verifying the position of the ETT, providing information about $CO_2$ production, pulmonary perfusion, alveolar ventilation, respiratory patterns, and the elimination of $CO_2$ from the anesthesia circuit and ventilator.

2. Capnography is a rapid and reliable method to detect life-threatening conditions, such as malposition of the ETT, ventilatory failure, circulatory failure, and defective breathing circuits.

3. With the sample patient you need to quickly rule out all potentially life-threatening conditions associated with a decrease in $EtCO_2$, including decreased cardiac output, cardiac arrest, ETT obstruction/malposition, ventilator malfunction, embolism, and oversedation. Call for help. Look at the patient's vital signs. Feel for a pulse. Take the patient off the ventilator and then hand-bag while listening for bilateral breath sounds. If you presume the patient to be in a low cardiac output state, turn off your anesthetics and start advanced cardiovascular life support (ACLS). If you presume a ventilatory problem, troubleshoot for the problem.

4. During ACLS resuscitation, exhaled $CO_2$ is a better guide to the presence of circulation than the EKG, pulse, or blood pressure. The effectiveness of the resuscitation can be measured by capnography. The capnogram is not susceptible to the mechanical artifacts associated with chest compressions. However, if high-dose IV epinephrine or bicarbonate is used, the $EtCO_2$ would not be an effective indicator to the resuscitation. A sudden increase in the $EtCO_2$ during the resuscitation is an early clue that spontaneous cardiac output has been restored.

## Bibliography

Barash PG, Cullen BF, Stoelting RK, et al. *Clinical Anesthesia*, 8th ed. Philadelphia: Lippincott Williams & Wilkins, 2017, pp. 710–13.

D'Mello J, Butani M. Capnography. *Indian J Anaesth*, 2002;**46**(4):269–78.

Gropper MA. *Miller's Anesthesia*, 9th ed. Philadelphia: Elsevier, 2020, pp. 1308–12.

**Chapter**

**4**

# Electrocardiogram (EKG)

Karl Wagner

## Sample Case

A 50-year-old male comes to the operating room (OR) for a laparoscopic cholecystectomy. His past medical history is significant for hypertension controlled with metoprolol and hydrochlorothiazide (HCTZ) and chronic smoking. He reports good functional capacity and is able to care for his lawn and house. He does not have an EKG on file. Should you delay the case in order to get an EKG?

## Clinical Issues

This patient overall enjoys good health and he is considered an ASA class 2. However, he has a few minor indicators of cardiovascular disease. He is an older male with chronic hypertension and he smokes.

## Mechanism of Function

1. The electrocardiogram (EKG) is a measurement of the electrical activity of the heart.
2. The waveforms generated by the electrical impulses of the conduction system give a glimpse into the function of the heart.
3. The measurements are time (seconds) on the $x$-axis and electromotive force (mV) on the $y$-axis.
4. The paper speed is 25 mm per second.
5. By convention, 1 mm corresponds to 0.04 seconds ($x$) or 0.1 mV ($y$).

**Table 4.1** EKG rate

| Rate | Diagnosis |
| --- | --- |
| 60–100 | Normal |
| <60 | Bradycardia |
| >100 | Tachycardia |

## How to Read an EKG

1. When reading the EKG (Fig. 4.1, Table 4.1) it is important to have a system/method for evaluation to ensure maximum diagnostic value.
2. Below is how I approach reading EKGs, but this was learned from reading other authors.

Rhythm: sinus or non-sinus
Regularity: regular or irregular

**P wave:** generated by atrial depolarization.

1. It should be 2.5 mm long and 2.5 mm high.
2. Best viewed in lead II and V1. Therefore, lead II is commonly monitored in the OR because it is the most sensitive for diagnosing arrhythmias.

**PR interval:** generated by the conduction of the electrical impulse through the atria and the AV node.

1. This should not be longer than 0.2 seconds (5 mm).
2. The duration and comparisons of the PR intervals give an insight into the depolarization of and conduction through the atria.

**Figure 4.1** A basic EKG. Drawing credit: J Lovich-Sapola, MD.

R

P

T

Q   S

|<--- PR interval --->|

QRS complex

|<------------ QT interval ------->|

3. First-degree heart block has a PR interval longer than 0.2 seconds. The shape of the wave is unchanged.
4. Second-degree heart blocks
   a. Mobitz Type 1 (Wenckebach): repeating cycles of lengthening PR intervals until there is a dropped beat.
   b. Mobitz Type 2: dropped beats with uniformly prolonged PR intervals.
5. Third-degree heart block is a complete dissociation of the atria and ventricles.
   a. There is not a QRS complex after every P wave.

**TKO:** Remember that second-degree type 2 and third-degree heart blocks require cardiac pacing.

**Q wave:** should not be longer than 0.03 seconds.
1. Greater than 0.03 seconds can be a sign of transmural infarction.
2. A prolonged Q wave is a sign of a post-infarction scar and not a sign of acute ischemia.

**QRS complex:** this is the time for ventricular depolarization and contraction.
1. Normal duration is up to 0.12 seconds.
2. Longer duration is a sign of hemi-block in the AV bundle of His.
3. Look for bundle branch blocks here as well.
   a. If there is an R and R′ in lead V1, then suspect a right bundle branch block (RBBB).
   b. If there is R and R′ in lead V6, then suspect a left bundle branch block (LBBB).

**ST segment:** this should be isoelectric.
1. If it is depressed, then there is myocardial ischemia.
2. If it is elevated, then there is myocardial necrosis.
3. This is measured by the computer on the monitors and we need to take them seriously! Our patients are usually asleep and cannot tell us if they have chest pain.
4. The most sensitive lead for diagnosis of ischemia is chest lead V5.
5. The next most sensitive is chest lead V4.

**T wave:** this depicts ventricular repolarization.
1. It should not be longer than 0.2 seconds.
2. It should be concordant with the total amplitude of the QRS complex.

**Axis:** normal values range between −30° and +110°.
1. Look at the total amplitude of lead I and lead aVf.
2. The vector of these two leads is where the axis lies.

The EKG is a diagnostic test for the heart. We monitor the EKG every day in the OR because we love the heart. We cannot always use a 12-lead EKG for continuous monitoring, however; we do use limb lead II to watch for arrhythmias and chest lead V5 to watch for ischemia. There are also other physiologic abnormalities that can cause EKG changes that will be mentioned in later sections. It is important to keep in mind that patients who are asymptomatic but do have chronic cardiac disease may have a normal EKG. Additionally, patients who have EKG abnormalities pre-operatively along with chronic cardiac disease have a higher risk associated with noncardiac surgery.

## KO Treatment Plan

1. The American College of Cardiology/American Heart Association Task Force developed practice guidelines for peri-operative cardiovascular evaluation and management of patients undergoing noncardiac surgery. These were updated in 2014.
   a. Pre-operative EKG is recommended for patients with known heart disease, arrhythmia, arterial disease, history of a stroke, or other significant structural heart disease.
      i. EKG is not recommended in these patients if they are undergoing a low-risk surgery.
   b. This patient does not meet any of the above criteria, therefore he does not need an EKG.
2. EKG is mandatory if the patient has a change in cardiac symptoms: shortness of breath, or chest pain

# Bibliography

Dubin D. *Rapid Interpretation of EKGs*, 6th ed. Tampa: COVER Publishing, 2000.

Fleisher, LA. *Evidence-Based Practice of Anesthesiology*. Philadelphia: Saunders, 2004, pp. 27–9.

Fleisher LA, Fleischmann KE, Auerbach AD, et al. 2014 ACC/AHA guideline on perioperative cardiovascular evaluation and management of patients undergoing noncardiac surgery. *Circulation*. 2014;**130**: e278–e333.

O'Keefe JH, Hammill SC, Freed MS, et al. *The Complete Guide to ECGs*, 2nd ed. Royal Oak, MI: Physicians' Press, 2002.

**Chapter 5**

# Blood Pressure Monitoring

Karl Wagner

## Sample Case

A one-month-old male comes to the operating room (OR) for a pyloromyotomy. He has been volume resuscitated and has normal electrolytes. He has a 24-gauge IV in his right hand. What kind of blood pressure monitoring would you like for this patient?

## Clinical Issues

One of the standards of anesthesia practice is to measure the blood pressure at least every 3–5 minutes. This can be done either noninvasively or invasively.

## Arterial Blood Pressure Definitions

1. Systolic arterial blood pressure (SBP): the peak left ventricular end-systolic pressure.
2. Diastolic blood pressure (DBP): the lowest arterial pressure during diastolic relaxation.
3. Pulse pressure: the difference between systolic and diastolic pressures.
4. Mean arterial pressure (MAP): the time-weighted average of arterial pressures during a pulse cycle:

$$MAP = (SBP + 2 \cdot DBP) / 3$$

## Noninvasive Blood Pressure (NIBP) Monitoring

1. Techniques
   a. Manual cuff
   b. Automatic cuff
2. Mechanism of function for the manual cuff
   a. The cuff is inflated with a manometer to a pressure that is high enough to stop the flow of blood.
   b. The pressure at which the flow intermittently returns is the SBP.
   c. The vessel is partially occluded, the flow at this point is turbulent, and the sounds heard are Korotkoff's sounds.
   d. When the flow becomes laminar again, the sounds stop and this correlates with the DBP.
   e. The bladder in the cuff should be large enough to cover 60% of the circumference of the arm and the width should be approximately 40% of the length of that limb segment.
3. Mechanism of function for the automatic cuff
   a. Used more commonly

b. The cuff is inflated above the systolic pressure and the flow of blood is stopped.
   c. The pressure in the cuff is decreased slowly, and once there is a return of blood flow through the artery, oscillations are detected.
   d. The MAP is the point at which the oscillations are at their maximum.
   e. The SBP and DBP are calculated values based on the mean and the rate of change in the oscillations.

4. Complications of NIBP monitoring
   a. The cuff, while measuring pressure, is preventing blood flow to the extremity.
      i. Patients have been reported to get compartment syndromes and neuropathies from overuse of the cuff.
      ii. Local skin abrasion and contusion
      iii. Avoid extremities with vascular abnormalities.
         (1) Dialysis shunts
         (2) Peripherally inserted central catheter line (PICC line)
      iv. Avoid extremities with significant lymphedema (e.g., from axillary lymph node resection).
      v. Avoid extremities with bone fractures or open injury to the skin.
   b. There is a change of 0.74 mm Hg in pressure for each centimeter the cuff is above (lower readings) or below (higher readings) the heart.
      i. Improper positioning may lead to inappropriate medical management.
   c. The cuff measures oscillations; any disturbance of the cuff or patient's arm during the reading can introduce error into the results.

## Invasive Arterial Blood Pressure Monitoring

1. Techniques
   a. Catheters are inserted intra-arterially.
   b. The most common arteries are the radial, brachial, axillary, femoral, and dorsalis pedis.
2. Mechanism of function

a. Pulse waves are transmitted along a column of saline to a transducer and the signal is converted into an electrical signal.

b. A waveform can be graphically displayed and used for analysis.

c. Waves can be amplified while traveling back and forth along the vessels (Fig. 5.1).

    i. This amplification also occurs in the tubing used to transmit the signal to the transducer.

    ii. This amplification can result in "whip," an increased systolic pressure reading if the system is under-damped.

    iii. If the system is over-damped it will read as an artificially low blood pressure.

    iv. Use short, noncompliant tubing with saline to conduct the impulse to the transducer; this will minimize error in the pressure readings.

d. The natural frequency of the measuring system is much higher than that of the vascular system and is thought to minimize error in readings because the system does not naturally increase its wave amplitude.

e. The system is described as "critically damped" when the readings are neither artificially high nor low, but are just right.

3. For complications of invasive arterial monitoring, see Chapter 6.

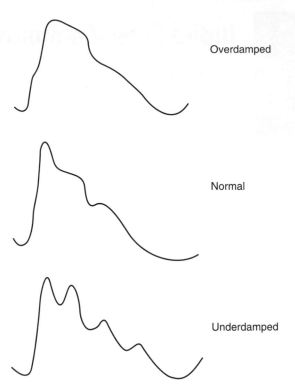

**Figure 5.1** Arterial line dampening. Drawing credit: James Lovich.

## KO Treatment Plan

Remember that this type of case is a medical emergency and not a surgical one. The patient is not an operative candidate until he has been adequately volume resuscitated. Once that occurs, then using a noninvasive blood pressure monitor is reasonable unless there are other variables or indications for an invasive line.

## Bibliography

Barash PG, Cullen BF, Stoelting RK, et al. *Clinical Anesthesia*, 8th ed. Philadelphia: Lippincott Williams & Wilkins, 2017, pp. 713–17.

Butterworth JF, Mackey DC, Wasnick JD. *Morgan & Mikhail's Clinical Anesthesiology*, 6th ed. New York: McGraw-Hill Education, 2018, pp. 81–90.

# Indications, Complications, and Waveforms for an Arterial Line, Pulmonary Artery Catheter (PAC), and Central Venous Pressure Monitor (CVP)

Chris P. Boutton and Jessica A. Lovich-Sapola

## Arterial Line

### Sample Case

A 62-year-old female is scheduled for a carotid surgery. She has a history of Raynaud's disease. Your colleague places a left radial arterial line for the surgery. You are called to the post-anesthesia care unit to evaluate the patient. Her left hand is blue.

### Clinical Issues

#### Indications

1. Continuous, real-time blood pressure monitoring
2. Planned pharmacologic or mechanical cardiovascular manipulation
3. Repeated blood samplings
   a. Arterial blood gas (ABG)
   b. Hematocrit
   c. Glucose
4. Failure of indirect arterial blood pressure measurement
5. Supplementary diagnostic information from the arterial waveform
   a. Arterial pulse contour analysis
      i. Systolic pressure variation
      ii. Pulse pressure variation
6. Patients in hypovolemic, cardiogenic, or septic shock, or with end organ disease
7. Patient with large fluid shifts
8. Procedures involving the use of prolonged deliberate hypotension or hypothermia
9. Patients with decreased left ventricular function or significant valvular disease
10. Patients with cor pulmonale: a condition that leads to right heart failure
    a. COPD, untreated obstructive sleep apnea, interstitial lung disease, primary pulmonary hypertension, and pulmonary thromboembolic disease

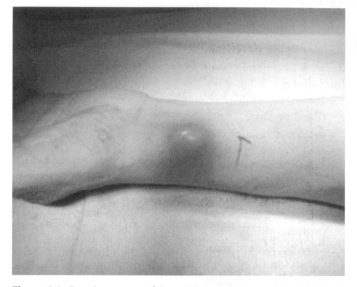

**Figure 6.1** Pseudoaneurysm of the radial artery. Photo credit: Lovich-Sapola, MD, MBA, FASA.

#### Complications

1. Distal ischemia secondary to thrombosis, proximal emboli, or prolonged shock
2. Pseudoaneurysm (Fig. 6.1)
3. Arteriovenous fistula
4. Hemorrhage
5. Hematoma
6. Infection
7. Skin necrosis
8. Peripheral neuropathy and damage to adjacent nerves
9. Misinterpretation of data
10. Cerebral air embolism secondary to retrograde flow with flushing

#### Patients at Increased Risk of Complications

1. Severe atherosclerosis
2. Diabetes mellitus
3. Low cardiac output
4. Intense peripheral vasoconstriction: Raynaud's disease
5. Patients with thromboangiitis obliterans (Buerger's disease)

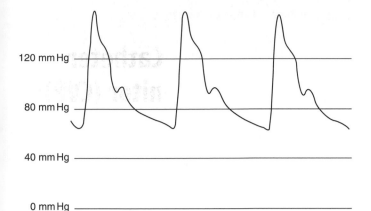

**Figure 6.2** Normal arterial line pressure tracing. Drawing credit: James Lovich.

## Normal Arterial Waveform (Fig. 6.2)

1. Systolic upstroke: ventricular ejection
2. Systolic peak pressure: maximum pressure experienced in the arterial system during systole. Represents the systolic blood pressure.
3. Systolic decline: rapid decline in arterial pressure as ventricular contraction comes to an end (aortic valve still open)
4. Dicrotic notch: secondary upstroke during the descending limb corresponding to transient increase in aortic pressure due to aortic valve closure. Systole is complete and diastole begins.
5. Diastolic runoff: gradual pressure decrease after aortic valve closure
6. End-diastolic pressure: lowest pressure experienced in the arterial system during diastole. Represents the diastolic blood pressure.

## Waveform Abnormalities

1. Aortic stenosis: pulsus parvus (narrow pulse pressure) and pulsus tardus (delayed upstroke)
2. Aortic regurgitation: bisferiens pulse (double peak) and wide pulse pressure
3. Hypertrophic cardiomyopathy: spike and dome (midsystolic obstruction)
4. Systolic left ventricular failure: pulsus alternans (alternating pulse pressure amplitude)
5. Cardiac tamponade: pulsus paradoxus (exaggerated decrease in systolic blood pressure during spontaneous inspiration)
6. Hypovolemia: exaggerated decrease in systolic blood pressure or pulse pressure during mechanical ventilation

## KO Treatment Plan

### Pre-operative Treatment

1. Raynaud's disease is the episodic vasospastic ischemia of the digits.
   a. Affects women more than men
   b. Characteristic digital blanching and cyanosis after cold exposure or sympathetic activation
   c. Vasodilation with hyperemia is often seen after rewarming and reestablishment of blood flow.

### Intra-operative Treatment

1. Protect the patient's hands and feet from cold exposure.
2. Maintain the patient's core body temperature.
3. Noninvasive blood pressure monitoring techniques are recommended over invasive techniques secondary to the increased risk of ischemic injury.
4. The risk–benefit ratio of radial arterial cannulation must be considered for each patient.
5. Consider using a larger artery, such as the brachial or femoral artery, if an arterial line is necessary.

### Post-operative Treatment

1. Evaluate the patient.
2. Warm the patient and her left extremity especially.
3. Determine if this is a Raynaud's event or ischemia secondary to the arterial line.
4. A stellate ganglion block may improve blood flow.
5. Pharmacologic agents such as calcium channel blockers or alpha blockers may be beneficial in some patients.
6. Vascular surgery should be consulted to evaluate the patient for a possible embolectomy.

# Central Venous Access and Central Venous Pressure Monitoring

## Clinical Issues

### Indications

1. CVP monitoring
2. Transvenous cardiac pacing
3. Required for the insertion of PACs
4. Temporary hemodialysis
5. Drug administration: drugs that are irritating to peripheral veins
   a. Vasoactive drugs
   b. Hyperalimentation
   c. Chemotherapy
   d. Prolonged antibiotic therapy
6. Rapid infusion of fluids: trauma, major surgery
7. Major surgery with large fluid shifts
8. Aspiration of a venous air embolus
9. Inadequate peripheral access
10. Sampling site for repeated blood testing

## Complications and Limitations

1. Mechanical injury: arterial, venous, nerve injury, and cardiac tamponade (catheter or wire shearing, loss of guidewire)

    a. Brachial plexus injury
    b. Stellate ganglion injury: Horner syndrome
    c. Hemothorax
    d. Chylothorax

2. Respiratory compromise: airway compression by a hematoma and pneumothorax
3. Arrhythmias
4. Thromboembolic events: venous or arterial thrombosis, pulmonary embolism, and catheter/guidewire embolism
5. Air embolism
6. Infectious: infection at site, catheter infection, blood stream infection, and endocarditis
7. Misinterpretation of data

## Waveform Components (Fig. 6.3)

1. a wave: end diastole; atrial contraction
2. c wave: early systole; isovolumic ventricular contraction, tricuspid motion toward the right atrium
3. v wave: late systole; systolic filling of the atrium
4. h wave: mid-to-late diastole; diastolic plateau
5. x descent: mid-systole; atrial relaxation, descent of the base, systolic collapse
6. y descent: early diastole; early ventricular filling, diastolic collapse

## Waveform Abnormalities by Diagnosis

1. Atrial fibrillation/flutter: loss of the a wave and prominent c wave
2. Atrioventricular dissociation: cannon a wave
3. Tricuspid regurgitation: tall systolic c–v wave and loss of x descent
4. Tricuspid stenosis: tall a wave and attenuation of y descent
5. Right ventricular ischemia and pericardial constriction: tall a and v waves, steep x and y descent, and M or W configuration (fusion of a prominent a and v wave)
6. Cardiac tamponade: dominant x descent and attenuated y descent
7. Respiratory variation during spontaneous or positive-pressure ventilation: measure pressures at end-expiration

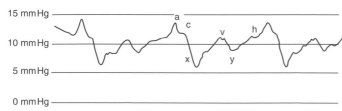

**Figure 6.3** Normal CVP waveform. Drawing credit: James Lovich.

## Waveform Abnormalities by Waveform

1. Loss of the a wave: atrial fibrillation/flutter
2. Cannon a waves: right ventricular hypertrophy, tricuspid/pulmonary stenosis, acute or chronic lung disease associated with pulmonary hypertension, and junctional or nodal rhythm
3. Large v waves: tricuspid regurgitation and right ventricular papillary muscle ischemia

# Pulmonary Artery Catheter (PAC)

## Sample Case

A 77-year-old female had a PAC placed for a routine triple-vessel coronary artery bypass grafting (CABG). The patient was transported to the intensive care unit (ICU). Upon arrival, you note significant hemoptysis. The patient was an easy intubation.

## Clinical Issues

### PAC Measurements

1. Cardiac output (CO)/cardiac index (CI)
2. Pulmonary artery pressure (PAP)
3. Central venous pressure (CVP)
4. Calculation of oxygen delivery
5. Assessment of cardiac work
6. Mixed venous oxygen saturation ($SVO_2$)
7. Pulmonary capillary wedge pressure (PCWP)
8. Systemic vascular resistance (SVR)

### Possible Indications

1. Cardiac

    a. Congestive heart failure (CHF)
    b. Low ejection fraction (EF)
    c. Left-sided, valvular heart disease
    d. CABG
    e. Aortic cross clamp
    f. Left ventricular assist device (LVAD) implantation

2. Pulmonary

    a. Chronic obstructive pulmonary disease (COPD)

        i. Pulmonary hypertension

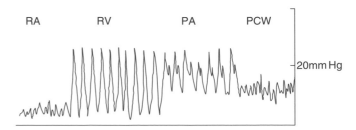

**Figure 6.4** Pressure tracing during the insertion of a PAC. Drawing credit: James Lovich.

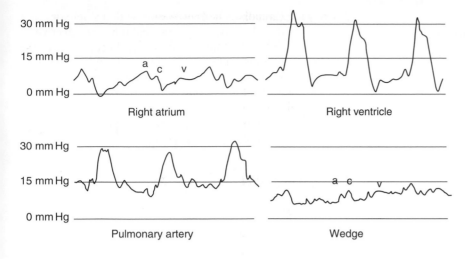

**Figure 6.5** PAC pressure tracings. Drawing credit: James Lovich.

b. Acute respiratory distress syndrome (ARDS)

3. Complex fluid management

    a. Shock

    b. Burns

    c. Acute renal failure

4. High-risk obstetrical care

    a. Eclampsia

    b. Placental abruption

5. Neurological

    a. Sitting craniotomy

    b. Venous air embolus

## Complications

1. Venous access and PAC placement

    a. Arterial puncture

    b. Arrhythmias

        i. Right bundle branch block

        ii. Complete heart block (if pre-existing LBBB)

        iii. Ventricular fibrillation/tachycardia

    c. Post-operative neuropathy

    d. Pneumothorax

    e. Air embolism

2. Catheter residence

    a. Catheter knots

    b. Infection

    c. Thrombophlebitis

    d. Thromboembolism

    e. Pulmonary infarct

    f. Endocarditis

    g. Valvular injury

    h. Pulmonary artery rupture

    i. Pulmonary artery pseudoaneurysm

3. Death

4. Misinterpretation of data

## Waveform Abnormalities by Diagnosis

1. Mitral regurgitation: tall regurgitant v waves, fusion of c and v waves, and obliteration of the x descent

2. Mitral stenosis: slurred early diastolic y descent, tall end-diastolic a wave

3. Ventricular septal defect (VSD): tall anterograde v wave

4. Myocardial ischemia: tall a wave when wedged

    a. Can lead to mitral regurgitation waveform when ischemia affects papillary muscles

5. Right ventricular ischemia: prominent a wave, prominent v wave (from ischemia-induced tricuspid regurgitation)

    a. One of the few times CVP may be higher than wedge pressure

    b. Described as having M or W configuration (tall a and v waves with interposed steep x and y descents)

### Waveform Abnormalities by Waveform

1. Large a wave: mitral stenosis, atrial myxoma, myocardial ischemia, and acute CHF

2. Large v waves: mitral regurgitation (papillary muscle dysfunction), CHF, myocardial ischemia, and VSD

## KO Treatment Plan

### Pulmonary Artery Rupture

1. Most life-threatening complication of the PAC

2. Uncommon: 0.03–0.2% of catheterized patients

3. Often avoidable with meticulous attention to insertion and monitoring techniques

    a. Avoid unnecessary catheter manipulation, excessive insertion distance, persistent or prolonged balloon inflation, and balloon inflation with liquid rather than air.

4. Mortality rate estimated at 41–70%
5. Occurs more commonly in females than males
6. Right pulmonary artery is more commonly injured: about 90% of cases
7. More common in patients undergoing cardiopulmonary bypass (CPB)
8. Increased risk of occurrence
   a. hypothermia
   b. anticoagulation
   c. age >60
   d. pulmonary hypertension
   e. distal PAC migration
   f. catheter balloon overinflation
   g. mitral stenosis
9. Mechanism of injury
   a. Balloon inflation
      i. Especially the over-wedged, distally placed catheter
      ii. Chronic erosion
10. Hallmark: hemoptysis
11. Other presenting signs and symptoms
    a. Hypotension
    b. Respiratory compromise
       i. Hypoxemia and dyspnea
    c. Hemothorax: visualized on a chest X-ray
12. Treatment
    a. Initially position the patient with the bleeding lung dependent until the lung is isolated.
    b. Stabilize the cardio-respiratory condition.
    c. Maintain adequate gas exchange.
       i. Endobronchial intubation with a single or double lumen endotracheal tube for selective unilateral lung ventilation and protection of the unaffected lung.
       ii. Positive end-expiratory pressure (PEEP) applied to the affected lung.
       iii. Bronchoscopy, chest X-ray, and/or transesophageal echocardiography can be used to localize the site of bleeding.
    d. Stop the bleeding.
       i. Reverse anticoagulation, unless on cardiopulmonary bypass.
       ii. Bronchial blocker may be placed into the bronchus to tamponade the bleeding and prevent contamination of the unaffected lung.
    e. PAC
       i. Withdraw the PAC a few centimeters. Leave it in the main pulmonary artery. Leaving it in place helps to monitor the pulmonary artery pressure and guide antihypertensive therapy targeted at reducing the bleed.
       ii. Do not inflate the balloon except under fluoroscopic guidance.
    f. Early pulmonary angiography can be used for diagnosis and treatment by embolization.
    g. The patient may require definitive surgical therapy, including oversewing the involved pulmonary artery or surgical ligation of the pulmonary artery with or without resection of the involved lung lobe or segment.

# Bibliography

Barash PG, Cullen BF, Stoelting RK, et al. *Clinical Anesthesia*, 8th ed. Philadelphia: Lippincott Williams & Wilkins, 2017, pp. 713–21.

Fleisher LA, Rosenbaum SH. *Complications in Anesthesia*, 3rd ed. Philadelphia: Elsevier, 2018, pp. 471–5.

Gropper MA. *Miller's Anesthesia*, 9th ed. Philadelphia: Elsevier, 2020, pp. 1157–90.

Hines RL, Marschall KE. *Stoelting's Anesthesia and Co-Existing Disease*, 7th ed. Philadelphia: Elsevier, 2018, pp. 257–8.

Kaplan, JA, Cronin B, Maus T. *Kaplan's Essentials of Cardiac Anesthesia for Cardiac Surgery*, 2nd ed. Philadelphia: Elsevier 2018, pp. 203–25.

Urschel JD, Myerowitz PD. Catheter-induced pulmonary artery rupture in the setting of cardiopulmonary bypass. *Annals of Thoracic Surgery*, 1993;**56**:586–9.

# Chapter 7

# False Measurements in Thermodilution Cardiac Output Readings

Wesley G. Dougall and Jessica A. Lovich-Sapola

## Clinical Issues

### Thermodilution Cardiac Output Monitoring

1. This is the clinical gold standard for measuring cardiac output.
2. Cardiac output is the total blood flow generated by the heart, which can be measured either from the blood entering into the aorta or into the pulmonary trunk.
3. Normal cardiac output in an adult ranges from 4 to 6.5 L/min.
4. The thermodilution method uses a thermal indicator.
5. The temperature of the patient's blood is measured continuously by a thermistor at the tip of the pulmonary artery catheter (PAC).
6. The injectate temperature is measured by a second thermistor at the injectate port.
7. To perform an accurate cardiac output reading, a fixed volume of iced or room-temperature fluid is injected as a bolus into the proximal central venous pressure (CVP) lumen of the PAC. The resulting change in pulmonary artery blood temperature is recorded by the thermistor at the catheter tip. Cardiac output is inversely related to the area under the $\Delta dT/t$ (change in temperature over time) curve.
8. An injectate volume of 10 mL is typically used in adults, whereas 0.15 mL/kg is recommended in children.
9. Three cardiac output measurements are usually taken in quick succession and averaged in order to improve result reliability.
10. The thermodilution technique measures right ventricular output and pulmonary artery blood flow. Following the trends of successive results is probably more clinically useful than any individual absolute value.

### Assumptions and Errors of Thermodilution Cardiac Output Measurements

1. Assumptions
   a. Flow is constant.
   b. Blood volume is constant (no rapid IV fluid administration).
   c. Pulmonary artery (PA) temperature is constant.
   d. There is no significant venous pooling.
   e. The volume of injectate must be correct.
   f. The temperature of injectate must be accurate.
   g. There are no intracardiac or pulmonary shunts.
   h. The tip of the PA catheter must be in the PA and not covered by fibrin or a thrombus.
   i. There is insignificant tricuspid or pulmonic valve regurgitation (higher levels of regurgitation result in either under- or overestimation of results depending on the severity of the regurgitation and the magnitude of the cardiac output).

2. Errors
   a. Right ventricular stroke output can vary by as much as 50% in patients receiving positive pressure mechanical ventilation, depending on where in the respiratory cycle the measurement is taken.
   b. The readings are also inaccurate if the PA catheter is wedged or if there is a thrombus covering the tip.
   c. The computer algorithm bases the cardiac output calculation on a specific injectate volume at a specific temperature, and assumes that no communication exists between the pulmonary and systemic circulations and there is no pooling of blood in either circulation (pulmonary and systemic outputs match).

### False Increase in Thermodilution Cardiac Output Readings

1. Smaller than expected injectate volume or central venous injection site within catheter introducer sheath
2. Higher than expected temperature of injectate
3. Fibrin or thrombus on thermistor resulting in its malfunction
4. The patient is in a very low cardiac output state.
   a. The slow transit results in significant heat absorption of the injectate from the surrounding tissues prior to it reaching the thermistor (and therefore a smaller temperature change is sensed).
5. Right-to-left and left-to-right intracardiac shunts
   a. The former results in diversion of some cold injectate to the left side of the heart and therefore less reaches the thermistor.

b. The latter results in left-sided blood mixing with and diluting the injectate in the right side, and therefore warms the injectate prematurely.

## False Decrease in Thermodilution Cardiac Output Readings

1. Larger than expected injectate volume
2. Lower than expected temperature of injectate

3. Inflation cycle of lower limb sequential compression devices (SCDs)
4. Either rapid or continuous infusion of intravenous fluid through the PAC (resulting in a cooling effect on the blood)
5. Immediately following cardiopulmonary bypass. At this stage there is an unstable thermal baseline due to redistribution of heat from the vasculature and vessel-rich tissues to the less perfused, cooler, core. This causes blood temperature fluctuations and unreliable results until equilibration is once again achieved.

## Bibliography

Fleitman J. Pulmonary artery catheterization: interpretation of hemodynamic values and waveforms in adults. In: Manaker S, Finlay G, eds. *UpToDate*. Waltham, MA. (accessed on October 20, 2021).

Gropper MA. *Miller's Anesthesia*, 9th ed. Philadelphia: Elsevier, 2020, pp. 1186–90.

Hensley FA, Martin DE, Gravlee GP. Monitoring the cardiac surgical patient. In: *A Practical Approach to Cardiac Anesthesia*, 4th ed. Philadelphia: Lippincott Williams & Wilkins, 2007, chapter 3.

Killu K, Oropello JM, Manasia Ar, et al. Effects of lower limb compression devices on the thermodilution cardiac output measurement. *Crit Care Med* 2007;**35**(5):1307–11.

Kolb B, Kapoor V. Cardiac output measurement. *Anesthesia and Intensive Care Medicine* 2019;**20**(3):193–201.

Nishikawa T, Dohi S. Errors in the measurement of the cardiac output by thermodilution.*Canadian J Anesthesia* 1993;**40**: 142–53.

van Grondelle A, Ditchey RV, Groves BM, et al. Thermodilution method overestimates low cardiac output in humans. *Am J Physiol Heart Circ Physiol* 1983;**245**: H690–2.

# Pulse Pressure Variation (PPV) for Goal-Directed Fluid Therapy

Jessica A. Lovich-Sapola

## Clinical Issues

1. Dynamic marker of the patient's preload reserve and their position on the Frank–Starling curve
2. Predictor of fluid responsiveness
3. Requires arterial blood pressure monitoring
4. Recommended to duplicate experimental conditions under which the indices were investigated
   a. Tidal volume 8–10 mL/kg
   b. Positive end-expiratory pressure ≥5 mm Hg
   c. Regular cardiac rhythm
   d. Normal intra-abdominal pressure
   e. Closed chest

## Pulse Pressure Variation for Fluid Therapy

1. PPV <13–17%: normal
2. PPV >13%: likely fluid responsive
3. PPV <9%: not fluid responsive
4. 9% < PPV < 13%: "gray zone"

## Indications

1. Critically ill patient
2. Patient in septic shock
3. After cardiac surgery
4. Liver failure

## Limitations

1. Extreme bradycardia
2. High respiratory rate
3. Arrhythmias/irregular heart rate
   a. Atrial fibrillation
4. Increased intra-abdominal pressure
5. Patient positioning
   a. Steep Trendelenburg
   b. Prone
   c. Lateral
6. Open thorax/open abdomen
7. Spontaneous ventilation
8. Low tidal volume ventilation
9. Low arterial compliance
   a. High-dose vasopressors
   b. Severe atherosclerosis
   c. Peripheral vascular disease
10. Right and/or left ventricular failure
11. Children
12. Ventilated, sedated, but not paralyzed
13. Pulmonary hypertension

## Bibliography

Gropper MA. *Miller's Anesthesia*, 9th ed. Philadelphia: Elsevier, 2020, pp. 1167–9.

# Chapter 9

# Types of Anesthesia Circuits

Karl Wagner

## Sample Case

A two-year-old female presents to the operating room for a repair of her club foot. Do you think that a circle system is appropriate for her?

## Clinical Issues

### Breathing Systems

1. Insufflation

   a. Most basic type of oxygen delivery

   b. Blowing of a gas across a patient's face

   c. This utilizes a high fresh gas flow and does not require direct contact between the patient and oxygen source.

   d. The FiO$_2$ delivered to the patient is dependent on the respiratory rate, tidal volume, and fresh gas flow.

   e. Advantages

      i. Useful for children who are afraid of having a mask on their face during an inhalational induction

      ii. Useful for patients who are covered with a drape during an operative intervention but are breathing spontaneously without an endotracheal tube or a laryngeal mask airway (LMA), to prevent carbon dioxide accumulation

      iii. A high fresh gas flow can prevent hypercarbia in the spontaneously breathing patient.

      iv. No rebreathing

      v. Can be used to maintain arterial oxygenation during short periods of apnea

   f. Disadvantages

      i. Not able to deliver anesthetic gases

      ii. Not able to scavenge with this system

      iii. Not able to control ventilation

      iv. The inspired gas contains unpredictable amounts of atmospheric gas.

      v. No conservation of exhaled heat or humidity

2. Simple face mask, face tent, venturi mask, and non-rebreather face mask

   a. Simple circuits that allow delivery of oxygen from the wall supply to the patient

   b. They may or may not have valves, and there can be variable amounts of rebreathing.

   c. A bag valve mask (i.e., the Ambu bag commonly used for resuscitation in the wards) differs in that it has a one-way valve to prevent rebreathing and delivers nearly 100% oxygen.

   d. Advantages

      i. They allow a greater increase in FiO$_2$ when comparing the face mask to insufflation.

      ii. They are lightweight and portable.

   e. Disadvantages

      i. They are not capable of scavenging waste.

      ii. Except for the Ambu bag, they all rely on spontaneous ventilation.

3. Mapleson circuits (Fig. 9.1)

   a. Semi-open system

   b. Allows delivery of oxygen and with some modifications can be used to deliver anesthetic gases

   c. The amount of rebreathing with the different types is dependent on

      i. Fresh gas flow

      ii. Minute ventilation

      iii. Mode of ventilation: spontaneously breathing or controlled ventilation

      iv. Tidal volume

      v. Respiratory rate

      vi. I:E ratio

      vii. Peak inspiratory flow rate

      viii. Volume of the reservoir tube

      ix. Volume of the breathing bag

   d. They are considered to be valveless, because the direction of flow is not limited by valves, although there is a pop-off pressure valve.

   e. Advantages

      i. Simple to use

      ii. Decreased resistance to respiratory flow since they do not have valves or an absorber

      iii. Lightweight

      iv. Not complicated

      v. Easily used while transporting patients

      vi. Inexpensive

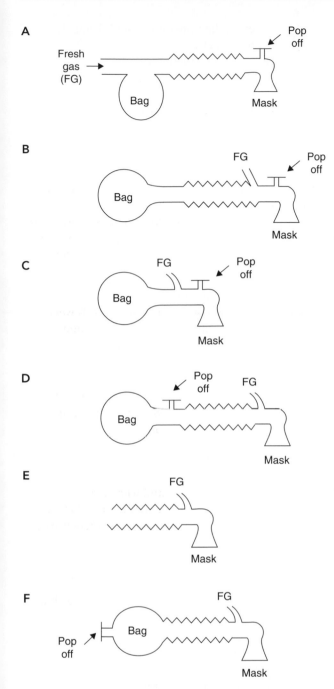

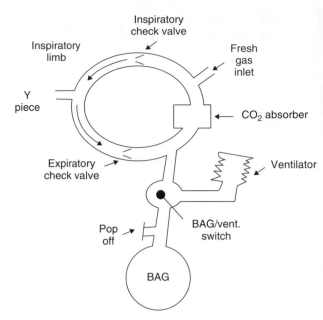

**Figure 9.2** Circle system. Drawing credit: K. Wagner, MD, FASA.

i. For your exam you may be asked to draw the different circuits, so be prepared to do so.

ii. The Mapleson A circuit is best used for a spontaneously ventilating patient.

iii. The Mapleson D circuit is best for controlled ventilation.

4. Circle system (Fig. 9.2)

   a. The circle system contains

      i. Inspiratory limb

      ii. Expiratory limb

      iii. One-way valves to ensure flow direction

      iv. $CO_2$ absorber

      v. Gas reservoir bag

      vi. Pop-off valve on the expiratory limb

   b. It is considered a semi-closed system (instead of a completely closed system) because there is not complete rebreathing.

      i. Some of the tidal volume during exhalation goes to the scavenging system.

      ii. The amount of volume that is sent through the scavenger is a function of the total fresh gas flow rate, pressure in the system, and minute ventilation.

      iii. Once a threshold pressure is reached, the gas volume is released to the scavenging system via a valve.

   c. Advantages

      i. Can be used to conserve heat and humidity

      ii. Uses low flows of fresh gas, thereby conserving volatile anesthetics

      iii. There is a $CO_2$ absorber.

**Figure 9.1** Mapleson-type circuit. Drawing credit: K. Wagner, MD, FASA.

      vii. Easy to sterilize

     viii. Ability to change the depth of anesthesia rapidly

      ix. Lack of rebreathing of exhaled gases, provided the fresh gas flow is adequate

   f. Disadvantages

      i. Do not conserve heat, humidity, or anesthetic gases

      ii. Require high fresh gas flows

      iii. Have no $CO_2$ absorbers

      iv. Limited ability to scavenge waste gases

   g. Modifications of the Mapleson circuit

   (1)  Prevents rebreathing of $CO_2$

   (2)  Allows partial rebreathing of other anesthetic gases

  iv.  Scavenging can easily be done to prevent contamination of the operating room.

   (1)  Because there is a scavenger built into the system, the exhaled gas can either be rebreathed or go out to the scavenger.

  v.  Good control of anesthetic depth

  vi.  They come in different sizes and tubing compliances.

   (1)  Remember that compliance is the change in volume per unit of pressure.

  vii.  Good for pediatric patients

   (1)  The pediatric population benefits from less compliant tubing so that the tidal volume delivered from the machine is not utilized in expanding the tubing but is being delivered to the patient.

   (2)  Heat conservation is critical in small children, as is volume control against dehydration; these are both accomplished with the circle system.

  d.  Disadvantages

  i.  These circuits are more complicated than the Mapleson type and are not as portable.

  ii.  There is an increase in resistance with the tubing and valves, which can increase the work of breathing in a spontaneously breathing patient.

## KO Treatment Plan

Assuming the patient requires general anesthesia, she would benefit from the conservation of heat and humidity provided by the circle system, which does not exist with the Mapleson-type circuits. We would use pediatric tubing that is smaller and less compliant than adult tubing.

## Bibliography

Barash PG, Cullen BF, Stoelting RK, et al. *Clinical Anesthesia*, 8th ed. Philadelphia: Lippincott Williams & Wilkins, 2017, pp. 679–81.

Butterworth JF, Mackey DC, Wasnick JD. *Morgan & Mikhail's Clinical Anesthesiology*, 6th ed. New York: McGraw-Hill Education, 2018, pp. 36–46.

Gropper MA. *Miller's Anesthesia*, 9th ed. Philadelphia: Elsevier, 2020, pp. 601–14.

# Sodium

Jennifer Eismon

## Hypernatremia

### Sample Case

A 42-year-old male from a group home, who is baseline non-verbal with mental retardation, is brought into the hospital for confusion, muscle weakness, lethargy, poor oral intake, and abdominal pain. The patient is found to have an abdominal hernia. His laboratory results reveal a sodium level of 157 mEq/L. The surgeon is concerned that the hernia is incarcerated and wants to operate immediately. What are your concerns? Would you like to order any more labs or tests? How would you treat the hypernatremia? Would you delay this surgery if it was an elective hernia repair? If this is emergent, what is your anesthetic plan?

### Clinical Issues

#### Definition of Hypernatremia

1. Sodium ($Na^+$) concentration >145 mEq/L
2. Produces a state of hyperosmolality
3. Maintenance of osmotic equilibrium in hypernatremia results in intracellular fluid volume contraction.
4. Mechanism

   a. Primary $Na^+$ gain
   b. $H_2O$ deficit

      i. Majority of cases are iatrogenic

         (1) Failure to provide water to a patient who is unconscious, lacks the thirst mechanism, or is unable to get water for themselves

      ii. Pre-operative hypernatremia is associated with increased 30-day peri-operative mortality.
      iii. ICU-acquired hypernatremia occurs in 30% of patients and is associated with increased mortality.
      iv. Risk factors for developing hypernatremia in the ICU

         (1) Sepsis
         (2) Decreased level of consciousness
         (3) Parenteral/enteral feeding
         (4) Hypertonic infusions
         (5) Osmotic and other diuretics
         (6) Mechanical ventilation

5. Less common than hyponatremia

#### Appropriate Response to Hypernatremia in an Awake, Otherwise Normal Patient

1. Increased water ($H_2O$) intake stimulated by thirst
2. Excretion of minimal volume

   a. Maximally concentrated urine reflecting antidiuretic hormone (ADH) secretion in response to an osmotic stimulus

#### Causes of Hypernatremia

1. $Na^+$ excess (urine $Na^+$ >20 mmol/L)

   a. Hyperaldosteronism
   b. Cushing's syndrome
   c. Iatrogenic administration of sodium bicarbonate or hypertonic saline

2. Water depletion (urine $Na^+$ variable)

   a. Renal loss: diabetes insipidus
   b. Insensible water loss
   c. Insufficient water intake

3. $Na^+$ deficiency with greater water deficiency

   a. Renal loss (urine $Na^+$ > 20 mmol/L)

      i. Osmotic diuresis caused by mannitol, glucose, urea

   b. Other loss (urine $Na^+$ <10 mmol/L) caused by vomiting, diarrhea, sweating, wound losses

#### Clinical Features of Hypernatremia

1. The severity of the clinical manifestations is determined by the acuity.

   a. Chronic hypernatremia is less symptomatic.

2. The major symptoms are neurologic and are related to the osmotic decrease in brain volume (brain cell shrinkage).

   a. Altered mental status: lethargy, confusion, irritability
   b. Advanced neurologic deficit: coma, seizures, intracerebral bleeding due to the rupture of cerebral veins as a result of brain shrinkage

3. Other symptoms

   a. Expanded intravascular volume: signs of hypervolemic hypernatremia

      i. Pleural effusion

ii. Ascites

iii. Peripheral edema

iv. Heart failure

b. Complaints of thirst or polyuria

c. Nausea and vomiting

d. Neuromuscular irritability: myoclonus, muscular tremor/rigidity, hyperactive reflexes, muscle weakness

### Diagnosis of Hypernatremia

1. History and physical examination

   a. List of current medications

   b. Mental and neurologic exam

   c. Determine which of the three categories of volume status in the hypernatremic state the patient has: hypovolemic, hypervolemic, or isovolemic.

   d. Establish water intake, access to water, and salt intake.

2. Look for signs and symptoms including thirst, diaphoresis, diarrhea, vomiting, polyuria, and features of extracellular fluid volume contraction.

3. Measure urine osmolality, sodium concentration, and the integrity of the ADH–renal system.

   a. Consult an expert to aid in the diagnosis of diabetes insipidus.

4. Measure urine solute concentration to confirm osmotic diuresis: glucose and urea.

### Treatment of Hypernatremia

1. Determine the volume status of the patient and if applicable stop the ongoing $H_2O$ loss by treating the cause and correcting the $H_2O$ deficit.

   a. Hypernatremia with hypervolemia: use of diuretics and hemodialysis may be necessary to lessen symptoms of volume overload.

   b. Free $H_2O$ deficit (in liters of $H_2O$) = ((plasma $Na^+$/140) − 1) × kg × 0.6 in males

      i. 0.5 should be used for the calculation in females.

      ii. Goal should be a $Na^+$ ≤145 mEq/L.

      iii. Replace half of the free water deficit in the first 24 hours and the remainder over the following 2–3 days.

      iv. Use 5% dextrose in water or 0.45% NaCl to correct the deficit.

      v. Monitor serum sodium every 1–2 hours to ensure a gradual correction.

2. The rate of $Na^+$ correction should not exceed 0.5 mEq/L per hour or 10–12 mEq/L per day.

3. If the rate of correction is too rapid, it may produce cerebral edema, seizures, and irreversible neurologic damage or death.

## KO Treatment Plan

### Pre-operative

1. The patient in the sample case gives you an intuitive reason for the hypernatremia: poor access to water, poor oral intake due to mental retardation, and perhaps a reliance on caregivers for oral intake. There is a good chance that this patient has hypovolemic hypernatremia.

2. Verify the cause of the hypernatremia by obtaining urine sodium and urine osmolality.

3. Treat the hypernatremia acutely.

   a. Restore blood pressure by giving fluid replacement with 0.9% NaCl.

   b. Once the patient's blood pressure is stabilized, address the water deficit.

4. If this is an elective case, postpone the case until the serum sodium approaches normal levels.

   a. *Miller's Anesthesia* recommends patients undergoing surgery to have $Na^+$ <150 mEq/L prior to anesthesia unless the patient has a therapeutic reason for hypernatremia.

   b. The goal of treatment is $Na^+$ <145 mEq/L.

5. Treat the patient's hypernatremia with fluid replacement and frequent serum sodium evaluation.

### Intra-operative

1. If this is an emergency and the decision has been made to proceed with the case

   a. Monitors

      i. Standard ASA monitoring

      ii. Pre-induction invasive arterial blood pressure monitoring

   b. IV access

      i. Obtaining central IV access is necessary to measure central venous pressure and aid in volume resuscitation.

      ii. If there is no need for central venous pressure monitoring, peripheral IV access would be acceptable.

   c. Regional versus general anesthesia: due to this patient's mental retardation and questionable cooperativeness, general anesthesia is indicated for this procedure rather than a primary regional anesthetic. However, consider incorporating a regional block technique for post-operative pain control.

      i. In an otherwise cooperative patient, regional anesthesia would be preferred in an emergent surgery on a hypernatremic patient secondary to the ability to monitor their mental status.

d. Induction

    i. Etomidate is a good choice for induction due to the patient's associated hypovolemia.

    ii. Consider a rapid sequence induction (RSI) using succinylcholine if the patient's mental status puts him at increased risk for aspiration.

        (1) Avoid succinylcholine if it is contraindicated.

        (2) Avoid RSI if the patient has an anticipated difficult airway.

e. Maintenance anesthesia

    i. Inhalational agent

    ii. Short-acting narcotics (to ensure a "quick" wake-up and lessen residual anesthesia) would be ideal due to this patient's lethargy and baseline mental status.

f. Other considerations

    i. Frequent electrolyte checks

## Post-operative

1. Follow-up plan: despite his lethargy, this patient after the procedure can be extubated (assuming he meets extubation criteria) and transferred to the ICU for further monitoring of his serum sodium every 1–2 hours, replacement of fluid deficits, and urinary volume output measurement.

2. Investigate how he became so dehydrated and verify his safety in his group home setting.

# Hyponatremia

## Sample Case

A 32-year-old female presents to the emergency department. She reports being a contestant in a water-drinking competition to win a car from a radio station. She complains of nausea, headache, lethargy, and confusion. What are your concerns? How will you diagnose and treat the problem? What would your anesthetic plan be if she requires anesthesia?

## Clinical Issues

### Definition of Hyponatremia

1. $Na^+$ concentration <135 mEq/L

   a. Mild: 130–134 mEq/L

   b. Moderate: 120–130 mEq/L

   c. Severe: <120 mEq/L

2. Most common electrolyte disorder

   a. Acute hyponatremia

      i. Frequent in the hospital setting (especially post-operative)

      ii. Psychogenic polydipsia

      iii. Use of MDMA (methamphetamine, "molly," "ecstasy")

b. Chronic hyponatremia

    i. Hyponatremic state that lasts greater than 48 hours

3. Hyponatremia is commonly caused by cellular edema with the presence of hypotonicity.

4. Acute onset of moderate to severe hyponatremia leads to significant peri-operative mortality. Postpone nonurgent surgery.

   a. Acute onset of hyponatremia during surgery is from absorption of $Na^+$ free irrigating solutions (e.g., TURP surgery).

5. Thirty-day mortality increases even in mild hyponatremia due to

   a. Major cardiac events

   b. Wound infection

   c. Pneumonia

### Diagnosis of Hyponatremia

1. History and physical examination

2. The diagnosis algorithm of hyponatremia includes assessing first the plasma osmolality, then the volume status, and finally the urine $Na^+$ concentration.

   a. Plasma osmolality: normal, high, low

      i. Normal ranges from 285 to 295 mOsm/kg: consider pseudohyponatremia (hyperlipidemia or hyperproteinemia)

      ii. >295 mOsm/kg: consider hyperglycemia or administration of hypertonic infusions (mannitol or glucose)

      iii. <285 mOsm/kg: plasma is hypotonic; the next step is evaluation of volume status

   b. Volume status: hypotonic hyponatremia has been diagnosed and can now be differentiated into three states based on volume status. Establish if the patient has hypovolemia, euvolemia, or hypervolemia.

      i. Once extracellular fluid volume status is established then narrow diagnosis further by checking the urine $Na^+$ concentration.

        (1) Hypovolemia established: check urine $Na^+$ concentration

          (a) >20 mEq/L: renal solute loss: consider diuretics, osmotic diuresis, Addison's disease (adrenal insufficiency), renal tubular acidosis, obstruction

          (b) <20 mEq/L: nonrenal solute loss: consider GI loss (vomiting and diarrhea), skin losses (sweating), third spacing (burns and pancreatitis)

        (2) Euvolemia established: check urine $Na^+$ concentration

(a) >20 mEq/L: SIADH, cerebral salt wasting, adrenal insufficiency, renal failure, hypothyroidism

(b) <20 mEq/L: water intoxication, decreased solute intake

(3) Hypervolemia established: check urine Na$^+$ concentration

(a) >20 mEq/L: consider acute and chronic renal failure

(b) <20 mEq/L: consider edematous states such as congestive heart failure, cirrhosis, nephrotic syndrome

3. Consult an expert to help establish a diagnosis and correct the underlying cause.

## Clinical Manifestations of Hyponatremia

1. Symptoms are primarily neurologic and severity is determined by the rapidity of serum Na$^+$ loss.
2. Symptoms are related to fluid shift leading to an increase in intracellular fluid volume – specifically, brain cell swelling or cerebral edema.

   a. Increasing severity of hyponatremia with falling Na$^+$ levels (Table 10.1)

## Treatment of Hyponatremia

1. Before treatment, consider whether the patient has acute versus chronic hyponatremia and if they are symptomatic. Substantial risk is inherent when too rapid of a correction causes a demyelination syndrome.
2. Therapy can be guided by the assessment of plasma osmolality:

   a. Treatment of isotonic hyponatremia should be directed at underlying hyperlipidemia and paraproteinemia.
   b. Treatment of hypertonic hyponatremia should be directed at correcting hyperglycemia and terminating hypertonic infusions.
   c. Treatment of hypotonic hyponatremia can be tailored based on volume status

      i. Hypovolemic hyponatremia: replace extracellular fluid volume with isotonic saline. This minimizes ADH release.

Table 10.1 Symptoms associated with hyponatremia levels

| Symptoms | Associated serum Na$^+$ (mEq/L) |
| --- | --- |
| Asymptomatic | ≥125, or chronic ≥115 |
| Anorexia, nausea, malaise | 120–124 |
| Headache, lethargy, confusion, agitation, obtundation | 110–119 |
| Stupor, seizures, coma | ≤109 |

ii. Hypervolemic hyponatremia: in chronic cases restrict water intake and optimize any underlying disease. Using cardiac failure as an example, consider ACE inhibitors and loop diuretics

3. Therapy can also be guided by hyponatremia that is asymptomatic versus symptomatic.

   a. Chronic hyponatremia: treat underlying cause instead of immediate Na$^+$ correction. This may entail fluid restriction, ADH antagonists, and loop diuretics.
   b. Symptomatic hyponatremia: treatment aggressiveness is based on severity of symptoms.

      i. Therapy is directed at raising extracellular fluid tonicity to shift water out of the intracellular space, alleviating cellular edema.
      ii. The rate of correction must be carefully monitored; too rapid a correction may produce central pontine myelinolysis (CPM), an osmotic demyelination syndrome associated with irreversible neurologic deficits which develop 2–6 days after treatment: dysarthria, dysphagia, incoordination, quadriplegia, coma.

         (1) Moderate symptoms: use hypertonic 3% saline at a rate of 1 mL/kg/h with the goal to increase Na$^+$ levels by 1 mEq/L/h over 3–4 hours. Frequently monitor electrolytes, osmolality, and fluid status.
         (2) Severe symptoms: occur usually in acute onset of hyponatremia (Na$^+$ levels <120 mEq/L)

            (a) Bolus 100 mL hypertonic 3% saline to increase Na$^+$ levels by 2–3 mEq/L. If there is no change in neurologic status, repeat every 10 minutes.
            (b) Once the patient has resolution of severe symptoms, proceed to using treatment guided by that of a moderate symptomatic patient.
            (c) If the patient does not have resolution of severe symptoms, consider hemodialysis.

TKO: Suggested rate of correction with hypertonic saline in stable symptomatic patients

1. 10 mEq/L in the first 24 hours
2. 20 mEq/L in the first 48 hours

TKO: To use 3% hypertonic saline

1. Calculate the amount of sodium to be administered by multiplying the target change in serum sodium by the patient's total body water (TBW).

   a. TBW = 0.6 × kg
   b. Example 70 kg male: 0.6 × 70 = 42

2. Example: to change the serum Na$^+$ in the first 24 hours by an equivalent of 10 mEq/L in a 70 kg male: 10 × 42 = 420 mEq.

3. 3% saline has an $Na^+$ concentration of 513 mEq/L, therefore 420/513 = 0.82 L or 820 mL, which should be given in the first 24 hours.

## KO Treatment Plan

### Pre-operative

1. The patient's hyponatremia is related to excessive water drinking that is not likely related to psychiatric illness.

   a. Patients with pure water excess appear euvolemic.

2. The patient should be transferred from the emergency department to the medical ICU.

   a. She should be electively intubated due to her mental confusion.

   b. Peripheral access should be obtained.

   c. Central access should be obtained to monitor central venous pressure and help establish her volume status.

   d. An arterial catheter should be placed for frequent serum laboratory tests.

   e. A Foley catheter should be inserted to closely monitor urine output.

   f. A chest X-ray should be obtained to rule out pulmonary edema.

3. Laboratory

   a. Serum $Na^+$ should be monitored as fluid restriction occurs along with measurement of urine output.

   b. The normal response to significant water ingestion is to excrete maximally dilute urine (urine osmolality less than 100 mOsm/kg).

   c. Usually, low blood urea nitrogen and serum uric acid concentration is the only laboratory evidence of increased TBW.

   d. Toxicology screen should be done to rule out the use of MDMA.

   i. MDMA can have the resulting side effect of significant hyponatremia.

4. The patient can be started on an infusion of hypertonic 3% saline for symptomatic hyponatremia.

   a. Patients with psychogenic polydipsia require fluid restriction and/or hypertonic 3% saline, depending on the presence of symptoms and acuity of the hyponatremia.

### Intra-operative

1. If this patient does need emergent surgery, meticulous attention should be paid to her volume status.

   a. 3% hypertonic saline should be infused along with serial monitoring of serum sodium concentrations.

   b. Pre-induction arterial line for frequent electrolyte measurements

   c. Central venous line to measure her volume status

   d. Careful titration of anesthetics secondary to her already confused and lethargic state

   e. She will require RSI secondary to her nausea and likely full stomach; she did drink a lot of water.

**TKO:** Delay any case until the patient's hyponatremia improves unless it is an absolute emergency. This patient should not go to the operating room for an elective case since it puts her at a significantly increased risk for morbidity and mortality.

### Post-operative

1. Close monitoring in the ICU
2. If she required an emergent surgery, delay extubation until her hyponatremia begins to resolve.

   a. Her pre-operative confusion and lethargy will not resolve until her serum sodium values are normalized.

## Bibliography

Barash PG, Cullen BF, Stoelting RK, et al. *Clinical Anesthesia*, 8th ed. Philadelphia: Lippincott Williams & Wilkins, 2017, pp. 398–404.

Gropper MA. *Miller's Anesthesia*, 9th edition. Philadelphia: Elsevier, 2020, pp. 4848–58.

Harring T, Deal N, Kuo D. Disorders of sodium and water balance. *Emerg Med Clin N Am* 2014;**32**:379–401.

Humes DH, Dupont HL, Gardner LB, et al. *Kelley's Textbook of Internal Medicine*, 4th ed. Philadelphia: Lippincott, Williams & Wilkins, 2000, pp. 1150–61.

Loscalzo J, Fauci AS, Kasper DL, et al. *Harrison's Principles of Internal Medicine*, 21st ed. New York: McGraw Hill Medical Publishing Division, 2022, pp. 1613–43.

Parsons P, Wiener-Kronish JP, Berra L, Stapleton RD. *Critical Care Secrets*, 6th ed. Philadelphia: Elsevier, 2018, pp. 321–6.

Seay N, Lehrich W, Greenberg A. Diagnosis and management of disorders of body tonicity: hyponatremia and hypernatremia – core curriculum 2020. *Am J Kidney Dis* 2020;**75** (2):272–86.

Winshall JS, Lederman RJ. *Tarascon Internal Medicine & Critical Care Pocketbook*, 3rd ed. Lompoc: Tarascon Publishing, 2004, pp. 146–9.

# Potassium

Jennifer Eismon

## Hyperkalemia

### Sample Case

A 65-year-old male patient with hypertension, diabetes, and chronic renal failure on hemodialysis presents for an elective left arm arteriovenous fistula grafting. The patient unfortunately missed his dialysis and his last $K^+$ was 6.7 mEq/L. The patient is asymptomatic. What are your concerns? What tests and labs do you want? Would you postpone the surgery? Would you demand hemodialysis first? Would you be less concerned if the patient was not on dialysis? If this case suddenly became an emergency, what is your anesthetic plan?

### Clinical Issues

#### Definition

Hyperkalemia is defined as potassium ($K^+$) concentration >5 mEq/L.

#### Causes of Hyperkalemia

1. Pseudohyperkalemia: artificially increased serum $K^+$ concentration

   a. Hemolysis
   b. Prolonged use of a tourniquet with or without fist clenching: releases $K^+$ from the ischemic muscle
   c. Marked leukocytosis: white cell count >70,000/cm$^3$ causes spurious hyperkalemia due to $K^+$ leakage from the cells when the specimen is allowed to clot.
   d. Thrombocytosis: platelet count >1,000,000/cm$^3$ can release $K^+$ from platelets during clotting.

2. Endogenous $K^+$: $K^+$ released from cells (Table 11.1)

**Table 11.1** Approximate intracellular and extracellular concentrations of electrolytes (mEq/L)

|  | Intracellular | Extracellular |
|---|---|---|
| Sodium (Na$^+$) | 12 | 150 |
| Potassium (K$^+$) | 150 | 4 |
| Chloride (Cl$^-$) | 4 | 115 |
| Phosphate (PO$_4$$^{3-}$) | 40 | 2 |

Adapted from VanPutte CL, Regan JL, Russo AF. *Seeley's Anatomy & Physiology*, 10th ed. New York: McGraw-Hill, 2014.

   a. Tumor lysis syndrome
   b. Rhabdomyolysis: elevated levels of serum creatinine kinase
   c. Exercise-induced hyperkalemia related to the degree of exertion
   d. Thermal and electrical burns

3. Exogenous $K^+$

   a. Increased $K^+$ intake: rarely a cause
   b. Iatrogenic $K^+$ administration
   c. Transfusions with near-expired blood products

      i. Increased $K^+$ content due to hemolysis

4. Renal conditions

   a. Renal insufficiency/chronic renal failure
   b. Acute oliguric renal failure: increased $K^+$ release from the cells (acidosis, catabolism) and decreased $K^+$ excretion
   c. Nephropathy due to

      i. Drug-induced interstitial nephritis
      ii. Lupus nephritis
      iii. Sickle cell disease
      iv. Diabetic nephropathy
      v. Obstructive uropathy
      vi. Post-renal transplantation

   d. Hyperkalemic distal (type 4) renal tubular acidosis: due to hypoaldosteronism or chloride shunt

5. Acidosis

   a. Metabolic acidosis: raises $K^+$ an average of 0.7 mEq/0.1 pH unit
   b. Respiratory acidosis: raises $K^+$ an average of 0.1 mEq/0.1 pH unit
   c. Diabetic ketoacidosis results in hyperkalemia from high extracellular fluid osmolality pulling both water and $K^+$ from the intracellular space. A consequence of

      i. Insulin deficiency
      ii. Hypertonicity from hyperglycemia

6. Drugs

   a. Succinylcholine

      i. Raises the $K^+$ level 0.5–0.7 mEq/L in otherwise normal patients

ii. Exaggerated release of $K^+$ from the cellular membrane can be seen when succinylcholine is used in patients who have

    (1) Massive trauma

    (2) Burns

    (3) Neuromuscular disease

b. β-blocker: elevates $K^+$

c. Severe digitalis toxicity: due to $Na^+/K^+$ ATPase pump inhibition, which reduces $K^+$ influx and increases extracellular $K^+$.

d. Angiotensin-converting enzyme inhibitor (ACEI): results in impaired aldosterone release, which in turn increases the $K^+$ in patients who are more susceptible. These include patients with:

  i. Diabetes

  ii. Renal insufficiency

  iii. Decreased effective circulation volume

  iv. Bilateral renal artery stenosis

  v. Concurrent use of $K^+$-sparing diuretics and nonsteroidal anti-inflammatory drugs (NSAIDs)

e. Heparin: inhibits aldosterone biosynthesis, therefore leading to renal sodium wasting and potassium retention

f. Cyclosporine: suppresses renin levels and may impair aldosterone secretion by directly interfering with tubular $K^+$ secretion

g. Prostaglandin synthetase inhibitors (indomethacin): reduce renin release and produce reversible hyporeninemic hypoaldosteronism

h. Medications that impair renal $K^+$ excretion

  i. Spironolactone: competitive mineralocorticoid antagonist

  ii. Amiloride or triamterene: blocks the principal cell apical $Na^+$ channel and thus $K^+$ excretion causing hyperkalemia via an aldosterone-independent mechanism.

  iii. Trimethoprim and pentamidine (antivirals): block distal nephron $Na^+$ reabsorption, which may contribute to elevated $K^+$ levels in patients with HIV being treated for *P. carinii* pneumonia.

7. Endocrine abnormalities

a. Primary adrenal insufficiency (Addison's) or congenital adrenal enzyme deficiency: both result in decreased aldosterone synthesis leading to renal sodium wasting and potassium retention.

b. Pseudohypoaldosteronism: a rare familial disorder which presents with hyperkalemia, metabolic acidosis, renal $Na^+$ wasting, hypertension, and increased renin and aldosterone levels.

c. Hyporeninemic hypoaldosteronism: results in mild increase in $K^+$ due to euvolemia or extracellular fluid volume expansion and suppressed renin aldosterone levels; seen in

  i. Mild renal insufficiency

  ii. Diabetic nephropathy

  iii. Chronic tubulointerstitial disease

8. Hyperkalemia periodic paralysis: a rare autosomal dominant disorder presenting with episodic paralytic attacks that results in shifts of $K^+$ from the cellular compartment.

a. Precipitated by

  i. Excitement

  ii. Cold

  iii. Fasting

  iv. Stress

  v. Infection

  vi. General anesthesia

9. Chronic hyperkalemia: associated with decreased renal $K^+$ excretion:

a. Impaired secretion

  i. Impaired $Na^+$ reabsorption

  ii. Increased chloride reabsorption

b. Diminished distal tubule solute delivery

  i. Protein malnourishment: low urea excretion

  ii. Extracellular fluid volume contraction: decreased distal tubule $Na^+Cl^-$ delivery

## Clinical Features of Hyperkalemia

**TKO:** The ECG nor the serum $K^+$ alone is an indication for urgency; rather clinical context should be considered instead; EKG effects are directly proportional to both absolute serum $K^+$ and rate of rise

1. Weakness, tingling, and paresthesias

2. Flaccid paralysis particularly of the lower extremities

3. Hypoventilation if respiratory musculature is involved

4. Renal ammoniagenesis

a. Increased $K^+$ inhibits renal production of ammonia and reabsorption in the thick ascending loop of Henle; therefore, net acid excretion is impaired, leading to metabolic acidosis exacerbating $K^+$ movement out of cells.

5. Cardiac toxicity: does not correlate well with the plasma concentration of $K^+$

a. Cardiac toxicity usually precedes neurologic toxicity.

b. Estimated EKG changes listed below with increasing severity of hyperkalemia:

  i. As $K^+$ levels approach 6–7 mEq/L

    (1) Increased T wave amplitude

    (2) Flattened P wave, prolonged PR interval, and widening of QRS complex with deepening of the S wave

    (3) AV conduction delay

    (4) Loss of P wave

(5) Progressive widening of the QRS complex and merging of T wave: resembles a sine-wave pattern

ii. As K$^+$ levels approach 10–12 mEq/L

(1) Ventricular fibrillation/flutter and asystole

## Diagnosis of Hyperkalemia

1. Obtain a history and physical examination including review of current medication therapy.
2. Check the serum chemistry.
   a. If the serum concentration of K$^+$ is elevated, treatment takes precedence over diagnosis.
   b. Obtain an EKG to ascertain if cardiac toxicity is occurring.
   c. Rule out pseudohyperkalemia or spurious laboratory values; check a complete blood count (CBC) and peripheral blood smear.
   d. Rule out transcellular K$^+$ shift.
      i. Review the clinical circumstances.
      ii. Determine the patient's acid–base status.
      iii. Check other labs, including
         (1) Creatinine kinase
         (2) Myoglobin
         (3) Urinalysis
         (4) Serum drug levels: digoxin
3. Rule out renal etiology of the hyperkalemia.
   a. GFR <20 mL/min
      i. Acute renal failure
      ii. Oliguria
      iii. K$^+$ load
         (1) Exogenous source
         (2) Endogenous source
   b. GFR >20 mL/min
      i. Measure plasma renin and aldosterone levels.
         (1) Low aldosterone and high renin suggest adrenal insufficiency: confirmed by measuring plasma cortisol
         (2) Low aldosterone and renin: hyporeninemic hypoaldosteronism
         (3) Normal aldosterone and renin: primarily a renal tubular defect

## Treatment of Hyperkalemia

1. Treatment action is determined by the severity of the patient's EKG changes and symptomatology.
   a. Nonemergent treatment
      i. Reduce K$^+$ intake: eliminate K$^+$-rich foods from the patient's diet.

ii. Increase K$^+$ output by promoting gastrointestinal loss with cation exchange resins which promote the exchange of Na$^+$ for K$^+$.
         a. Onset 1–2 hours
         b. Duration 4–6 hours
      iii. Intravenous diuretics: loop and thiazide diuretics
      iv. Consider dialysis in a patient with renal failure.
      v. Avoid medication that can interfere with K$^+$ elimination.
   b. Emergent treatment goals
      i. Protect the myocardium.
         (1) Calcium chloride given in a central line or calcium gluconate in a peripheral vein
            (a) The onset of the effect is within minutes, but the duration is short-lived (30–60 minutes).
            (b) The dose should be repeated every 5–10 minutes as necessary.
            (c) Avoid in suspected digitalis toxicity.
      ii. Shift K$^+$ into cells temporarily.
         (1) Give sodium bicarbonate 50 mEq IV over 5 minutes.
            (a) Note that a patient in end-stage renal failure may not respond.
         (2) D50 plus insulin IV
            (a) Onset 10–20 minutes
            (b) Duration 4–6 hours
         (3) Albuterol (nebulized β$_2$-adrenergic agonist): promotes cellular K$^+$ uptake and can lower K$^+$ by 0.5–1.5 mEq/L.
            (a) Onset in 30 minutes
            (b) Duration 2–4 hours
      iii. Continue with nonemergent treatments as listed above once the myocardium is stabilized.

# KO Treatment Plan

## Pre-operative

1. The ideal goal K$^+$ level is below 5 mEq/L prior to surgery.
   a. If the patient is symptomatic, the surgery should be postponed.
      i. Keep in mind that clinical signs and symptoms do not correlate predictably with K$^+$ serum concentrations.
   b. Acute hyperkalemia
      i. The surgery should be postponed and treatment should be initiated immediately.

c. Many authors describe thresholds for postponing surgery varying from 5.5 to 5.9 mEq/L.

d. Some studies suggest that this may be an arbitrary number when dealing with patients who have chronic hyperkalemia. Chronic hyperkalemia does not automatically contraindicate surgery.

  i. First determine whether the hyperkalemia is chronic or acute.

  ii. If the patient has chronic hyperkalemia, determine the etiology and decide if the patient's $K^+$ is at baseline.

  iii. Consider the length and type of surgery proposed.

e. The patient with chronic renal failure on hemodialysis should have hemodialysis the day prior to any elective surgery.

  i. In this sample case, despite the patient having asymptomatic hyperkalemia, since the surgery is elective it should be postponed until after hemodialysis.

2. Pre-operative tests

a. Serum $K^+$ and electrolyte panel

b. EKG

  i. If the patient does have cardiac changes, start treatment to lower $K^+$ immediately.

### Intra-operative

1. In an emergent surgery, start treatment for hyperkalemia immediately and proceed to the operating room.

a. Central IV access and an arterial line should be obtained for medication administration and monitoring of hemodynamics and serial labs.

2. Induction medications

a. Avoid succinylcholine.

  i. It raises the $K^+$ level 0.5–0.7 mEq/L.

b. Use etomidate if the patient is hemodynamically unstable; otherwise use propofol.

3. Maintenance of anesthesia

a. Isoflurane: safer than sevoflurane due to the theoretical nephrotoxicity

b. Avoid acidemia, hypoventilation, and lactated ringer's IV solution.

4. Monitors

a. Standard ASA monitors should be applied.

b. Consider placing transcutaneous defibrillator pads to treat ventricular fibrillation, which could occur secondary to the hyperkalemia.

c. Place an arterial line for frequent blood draws.

### Post-operative

1. Patient should be transported with standard ASA monitors and supplemental oxygen to the ICU for close observation.

2. Frequent blood draws to monitor serum $K^+$

3. Continue therapy to lower the serum $K^+$.

4. Investigate the causes of hyperkalemia.

# Hypokalemia

## Sample Case

A 28-year-old female model presents for elective plastic surgery: breast augmentation, facial contouring with liposuction, and labial rejuvenation. She states that she has no medical problems and is 5'10" and 105 lbs. She does not take any medications. Pre-operative chemistry indicates a $K^+$ of 2.8 mEq/L and she is tachycardic at a rate of 109 bpm. Her other vital signs are within normal limits. What are your concerns? What should you suspect as the etiology of hypokalemia in this patient? Would you postpone the surgery? What would your anesthetic plan entail if this case was an emergency?

## Clinical Issues

Definition: hypokalemia is defined as a serum $K^+$ concentration <3.5 mEq/L.

### Causes of Hypokalemia

1. Redistribution of $K^+$ into the cells: extracellular to intracellular

a. Metabolic alkalosis: decreases serum $K^+$ by 0.3 mEq/L for each 0.1 unit increase in pH.

b. Drugs

  i. Insulin therapy: stimulates $K^+$ uptake by muscle and liver cells

  ii. Epinephrine and selective $\beta_2$-adrenergic agonist: catecholamine release and administration of $\beta_2$-adrenergic agonist directly induces cellular uptake of $K^+$ and promotes insulin secretion by pancreatic beta cells.

    (1) $\beta_2$-adrenergic agonist: pressors, bronchodilators, tocolytic agents

  iii. Glue-sniffing: toluene abuse

  iv. Drug intoxication: verapamil, chloroquine, methylxanthines, and barium

  v. Stress-induced catecholamine activity

  vi. Lithium overdose

c. States of rapid cell proliferation sequester extracellular $K^+$.

  i. Correction of megaloblastic anemia with vitamin $B_{12}$ therapy induces red blood cell production that avidly extracts $K^+$ from the extracellular fluid.

  ii. Granulocyte-macrophage colony stimulating factor: stimulates white blood cell production

iii. Acute leukemia and Burkitt's lymphoma

d. Hypokalemic periodic paralysis

   i. Rare familial hereditary disorder: results in intracellular shift of $K^+$ spontaneously or induced by carbohydrate-rich diet or excessive sugar intake.

e. Thyrotoxicosis: thyroid hormone stimulates cellular uptake of $K^+$.

f. Hypothermia

g. Delirium tremens

2. Potassium depletion

a. Decreased dietary intake of $K^+$

   i. Starvation: "tea and toast" diet of the elderly, anorexia nervosa, and bulimia

   ii. Clay ingestion: white clay binds intestinal $K^+$.

   iii. Alcoholism

b. Extrarenal: urine $K^+$ <20 mEq/day

   i. Gastrointestinal loss

     (1) Diarrhea

     (2) Laxative abuse: test stool and urine for phenolphthalein derivatives and consider proctoscopy for confirmation of melanosis coli.

     (3) Villous adenomas, VIPomas (vasoactive intestinal peptide tumors), and nonbeta cell pancreatic islet tumor: create profuse diarrhea.

     (4) Intestinal bypass or fistula

     (5) Vomiting and gastric suctioning: chloride depletion contributes to hypokalemic metabolic alkalosis.

   ii. Integumentary loss

c. Renal: urine $K^+$ >20 mEq/day

   i. Drugs

     (1) Diuretics

     (2) High-dose steroids

     (3) Penicillin derivatives

     (4) Hypomagnesemia-inducing drugs: amphotericin B, aminoglycosides, cisplatin, foscarnet

       (a) Hypokalemia is resistant to correction unless magnesium replacement occurs first.

   ii. Renal tubular acidosis (RTA): seen clinically as metabolic acidosis, renal $K^+$ wasting, and hypokalemia

     (1) Distal RTA (type I): seen most often

     (2) Proximal RTA (type II): common during usage of high-dose bicarbonate

iii. Diabetic ketoacidosis: several components lead to hypokalemia.

   (1) Delivery of beta hydroxybutyrate to collecting ducts and $K^+$ loss

   (2) Uncontrolled hyperglycemia leads to $K^+$ depletion from osmotic diuresis.

   (3) Treatment with insulin leads to decreased $K^+$ by stimulation of $Na^+/H^+$ anti-porter secondary to the $Na^+/K^+$ ATPase pump.

iv. Mineralocorticoid excess

   (1) Primary hyperaldosteronism: characterized by low renin and hypertension

     (a) Conn's syndrome (adrenal adenoma)

     (b) Adrenocortical hyperplasia

     (c) Carcinoma

   (2) Secondary hyperaldosteronism: characterized by high renin and hypertension

     (a) Malignant hypertension

     (b) Renin-secreting tumors

       (i) Renal cell carcinoma

       (ii) Ovarian carcinoma

       (iii) Wilm's tumor

     (c) Renal artery stenosis

   (3) Circumstances producing mineralocorticoid excess

     (a) Inhibition of 11β-hydroxysteroid dehydrogenase: an enzyme necessary for the conversion of cortisol

       (i) Glycyrrhizic acid: found in licorice and chewing tobacco

       (ii) Carbenoxolone

     (b) Cushing's syndrome

v. Rare familial syndromes that produce hypokalemia

   (1) Bartter's syndrome

   (2) Gitelman syndrome

   (3) Liddle syndrome

### Clinical Features of Hypokalemia

1. Noncardiac symptoms

a. $K^+$ <3 mEq/L: symptoms are unlikely if $K^+$ is above this value.

   i. Fatigue

   ii. Myalgia

   iii. Muscular weakness of the proximal lower extremities

   iv. Constipation and intestinal ileus

   v. $K^+$ depletion manifests as polydipsia and polyuria.

vi. Glucose intolerance from decreased $K^+$ due to impaired insulin secretion or peripheral insulin resistance

b. Severe hypokalemia: <2 mEq/L

  i. Progressive weakness
  ii. Hypoventilation due to respiratory involvement
  iii. Complete paralysis
  iv. Increased risk of rhabdomyolysis: due to impaired muscle metabolism and blunted hyperemic response to exercise

2. Cardiac symptoms due to hypokalemia

a. Cardiac symptoms due to delayed ventricular repolarization: does not correlate well with specific plasma $K^+$ concentration.

b. Cardiac problems frequently involve

  i. Arrythmias
  ii. Atrial fibrillation
  iii. Premature ventricular contraction (PVC)

c. Early hypokalemia: $K^+$ <3 mEq/L

  i. Flattening or inversion of T wave
  ii. Prominent U wave: more than 1 mm
  iii. ST segment depression
  iv. Prolonged QT interval
  v. Hypokalemia predisposes patients to digitalis toxicity.

d. Increasing severity of hypokalemia

  i. Prolonged PR interval
  ii. Decreased voltage
  iii. Widening of QRS
  iv. Increased risk of ventricular arrhythmia

## Diagnosis of Hypokalemia

1. Patient's history

a. Exclude diuretic use, laxative abuse, and dietary causes.

2. Medical exam: determine if there is hypertension, features of Cushing's, and edema.

3. Laboratory workup

a. Exclude marked leukocytosis by obtaining a CBC.

  i. Acute myeloid leukemia: white blood cells uptake plasma $K^+$, leading to a low $K^+$ concentration.

b. Pseudohypokalemia: prevented by storing blood samples on ice

c. Determine acid–base disturbances

  i. Arterial blood gas (ABG) sample
  ii. Urine $K^+$ and $Cl^-$
  iii. Renin and aldosterone levels
  iv. Serum magnesium level

d. Determine if the cause is renal.

  i. In the presence of renal $K^+$ loss, urine $K^+$ >20 mEq/day, metabolic alkalosis, and a urine $Cl^-$ is invaluable to differentiate etiology.

    (1) Urine $Cl^-$ >10 mEq/day suggests etiology of mineralocorticoid or glucocorticoid excess production.
    (2) Urine $Cl^-$ <10 mEq/day suggests a functioning kidney: hypokalemia is due to $K^+$ loss from the skin, GI tract, or from vomiting, or remote diuretic use.

  ii. The presence of renal $K^+$ loss, urine $K^+$ >20 mEq/day, and metabolic acidosis suggests RTA.
  iii. Extrarenal etiology is suggested when urine $K^+$ is <20 mEq/day.

**Treatment of Hypokalemia:** total body $K^+$ deficit correlates poorly with serum levels.

1. Identify the etiology and correct the underlying disorder.
2. Asymptomatic or minor symptoms (potassium of 2.5–3.5 mEq/L)

a. Give oral potassium replacement therapy: $K^+ Cl^-$ 20–40 mEq PO q 4–6 hours.
b. Encourage $K^+$-rich foods such as dried fruits, nuts, lima beans, tomatoes, carrots, potatoes, bananas, oranges, ground beef, lamb, and veal.

  i. 1 inch banana or 1 oz orange juice: 1.6 mEq $K^+$

3. Cardiac manifestations or significant symptoms are present

a. More aggressive therapy is warranted.
b. If the potassium level is <2.5 mEq/L, IV potassium replacement therapy should be given.

  i. IV supplementation: maximum 20–40 mEq/h, ideally through central access with continuous cardiac monitoring
  ii. Hospital admission or emergency room observation is indicated.
  iii. Repeat serum $K^+$ level measurement every 1–3 hours.

4. Serum $K^+$ levels are difficult to replenish with coinciding hypomagnesemia. Therefore, magnesium may need to be replaced prior to correcting $K^+$.
5. If the patient is manifesting cardiac arrhythmias

a. Appropriate pharmacologic therapy should be initiated.
b. Place cardiac monitoring.
c. Establish intravenous access.
d. Assess respiratory status.
e. Cardiac pacing should be considered in scenarios of severe bradycardia.

6. An internist or a nephrologist should be consulted for admission or follow-up care.

## KO Treatment Plan

### Pre-operative

1. Case delay

    a. According to *Miller's Anesthesia*, the decision to proceed with surgery is multifactorial and consideration should be given for the urgency of surgery, the level of abnormality, and what those effects are clinically.

    b. Proceeding with anesthesia is also dependent on the clinical setting.

        i. If the patient is having cardiac dysrhythmias, surgery should be postponed.

        ii. Is hypokalemia acute or chronic?

            (1) In the acute setting it is ideal to postpone surgery, especially in the face of cardiac dysrhythmias

            (2) In the setting of chronic depletion of $K^+$ without cardiac changes, it may be reasonable to proceed with surgery and plan to replace $K^+$ intra-operatively.

2. Labs and tests

    a. Obtain serum magnesium: replacement of $K^+$ can be inhibited by hypomagnesemia.

    b. EKG: rule out cardiac dysrhythmias.

    c. Urine $K^+$: rule out renal involvement.

3. In regard to the patient being underweight, tachycardic, and having low serum $K^+$, you should determine if she uses or abuses diuretics and/or laxatives, and whether she has an eating disorder that could contribute to her presentation. Express to the patient your concern for intra-operative cardiac dysrhythmias and complications her low serum $K^+$ has for her anesthetic management. As an aside, she could be taking other diet and weight-loss aids with amphetamine derivatives that can make her more susceptible to cardiac events. If she denies the above scenario, you should investigate other causes for her low serum $K^+$.

### Intra-operative

1. Emergent surgery in a hypokalemic patient

    a. Proceed with anesthesia once the patient is hemodynamically stable.

    b. Use invasive blood pressure monitoring.

    c. Check electrolytes frequently.

    d. Continue treatment of the hypokalemia in the operating room.

2. Nonemergent surgery

    a. In the case scenario given, it is reasonable to proceed with surgery assuming no cardiac manifestations are present; however, investigation of underlying disorders should be made.

    b. I would perform general anesthesia with endotracheal intubation due to surgery length and plan $K^+$ replacement to be initiated through a peripheral IV.

        i. Correcting $K^+$: the infusion rate should not exceed 20 mEq/h unless the patient exhibits paralysis or malignant ventricular arrhythmia.

2. Induction

    a. After standard ASA monitors are placed and preoxygenation occurs, induction can be carried out with fentanyl, propofol, and rocuronium assuming she has a good airway evaluation.

    b. Avoid sympathomimetics, such as ketamine, due to her resting tachycardia.

3. Maintenance

    a. The patient can be maintained on volatile anesthetics along with narcotics when necessary.

## Post-operative

1. A plan for follow-up care and oral supplementation of her $K^+$ level should be arranged with her primary care physician.

2. She should be counseled on the gravity of using diuretics and laxatives for weight loss.

## Bibliography

Barash PG, Cullen BF, Stoelting RK, et al. *Clinical Anesthesia*, 8th ed. Philadelphia: Lippincott Williams & Wilkins, 2017, pp. 404–9.

Gropper MA. *Miller's Anesthesia*, 9th ed. Philadelphia: Elsevier, 2020, pp. 4848–58.

Humes HD, DuPont HL, Gardner LB, et al. *Kelley's Textbook of Internal Medicine*, 4th ed. Philadelphia: Lippincott Williams & Wilkins, 2000, pp. 1162–71.

Loscalzo J, Fauci AS, Kasper DL, et al. *Harrison's Principles of Internal Medicine*, 21st ed. New York: McGraw Hill Medical Publishing Division, 2022, pp. 1643–74.

Olson RP, Schow AJ, McCann R, et al. Absence of adverse outcomes in hyperkalemic patients undergoing vascular access surgery. *Can J Anesth* 2003;50:553–7.

Palmer BF. Approach to fluid and electrolyte disorders and acid–base problems. *Prim Care* 2008;35(2):195–213.

VanPutte CL, Regan JL, Russo AF. *Seeley's Anatomy & Physiology*, 10th ed. New York: McGraw-Hill, 2014, p. 989.

Winshall JS, Lederman RJ. *Tarascon Internal Medicine & Critical Care Pocketbook*, 3rd ed. Lompoc: Tarascon Publishing, 2004, pp. 149–51.

# Chapter 12

# Calcium

Melvyn J. Y. Chin, Brian M. Sapola, and Jessica A. Lovich-Sapola

## Sample Case

A 25-year-old otherwise healthy male was involved in a motorcycle accident resulting in multiple long bone and pelvic fractures, and blood in his pelvis and abdomen. Massive blood loss occurred in the operating room, and the patient was rapidly transfused with 15 units of packed red blood cells (pRBC), 12 units of fresh frozen plasma (FFP), and two 6-packs of platelets. Despite the fluid resuscitation, the patient remained hypotensive. The astute resident in the case noted that the ionized calcium level on the last arterial blood gas was low and promptly administered 1 g of intravenous calcium chloride. The blood pressure rapidly improved. Why was the patient's calcium low? Why did treating the hypocalcemia improve the blood pressure?

## Clinical Issues

1. Total serum calcium = protein-bound (40%) + chelated fraction (10%) + ionized fraction (50%)
2. Ionized calcium is the physiologically active form of calcium.
   a. Even if total serum calcium is low, it may not be clinically significant if the ionized calcium level is within the normal range.
3. Calcium is essential for
   a. Normal muscle function: excitation–contraction coupling
   b. Generation of cardiac pacemaker activity and cardiac action potential
   c. Cardiac contractility
   d. Neurotransmitter release
   e. cAMP and phosphoinositide function
   f. Membrane and bone structure
4. Main regulators of serum calcium
   a. Parathyroid hormone, calcitriol, and vitamin D
   b. Calcitonin
   c. Homeostasis of calcium is maintained by processes in the intestinal tract (absorption vs. secretion), bones (resorption vs. deposition), and kidneys (absorption vs. excretion).
5. Correction for hypoalbuminemia
   a. Add 1 mg/dL to the serum calcium level for every 1 g/dL of albumin concentration below 4.0 g/dL.

## Hypocalcemia

### Definition

1. Ionized calcium <1.0 mmol/L or 4.0 mg/dL
2. Total serum calcium <2.1 mmol/L or 8.5 mg/dL

### Causes of Hypocalcemia

1. Parathyroid hormone (PTH) deficiency
   a. Parathyroid gland damaged or removed
   b. Parathyroid suppression from
      i. Severe hypomagnesemia
      ii. Burns
      iii. Sepsis
      iv. Pancreatitis
2. Vitamin D deficiency
3. Hyperphosphatemia: renal failure, tumor lysis, rhabdomyolysis
4. Renal failure: results in hyperphosphatemia and decreased calcitriol
5. Citrate toxicity: from massive transfusions (citrate added to banked blood as an anticoagulant preservative binds to calcium, decreasing the ionized calcium concentration)
6. Acute alkalemia
7. Post-cardiopulmonary bypass
8. Acute pancreatitis

### Clinical Manifestations of Hypocalcemia

1. Cardiovascular
   a. ECG changes
      i. Dysrhythmias: heart block in severe cases
      ii. QT prolongation
   b. Heart failure
   c. Hypotension
   d. Digitalis insensitivity
   e. Impaired β-adrenergic action
2. Neuromuscular
   a. Tetany:
      i. Chvostek's sign: tapping on the facial nerve elicits a contraction of facial muscles.

ii. Trousseau's sign: inflating a blood pressure cuff to 20 mm Hg above systolic blood pressure causing radial and ulnar nerve ischemia producing carpal spasms.

b. Muscle spasm

c. Papilledema

d. Seizure

e. Weakness

f. Fatigue

g. Paresthesia: around the mouth or fingertips

h. Irritability

i. Mental status changes

3. Respiratory

a. Apnea

b. Laryngeal spasm: can be seen in the immediate post-operative period after thyroidectomy or parathyroidectomy surgery.

c. Bronchospasm

4. Psychiatric

a. Anxiety

b. Dementia

c. Depression

d. Psychosis

## Treatment

1. Symptomatic and acute: seizures, laryngospasm, tetany, and cardiovascular depression

a. Intravenous calcium

b. Magnesium must also be replaced if it is low.

i. Citrate binds and chelates bivalent ($2+$) metal cations such as calcium ($Ca^{2+}$) and likely magnesium ($Mg^{2+}$).

c. Correct metabolic and/or respiratory alkalosis

2. Asymptomatic and less acute

a. Treat the underlying cause.

b. Oral calcium supplements

c. Oral vitamin D

## KO Treatment Plan

### Pre-operative

1. Identify the underlying cause of hypocalcemia.

2. Treat the hypocalcemia.

a. Administer calcium

i. Intravenous infusion of 10% calcium chloride or calcium gluconate

ii. Oral administration of 500–1000 mg elemental calcium every 6 hours

b. Administer vitamin D

i. Ergocalciferol 1200 µg/day

ii. Dihydrotachysterol 200–400 µg/day

iii. 1,25-dihydroxycholecalciferol 0.25–1.0 µg/day

3. Monitor the electrocardiogram for dysrhythmias and prolonged QT.

4. Monitor for hypomagnesemia and treat if necessary.

5. Symptomatic hypocalcemia must be treated prior to proceeding to the operating room.

### Intra-operative

1. Once in the operating room, try to avoid things that will continue to decrease the calcium level.

a. Avoid hyperventilation.

b. Avoid the administration of bicarbonate.

2. Hypocalcemia can occur with massive transfusion of pRBC or FFP because the citrate preservative in the blood product chelates the calcium in the blood.

a. The hypocalcemia can then result in hypotension secondary to the resulting poor cardiac function.

3. Repleting the calcium improves the contractility of the heart, which in turn increases the patient's blood pressure.

4. An arterial line can be placed for close intra-operative blood pressure monitoring and frequent serum calcium blood draws.

## Hypercalcemia

### Definition

1. Ionized calcium >1.5 mmol/L

2. Total serum calcium >10.5 mg/dL: customarily defined in terms of total serum calcium

### Causes

Ninety percent of cases are caused by malignancy (most common in inpatients) and primary hyperparathyroidism (most common in outpatients).

1. Hyperparathyroidism

2. Malignancy

a. Bone destruction from metastasis

b. Hormone-secreting malignant tissue

c. Hematologic malignancies

3. Vitamin D intoxication

4. Sarcoidosis and other granulomatous diseases

5. Hyperthyroidism

6. Immobilization

7. Milk-alkali syndrome

8. Drugs

a. Thiazide diuretics

b. Lithium

## Clinical Manifestations

1. Mild to moderate hypercalcemia (11–13 mg/dL)
   a. Lethargy
   b. Anorexia
   c. Nausea
   d. Polyuria
   e. At this level, some patients may even be asymptomatic.

2. Severe hypercalcemia (>13 mg/dL)
   a. Neuromuscular
      i. Muscle weakness: should receive decreased doses of nondepolarizing muscle relaxants.
      ii. Depression
      iii. Impaired memory
      iv. Emotional lability
      v. Lethargy
      vi. Stupor
      vii. Coma (usually occurs at 15–18 mg/dL)
   b. Cardiovascular
      i. Hypertension
      ii. Dysrhythmias
      iii. Widening QRS complex
      iv. Short QT interval
      v. Heart block
      vi. Cardiac arrest
      vii. Digitalis sensitivity
   c. Other
      i. Calcification in kidneys, skin, vessels, lungs, heart, and stomach
      ii. Renal insufficiency: hypercalcemia impairs renal concentrating ability and excretory capacity for calcium.

## KO Treatment Plan

### Pre-operative

1. Administration of normal saline to dilute plasma calcium and promote diuresis.
   a. Hypercalcemia is usually associated with hypovolemia.
   b. Normal saline restores the intravascular volume and increases urinary excretion of calcium.
   c. Normal saline should be started at rates of 200–300 mL/h.
   d. Once volume depletion is corrected, start loop diuretics.

2. Diuresis
   a. Along with fluid therapy, loop diuretics (furosemide) further enhance calcium excretion by increasing tubular sodium.
      i. The sodium ions compete with calcium ions for reabsorption in the proximal renal tubules and loop of Henle.
   b. The goal urine output should be 200–300 mL/h.

3. Bisphosphonates (i.e., pamidronate 30–90 mg IV)
4. Calcitonin (2–8 U/kg IV, SQ, or IM every 6–12 hours)
5. Phosphate: risk of ectopic calcification: renal damage, fatal hypocalcemia
6. Glucocorticoids: active only in certain malignancies
7. Dialysis: useful in renal failure
8. Increasing physical activity
9. Treat underlying cause.
10. Ideally, surgery should be postponed until the calcium level is normalized.

### Intra-operative

1. If the surgery is an emergency, then you must try to treat the hypercalcemia as quickly as possible intra-operatively: maintenance of hydration and urine output.
2. Monitors:
   a. Closely monitor the EKG for cardiac conduction abnormalities.
   b. Consider placing the following monitors:
      i. Arterial line for frequent blood samples
      ii. Central line and central venous pressure monitor to assess volume status/fluid resuscitation.
      iii. Foley catheter to monitor urine output.
3. Dosing of muscle relaxants should be guided by neuromuscular monitoring.
   a. Patients should receive a decreased dose of nondepolarizing muscle relaxants, especially if muscle weakness, hypotonia, or loss of deep tendon reflexes is present.

## Bibliography

Barash PG, Cullen BF, Stoelting RK, et al. *Clinical Anesthesia*, 8th ed. Philadelphia: Lippincott Williams & Wilkins, 2017, pp. 409–12.

Braunwald E, Fauci A, Kasper D, et al. *Harrison's Principles of Internal Medicine*, 15th ed. New York: McGraw-Hill, 2001, pp. 2194–5, 2209–26.

Goldman L, Ausiello D. *Cecil Medicine*, 23rd ed. Philadelphia: Saunders Elsevier, 2008, chapter 266.

Gropper MA. *Miller's Anesthesia*, 9th ed. Philadelphia: Elsevier, 2020, pp. 1017–1020, 1488–9, 1505–7.

Hensley F, Martin D, Gravlee G. *A Practical Approach to Cardiac Anesthesia*, 4th ed. Philadelphia: Lippincott Williams & Wilkins, 2008, pp. 232–3.

Hines M. *Stoelting's Anesthesia and Co-Existing Disease*, 7th ed. Philadelphia: Elsevier, 2018, pp. 416–18.

Sihler KC, Napolitano LM. Complications of massive transfusion. *Chest* 2010;**137**(1):209–20.

Winshall J, Lederman R. *Tarascon Internal Medicine & Critical Care Pocketbook*, 3rd ed. Lompoc: Tarascon Publishing, 2004, pp. 63–4.

Zakharchenko M, Leden P, Rulíšek J, et al. Ionized magnesium and regional citrate anticoagulation for continuous renal replacement therapy. *Blood Purif* 2016;**41**:41–7.

Chapter

# Magnesium

Melvyn J. Y. Chin, Brian M. Sapola, and Jessica A. Lovich-Sapola

## Sample Case

A 27-year-old female, G1P0 at 39 weeks gestational age, is currently receiving a magnesium sulfate infusion for pre-eclampsia. You are consulted for a possible cesarean section. You begin to interview her and notice that she is lethargic and has a hard time staying awake. You promptly check her deep tendon reflexes and notice that they are hyporeflexic. You immediately notify the obstetrician of your findings. What are the next steps you should take? What are your concerns? How would this affect your anesthetic management of this patient?

## Clinical Issues of Magnesium

1. Ionized magnesium is the physiologically active form of magnesium.
2. Normal level of magnesium is 1.8–2.5 mg/dL
3. Magnesium is essential for
   a. Various enzymatic reactions
      i. DNA and protein synthesis
      ii. Energy metabolism
      iii. Glucose utilization
      iv. Fatty acid synthesis and breakdown
   b. Regulation of
      i. Sodium–potassium pumps
      ii. Ca–ATPase enzymes
      iii. Adenylate cyclase
      iv. Proton pumps
      v. Slow calcium channels: contributes to maintenance of normal vascular tone and prevention of vasospasm.
      vi. Parathyroid hormone (PTH) secretion and sensitivity to PTH and vitamin D
      vii. Membrane excitability
   c. Membrane and bone structure
4. Main regulators of serum magnesium
   a. Absorbed through the gastrointestinal (GI) tract
   b. Filtered, reabsorbed, and excreted by the kidneys

## Magnesium Therapy Indications

1. Premature labor: tocolysis
2. Pre-eclampsia and eclampsia: anticonvulsant (therapeutic magnesium levels range from 5.0 to 7.0 mg/dL)

3. Tetanus and pheochromocytoma: blocks the release of catecholamines from adrenergic nerve terminals and adrenal glands.
4. Cardiology
   a. Improves myocardial oxygen supply and demand
   b. Reduces the incidence of dysrhythmias in post-myocardial infarction (MI) patients and in congestive heart failure (CHF) patients
   c. Decreases short-term mortality after an acute MI
   d. Treatment for torsades de pointes ventricular tachyarrhythmia
5. Respiratory
   a. Asthma management: contributes to smooth muscle relaxation of the bronchioles.

## Hypermagnesemia

### Definition

1. Magnesium level >2.5 mg/dL
2. Typically asymptomatic at levels between 2.5 and 5.0 mg/dL
3. Less common than hypomagnesemia because a magnesium load is usually quickly excreted in a patient with normal renal function

### Causes

1. Majority of cases are iatrogenic: administration of magnesium in antacids, laxatives, enemas, parenteral nutrition, or infusions: especially in the setting of renal failure.
2. Other rare causes
   a. Hypothyroidism
   b. Addison's disease
   c. Lithium toxicity

### Clinical Manifestations

1. Magnesium levels of 5–7 mg/dL (the therapeutic level for the treatment of pre-eclampsia/eclampsia)
   a. Lethargy
   b. Drowsiness
   c. Flushing
   d. Nausea

e. Vomiting

f. Diminished deep tendon reflexes (DTRs)

2. Magnesium levels above 7.0–12 mg/dL

a. Cardiovascular effects

i. Hypotension: direct vasodilation

ii. Dysrhythmia

iii. Increased QRS duration

iv. Prolonged PR and QT intervals

v. Depressed myocardial performance

b. Neuromuscular

i. Muscle weakness

(1) Hypermagnesemia antagonizes the release and effect of acetylcholine at the neuromuscular junctions.

(2) Potentiates the action of depolarizing and nondepolarizing muscle relaxants and decreases the potassium release in response to succinylcholine.

(a) Muscle relaxants should be carefully titrated by assessing the degree of neuromuscular blockade (i.e., use of a nerve stimulator).

(3) May precipitate severe muscle weakness in Eaton–Lambert syndrome or myasthenia gravis patients

ii. Somnolence

iii. Loss of DTRs

c. Respiratory effects

i. Depressed respiration and apnea from muscle weakness and/or paralysis

ii. Bronchodilator effects

3. Magnesium levels above 12 mg/dL

a. Hypotension

b. Bradycardia

c. Diffuse vasodilation

d. Paralysis

e. Coma

f. Significant respiratory depression

g. Complete heart block

h. Cardiac arrest

## Treatment of Hypermagnesemia

1. Stop or treat the underlying cause.

2. Forced diuresis with saline followed by a loop diuretic

3. Intravenous calcium

4. Hemodialysis

## KO Treatment Plan

### Pre-operative

1. Identify and treat the underlying cause.

a. This usually means stopping the magnesium-containing preparation.

b. Draw a magnesium level.

2. Magnesium is quickly excreted by the kidneys.

a. Further diuresis can be induced with an infusion of normal saline and/or IV furosemide.

3. IV calcium (5–10 mEq) will antagonize the neuromuscular and cardiac toxicity of hypermagnesemia.

4. Renal failure or life-threatening situations may require hemodialysis.

5. Nonurgent surgeries should be delayed until the patient's significant symptoms have resolved.

### Intra-operative

1. Consider invasive cardiovascular monitoring

a. Measure and treat the associated hypotension and vasodilation.

b. Guide fluid resuscitation.

c. Guide the forced diuresis.

2. Avoid acidosis: it exaggerates hypermagnesemia.

3. Muscle relaxant

a. Magnesium enhances the action of nondepolarizing muscle relaxants.

b. Magnesium prolongs the action of depolarizing muscle relaxants.

c. Decreased initial and subsequent doses, especially in patients with muscle weakness

i. Use your peripheral nerve stimulator as a guide.

4. If the sample patient requires an emergent cesarean section

a. Regional anesthesia is preferred.

i. Use an existing epidural or place a spinal.

b. If a general anesthetic is required, a rapid sequence induction should be performed. Reductions in the doses of induction and paralytic agents should be considered.

c. Arterial and central venous lines may be necessary to adequately measure and treat the associated hypotension, and for frequent blood samples.

d. An attempt can be made at forced diuresis.

i. Be careful to closely follow the volume status in a pre-eclamptic patient.

e. The patient may require prolonged ventilation.

## Post-operative

1. Hypermagnesemia and its associated skeletal muscle weakness often leads to difficulty in weaning from mechanical ventilation.
2. Patients often require a stay in the ICU until the hypermagnesemia is corrected.

# Hypomagnesemia

## Definition

1. Magnesium level <1.8 mg/dL
2. Symptoms are rare at levels between 1.5 and 1.7 mg/dL.
3. Symptoms often occur when the magnesium level is <1.2 mg/dL.

## Causes

1. Renal loss
   a. Volume expansion
   b. Hypercalcemia
   c. Osmotic diuresis: diabetes mellitus
   d. Renal disease with magnesium wasting: advanced renal disease may lead to magnesium retention.
   e. Drugs
      i. Loop diuretics
      ii. Aminoglycosides
      iii. Cisplatin
      iv. Cyclosporine
      v. Amphotericin B
      vi. Ethanol
         (1) Hypomagnesemia is prevalent in alcoholics: seen in about 30% of alcoholics admitted to the hospital.

2. GI loss/decreased intestinal absorption
   a. Vomiting
   b. Prolonged nasogastric suctioning
   c. GI or biliary fistulas
   d. Intestinal drains
   e. Diarrhea: Crohn's disease and ulcerative colitis

3. Massive blood infusion
   a. Citrate is used as a blood preservative through anticoagulation by chelating and inactivating factor IV (calcium).
   b. Citrate binds bivalent metal cations (e.g., $Ca^{2+}$ and $Mg^{2+}$) which contributes to low ionized calcium and likely low ionized magnesium after massive infusion of blood products containing citrate.

## Clinical Manifestations

Usually seen at magnesium levels <1.2 mg/dL.
1. Cardiovascular

   a. ECG changes
      i. Arrhythmias: ventricular tachycardia, torsades de pointes, and ventricular fibrillation
      ii. PR and QT prolongation
      iii. U waves
      iv. Nonspecific T wave changes

   b. Heart failure
   c. Hypotension
   d. Aggravates digoxin toxicity
   e. Coronary artery spasm

2. Neuromuscular/psychiatric
   a. Muscle spasm
      i. Chvostek's sign: tapping on the facial nerve elicits a contraction of facial muscles.
      ii. Trousseau's signs: inflating a blood pressure cuff to 20 mm Hg above the systolic blood pressure causing radial and ulnar nerve ischemia producing carpal spasms.

   b. Muscle weakness
   c. Lethargy
   d. Paresthesias
   e. Seizures
   f. Depression
   g. Confusion
   h. Coma
   i. Tetany

3. Endocrine
   a. Decreases parathyroid hormone (PTH) secretion and impairs end-organ responsiveness (i.e., bone, kidney, intestine) to PTH.
      i. Associated with hypocalcemia.
   b. Hypokalemia
      i. Renal potassium wasting: the sodium–potassium pump is magnesium-dependent.

## Treatment

1. Depends on the severity of the deficiency
   a. Treat patients with
      i. Cardiac arrhythmias and seizure
      ii. Associated severe hypocalcemia or hypokalemia
      iii. Severe hypomagnesemia <1.4 mg/dL
         (1) Treat with intravenous magnesium as a bolus.
         (2) Repeat the bolus dose until symptoms resolve.
         (3) Once symptoms resolve, continue a slower infusion for a few days.
   b. Mild cases
      i. Oral magnesium salts

## KO Treatment Plan

### Pre-operative

1. Identify and treat the underlying cause.

   a. 24-hour urinary magnesium excretion will help separate renal from nonrenal causes of hypomagnesemia.

      i. Hypomagnesemia coupled with high urinary excretion of magnesium (>3–4 mEq/day) suggests a renal etiology.

2. Mild hypomagnesemia (magnesium level 1.5–1.8 mg/dL)

   a. Oral magnesium replacement is effective.

3. Moderate to severe (magnesium level <1.2 mg/dL)

   a. Parenteral magnesium is usually needed (usually in the form of IV magnesium sulfate 2 g over the first hour, with a cumulative dose of up to 6 g over 24 hours).

4. A nonemergent anesthetic should be delayed if the patient is displaying significant signs or symptoms: cardiac arrhythmias or seizures.

### Intra-operative

1. Anticipate ventricular arrythmias and be prepared to treat them.
2. Guide muscle relaxation with a peripheral nerve stimulator.

   a. Hypomagnesemia is associated with both muscle weakness and excitation.

3. Prepare for possible prolonged ventilation secondary to the associated impairment of respiratory muscle power.
4. Be prepared for seizures.
5. Avoid fluid loading, particularly with sodium-containing solutions.
6. Avoid the use of diuretics: renal excretion of magnesium passively follows sodium excretion.

## Bibliography

Barash PG, Cullen BF, Stoelting RK, et al. *Clinical Anesthesia*, 8th ed. Philadelphia: Lippincott Williams & Wilkins, 2017, pp. 414–15.

Braunwald, E, Fauci A, Kasper D, et al. *Harrison's Principles of Internal Medicine*, 15th ed. New York: McGraw-Hill, 2001, pp. 2197–8.

Goldman L, Ausiello D. *Cecil Medicine*, 23rd ed. Philadelphia: Saunders Elsevier, 2008, chapter 120.

Gropper MA. *Miller's Anesthesia*, 9th ed. Philadelphia: Elsevier, 2020, pp. 1489–90, 1507–8.

Hines M. *Stoelting's Anesthesia and Co-Existing Disease*, 7th ed. Philadelphia: Elsevier, 2018, pp. 418–19.

Sihler KC, Napolitano LM. Complications of massive transfusion. *Chest* 2010;**137**(1):209–20.

Winshall J, Lederman R. *Tarascon Internal Medicine & Critical Care Pocketbook*, 3rd ed. Lompoc: Tarascon Publishing, 2004, p. 151.

Zakharchenko M, Leden P, Rulíšek J, et al. Ionized magnesium and regional citrate anticoagulation for continuous renal replacement therapy. *Blood Purif* 2016;**41**:41–7.

# Intravenous Anesthetics

Varun Dixit and Jessica A. Lovich-Sapola

## Clinical Issues

### Properties of the Ideal IV Anesthetic

#### Physical Properties

1. Long shelf life
2. Water-soluble
3. Drug compatibility and stability in solution
4. No pain on injection, venous irritation, or local tissue damage from extravasation
5. Nonteratogenic
6. Analgesic
7. Amnestic
8. Hypnotic

#### Pharmacological Properties

1. Rapid and smooth onset
2. Lack of cardiovascular and respiratory depression
3. Rapid metabolism to pharmacologically inactive metabolites
4. No histamine release or hypersensitivity reactions
5. Rapid emergence without excitation or delirium
6. Antiemetic properties
7. No accumulation with infusion

**TKO:** You will be asked which IV anesthetic you plan to use and why. There is usually no single correct answer. Just pick one and defend it!

## Propofol

1. Physical attributes

   a. Insoluble in water
   b. Highly lipid-soluble
   c. Prepared in the form of an emulsion
   d. Stable at room temperature
   e. Not light-sensitive
   f. Formulations can support bacterial growth and therefore should be used within 6 hours of opening.

2. Mechanism of action

   a. Primarily a hypnotic
   b. Exact mechanism and location of propofol action is unclear; there may be multiple actions

       i. May prolong opening of chloride channels to maintain the neuron in a hyperpolarized state and prevent action potentials, similarly to a benzodiazepine
       ii. May also act to inactivate sodium channels in addition to potentiating chloride channels
       iii. May decrease the rate of dissociation of GABA from the GABA-A receptor, but may also bind to the receptor directly in some cells
       iv. It is still unclear whether one, some, or all of these actions of propofol actually induce the wanted and noticeable effects.
       v. The studies have involved mostly rodent models and it has not been determined how well the recent findings will translate to human brains.

3. Metabolism

   a. Rapidly metabolized in the liver to water-soluble compounds
   b. Water-soluble compounds are then excreted by the kidneys.
   c. Kidneys and lungs have extra-hepatic metabolism.

4. Pharmacokinetics

   a. Elimination half-life is 4–7 hours.
   b. Clearance is 20–30 mL/kg/min.
   c. Large volume of distribution at steady state

5. Effects

   a. Central nervous system (CNS)

       i. Rapid onset of hypnosis after doses of 2.5 mg/kg (one arm–brain circulation) with a peak effect seen at 90–100 seconds
       ii. Sense of well-being noted after administration secondary to an increase in dopamine concentrations
       iii. Induction dose affected by age, decreasing with increasing age
       iv. Decreases

         (1) Cerebral metabolic oxygen consumption ($CMRO_2$)
         (2) Cerebral blood flow (CBF)
         (3) Intracranial pressure (ICP)
         (4) Intraocular pressure

(5) Cerebral perfusion pressure (CPP) if the propofol causes a significant drop in systemic blood pressure

b. Respiratory

  i. Apnea with the induction dose

  ii. Maintenance infusion causes a decreased tidal volume (TV) and increased respiratory rate (RR)

  iii. Reduced ventilatory response to hypoxia and carbon dioxide

  iv. Causes bronchodilation in patients with chronic obstructive pulmonary disease (COPD)

  v. Potentiates hypoxic pulmonary vasoconstriction

c. Cardiovascular

  i. Decreases

    (1) Systolic blood pressure (SBP)

    (2) Diastolic blood pressure (DBP)

    (3) Mean arterial blood pressure (MAP)

    (4) Cardiac output (CO)

    (5) Cardiac index (CI)

    (6) Stroke index (SI)

    (7) Systemic vascular resistance (SVR)

  ii. Usually no change in heart rate.

    (1) Marked drop in cardiac filling can result in a vagally mediated reflex bradycardia.

    (2) No reflex tachycardia

6. Uses

a. Induction of general anesthesia (dose 1–2.5 mg/kg IV)

b. Maintenance of general anesthesia (dose 50–150 μg/kg/min IV)

c. Sedation (25–75 μg/kg/min IV)

7. Side effects

a. Pain on injection.

  i. Pain can be reduced by using a large vein, utilizing IV lidocaine, and avoiding the back of the hand.

b. Myoclonus (rare)

c. Apnea (with a bolus)

d. Reduction in blood pressure

e. Anaphylactoid reactions

  i. A history of an egg allergy is not an absolute contraindication secondary to propofol.

  ii. Egg lecithin that is extracted from yolk to be used as the propofol emulsifier is not as allergenic as egg white (albumin), which is the most common cause of patient egg allergy.

f. Thrombophlebitis of the vein into which it is injected (rare)

g. Propofol infusion syndrome: rare and often fatal syndrome most commonly described in critically ill children and adults undergoing a prolonged propofol infusion at high doses.

  i. Symptoms include cardiomyopathy, rhabdomyolysis, severe metabolic acidosis, hyperkalemia, hepatomegaly, and renal failure.

  ii. Mechanism is impaired fatty acid metabolism and lack of glucose.

  iii. Treatment is supportive.

8. Special characteristics

a. Antiemetic (dose 10–20 mg IV, infusion 10 μg/kg/min IV)

b. Rapid emergence and return of psychomotor function

c. Rapid recovery following prolonged infusion

d. Safe in malignant hyperthermia-susceptible patient

e. Most commonly used induction agent

f. Subhypnotic dose can be used to treat pruritus induced by spinal opiates

g. Anticonvulsant properties

# Etomidate

1. Physical attributes

a. Imidazole derivative

b. Water-soluble in acidic solutions

c. Lipid-soluble at physiologic pH

2. Mechanism of action

a. Depresses the reticular activating system

b. Mimics the inhibitory effects of GABA

c. May have disinhibitory effects on parts of the nervous system that control extrapyramidal motor activity

3. Metabolism

a. Hepatic microsomal enzymes and plasma esterases rapidly hydrolyze etomidate to an inactive metabolite.

b. The metabolites are then excreted by the kidneys (85%) and bile (13%).

c. A small amount (2%) is excreted without being metabolized.

4. Pharmacokinetics

a. Elimination half-life is 2.9–5.3 hours.

b. Highly protein-bound

c. Rapid onset of action

d. Redistribution is responsible for decreasing plasma concentration to awakening levels.

5. Effects

a. CNS

  i. Hypnosis

  ii. No analgesic activity

  iii. Decreases

    (1) CBF

(2) $CMRO_2$

(3) ICP

(4) Intraocular pressure

    iv. CPP is maintained or increased.

    v. Cerebral protection

    vi. Associated with grand mal seizures and increased activity in epileptogenic foci

b. Respiratory

    i. Minimal respiratory depression

    ii. May not totally ablate the sympathetic response to direct laryngoscopy and intubation

c. Cardiovascular

    i. Hemodynamic stability

    ii. Almost no change in

        (1) Heart rate (HR)

        (2) MAP

        (3) Mean pulmonary pressure

        (4) Central venous pressure (CVP)

        (5) Stroke volume (SV)

        (6) CI

        (7) SVR

    iii. Does not release histamine

d. Endocrine

    i. Induction dose transiently inhibits enzymes involved in the synthesis of cortisol and aldosterone.

    ii. Infusion for sedation results in consistent adrenocortical suppression with increased mortality in the critically ill patient.

6. Uses

a. Induction of patients

    i. With cardiovascular disease

        (1) History of cerebral vascular accident

        (2) Cardioversion

        (3) Aortic surgery

    ii. With reactive airway disease

    iii. Neurosurgical patients

        (1) Increased ICP

    iv. Trauma patients with hypovolemia

    v. Electroconvulsive therapy (ECT)

    vi. Retrobulbar block

7. Side effects

a. Inhibition of cortisol and aldosterone synthesis

b. Pain on injection

c. Superficial thrombophlebitis

d. Myoclonus

e. Nausea and vomiting

8. Special characteristics

a. Hemodynamic stability

b. Minimal respiratory depression

c. Cerebral protection

d. Rapid onset and termination of effect

# Ketamine

1. Physical attributes

a. Phencyclidine derivative

c. Partially water-soluble

d. Highly lipid-soluble

e. Low molecular weight

f. Near physiologic pH

g. Can be used in intravenous, intramuscular, oral, nasal, and rectal routes.

2. Mechanism of action

a. Inhibits N-methyl-D-aspartate (NMDA) channels and neuronal hyperpolarization-activated cationic ($HCN_1$) channels

3. Metabolism

a. Hepatic microsomal enzymes

b. The metabolites are then conjugated into water-soluble glucuronide derivatives that are excreted in the urine.

4. Pharmacokinetics

a. Elimination half-life is 2.5–2.8 hours.

b. Rapidly crosses the blood–brain barrier

5. Effects

a. CNS

    i. Unconsciousness

    ii. Dissociate anesthesia

    iii. Increased

        (1) $CMRO_2$

        (2) Cerebral metabolism

        (3) CBF

        (4) ICP when given alone

            (a) When combined with a benzodiazepine and controlled ventilation ketamine is not associated with increased ICP.

    iv. Maintains corneal, cough, and swallow reflexes, but may still be at risk for aspiration.

    v. Profound analgesia

    vi. Pupils dilate

    vii. Nystagmus

    viii. Increased muscle tone

    ix. May prevent opioid-induced hyperalgesia due to NMDA receptor antagonism

b. Respiratory

i. Minimal effect on the central respiratory drive
ii. Unaltered response to $CO_2$
iii. Bronchodilation

c. Cardiovascular

i. Stimulates the sympathetic nervous system
ii. Systemic release of catecholamines, inhibits vagal tone, and causes norepinephrine reuptake inhibition
iii. Increased

(1) CO
(2) HR
(3) Blood pressure (BP)
(4) $O_2$ consumption

iv. Sympathetic stimulation can be blunted by use of a benzodiazepine and the use of a continuous infusion.

6. Uses

a. Good choice for induction and maintenance of anesthesia in patients with:

i. Reactive airway disorders
ii. Healthy trauma with unknown blood loss
iii. Cardiac tamponade
iv. Restrictive pericarditis
v. Congenital heart disease, especially for right-to-left shunt
vi. Septic shock
vii. Hemodynamic compromise based on hypovolemia or cardiomyopathy
viii. ASA class IV patients with respiratory and cardiovascular system disorders (excluding ischemic heart disease)
ix. Remote location: dressing changes, radiation therapy, dental work
x. Treatment of opioid-resistant chronic pain

(1) Cancer pain
(2) Neuropathic pain
(3) Ischemic pain
(4) Fibromyalgia

xi. Pediatric patients

7. Side effects

a. Increased lacrimation and salivation which can further increase the risk of laryngospasm
b. Increased skeletal muscle tone
c. Emergence reactions

i. Excitement
ii. Confusion
iii Hallucinations: treat with benzodiazepines
iv. Vivid dreaming

d. Not recommended

i. Open eye injury: increases intraocular pressure
ii. Significant coronary artery disease (CAD)
iii. Vascular aneurysm
iv. Schizophrenia
v. Patient with increased ICP or an intracranial mass lesion (when used as the sole anesthetic)

8. Special characteristics

a. Minimal hemodynamic changes
b. Profound analgesia and amnesia
c. The patient maintains the cough, corneal, and swallow reflexes.
d. Bronchodilation
e. Dissociative anesthesia
f. Post-operative analgesia
g. Patients who have been critically ill for a prolonged period may have exhausted their catecholamine stores and may be subject to the circulatory depressant effects of ketamine.
h. Ketamine affects mood.
i. Treatment of severe, treatment-resistant depression with suicidal ideation

# Dexmedetomidine (Precedex)

1. Mechanism of action

a. Selective $\alpha_2$ adrenergic receptor agonist in locus coeruleus and dorsal spinal cord
b. Sedative properties

2. Metabolism

a. Rapid redistribution
b. Relatively short half-life
c. Metabolized by the liver by the CYP450 system and through glucuronidation
d. Nearly all metabolites are excreted in the urine

3. Pharmacokinetics

a. Complete biotransformation by glucuronidation, hydroxylation, and methylation
b. Slowed in hepatic impairment but no effect in renal disease or advanced age

4. Effects

a. CNS

i. Sedation: endogenous sleep-promoting pathways
ii. Mimics natural sleep pattern
iii. Reduced delirium in ICU
iv. Analgesia while preserving respiratory function
v. Useful in neurosurgery with neuro-monitoring since cortical evoked potentials are maintained
vi. Decreases

(1) CBF
(2) $CMRO_2$

(3) ICP

b. Respiratory

  i. Reduces minute ventilation but no change in arterial oxygenation or pH

c. Cardiovascular

  i. Hypotension and bradycardia which is dose-related

    (1) Decreases

      (a) SV

      (b) CO

    (2) Increasing concentration leads to increases in

      (a) MAP

      (b) CVP

      (c) Pulmonary arterial wedge pressure (PAWP)

      (d) SVR

5. Uses

a. Anxiolytic

b. Sedation

c. Analgesia

d. Procedural sedation

  i. ICU

  ii. Pediatric patients

  iii. Remote location

  iv. Invasive procedures

  v. Awake craniotomy

  vi. Intubations

  vii. Carotid endarterectomies

  viii. Bariatric surgery due to opioid-sparing effect

e. Addiction treatment

  i. Alcohol withdrawal

  ii. Cocaine intoxication

f. Treatment and prevention of emergence delirium after an inhalational anesthetic

6. Side effects

a. Risks of hypotension, bradycardia, and sinus arrest

  i. Increased risk with patients with hypovolemia, diabetes mellitus, chronic hypertension, and the elderly

b. Hypertension is seen with large boluses and loading dose.

c. Dry mouth

7. Special characteristics

a. Relative contraindication with advanced heart block or severe ventricular dysfunction

b. Relative contraindication in pregnancy (Category C)

c. Tolerance and tachyphylaxis can occur with prolonged exposure greater than 24 hours.

# Bibliography

Barash PG, Cullen BF, Stoelting RK, et al. *Clinical Anesthesia*, 8th ed. Philadelphia: Lippincott Williams & Wilkins, 2017, pp. 486–502.

Butterworth JF, Mackey DC, Wasnick JD. *Morgan & Mikhail's Clinical Anesthesiology*, 6th ed. New York: McGraw-Hill Education, 2018, pp. 171–85.

Gropper MA. *Miller's Anesthesia*, 9th ed. Philadelphia: Elsevier, 2020, pp. 638–79.

Sedwick C. Propofol's paradox explained. *J Gen Physiol* 2018;**150**(9):1231–2.

Trapani G, Altomare C, Liso G, et al. Propofol in anesthesia: mechanism of action, structure–activity relationships, and drug delivery. *Curr Med Chem* 2000;7(2):249–71.

# Inhalational Anesthetics

Jessica A. Lovich-Sapola and Andrew M. Bauer

## Clinical Issues

### Factors that Influence the Choice of an Inhaled Agent

1. Speed of induction and emergence
2. Suitability for inhalational induction
3. Effects on physiology: cardiovascular, intracranial pressure
4. Coexisting diseases: obesity, pneumothorax
5. Cost

### Isoflurane

1. Facts
    a. Low minimum alveolar concentration (MAC): 1.2
    b. Halogenated methyl ether
    c. Clear
    d. Nonflammable
    e. Liquid at room temperature
    f. Systemic and coronary vasodilator

2. Advantages
    a. Lowest cost of the halogenated anesthetics
    b. Nonflammable
    c. Minimal cardiac depression: cardiac output is maintained by a rise in heart rate.
    d. Reverses bronchospasm
    e. Skeletal muscle relaxant

3. Disadvantages
    a. High blood and lipid solubility
        i. Slower onset and emergence
        ii. May be more of an issue in morbidly obese patients and long cases
    b. Pungent odor may not be well tolerated for inhalational inductions.
    c. May produce tachycardia
    d. Sometimes avoided in patients with significant coronary artery disease because of the theoretical risk of coronary steal syndrome: dilation of the normal coronary arteries with resultant diversion of blood away from the fixed stenotic lesion.

    e. Not tolerated well in patients who are severely hypovolemic due to its vasodilating effects
    f. Malignant hyperthermia trigger

### Sevoflurane

1. Facts
    a. Relatively low MAC: 2.0
    b. Completely fluorinated methyl isopropyl ether
    c. Intermediate cost between isoflurane and desflurane
    d. Low blood solubility but high lipid solubility

2. Advantages
    a. More rapid induction than isoflurane
    b. Sweet relatively nonpungent odor with minimal airway irritation
        i. Best choice for inhalational induction
        ii. Well suited to pediatric anesthesia
        iii. Reverses bronchospasm: potent bronchodilator
    c. Faster emergence when compared to isoflurane
    d. Less decrease in systemic vascular resistance and arterial blood pressure when compared to isoflurane and desflurane
    e. Skeletal muscle relaxant

3. Disadvantages
    a. May start to accumulate over a long case, especially in an obese patient
    b. Potential for emergence delirium
        i. Some clinicians will change to isoflurane after induction.
    c. Cardiac output is not well maintained secondary to the minimal rise in heart rate compared to isoflurane and desflurane.
        i. Mild myocardial depressant
    d. May prolong QT
    e. Contraindicated in patients with severe hypovolemia and intracranial hypertension
    f. Malignant hyperthermia trigger
    g. Potential nephrotoxicity if given at flow rates less than 2 liters
        i. Formation of compound A

h.  Can form carbon monoxide during exposure to dry $CO_2$ absorbents, and an exothermic reaction has occurred and resulted in fires

# Desflurane

1.  Facts

    a.  High MAC: 6.0
    b.  Fluorinated methyl ether

2.  Advantages

    a.  Very low solubility in blood and lipid

        i.   Fast induction and emergence
        ii.  Less residual anesthetic in peripheral tissues in obese patients and after long cases

    b.  Near-absent metabolism
    c.  Skeletal muscle relaxant

3.  Disadvantages

    a.  Expensive
    b.  Most pungent: may cause coughing, bronchospasm, laryngospasm, salivation, and breath holding

        i.    Unsuitable for inhalational inductions
        ii.   Not a good choice for pediatric anesthesia
        iii.  Not suitable for patients with significant pulmonary disease

    c.  A rapid increase in the desflurane concentration level or high levels alone can result in tachycardia, hypertension, myocardial ischemia, and elevated catecholamine levels.
    d.  Malignant hyperthermia trigger
    e.  Contraindicated in patients with severe hypovolemia and intracranial hypertension
    f.  Requires a heated, pressurized vaporizer

        i.   Requires electrical power
        ii.  Requires more servicing

    g.  Degrades to form carbon monoxide in extremely dry $CO_2$ absorbers to a greater extent than the other volatile anesthetics.

# Nitrous Oxide

1.  Facts

    a.  Very high MAC: 104%
    b.  Only inorganic anesthetic gas
    c.  Colorless
    d.  Essentially odorless
    e.  Gas at room temperature
    f.  Stored as a liquid under pressure
    g.  NMDA receptor antagonist

2.  Advantages

    a.  Inexpensive

    b.  Very low solubility in blood and lipids

        i.  Allows the use of less halogenated agent when used in combination

    c.  Rapid induction and recovery
    d.  Can speed induction of other anesthetics

        i.  Concentration effect

            (1)  Combination of low solubility and high inhaled partial pressures
            (2)  Increases the blood concentration of nitrous oxide
            (3)  Speeds induction
            (4)  Diffusion hypoxia

                (a)  Occurs during emergence if low $FiO_2$ used
                (b)  Opposite of concentration effect: rapid diffusion of nitrous oxide from the blood to the alveoli decreases the alveolar $PO_2$

        ii.  Second gas effect when used with a volatile agent

            (1)  Same principle as the concentration effect
            (2)  Rapid diffusion of nitrous oxide from the alveoli to the blood increases the alveolar concentration of the volatile agent.

    e.  Not a trigger for malignant hyperthermia; therefore, may be used as an adjunct to intravenous anesthesia in these patients.
    f.  Nonexplosive and nonflammable
    g.  Minimal cardiovascular effects
    h.  Minimal change in minute ventilation: increased respiratory rate and decreased tidal volume
    i.  Analgesic effect

3.  Disadvantages

    a.  Very high MAC (104%): cannot be used as sole agent
    b.  Will expand gas-filled spaces

        i.    Do not use in patients with a pneumothorax, pneumocephalus, pulmonary hypertension, or intestinal obstruction.
        ii.   Do not use in certain eye or inner ear surgeries.

            (1)  Discuss with the surgeon if it is appropriate to use.

        iii.  Use clinical judgment for laparoscopy or bowel surgery.
        iv.   Do not use in cases that are high risk for a venous air embolism.

    c.  Capable of supporting combustion
    d.  Increased risk of post-operative nausea and vomiting
    e.  Does not produce skeletal muscle relaxation like the other volatile anesthetics.
    f.  Potential toxic effect on cell function

    i.   Inactivation of vitamin $B_{12}$

    ii.  Effect on embryonic development

## Xenon

1. Facts

    a.  Low potency (MAC 71%)

    b.  Noble gas

    c.  Odorless

    d.  Nonexplosive

    e.  NMDA receptor antagonist

2. Advantages

    a.  Inert element

    b.  Minimal cardiovascular effects

    c.  Low blood solubility

    d.  Rapid induction and recovery

    e.  Does not trigger malignant hyperthermia

    f.  Environmentally friendly

    g.  Nonexplosive

    h.  Protective against neuronal ischemia

3. Disadvantages

    a.  High cost

    b.  Limited availability

    c.  Low potency

**TKO:** It is important not only to choose an anesthetic but also to be able to explain why you chose it on the day of your exam!

## Bibliography

Barash PG, Cullen BF, Stoelting RK, et al. *Clinical Anesthesia,* 8th ed. Philadelphia: Lippincott Williams & Wilkins, 2017, pp. 459–82.

Butterworth JF, Mackey DC, Wasnick JD. *Morgan & Mikhail's Clinical Anesthesiology,* 6th ed. New York: McGraw-Hill Education, 2018, pp. 149–70.

**Chapter**

# 16

# Hypoxemia and Hypercarbia

Emma Fu and Jessica A. Lovich-Sapola

## Hypoxemia

### Sample Case

A 47-year-old female presents for an open reduction and internal fixation (ORIF) of the left femur after an automobile accident. Her past medical history is significant for hypertension. She has been a one-pack-per-day smoker for the past 20 years. The patient's oxygen saturation is 93% on 2 L nasal cannula. What pre-operative tests would you like? Why? How will her low oxygen saturation affect your anesthetic plan?

### Clinical Issues

**Definition of Hypoxemia:** deficiency in the concentration of dissolved oxygen in the arterial blood, secondary to either low oxygen saturation or low partial pressure of oxygen, which can be caused by alveolar hypoventilation, diffusion impairment, ventilation–perfusion (V/Q) mismatch, and/or right-to-left shunt.

**Definition of Hypoxia:** abnormally low oxygen availability to the body or to a specific tissue/organ, which will cause signs of ischemia (whereas hypoxemia may not cause symptoms).

#### Classification of Hypoxemia

##### Pathophysiological Mechanism of Classification

1. Decreased inspired oxygen
   a. Mechanical failure of the anesthesia apparatus to deliver oxygen to the patient
   b. Disconnection from the oxygen supply is the most common form of mechanical failure. This usually occurs at the junction of the endotracheal tube and the elbow connector of the circuit.
   c. Empty or depleted oxygen cylinder
   d. Gas pressure failure
   e. Crossing of pipelines
   f. Crossing of tanks
   g. Fracture or sticking of flow meters
   h. Transposition of rotameter tubes
   i. Improper oxygen sensor calibration
2. Impaired diffusion
3. Hypoventilation
   a. Esophageal intubation

b. Endotracheal tube kinking, blockage with secretions, and herniated or ruptured cuff all lead to increased airway resistance and hypoventilation.
   c. Right main-stem intubation
   d. Respiratory depression or failure secondary to anesthetic medications and paralysis
   e. Ventilator failure
4. Ventilation–perfusion (V/Q) mismatch
   a. Asthma
   b. Chronic obstructive pulmonary disease (COPD)
5. Shunt
   a. Intracardiac shunt
      i. Patent foramen ovale
      ii. Tetralogy of Fallot
   b. Pulmonary embolism
6. Intrapulmonary derangements
   a. Pneumonia
   b. Atelectasis
   c. Edema
   d. Acute respiratory distress syndrome (ARDS)
   e. Interstitial lung disease
7. Hypercarbia

##### Structural-Anatomic Classification

1. Alveoli
   a. Pulmonary edema
   b. Acute lung injury/pulmonary contusion
   c. ARDS
   d. Pulmonary hemorrhage
   e. Pneumonia
2. Interstitium
   a. Pulmonary fibrosis
   b. Viral pneumonia
   c. Allergic alveolitis
3. Heart and pulmonary vasculature
   a. Pulmonary embolism
   b. Intracardiac or intrapulmonary shunt
   c. Congestive heart failure (CHF)

4. Airways
   a. Asthma
   b. COPD
   c. Mucus plugging
   d. Right main-stem intubation
5. Pleura
   a. Pneumothorax
   b. Pleural effusion

Hypoxemia from V/Q mismatch is responsive to supplemental oxygen, while hypoxemia from right-to-left shunt is not responsive to supplemental oxygen. The cause can then be easily determined with the application of supplemental oxygen. Hypoventilation can be ruled out if the patient is not hypercapnic or acidemic. Impaired diffusion is usually a rare cause of hypoxemia because the red blood cell has plenty of time to traverse the capillary bed for the diffusion of oxygen even in the presence of intrinsic lung disease. Equilibrium is typically reached within the first one-third of the bed, and the remaining two-thirds contribute to this large safety factor. Most patients with acute hypoxic respiratory failure have a combination of V/Q mismatch and right-to-left shunt.

## KO Treatment Plan

### Pre-operative

1. When evaluating this patient, it is important to think about the full differential diagnosis prior to the induction of anesthesia.
2. Think about the possible chronic causes of hypoxia, including COPD.
3. Think about the possible acute causes, including a pulmonary/cardiac injury secondary to the accident.
4. Also, consider over-sedation as the cause of hypoxia.
5. Would her saturations improve with increased oxygen and albuterol, or does she need a chest tube?
6. Since this is a trauma, you should work quickly. Listen to cardiac and breath sounds. Access her vital signs. Is she responsive? Where does she have pain?

From sample case stem: what pre-operative tests would you like? Why?

1. I would get a portable chest X-ray if it was not already done in the emergency room. This would help evaluate for possible pulmonary causes.
2. An EKG can be done to help rule out a cardiac cause for the hypoxemia.
3. I would also consider a baseline arterial blood gas (ABG) to help narrow down my differentials for hypoxia in this patient.

### Intra-operative

How will her low oxygen saturation affect your anesthetic plan?

1. Apply the standard ASA monitors.
2. Preoxygenate the patient.

3. Apply in-line stabilization (to protect the cervical spine in case there is any injury secondary to the trauma).
4. Assuming the airway is normal, perform a rapid sequence induction using propofol and succinylcholine. (Etomidate or ketamine can also be used. It does not matter which induction agent you use as long as it is safe, you understand the proper dosing, and you can provide reasons for why you are using it.)
5. Apply cricoid pressure during induction (unless there is a known cervical injury).
6. Intubate
7. Listen for bilateral breath sounds and verify end-tidal carbon dioxide (ETCO$_2$) prior to releasing cricoid pressure.
8. Maintain anesthesia with a combination of oxygen and sevoflurane. I would use sevoflurane because it is less irritating to the airways. You can use any volatile anesthetic, but have a reason for your choice.
9. I would not use nitrous oxide secondary to her hypoxia and the risk of potentially expanding a small pneumothorax induced by the trauma.
10. Obtain an ABG.

### Intra-operative Acute Hypoxia

1. Check the color of the patient.
2. Check for a pulse.
3. Check all vital signs.
4. Check for ETCO$_2$.
5. Take the patient off the ventilator and hand-bag with 100% O$_2$.
6. Call for help.
7. Check the O$_2$ monitor, peak airway pressure, and capnograph waveform.
8. Listen to the chest for bilateral breath sounds. Note chest rise.
   a. Unilateral breath sounds: endotracheal tube (ETT) is too deep, pneumothorax, tension pneumothorax
   b. Wheezing: give aerosolized albuterol
   c. If you think that the patient has bronchospasm, deepen the anesthetic. If deepening the anesthetic does not treat the bronchospasm, give IV epinephrine.
9. Evaluate the ETT. Rule out kinking, mucus plug, and herniated cuff. Pass the suction catheter or fiber optic scope. Check for proper placement and position.
10. Order a chest X-ray.

### Tension Pneumothorax

1. Presentation
   a. Unilateral absence of breath sounds
   b. Tracheal deviation
   c. Unexplainable hypotension

d. Distended neck veins

2. Treatment

   a. Find the second intercostal space on the side of the pneumothorax.
   b. Find the midclavicular line.
   c. Insert a 14-gauge angiocatheter into this space over the top of the rib.
   d. Listen for a decompressive air rush.
   e. Leave the angiocatheter in place.
   f. Place a chest tube.

### Post-operative

1. Plan on extubating if she meets the extubation criteria (covered in Chapter 17).
2. Understand that a pulmonary contusion may not be evident early on after the injury but may develop a few hours later. A normal chest X-ray pre-operatively does not rule out pulmonary injury. If the patient had worsening oxygenation during the surgery, a repeat chest X-ray may be warranted.

# Hypercarbia

## Clinical Issues

**Definition of Hypercarbia:** Also known as hypercapnia. Partial pressure of carbon dioxide in arterial blood >45 mm Hg (at sea level).

### Causes of Hypercarbia

1. Increased production of $CO_2$

   a. Tourniquet release
   b. Aortic cross-clamp release
   c. Malignant hyperthermia
   d. Sepsis
   e. Thyrotoxicosis
   f. Fever
   g. Metabolic acidosis

2. Decreased removal of $CO_2$

   a. Decreased minute ventilation (won't or can't breathe)
   b. Airway obstruction
   c. Increased dead space

3. Rebreathing of $CO_2$ due to mechanical malfunction

   a. Faulty valves
   b. Exhausted $CO_2$ absorber
   c. Low fresh gas flows

4. Iatrogenic

   a. Sodium bicarbonate administration
   b. Increased $CO_2$ during laparoscopic procedures

# Bibliography

Broaddus VC, Ernst JD, King TE, et al. *Murray & Nadel's Textbook of Respiratory Medicine*, 7th ed. Philadelphia: Elsevier, 2022, chapters 44–45.

Gropper MA. *Miller's Anesthesia*, 9th ed. Philadelphia: Elsevier, 2020, pp. 354–83.

# Indications for Intubation and Extubation

Emma Fu and Jessica A. Lovich-Sapola

## Indications for Intubation

### Sample Case

You are called to the medical intensive care unit to intubate a patient. He weighs 236 kg (520 lb). He has obstructive sleep apnea and pneumonia. He has no allergies. He is on bi-pap and his oxygen saturation is 87%. The patient is refusing to be intubated.

Labs: pH 7.18, $PCO_2$ 70 mm Hg, $PO_2$ 60 mm Hg, oxygen saturation is 93.7%, base excess 8.4 mmol/L, and bicarbonate 43.6 mmol/L

### Clinical Issues

#### Indications for Intubation

1. Mechanical function
   a. Respiratory rate (RR) >35
   b. Vital capacity (VC) <15 mL/kg (adult)
   c. VC <10 mL/kg (child)
   d. Negative inspiratory force (NIF) <20–25 cm $H_2O$

2. Gas exchange function
   a. $PaO_2$ <60 on a $FiO_2$ of 50%
   b. $PaCO_2$ ≥55 (unless chronically elevated $CO_2$)
   c. P/F ratio < 150 on Fio2 of 100%)
   d. Dead space ventilation/tidal volume (Vd/Vt) ratio ≥0.6 (normal = 0.3)

3. Unstable vital signs
   a. Desaturation
   b. Bradycardia
   c. Hypotension
   d. Increasing respiratory rate

4. Symptoms of impending airway obstruction
   a. Increased secretions
   b. Stridor
   c. Dyspnea
   d. Dysphagia
   e. Progressive hoarseness

5. Inability of the patient to protect the airway from aspiration
   a. Agitation
   b. Airway burns

   c. Trauma
      i. Oral or nasal bleeding
      ii. Full stomach
   d. Neurologic injury
   e. General anesthesia

#### Complications of Intubation

1. Malposition of the endotracheal tube
   a. Esophageal
   b. Bronchial
   c. Laryngeal cuff

2. Airway trauma
   a. Dental
   b. Lip
   c. Tongue
   d. Mucosal laceration
   e. Dislocated mandible
   f. Retropharyngeal dissection

3. Physiologic reflexes
   a. Hypoxia
   b. Hypercarbia
   c. Hypertension
      i. Systemic
      ii. Intracranial
      iii. Intraocular
   d. Tachycardia
   e. Laryngospasm

4. Fire or explosion

## KO Treatment Plan

1. Despite the fact that this patient is refusing to be intubated, he is clearly hypercarbic and cannot be expected to make appropriate decisions for his medical care.
2. Begin by completing an airway examination and paying attention to any signs of a difficult airway.
3. Although an awake fiber-optic intubation would have been a preferred choice, it is out of the question secondary to the fact that he is refusing the intubation and is not cooperative.
4. This patient will have to be intubated with some sedation.

5. Suction, as his NPO status is unknown, a free-flowing intravenous (IV) line and all emergency airway equipment (including fiber-optic scope) should be available.
6. Call the ear, nose, and throat (ENT) physicians for backup, in case he requires an emergent tracheotomy.
7. The patient should be preoxygenated and a nasal canula should be worn during intubation to maintain oxygen insufflation.
8. A GlideScope is a good option for this patient.
9. Position the patient in the bed, ensuring a good sniffing position, and use 4% aerosolized lidocaine spray as it would help the GlideScope to be less stimulating to the patient compared with direct laryngoscopy.
10. Once all of the required equipment is verified, give minimal IV sedation using midazolam and etomidate (again, any drug can be used, just be able to justify its use).
11. Sedation should be done slowly since he is probably tired from the work of breathing.
12. An apneic patient could be a dead patient so it is advisable to try to maintain spontaneous respirations.
13. Once the endotracheal tube is in place, verify placement with auscultation and end-tidal $CO_2$.

# Indications for Tracheal Extubation

## Clinical Issues

### Indication for Extubation

1. Subjective criteria
   a. Resolution of acute disease
   b. Adequate cough
   c. Patient should be awake, alert, and following commands.
   d. Cooperative
   e. Glasgow Coma Scale (GCS) ≥13
   f. No continuous sedation infusions
   g. Sustained hand grip
   h. Sustained head lift >5 seconds
   i. Able to tolerate spontaneous ventilation without excessive tachypnea, tachycardia, or obvious respiratory distress
   j. Acceptable electrolytes
   k. Appropriate gag reflex and cough
   l. Able to protect airway from aspiration
   m. Clear oropharynx: no active bleeding or secretions
   n. Adequate pain control
   o. Minimal end-expiratory concentration of inhaled anesthetics

2. Objective criteria
   a. Vital signs
      i. Respiratory rate <30–35 breaths/min
      ii. Stable blood pressure with minimal or no ionotropic support
      iii. Heart rate ≤140 beats/min
      iv. Afebrile (temperature <38 °C)
   b. Gas exchange function
      i. Arterial blood gas (ABG) on 40% $FiO_2$ and PEEP ≤ 5–10 cm $H_2O$
         (1) $PaO_2$ ≥60 mm Hg
         (2) $PaCO_2$ <55
      ii. $PaO_2/FiO_2$ (P/F ratio) ≥150–300 mm Hg
      iii. Maintenance of a normal pH (>7.30)
   c. Mechanical function
      i. Forced vital capacity (FVC) >10 mL/kg
      ii. Forced expiratory volume in 1 second ($FEV_1$) >10 mL/ kg
      iii. Tidal volume ($V_T$) ≥6 mL/kg
      iv. Negative inspiratory force (NIF) >−20 cm $H_2O$
      v. VC ≥15 mL/kg
      vi. Vd/Vt ratio ≤0.6*
      vii. Rapid shallow breathing index (RSBI) (f/Vt) ≤60–100 breaths/min
   d. Adequate hemoglobin (≥8–10 g/dL)
   e. No significant respiratory acidosis
   f. T1/T4 ratio >0.7–0.8 if paralytics were used

### Complications Associated with Extubation

1. Laryngospasm and bronchospasm
2. Hypoventilation
3. Hemodynamic changes
4. Coughing, straining
5. Negative-pressure pulmonary edema
6. Aspiration
7. Airway trauma
   a. Edema and stenosis
      i. glottic, supraglottic, or tracheal
   b. Hoarseness
      i. Vocal cord granuloma
      ii. Vocal cord paralysis
      iii. Paradoxical vocal cord motion
   c. Laryngeal malfunction
   d. Arytenoid dislocation

# Bibliography

Barash PG, Cullen BF, Stoelting RK, et al. *Clinical Anesthesia*, 8th ed. Philadelphia: Lippincott Williams & Wilkins, 2017, pp. 770–90.

Butterworth JF, Mackey DC, Wasnick JD. *Morgan & Mikhail's Clinical Anesthesiology*, 6th ed. New York: McGraw-Hill Education, 2018, pp. 324–36.

Gropper MA. *Miller's Anesthesia*, 9th ed. Philadelphia: Elsevier, 2020, pp. 1373–412, 2483.

Hines RL, Jones SB. *Stoelting's Anesthesia and Co-Existing Disease*, 8th ed. Philadelphia: Elsevier, 2021, pp. 1–18.

# The Difficult Airway

Mariam Naeem Ibrahim, Jeffrey A. Brown, and Jessica A. Lovich-Sapola

## Sample Case

A 53-year-old male is emergently brought to the operating room for repair of a bleeding gastric ulcer. The patient is sedated from a previous upper endoscopy performed to diagnose the bleeding. The patient weighs 133 kg, has a bull neck, and has a known difficult airway. The patient's heart rate is 140 and his blood pressure is 90/60 mm Hg. He is breathing spontaneously and has an oxygen saturation of 94% on room air. The surgeon is waiting. What is your plan?

## Clinical Issues

### Definition of a Difficult Airway

1.  A difficult airway is a clinical situation in which a conventionally trained anesthesiologist experiences difficulty with face mask ventilation of the upper airway via a mask, difficulty with tracheal intubation, or both.
2.  The difficult airway represents a complex interaction between patient factors, the clinical setting, and the skill of the practitioner (Fig. 18.1).

### Incidence

1.  The incidence of cannot intubate/cannot oxygenate has been estimated to range from 0.01 to 2 per 10,000 patients.
2.  Difficult laryngoscopy occurs in about 1–18% of surgical cases, but the majority of these patients are successfully intubated. Unsuccessful intubation with direct laryngoscopy occurs at a rate of 5–35 per 10,000 anesthetics.
3.  The incidence of failed intubations ranges from 0.05% to 0.35%; the low and high ends of this range are associated with elective surgical and obstetric patients, respectively.
4.  Difficult and failed airway accounts for 2.3–16.6% of anesthetic deaths.

### Criteria for Difficult Mask Ventilation

1.  Inability for one anesthesiologist to maintain oxygen saturation >92%
2.  Significant gas leak around facemask
3.  Need for >4 L/min gas flow or use of fresh gas flow button more than twice
4.  No chest movement
5.  Two-handed mask ventilation needed
6.  Change of operator required

## Predictors of Difficult Mask Ventilation

1.  Beard
2.  Obesity, BMI greater than or equal to 30 kg/m$^2$
3.  Lack of teeth or edentulousness
4.  Obstructive sleep apnea or history of snoring
5.  Age >55
6.  Male gender
7.  Mallampati classification 3 or 4
8.  Piercing of the tongue, lip, cheek, and chin

## Predictors of Difficult Laryngoscopy

1.  Long upper incisors
2.  Prominent overbite
3.  Inability to protrude mandible
4.  Small mouth opening
5.  Mallampati classification 3 or 4
6.  High, arched palate
7.  Short thyromental distance
8.  Short, thick neck
9.  Limited cervical mobility

## Supraglottic Airway (SGA) Failure Risk Factors

1.  Trismus
2.  Mass lesion
3.  Male gender
4.  Age >45
5.  Short thyromental distance
6.  Reduced cervical range of motion

## Pathological States Associated with Difficult Airway Management

1.  Congenital
    a.  Pierre Robin syndrome: micrognathia, macroglossia, glossoptosis, cleft palate
    b.  Treacher Collins syndrome: malar and mandibular hypoplasia, microstomia, choanal atresia
    c.  Down's syndrome: macroglossia, atlantoaxial instability
    d.  Klippel–Feil syndrome: restricted cervical range of motion secondary to cervical vertebrae fusion
    e.  Cretinism: macroglossia, compression or deviation of larynx/trachea by goiter

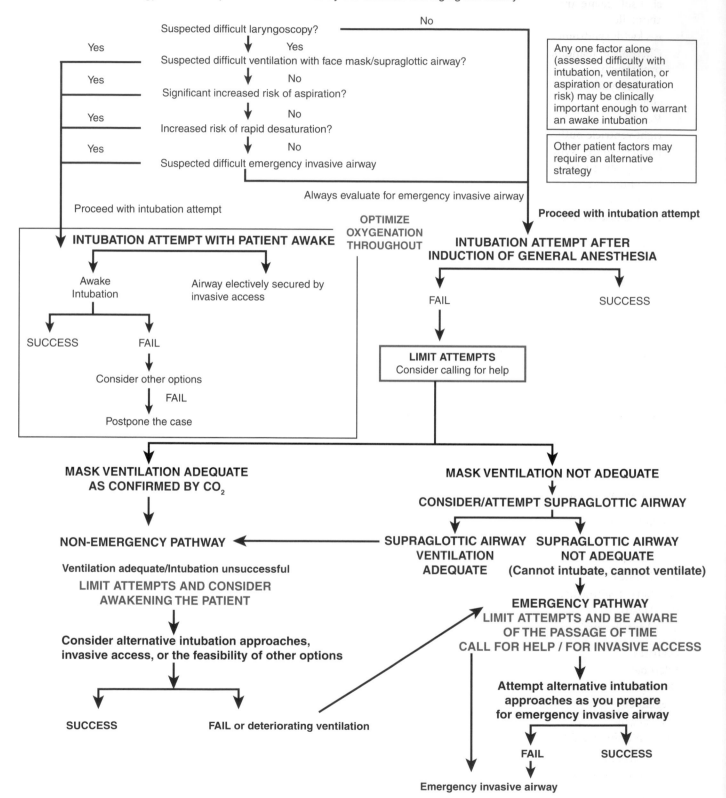

**Figure 18.1** ASA: difficult airway algorithm. Reprinted from Apfelbaum JL, Hagberg CA, Connis RT, et al. 2022 American Society of Anesthesiologists Practice Guidelines for Management of the Difficult Airway. *Anesthesiology* 2022;136:31–81 with permission.

f. Cri du Chat syndrome: micrognathia, laryngomalacia, stridor

g. Alport syndrome: maxillary hypoplasia, prognathism, cleft soft palate, tracheobronchial cartilaginous anomalies

h. Beckwith syndrome: macroglossia

i. Cherubism: mandibular and maxillary fibrous overgrowth

j. Meckel syndrome: microcephaly, micrognathia, cleft epiglottis

k. Von Recklinghausen disease: tumors of the larynx and right ventricle outflow tract

l. Hurler/Hunter syndrome: stiff joints, upper airway obstruction due to infiltration of lymphoid tissue, abnormal tracheobronchial cartilages

m. Pompe disease: macroglossia, muscle deposits

2. Infection
   a. Croup
   b. Ludwig's angina
   c. Intraoral/retropharyngeal abscess
   d. Epiglottitis
   e. Papillomatosis

3. Arthritis
   a. Rheumatoid arthritis
   b. Ankylosing spondylitis

4. Benign tumors
   a. Lipoma
   b. Adenoma
   c. Goiter
   d. Cystic hygroma

5. Malignancy of the tongue/larynx/thyroid
6. Injury
   a. Facial
   b. Cervical
   c. Laryngeal/tracheal
   d. Head
   e. Acute burns

7. Diabetes
8. Scleroderma
9. Obesity
10. Pregnancy
11. Acromegaly
12. Anatomic abnormalities
    a. Micrognathia
    b. Limited jaw motion

13. History of head and neck radiation

# Criteria Commonly Used to Predict a Difficult Airway

1. History
   a. History of a previous difficult intubation
   b. Burns
   c. Edema
   d. Bleeding
   e. Airway stenosis
   f. Gastroesophageal reflux
   g. Poor dentition
   h. Radiation treatments

2. Physical exam
   a. General
      i. Massive obesity
      ii. Cervical collar
      iii. Traction device
      iv. External trauma
      v. Current respiratory difficulty/stridor
      vi. Pregnancy
   b. Patency of nares
      i. Masses
      ii. Deviated nasal septum
   c. Mouth opening and temporomandibular joint movement
      i. Less than two finger breadths (3 cm)
   d. Teeth
      i. Prominent incisors
      ii. Overbite
      iii. Loose teeth
   e. Palate
      i. High arch
      ii. Narrow mouth
   f. Tongue
      i. Macroglossia
      ii. Retrognathia causing difficult tongue displacement
   g. Prognathism
      i. There is increased risk of a difficult intubation if the patient cannot protrude the lower jaw beyond the upper incisors.
   h. Thyromental distance less than 6–6.5 cm (3 finger breadths)
   i. Neck

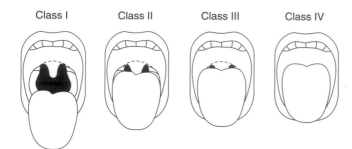

Figure 18.2 Mallampati score. This figure was published in *Evidence-Based Practice of Anesthesiology*, 3rd ed. Lee A. Fleisher, Chapter 15, Figure 15.2. Copyright © 2013, 2009, 2004 by Saunders, an imprint of Elsevier Inc. Reprinted with permission.

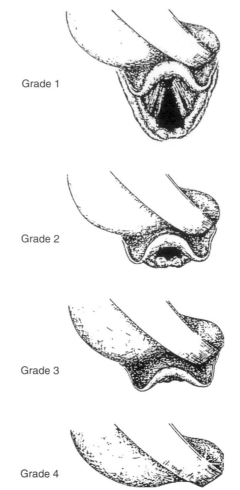

    i. Short and thick

    ii. Neck circumference >43 cm (17 in.)

    iii. Atlanto-occipital extension less than 35 degrees

    iv. Neck range of motion, angle created when neck fully flexed and then fully extended <80 degrees

3. Specific tests

    a. Mallampati score of 3 or higher (Fig. 18.2)

    b. Laryngoscopic grades (Fig. 18.3) 2b and 3 are associated with a higher incidence of failed intubation. Grade 4 – consider an alternate method of intubation.

    c. Sternomental distance when head fully extended and mouth closed <12.5 cm

    d. Upper lip bite test (lower incisors can bite upper lip above vermillion line – class 1; below vermillion line – class 2; cannot bite upper lip at all – class 3)

    e. Radiographic assessment

        i. Lateral cervical films

        ii. CT scan: trachea and mediastinal tumors

        iii. Flow-volume loop test to evaluate intra- and extrathoracic obstructive lesions

    f. Predictors of difficult airway in diabetics

        i. Positive prayer sign: gap between palms

        ii. Palm print test

**TKO:** No single test can provide a high index of sensitivity and specificity. You must use a combination of tests. However, a difficult airway may not always be predicted. You must always be prepared for an unexpected difficult airway.

## Treatment Techniques for a Difficult Airway

1. Laryngeal manipulation

    a. Backward pressure

    b. Upward pressure

    c. Rightward pressure

    d. Optimal laryngeal manipulation

    e. Conventional cricoid pressure

2. Stylet

Figure 18.3 Laryngoscopic grades. Cormack–Lehane grading system. Grade 1 is visualization of the entire laryngeal aperture; grade 2A is partial visualization of the vocal cords; grade 2B is visualization of only the posterior commissure of the vocal cords or arytenoid cartilages; grade 3A is visualization of only the epiglottis (epiglottis can be lifted); grade 3B is visualization of only the epiglottis (epiglottis cannot be lifted off the posterior pharynx); and grade 4 is visualization of only the soft palate. Bottom: Cook grading system. *Easy*, the laryngeal inlet is visible; *Restricted*, the posterior glottic structures are visible and the epiglottis can be lifted; *Difficult*, the epiglottis cannot be lifted, or no laryngeal structures are visible. This figure was published in *Hagberg and Benumof's Airway Management*, 4th edition. Carin A. Hagberg, Carlos A. Artime, Michael F. Aziz. Chapter 8, figure 8.3. Copyright 2018 by Elsevier Inc. Reprinted with permission.

3. Reposition the patient.

4. Operator change

5. Change the length and type of laryngoscope blades.

6. Change the size of the ETT.

7. Use adjuncts: oral/nasal airways, suction, gum elastic bougie (consider for laryngoscopic views 2b and 3a – helps to lift up the epiglottis)

8. Intubating laryngeal mask airway (LMA)

    a. The LMA classic has a reported success rates of 95.3–99.8%.

9. Video-assisted laryngoscopy

10. Flexible or rigid fiber-optic scope intubation

11. Nasotracheal intubation
12. Blind nasal intubation (consider for grade 3b and 4): successful in only 50% of cases and has an increased risk of bleeding and trauma.
13. Lighted stylets, or lighted optical stylets
14. Esophageal tubes with laryngeal openings (risk of esophageal rupture)
15. Transtracheal jet ventilation (TTJV)
16. Cricothyrotomy (percutaneous/needle, bougie-scalpel method, or surgical)
17. Surgical tracheostomy

## KO Treatment Plan

There are two key branch points regarding the ASA algorithm for difficult airways: anticipated and unanticipated.

### Anticipated Difficult Airway

1. Keep the patient breathing spontaneously.
2. Flexible scope intubation of the trachea in an awake, spontaneously ventilating, and cooperative patient is the gold standard for the management of the difficult airway – if failed, consider regional/local anesthesia or canceling the case. If neither is possible, proceed down the alternative noninvasive tracheal intubation techniques or invasive airway access, based on expertise experience and clinical judgment.

### Unanticipated Difficult Airway

1. The algorithm path branches at two key points: either mask ventilation is successful or it is not.
2. If mask ventilation is successful, the airway may still be urgent but is no longer emergent and options for securing it can be quickly implemented.
3. If both direct laryngoscopy and mask ventilation are not successful, the ASA's algorithm is very clear that the next step is placement of an LMA.
4. If this provides adequate ventilation, then go back on the urgent, nonemergent pathway.
5. If the LMA placement is not successful or fails to sustain the patient adequately, enter the emergency pathway and an alternative means for noninvasive ventilation should quickly be instituted (these include an intubating LMA, fiber-optic intubation, bougie, lighted stylet, optical stylets, esophageal tubes for blind oral or nasal intubation).
6. At any juncture, the decision to awaken the patient should be considered based on adequacy of ventilation, risk of aspiration, risk of proceeding with intubation attempts or surgical procedure.
7. Five criteria for transtracheal invasive airway include: cannot intubate, cannot ventilate, cannot awaken patient, SGA failure, and clinically significant hypoxemia has ensued. Transtracheal invasive airway includes cricothyrotomy, transtracheal jet ventilation (TTJV), surgical cricothyroidotomy, and tracheostomy.

8. Percutaneous emergency airway access (PEAA) is a form of cricothyrotomy known to anesthesiologists.
9. Retrograde wire intubation (RWI) is a form of an invasive airway technique that was previously part of the emergency pathway of the difficult airway algorithm. Newer recommendations suggest that this could be utilized in the nonemergent pathway when intubation is unsuccessful but mask ventilation is adequate. Since it takes several minutes to accomplish, it is contraindicated in an emergent cannot intubate/cannot ventilate scenario.
10. There are rare extreme circumstances where one might consider invasive methods first, such as severe craniofacial abnormalities from a trauma patient with blood and edema obscuring the airway.
    a. In these instances, a surgical airway might be the first option.
11. Some texts state that secretions and blood in the airway may prevent successful fiber-optic intubation.
    a. If these secretions are too great and visualization is not possible, then the key is whether the patient is hypoxic or not.
    b. If there is time, a retrograde intubation may be performed. If not, then an invasive airway must be obtained.

### Sample Case KO Treatment Plan

In the sample case above there are several issues to consider. The patient has a known difficult airway, is at risk for aspiration, and may not be cooperative with an awake fiber-optic intubation. The patient is breathing spontaneously. He should remain breathing spontaneously until his airway is secured. If the sedation given for the endoscopy is not too great, and the secretions and blood in the airway are easily dealt with, then an awake fiber-optic intubation should be the first choice. An awake intubation after topicalization with a video laryngoscope may be another option. If these methods cannot be performed, the choices are limited to invasive means to secure the airway (i.e., awake tracheostomy). In any case, backup methods such as an LMA should be immediately available.

### TKO

1. You will almost always have a difficult airway scenario on your oral board examination. Be prepared!
2. The LMA and video laryngoscope have revolutionized airway management, both difficult and elective. You can be sure that the board expects you to know its roles in the difficult airway.
3. Fiber-optic intubations are most useful in an elective setting, not as an emergency backup.
4. Airway trumps everything else! Remember the ABCs! Whatever methods you choose, once you are on the difficult airway path, keep the patient breathing spontaneously until the airway is secured.

5. Call for help early. A wise anesthesiologist recognizes that a colleague who is skilled in the performance of a surgical airway is the one best suited to do it. However, if pushed, do not allow life-threatening or brain-threatening hypoxia to stand between you and the knife.

## Bibliography

Apfelbaum JL, Hagberg CA, Connis RT, et al. 2022 American Society of Anesthesiologists practice guidelines for management of the difficult airway. *Anesthesiology* 2022;**136**:31–81.

Barash PG, Cullen BF, Stoelting RK, et al. *Clinical Anesthesia*, 8th ed. Philadelphia: Lippincott Williams & Wilkins, 2017, pp. 791–7.

Fleisher, LA. *Evidence-Based Practice of Anesthesiology*, 3rd ed. Philadelphia: Saunders Elsevier, 2013.

Hagberg CA, Artime CA, Aziz MF. *Hagberg and Benumof's Airway Management*, 4th ed. Philadelphia: Elsevier, 2018, chapters 8 and 10.

Gropper MA. *Miller's Anesthesia*, 9th ed. Philadelphia: Elsevier, 2020, pp. 1373–409.

Gupta S, Sharma R, Jain D. Airway assessment: predictors of difficult airway. *Indian J Anesth* 2005;**49**(4):257–62.

# Chapter 19

# Breathing Difficulties

Augusto Torres and Jessica A. Lovich-Sapola

## Dyspnea

### Sample Case

A 75-year-old female is experiencing difficulty breathing in the post-anesthesia care unit after an open colectomy. She has a history of congestive heart failure. Estimated blood loss was 250 mL. Total intravenous fluids administered were 4.5 L of Lactated Ringer's throughout the three-hour case. She is breathing 34 times per minute and appears uncomfortable.

### Clinical Issues

#### Definitions

1. Dyspnea

    a. The sensation of breathlessness and the patient's reaction to that sensation.

    b. Dyspnea occurs when the requirement for ventilation is greater than the person's ability to respond appropriately.

    c. Quantified by:

        i. the amount of physical activity required to produce adequate ventilation

        ii. the level of activity possible

        iii. the ability to manage daily activities

2. Tachypnea

    a. Increased respiratory rate. Typical respiratory rate for adults is 12–20 breaths per minute.

#### Differential Diagnosis of Acute Dyspnea

1. Pulmonary

    a. Aspiration

    b. Mucous plug

    c. Pulmonary embolism

    d. Foreign body

    e. Asthma

    f. COPD exacerbation

    g. Pneumonia

    h. Pleural effusion

    i. Anaphylaxis

    j. Noncardiogenic edema

    k. Neoplasm

2. Cardiac

    a. Pulmonary edema

    b. Myocardial infarction

    c. Cardiac tamponade

    d. Valvular heart disease

    e. Arrythmia

3. Other factors

    a. Residual anesthetic or muscle relaxant

    b. Sepsis

    c. Thyroid disease

    d. Anemia

    e. Psychogenic

### KO Treatment Plan

1. Administer supplemental oxygen.

2. Monitor the patient closely with pulse oximetry.

3. Assess the patient's mental status.

4. Obtain a chest X-ray to evaluate for an intrapulmonary or cardiac process.

5. Obtain an EKG to investigate for an acute coronary event or arrythmia.

6. Obtain an arterial blood gas (ABG) to evaluate the patient's oxygenation and ventilatory status.

7. Consider a diuretic if fluid overload is suspected.

## Wheezing and Stridor

### Sample Case

A four-year-old male presents to the emergency department with difficulty breathing. Prior outpatient treatment for newly diagnosed asthma with albuterol nebulizers and corticosteroids has not improved the symptoms. An otolaryngologist wishes to take the patient to the operating room for removal of a possible foreign body.

### Clinical Issues

#### Definitions

1. Wheezing

    a. Expiratory sound produced by turbulent gas flow through narrowed bronchial airways

    b. Acute wheezing is a medical emergency.

    c. Chronic wheezing

        i. Common with COPD

ii.  Gas flow obstruction secondary to:
    (1)  Smooth muscle contraction
    (2)  Secretions
    (3)  Mucosal edema

2.  Stridor
    a.  High-pitched respiratory sound resulting from turbulent upper-airway gas flow
    b.  Often mistaken for wheezing

3.  Asthma
    a.  A disease characterized by recurrent episodes of lower airway obstruction and chronic inflammation.
    b.  An exaggerated bronchial response to stimuli exists that would have little or no effect on a nonasthmatic patient.

## Differential Diagnosis of Wheezing

1.  Asthma
2.  Pneumonia
3.  COPD
4.  Pulmonary edema
5.  Aspiration
6.  Foreign body
7.  Pneumothorax
8.  Mucous plug
9.  Upper-airway obstruction which sounds like wheezing (croup, epiglottitis, congenital anomalies, tumors, foreign body)
10. Pulmonary embolism

## Other Causes of Wheezing

1.  Anaphylaxis
2.  Transfusion reaction

## Differential Diagnosis of Stridor

1.  Vocal cord paralysis (congenital or acquired)
2.  Laryngomalacia (may present at birth)
3.  Laryngocele
4.  Infection: croup and epiglottitis
5.  Craniofacial abnormalities
6.  Foreign body in the airway
7.  Cyst or mass in the airway
8.  Tracheomalacia
9.  Vascular ring

## Classification of Stridor

1.  Inspiratory stridor: glottic or supraglottic airway obstruction; upper-airway obstruction
2.  Expiratory stridor: obstruction at distal trachea or mainstem bronchi; lower airway obstruction
3.  Biphasic stridor: obstruction at or just below level of the glottis; midtracheal obstruction

## Causes of Stridor

1.  Supraglottic airway
    a.  Choanal atresia
    b.  Cyst
    c.  Mass
    d.  Large tonsils
    e.  Large adenoids
    f.  Craniofacial abnormalities

2.  Larynx
    a.  Laryngomalacia
    b.  Vocal cord paralysis
    c.  Subglottic stenosis
    d.  Laryngocele
    e.  Laryngeal cancer
    f.  Infection (croup, epiglottitis)

3.  Subglottic airway
    a.  Tracheomalacia
    b.  Vascular ring
    c.  Foreign body
    d.  Infection (croup, epiglottitis)

## Clinical Signs Associated with Stridor

1.  Noisy upper-airway breathing
2.  Wheezing
3.  Cyanosis
4.  Chest retractions
5.  Nasal flaring

# KO Treatment Plan

## Pre-operative

Determining whether the patient has poorly controlled asthma or an unrecognized aspirated foreign body which has caused a post-obstructive pneumonia may be difficult.

1.  History
    a.  Asthma
        i.    Gradual onset of respiratory problems
        ii.   Last asthma attack
        iii.  Determine if the patient has ever been hospitalized for his asthma. If he was hospitalized, did he ever require endotracheal intubation?
        iv.   Frequency of rescue inhaler use versus daily inhaler control

    b.  Foreign body
        i.    Sudden onset of symptoms
        ii.   Choking while eating or playing
        iii.  Persistent cough

iv. Wheezing that does not respond to medical treatment

2. Physical exam

   a. Stridor: respiratory noise heard best in neck or lung fields
   b. Wheezing: bilateral vs. unilateral
   c. Chest retractions
   d. Persistent cough
   e. Pulse oximetry
   f. May require direct laryngoscopy or bronchoscopy for definite diagnosis

3. A chest X-ray to evaluate for pneumonia or an aspirated foreign body. If a bronchial foreign body is not radio-opaque, chest X-ray may reveal hyperinflation of a lung field caused by air trapping distal to the obstructing foreign body. A ball-valve effect of the obstructing foreign body causes this unilateral of localized hyperinflation.

4. Treatment of acute asthma

   a. Supplemental oxygen
   b. Sympathomimetics

      i. Selective β2 agonists
         (1) Albuterol meter dose inhaler or aerosol (first-line treatment)
         (2) Terbutaline
         (3) Metaproterenol

      ii. Mixed β1 and β2 agonists: β1 can have undesirable cardiac effects
         (1) Epinephrine: can be used to treat severe asthma attacks (also an alpha agonist)
         (2) Isoproterenol
         (3) Ephedrine

   c. Corticosteroids: decrease mucosal edema and prevent the release of bronchoconstricting substances
   d. Anticholinergic (supplements B-agonist therapy)

      i. Atropine
      ii. Ipratropium

   e. Extremely severe asthma exacerbation may necessitate endotracheal intubation
   f. Chronic asthma treatment includes mast cell stabilizers, methylxanthines, and leukotriene modifiers.

### Intra-operative

1. The goal of the induction of anesthesia is to depress airway reflexes to avoid bronchospasm in response to endotracheal intubation.
2. If IV access is not present, a careful inhalational induction with a nonirritating inhaled anesthetic such as sevoflurane is recommended.

   a. Once IV access is obtained, the sympathetic response to direct laryngoscopy can be blunted by IV narcotics and lidocaine 1.5 mg/kg.

3. Propofol as an induction agent has a decreased incidence of wheezing compared to other induction agents. Therefore, it is the preferred induction agent in hemodynamically stable, wheezing patients.
4. Ketamine has a sympathomimetic effect that may produce smooth muscle relaxation and decreased wheezing. This is a good choice if the patient is actively wheezing or is hemodynamically unstable.
5. Use of muscle relaxation in the setting of a possible aspirated airway foreign body is controversial. A discussion with the otolaryngologist is warranted.

## Laryngospasm

### Sample Case

A four-year-old female is scheduled for a tonsillectomy. During the inhalational mask induction your resident decides to work on the IV. You are suddenly not able to ventilate. How do you treat this? What is the cause?

### Clinical Issues

#### Definition of Laryngospasm

1. Reflex closure of the upper airway secondary to glottic musculature spasm

   a. The involuntary spasm of the laryngeal musculature results from stimulation of the superior laryngeal nerve.

2. The false cords and the epiglottic body close firmly together.
3. Hypoxia and hypercarbia result in a less vigorous glottic closure; therefore, the unsuccessful treatment of hypoxia will usually result in a spontaneous reversal of the laryngospasm.

#### Risk Factors for Laryngospasm

1. Stimulation of the patient while in a light plane of anesthesia: the likely cause for this sample case.

   a. Can occur at any point during the case
   b. Most common during the induction of anesthesia and the wake up

2. Foreign objects: oral and nasal airway
3. Secretions, blood, and/or vomitus irritating the vocal cords
4. Children are at an increased risk compared to adults.
5. Recent upper respiratory tract infection (URI). This is especially relevant in children.
6. Airway surgery
7. Airway pathology

### Associated Complications of Laryngospasm

1. Hypoxia
2. Noncardiogenic pulmonary edema can result if there is continued spontaneous ventilation against the closed vocal cords.
3. Cardiac arrest and death

## KO Treatment Plan

1. Place the patient on 100% oxygen.
2. Remove the irritating factor; in this case, stop the attempt at an IV placement.
3. Apply a jaw thrust.
4. Apply continuous positive pressure ventilation via a tight mask fit.
5. Increase the depth of anesthesia with a nonirritating inhalational agent or IV agent, such as fentanyl or propofol.
6. Give IV or topical lidocaine.
7. Call for help if these first few techniques do not immediately break the laryngospasm.
8. Give a rapid-acting muscle relaxant such as succinylcholine. A dose of 10–50 mg IV, IM, or sublingual (SL) is usually appropriate depending on the patient's weight.
9. Attempt to intubate if the above techniques do not break the laryngospasm!
10. As discussed above, hypoxia usually results in less vigorous glottic closure and therefore reversal of the laryngospasm.

## Bronchospasm

## Clinical Issues

### Definition of Bronchospasm

1. Spasm of the smooth muscle, resulting in narrowing of the bronchi secondary to a trigger

2. Sudden constriction of the bronchioles, triggered by an irritating stimulus
3. The resulting bronchiole constriction and inflammation causes narrowing of the airways and an increase in mucus production.
4. Most common in asthmatics

### Differential Diagnosis of Bronchospasm

1. Kinked ETT
2. Solidified secretion or blood
3. Pulmonary edema
4. Tension pneumothorax
5. Aspiration pneumonitis
6. Pulmonary embolism
7. Endobronchial intubation
8. Persistent cough or strain
9. Negative pressure expiration

### Symptoms of Intra-operative Bronchospasm

1. Wheezing
2. Increasing peak airway pressures
3. Decreasing exhaled tidal volumes
4. Slowly rising waveform on the capnograph

### Prevention and Treatment of Bronchospasm

1. Avoid manipulation of the airway in lightly anesthetized patients.
2. Use bronchodilating anesthetics.
3. Avoid histamine-releasing medications.
4. Deepen the anesthetic: IV propofol or ketamine or sevoflurane.
   a. Barbiturates, benzodiazepines, etomidate, and opioids have not been proven effective to treat bronchospasm.
5. Administer beta-agonist such as albuterol.
6. Administer low doses of epinephrine to break through persistent bronchospasm.

## Bibliography

Barash PG, Cullen BF, Stoelting RK, et al. *Clinical Anesthesia*, 8th ed. Philadelphia: Lippincott Williams & Wilkins, 2017, pp. 1030, 1035, 1364–5, 2554, 2566–8.

Butterworth JF, Mackey DC, Wasnick JD. *Morgan & Mikhail's Clinical Anesthesiology*, 6th ed. New York: McGraw-Hill Education, 2018, pp. 335.

Goldman L. *Cecil Medicine*, 23rd ed. Philadelphia: Saunders, 2007, chapter 87.

Gropper MA. *Miller's Anesthesia*, 9th ed. Philadelphia: Elsevier, 2020, p. 1677.

Marx JA. *Rosen's Emergency Medicine: Concepts and Clinical Practice*. Philadelphia: Mosby, 2006, chapter 167.

Stoelting RK, Dierdorf SF. *Anesthesia and Co-existing Disease*, 4th ed. Philadelphia: Churchill Livingstone, 2002, pp. 193–204.

Walls R, Hockinberger R, Gausche-Hill M, et al. *Rosen's Emergency Medicine: Concepts and Clinical Practice*, 9th ed. Philadelphia: Elsevier, 2018, chapter 22.

# Obstructive Sleep Apnea

Mandeep Singh

**Chapter 20**

## Sample Case

A 54-year-old male is scheduled for a left knee arthroscopy for anterior cruciate ligament (ACL) reconstruction at an ambulatory center. The patient reports that a tooth was dislodged during a previous cholecystectomy. The patient has a past medical history significant for severe obstructive sleep apnea (OSA), where his previous sleep study indicated an apnea–hypopnea index (AHI) of 65 events per hour, minimum oxygen saturation 65% and mean oxygen saturation of 80%, and the patient spent 30% of total sleep time below oxygen saturation of 90%. The sleep study was done two years ago, and he gained some more weight due to the knee injury and limited physical activity. While he was advised to use positive airway pressure therapy, details of the machine settings were not known as he stopped using the machine a few months after the second therapeutic sleep study. He continues to snore loudly, his wife has observed him to have multiple "breathing stops" while asleep, he uses the bathroom 4–5 times per night, and is always found to be "sleepy" during the day. The patient has hypertension that is well controlled on a β-blocker and an ACE inhibitor. He has a blood pressure of 155/84 mm Hg, heart rate of 105, respiratory rate of 20, neck circumference of 45 cm, a temperature of 35.6 °C, and current BMI of 48 kg/m$^2$. His hematocrit is 49% and serum bicarbonate is 30 mmol/L. Is this patient a candidate for an outpatient surgery? How would you induce anesthesia? Would you prefer to do a regional or general anesthetic? Are you concerned that he is a difficult intubation? How would you manage his post-operative pain? Will he need special post-operative monitoring?

## Clinical Issues

### Sleep Disordered Breathing and OSA: Clinical Definitions

1.  Sleep disordered breathing (SDB) is a group of disorders characterized by abnormalities of respiratory patterns during sleep. The abnormal breathing patterns during sleep are broadly grouped as follows.

    a.  OSA disorders

        i.   OSA is the most common
        ii.  Characterized by episodes of apnea or hypopnea during sleep
        iii. Resulting in varying severity of hypoxemia with or without hypercapnia

        iv.  The obstructive apnea or hypopnea is caused by repeated episodes of complete or partial closure of the pharynx, accompanied with hypoventilation and desaturation, and terminated by cortical arousal.
        v.   Classic symptoms include loud snoring, sudden awakenings with a choking sensation, witnessed apneas by bed partner, frequent vivid dreams, nocturia, and excessive daytime sleepiness.

    b.  Central sleep apnea (CSA) disorders

        i.   Less common than OSA
        ii.  Do not result from airway obstruction
        iii. Occur when the brain fails to send appropriate signals to the respiratory muscles to stimulate a regular breathing pattern
        iv.  Symptoms include chronic fatigue, excessive daytime sleepiness, cognitive impairment, and inability to fall asleep.

    c.  Sleep-related hypoventilation disorders

        i.   Reduced air enters the lung alveoli during sleep.
        ii.  Results in low oxygen blood levels and elevated carbon dioxide
        iii. Often seen in patients with chronic obstructive pulmonary disease (COPD), pulmonary hypertension, and morbid obesity
        iv.  Symptoms include morning headache, restless sleep, daytime tiredness, and difficulty concentrating.

    d.  Sleep-related hypoxemia disorder

        i.   Low level of blood oxygen
        ii.  Levels of carbon dioxide do not rise high enough to be diagnosed as sleep-related hypoventilation disorder.

2.  The polysomnogram (PSG), classically the gold standard for the definitive diagnosis of OSA, requires an overnight polysomnography or sleep study.
3.  The AHI is calculated as the average number of abnormal breathing events per hour of sleep.

    a.  OSA severity is determined by AHI cutoffs.

        i.   Mild: 5–15 events per hour

ii. Moderate: ≥15–30 events per hour

iii. Severe: ≥30 events per hour

4. Treatment:

    a. Conservative options:

        i. Weight loss

        ii. Avoidance of alcohol

        iii. Avoidance of sedatives

        iv. Supine posture

    b. Therapeutic options:

        i. Continuous airway pressure (CPAP) or related modes of positive airway pressure (PAP) therapy

        ii. Dental appliances

        iii. Invasive options such as upper-airway or bariatric surgery

## Peri-operative Concerns

1. Increased risk for difficult intubation and mask ventilation

2. Post-operative hypoxemia

3. Post-operative airway obstruction requiring the need for reintubation

4. Increased risk of cardiovascular and respiratory complications such as myocardial injury, cardiac death, congestive heart failure, thromboembolism, atrial fibrillation, stroke, ICU admission, and longer duration of hospital stay

5. Increased association with opioid-related ventilatory depression and death

## Pathophysiology of OSA during the Peri-operative Period

1. All central nervous system (CNS) depressant drugs (inhaled agents, hypnotics, narcotics) and neuromuscular blocking agents cause (to varying degrees) relaxation of pharyngeal muscles.

2. Relaxation of pharyngeal muscles predisposes the OSA patient to airway collapse and obstruction.

3. CNS depressants also impair the arousal state (which would terminate apneic episodes), which predisposes the patient to hypoxemia and hypercarbia.

4. Patients with long-standing OSA may present with signs and symptoms of significant comorbidities including morbid obesity, metabolic syndrome, uncontrolled or resistant hypertension, arrhythmias, cerebrovascular disease, and heart failure.

5. Pre-operative assessment should rule out the presence of significant nocturnal hypoxemia, hypercarbia, and polycythemia.

6. Obesity hypoventilation syndrome (OHS), pulmonary hypertension, and cor pulmonale should be ruled out in OSA patients.

7. Compared to no OSA, the likelihood of post-operative respiratory failure has been found to be over 10-fold in patients with OHS with OSA.

8. Serum bicarbonate level of 28 mmol/L or more indicates metabolic compensation for chronic hypercapnia, and is a useful screening tool for OHS.

9. Transthoracic echocardiography can be useful in patients suspected to have severe pulmonary hypertension, for high-risk surgeries.

## KO Treatment Plan

### Pre-operative

1. A thorough history and physical examination regarding the nature and severity of OSA symptoms should be sought. As OSA remains undiagnosed in the majority of surgical patients, many will be identified to be at risk for OSA during the pre-operative screening. Previous consultation with a sleep physician and sleep reports should be reviewed, if possible.

2. There is insufficient evidence to support canceling or delaying surgery, unless there is evidence of uncontrolled systemic disease or additional problems with ventilation or gas exchange, such as hypoventilation syndromes, severe pulmonary hypertension, or resting hypoxemia in the absence of other cardiopulmonary disease.

3. The sleep study data of this patient is concerning. This patient not only has severe OSA (AHI >30 events per hour), but also moderate to severe hypoxemia as indicated by low mean and minimum oxygen saturation, and significant percentage of total sleep time spent below oxygen saturation of 90%. Given his high BMI and serum bicarbonate 30 mmol/L, he is at risk of untreated OHS.

4. Patients with OSA are known to be at risk for difficult intubation, and the fact that a tooth was dislodged during the previous surgical procedure suggests that this patient may have been a difficult intubation. One cannot guarantee that regional anesthesia can be successfully performed, nor can it be assumed that a peripheral nerve block will be successful; therefore, one must have contingency plans for a general anesthetic.

5. A thorough cardiac and pulmonary exam to evaluate for presence of pulmonary hypertension and cor pulmonale should be performed.

6. Given this patient's BMI, history of severe OSA, possible OHS, and probable history of difficult intubation, one can make a strong argument that it would be most prudent to obtain a sleep medicine consult to optimize before surgery, and he may need to be placed on advanced modes such as bi-level positive airway pressure (BIPAP). Moreover, a discussion with the surgeon needs to occur to consider performing this procedure on an inpatient basis. A monitored bed will need to be arranged in the post-operative period.

7. Pre-operative screening is used for suspected patients who may not have a sleep study available at the time of surgery.

a. Validated screening tools can be utilized.

   i. STOP-Bang questionnaire

     (1) Most popular

     (2) Concise

     (3) Easy to use

     (4) Consists of eight easily administered questions with the acronym STOP-Bang

     (5) It includes four yes/no questions with a mnemonic.

       (a) **S** – Snoring

       (b) **T** – Tiredness

       (c) **O** – Observed you stop breathing

       (d) **P** – blood **Pressure**

     (6) It includes four questions on demographic data.

       (a) **BMI** ($>35$ kg/m$^2$)

       (b) **Age** ($>50$ years)

       (c) **Neck** circumference ($>40$ cm)

       (d) **Gender** (male)

     (7) Risk

       (a) Score 0–2: low risk of OSA

       (b) Score 3–4: intermediate risk of OSA

       (c) Score 5–8: high risk of OSA

The STOP-Bang score for this patient is 5, consistent with high risk of OSA.

   ii. Berlin Questionnaire

   iii. Perioperative Sleep Apnea Prediction (P-SAP) score

## Intra-operative

1. Regional anesthesia as well as multimodal analgesia by facilitating additive and synergistic analgesic effects are both strongly recommended interventions to reduce peri-operative complications. Utilize regional anesthesia whenever possible for OSA patients. Neuraxial anesthesia (spinal or epidural) combined with adductor canal block should be the primary anesthetic plan. Patients with OSA are still at risk for airway obstruction and apnea following neuraxial opioids. Intrathecal opioids should be avoided in suspected high-risk, untreated moderate to severe OSA patients and those with hypoventilation syndromes.

2. Your contingency plan should be a general anesthetic (GA) if the regional anesthetic is unsuccessful or a high spinal develops. You should always be prepared for a difficult intubation by having a fiber-optic bronchoscope, GlideScope, bougie, and LMA and/or intubating LMA available. Adequate preoxygenation, head-elevated body position, and measures to decrease the risk of aspiration of gastric acid, such as pre-operative proton-pump inhibitors, antacids, and rapid sequence induction with cricoid pressure, should be considered. If GA is required, propofol, dexmedetomidine, remifentanil, and sevoflurane/desflurane are all good choices since they promote a rapid recovery.

3. Ensure that the patient's muscle relaxation is fully reversed with neostigmine or sugammadex, and neuromuscular quantitative monitoring is recommended to objectively determine the quality of reversal at the time of extubation.

4. Extubation should be performed in an awake, fully conscious patient with no neuromuscular blockade, who is able to obey commands and maintain a patent airway.

## Post-operative

1. Discuss a possible femoral nerve or adductor canal block with the patient. If successful, this may eliminate the need for high doses of intravenous narcotics.

2. Monitor the patient closely in the post-anesthesia care unit (PACU). The occurrence of recurrent respiratory events in the PACU is an indication for continuous post-operative monitoring and interventions such as use of CPAP.

3. Recurrent PACU respiratory events are defined as

   a. Episodes of apnea for 10 seconds or more

   b. Bradypnea fewer than 8 breaths per minute

   c. Pain–sedation mismatch

   d. Repeated oxygen desaturation to less than 90%

4. Patients with suspected OSA (i.e., scored as high-risk on screening questionnaires or diagnosed OSA with coexisting conditions) and who develop recurrent PACU respiratory events post-operatively are at increased risk of post-operative respiratory complications.

5. Patients should be encouraged to wear their CPAP during all periods of sleep. If they are sleeping during the day, they should be wearing their CPAP.

## Bibliography

Adesanya AO, Lee W, Greilich NB, Joshi GP. Perioperative management of obstructive sleep apnea. *Chest* 2010;**138**(6):1489–98.

American Academy of Sleep Medicine (AASM). *The International Classification of Sleep Disorders – Third Edition (ICSD-3).* 2014. www.aasmnet.org (accessed May 30, 2015).

Bady E, Achkar A, Pascal S, Orvoen-Frija E, Laaban JP. Pulmonary arterial hypertension in patients with sleep apnoea syndrome. *Thorax* 2000;**55**(11):934–39.

Balachandran JS, Masa JF, Mokhlesi B. Obesity hypoventilation syndrome: epidemiology and diagnosis. *Sleep Med Clin* 2014;**9**(3):341–7.

Berry RB, Brooks R, Garnaldo CE, et al. *The AASM Manual for the Scoring of Sleep and Associated Events: Rules, Terminology and Technical Specification, Version 2.0.* Darien: AASM, 2012.

Bradley TD, Floras JS. Obstructive sleep apnoea and its cardiovascular consequences. *Lancet* 2009;**373**(9657):82–93.

Chau EH, Lam D, Wong J, Mokhlesi B, Chung F. Obesity hypoventilation syndrome: a review of epidemiology, pathophysiology, and perioperative considerations. *Anesthesiology* 2012;**117**(1):188–205.

Chung F, Yegneswaran B, Liao P, et al. STOP questionnaire: a tool to screen patients for obstructive sleep apnea. *Anesthesiology* 2008;**108**(5):812–21.

Chung F, Subramanyam R, Liao P, et al. High STOP-Bang score indicates a high probability of obstructive sleep apnoea. *Br J Anaesth* 2012;**108**(5):768–75.

Chung F, Yang Y, Brown R, Liao P. Alternative scoring models of STOP-bang questionnaire improve specificity to detect undiagnosed obstructive sleep apnea. *J Clin Sleep Med* 2014;**10**(9):951–8.

Chung F, Abdullah HR, Liao P. STOP-Bang questionnaire: a practical approach to screen for obstructive sleep apnea. *Chest* 2016;**149**(3):631–8.

Chung F, Memtsoudis SG, Ramachandran SK, et al. Society of Anesthesia and Sleep Medicine guidelines on preoperative screening and assessment of adult patients with obstructive sleep apnea. *Anesth Analg* 2016;**123**(2):452–73.

Eckert DJ, White DP, Jordan AS, Malhotra A, Wellman A. Defining phenotypic causes of obstructive sleep apnea: identification of novel therapeutic targets. *Am J Respir Crit Care Med* 2013;**188**(8):996–1004.

Gali B, Whalen FX, Schroeder DR, Gay PC, Plevak DJ. Identification of patients at risk for postoperative respiratory complications using a preoperative obstructive sleep apnea screening tool and postanesthesia care assessment. *Anesthesiology* 2009;**110**(4):869–77.

Iber C, Cheeson A, Quan SFAS. *The AASM Manual for the Scoring of Sleep and Associated Events, Rules, Terminology and Technical Specifications*. Darien: AASM, 2007.

Kaw R, Bhateja P, Paz Y, et al. Postoperative complications in patients with unrecognized obesity hypoventilation syndrome undergoing elective non-cardiac surgery. *Chest* 2016;**149**(1):84–91.

Memtsoudis SG, Cozowicz C, Nagappa M, et al. Society of Anesthesia and Sleep Medicine guideline on intraoperative management of adult patients with obstructive sleep apnea. *Anesth Analg* 2018;**127**(4):967–87.

Netzer NC, Hoegel JJ, Loube D, et al. Prevalence of symptoms and risk of sleep apnea in primary care. *Chest* 2003;**124**(4):1406–14.

Ramachandran SK, Kheterpal S, Consens F, et al. Derivation and validation of a simple perioperative sleep apnea prediction score. *Anesth Analg* 2010;**110**(4):1007–15.

Singh M, Liao P, Kobah S, et al. Proportion of surgical patients with undiagnosed obstructive sleep apnoea. *Br J Anaesth* 2013;**110**(4):629–36.

Subramani Y, Singh M, Wong J, et al. Understanding phenotypes of obstructive sleep apnea: applications in anesthesia, surgery, and perioperative medicine. *Anesth Analg* 2017;**124**(1):179–91.

# Post-operative Mechanical Ventilation

Konstantinos Alfaras-Melainis and Jessica A. Lovich-Sapola

## Clinical Issues

Mode of ventilation is the most basic ventilator setting. Terminology varies among manufacturers.

The type of mechanical breath determines the flow, pressure, and volume given by the ventilator. There are two basic types of breaths:

1. Volume set breaths: provide selected tidal volume
2. Pressure set breaths: maintain a constant airway pressure during inspiration

## Volume-Controlled Ventilation (VCV)

1. The ventilator cycles from expiration to inspiration after a fixed time interval.
2. The interval determines the respiratory rate.
3. Fixed tidal volume and fixed rate; therefore, fixed minute ventilation
4. Pressure depends on lung resistance
5. Works independently of the patient's effort

    a. The patient cannot breathe spontaneously.
    b. Best used for patients with little or no respiratory effort

        i. Sedated
        ii. Paralyzed

6. Advantage

    a. Ability to deliver a set tidal volume

7. Disadvantages

    a. Higher airway pressures at the end of inspiration
    b. Constant inspiratory flow can lead to uneven alveolar filling.

8. The parameters that may be set by the clinician during VCV include:

    a. Tidal volume
    b. Respiratory rate
    c. Inspiratory time (TI) to expiratory time (TE) ratio (I:E ratio)
    d. Positive end-expiratory pressure (PEEP)
    e. $FiO_2$
    f. Pressure limit (Pmax)

## Assist-Control Ventilation (ACV)

1. Positive-pressure mechanical ventilation
2. Many sources call it CMV (continued mandatory ventilation).
3. It may be used with volume- or pressure-controlled breaths.
4. The patient can initiate each mechanical breath: assisted ventilation.
5. The ventilator provides machine breaths at a pre-selected rate: controlled ventilation.

    a. If no spontaneous effort is detected, the machine functions as if it is in control mode.

6. Advantages

    a. Comfortable for the patient with minimal work of breathing
    b. Can make adjustments to correct $CO_2$ levels

7. Disadvantages

    a. Occur primarily in patients who are spontaneously breathing rapidly

        i. Increased frequency of machine breaths can lead to overventilation, hyperventilation, and respiratory alkalosis.

            (1) Auto-PEEP

    b. Volume-cycled ventilation can lead to barotrauma.

8. The parameters that may be set by the clinician during VCV include:

    a. Breath type (volume control, pressure control)
    b. Respiratory rate
    c. $FiO_2$
    d. PEEP

## Intermittent Mandatory Ventilation (IMV)

1. Delivers periodic volume-cycled breaths at a pre-selected rate
2. Allows spontaneous ventilation between machine breaths

    a. Each spontaneous breath does not trigger a machine breath.

3. If the spontaneous breath triggers the scheduled machine breath, it is called synchronized IMV (SIMV).

    a. The machine breaths are synchronized to coincide with spontaneous lung inflations.

4. Can be used for tachypneic patients with incomplete exhalation during ACV

5. Advantage

    a. Spontaneous breathing promotes alveolar emptying, reducing intrinsic PEEP and air trapping.

6. Disadvantages

    a. Increases the work of breathing

        i. Spontaneous ventilation occurs against a high-resistance circuit.

        ii. Could lead to respiratory muscle fatigue

    b. Reduced cardiac output in patients with left-ventricular dysfunction

7. The parameters that may be set by the clinician during IMV include:

    a. Mandatory respiratory rate
    b. Mandatory breath type
    c. Spontaneous breath type
    d. FiO$_2$
    e. PEEP

## Pressure-Controlled Ventilation (PCV)

1. Pressure-cycled ventilation

    a. Peak airway pressure is set.
    b. Mandatory rate is set.

2. Lower peak airway pressure compared to volume-cycled ventilation

3. The ventilation is completely controlled by the machine and not the patient.

4. The inspiratory flow rate decreases exponentially during lung inflation.

    a. Reduces peak airway pressures
    b. May improve gas exchange and oxygenation

5. Advantages

    a. Decreased risk of barotraumas and volutrauma due to the ability to control the peak alveolar pressure
    b. Lower peak pressure for the same volume
    c. More comfortable for the patient compared to VCV

6. Disadvantage

    a. Inflation volumes vary. As lungs fill, they become less compliant, which leads to less flow to maintain pressure.

7. The parameters that may be set by the clinician during PCV include:

    a. Peak inspiratory pressure (PIP)
    b. Respiratory rate
    c. Inspiratory time or I:E ratio
    d. PEEP
    e. FiO$_2$
    f. Pmax

## Pressure-Controlled Ventilation – Volume Guaranteed (PCV-VG)

1. Controlled ventilation mode combining the advantages of VCV and PCV

2. Delivers the preset tidal volume (TV) with a decelerating flow at the lowest possible PIP

3. Preset inspiratory time

4. Preset respiratory rate

5. Advantages

    a. Useful for patients with low compliance and during surgery in which lung compliance is likely to vary
    b. Offers the benefits of PCV with consistent TV

6. The parameters that may be set by the clinician using PCV-VG include:

    a. TV
    b. Respiratory rate
    c. I:E ratio
    d. PEEP
    e. Pmax

## Pressure-Support Ventilation (PSV)

1. Flow-limited mode of ventilation

2. Pressure-augmented breathing

    a. Peak airway pressure is set.

3. Allows the patient to determine the inflation volume and respiratory cycle duration

4. Used to augment the TV of spontaneously breathing patients and to overcome any increased inspiratory resistance from the endotracheal tube, breathing circuit, and ventilator

5. Should not be used to provide full ventilatory support

6. At the onset of each spontaneous breath, the negative pressure generated by the patient opens a valve that delivers the inspired gas at a pre-selected pressure (usually 5–10 cm H$_2$O).

7. When the patient's inspiratory flow rate falls below 25% of the peak inspiratory flow, the augmented breath is terminated.

    a. This allows the patient to dictate the duration of lung inflation and the inflation volume.

8. Indications

a. Augment inflation volumes during spontaneous respiration

b. Used to overcome the resistance of breathing through the ventilator

c. Used for weaning the patient from mechanical ventilation

d. Increases patient comfort

e. Can be used in combination with IMV to decrease the work of breathing imposed by the breathing circuit and machine

9. Can be used noninvasively through a specialized face or nasal mask

a. Use pressures of 20 cm $H_2O$

10. Advantages

a. Useful for weaning from mechanical ventilation

b. Comfortable mode for the patient

c. Patient has better control over inspiratory flow rate and respiratory rate

d. Can be used with SIMV, spontaneous ventilation, and bilevel modes

11. Disadvantages

a. Not designed to provide full or near-full ventilatory support

b. Poor choice for patients with increased airway resistance

c. Does not decrease auto-PEEP.

12. The parameters set by the clinician using PSV-VG include:

a. Pressure support level

b. $FiO_2$

c. PEEP

## Positive End-Expiratory Pressure

1. The alveolar pressure at end-expiration is above the atmospheric pressure.

2. A pressure-limiting valve is placed in the expiratory limb of the ventilator circuit.

a. Positive pressure is applied during expiration.

3. Without PEEP, the distal airspaces would tend to collapse at the end of expiration.

a. This alveolar collapse impairs gas exchange.

b. PEEP prevents the alveoli from collapsing at end-expiration and can open alveoli that have already collapsed.

4. Improves gas exchange (decreases intrapulmonary shunt) and makes the lungs less stiff (increases lung compliance)

5. Physiologic effect

a. Cardiac filling and cardiac output are hampered due to pressure in the thoracic cavity having a negative effect on venous return.

b. Increased alveolar pressure causes higher partial pressure of oxygen at the alveoli.

6. Indications

a. Toxic levels of inhaled oxygen are required.

i. The addition of PEEP can increase arterial and systemic oxygenation and allow the reduction of the inhaled oxygen to less toxic levels.

b. Low-volume ventilation

c. Obstructive lung disease

7. Benefits

a. Increase in functional residual capacity (FRC)

b. Improved lung compliance

c. Correction of ventilation–perfusion abnormalities

d. Improved oxygenation

8. Adverse effects

a. Barotrauma

i. Pneumothorax

ii. Pneumomediastinum

iii. Pneumopericardium

iv. Spontaneous emphysema

b. Decreased venous return

c. Decreased cardiac output

## Noninvasive Ventilation

Noninvasive ventilation (NIV) refers to the delivery of positive-pressure ventilation through a noninvasive interface.

1. Short trial of NIV can be tried for:

a. Acute hypercapnic respiratory failure due to an acute exacerbation of chronic obstructive pulmonary disease

b. Acute cardiogenic pulmonary edema

c. Oxygenation before and during intubation

d. Intubation refusal or palliation

2. Patients less likely to benefit

a. Acute hypoxemic nonhypercapnic respiratory failure due to conditions other than acute cardiogenic pulmonary edema

b. Acute respiratory failure due to asthma exacerbation

c. Post-extubation, post-operative, or chest trauma-induced acute respiratory failure

3. Some of the contraindications for NIV

a. Need for emergent intubation

b. Nonrespiratory organ failure that is life-threatening

c. Facial trauma/surgery

d. Significant airway obstruction

e. Inability to protect airway

f. Recent esophageal or gastric anastomosis

Trials of NIV should be short.

## Continuous Positive Airway Pressure (CPAP)

1. Spontaneous breathing in which positive pressure is maintained throughout the respiratory cycle

   a. Positive pressure is applied during inspiration and expiration during spontaneous breathing.

2. The patient does not have to generate a negative airway pressure to receive the inhaled gas.

   a. This eliminates the extra work involved in generating a negative airway pressure to inhale.

3. CPAP can also be delivered through a ventilator machine.
4. Indications

   a. Nonintubated patients

      i. Nasal and face masks
      ii. The patient should be awake and alert.
      iii. Pressures should not exceed 15 cm $H_2O$.

   b. Obstructive sleep apnea
   c. Acute respiratory failure (to postpone intubation)
   d. Acute exacerbation of chronic obstructive pulmonary disease
   e. Cardiogenic pulmonary edema

5. APRV (airway pressure release ventilation) is a variation of CPAP on the ventilator. It releases pressure temporarily on exhalation, resulting in higher average airway pressures.

## Bilevel Positive Airway Pressure (BPAP)

1. Noninvasive positive-pressure ventilation
2. Preset inspiratory positive airway pressure (IPAP) and expiratory positive airway pressure (EPAP)
3. TV correlates with the difference between the IPAP and the EPAP.

4. A backup respiratory rate can be set with most BPAP devices.
5. Indications are similar to CPAP.

   a. Advantages over CPAP

      i. Active ventilation (provides inspiratory pressure support)
      ii. A lower mean airway pressure when treating obstructive sleep apnea (more comfortable)
      iii. More rapid improvement of respiratory acidosis
      iv. Compensation for minor air leaks

   b. Disadvantages compared to CPAP

      i. Potential for patient–ventilator asynchrony
      ii. Potential for persistent hypoventilation (severe obstruction, ineffective triggering, central apnea)

## High-Flow Nasal Cannula (HFNC)

1. Does not provide sufficient PEEP or decrease work of breathing like other NIV
2. Two parameters need to be set

   a. flow rate
   b. $FiO_2$

3. Indications are not absolute, with most data coming from observational studies

   a. For patients with severe nonhypercapnic hypoxemic respiratory failure as an alternative of other high-flow oxygen systems and noninvasive ventilation
   b. Post-extubation support
   c. Post-operative respiratory failure
   d. Preoxygenation prior to intubation
   e. Patients undergoing weaning trials and bronchoscopy

## Bibliography

Butterworth JF, Mackey DC, Wasnick JD. *Morgan & Mikhail's Clinical Anesthesiology*, 6th ed. New York: McGraw-Hill Education, 2018, pp. 1329–52.

Duke J. *Anesthesia Secrets*, 2nd ed. Philadelphia: Hanley & Belfus, 2000, p. 106.

Hyzy RC, Jia S. Modes of mechanical ventilation. In: TW Post (ed.) *UpToDate*, Waltham (accessed September 2021).

Kreit J. *Mechanical Ventilation: Physiology and Practice*, 2nd ed. Pittsburgh: Oxford University Press, 2018, pp. 75–81

Marino PL. *The ICU Book*, 4th ed. Philadelphia: Williams & Wilkins, 2014, pp. 760–75.

Miller RD, Fleisher LA, Johns RA, et al. *Anesthesia*, 7th ed. New York: Churchill Livingstone, 2010, pp. 2880–4.

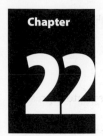

# Chapter 22

# High-Frequency Ventilation

Ryan J. Gunselman and Donald M. Voltz

## Sample Case

A famous vocalist presents to the operating room for removal of a vocal cord lesion. The surgeon is concerned about further damage to this patient's vocal cords and requests that the patient not be intubated. Given the shared nature of the airway and assuming the patient is otherwise healthy, how would you manage the anesthesia and the airway for this case? One suggestion by the surgeon is to use high-frequency jet ventilation. How is this managed and what are your concerns with this form of ventilation? Are there any patients for whom this type of ventilation is not appropriate? What additional monitoring is required to perform this type of ventilation?

## Clinical Issues

### Forms of High-Frequency Ventilation

1. High-frequency positive-pressure ventilation

   a. Delivers a small tidal volume

   b. Rate of 60–120 breaths/min

2. High-frequency jet ventilation (HFJV)

   a. Small cannula at or in the airway

   b. Pulsed jet of high-pressure gas is delivered

   c. Set frequency of 120–600 times/min (2–10 Hz)

3. High-frequency oscillation

   a. Piston creates to-and-fro gas movement in the airway at rates of 180–3000 times/min (3–50 Hz)

### Definition of High-Frequency Jet Ventilation

1. HFJV is a method of ventilation in patients requiring surgery of the larynx when an endotracheal intubation may obscure or interfere with the intended procedure.

2. HFJV has also been used

   a. As mode of ventilation in patients when a conventional endotracheal tube could not be placed.

   b. In neonatal patients with significant pulmonary disease when conventional ventilation is not successful.

3. This technique is usually performed using some type of high-flow oxygen source, tubing, and a narrow conduit (e.g., needle, bronchoscope) to deliver oxygen flows into the patient's trachea.

4. HFJV is most commonly used in procedures in which access to the larynx or trachea is required by the surgeon (i.e., excision/laser of tumors, polyps).

5. This technique stems from the clinical application of *Bernoulli's principle*, which is elaborated on below.

6. In addition to patients undergoing laryngeal surgery, HFJV has been utilized as a bridge to definitive, surgical airway control in patients who cannot be ventilated or intubated due to an anatomic or pathologic airway condition.

   a. Although the principles are the same in these two situations, the specialized ventilators typically used in airway surgery are often not present for emergency airway control, necessitating higher vigilance to avoid complications or injury to the patient.

### Principles Behind the HFJV Technique

1. *Bernoulli's principle*: as the velocity of a fluid (liquid or gas) increases, the pressure decreases.

2. *Venturi effect*: as a fluid flows through a narrowed orifice, the velocity of the fluid increases with a concomitant decrease in the pressure.

   a. This change in fluid velocity and pressure stems from *Bernoulli's principle*.

**TKO:** The clinical application of these two mechanisms using specialized ventilators and endotracheal delivery devices allows for HFJV.

### Mechanism of HFJV

1. With the jet delivery of oxygen through a specialized cannula placed in the patient's airway (i.e., larynx, trachea, distal airways) at a very high rate, one is able to deliver oxygen into the trachea.

   a. HFJV provides a tidal volume less than the anatomic dead space at rates significantly more rapid than normal.

      i. Delivery of a pulse of gas from a high-pressure source (50 psi)

   b. Frequencies are stated as cycles per minute or second (Hz).

      i. Goal rate is 100–400 breaths/min.

      ii. Inspiration accounts for 20–30% of the cycle.

2. Unlike conventional ventilation, the delivery of oxygen is at a lower pressure and therefore does not allow for traditional tidal volume excursion of the lungs and thoracic cage. Oxygen is distributed throughout the alveolar space by diffusion.

   a. HFJV delivers a small tidal volume with high gas flow rates and therefore lower maximum, mean, and transpulmonary airway pressures than with conventional positive-pressure ventilation.

3. Despite the name "jet ventilation," removal of carbon dioxide is not as efficient as with conventional ventilation and occurs by the passive recoil of the chest and lungs, with some assistance from intra-abdominal pressure.

   a. When the jet is active, a volume of oxygen is entrained, allowing for chest wall expansion, followed by elastic recoil of the chest wall when the jet flow is terminated.

      i. One important component of HFJV is the passive recoil of the chest wall and the exhalation of gas through the proximal airways.

   b. Despite oxygen diffusions into the alveoli, the alveolar ventilation is less than with conventional ventilation, resulting in carbon dioxide retention.

4. When this technique is applied in an emergency situation, if a patient does not have a patent supraglottic or glottic area, air trapping and hyper-expansion of the lungs can occur, resulting in a progressive decrement to ventilation as well as to hemodynamic compromise due to escalating intrathoracic pressures.

   a. The problem with air trapping can also occur during airway surgery when HFJV is utilized if the egress of gas is impeded, resulting in

      i. Hyper-expansion of the lungs
      ii. Potential barotraumas
      iii. Hemodynamic collapse
      iv. Inability to ventilate as well as oxygenate the patient

## Cautions of High-Frequency Ventilation

1. Inadequate humidification of the delivered gas

   a. Tracheal mucosal damage
   b. Thickened secretions

2. Patient requires total intravenous anesthetics
3. Barotrauma
4. Alveolar overdistension
5. Injection injury
6. Tension pneumothorax
7. Should never be used if expiratory outflow of gas is impeded

## Indications for High-Frequency Ventilation

1. Electively: to facilitate surgical procedures of the upper airway

   a. Provides for better exposure
   b. Decreases the risk of fire when the laser is utilized

2. Technique to provide adequate oxygenation and alveolar ventilation during rigid bronchoscopy and laryngeal surgery

   a. Bronchoscopy
   b. Tracheal reconstruction
   c. Laser resection of a bronchial lesion
   d. Open thoracic surgery

3. Emergently: a surgical airway technique to allow for oxygenation and some ventilation in a patient who cannot be intubated or ventilated by traditional means until a more definitive airway can be established

   a. ASA difficult airway algorithm
   b. Anesthesiology personnel may utilize transtracheal jet ventilation (TTJV) until a cricothyroidotomy or tracheotomy can be performed.

4. Respiratory failure

   a. Massive air leak from a fistula tract
   b. Pulmonary fibrosis
   c. Pulmonary hemorrhage

5. Adult and infant respiratory distress syndrome

## Jet Ventilator Setups

1. There are two ventilator sources that can be utilized.

   a. Standard anesthesia machine

      i. The HFJV circuit can be attached to standard ventilator tubing and conventional intermittent positive-pressure ventilation can be utilized.

         (1) Limited utility, often unable to generate high enough flow velocities to be effective

      ii. The HFJV circuit can be attached directly to the common gas outlet and the practitioner can manually deliver bursts of high velocity by using the flush button.

         (1) Higher velocities can be generated, allowing for effective oxygenation; however, this requires constant attention to airway pressures, leads to the accumulation of carbon dioxide, and is not "hands-free."

         (2) Measurement of airway pressure can be difficult and inaccurate (possibly through the side port).

(3) Due to the lack of specialized equipment, this ventilation source is often the choice only in an emergency situation.

b. Microcomputer-controlled jet ventilator (preferred)

i. Most commonly used in planned ear, nose, and throat (ENT) procedures, this can also be used in emergent situations if readily accessible and the anesthesiology provider is familiar with its use.

ii. Pressures can be monitored accurately and adjusted as needed to help reduce complications and improve oxygenation/ventilation.

iii. After the initial setup, this can be a relatively "hands-off" technique due to the ability to set alarms and pressure limits in the system.

(1) HFJV requires more vigilance than conventional ventilation since the positioning of the cannula and the delivery of oxygen are both more tenuous than with conventional ventilators.

(2) In addition, the airway is being shared with the surgical team, requiring both to be cognizant of the complications and treatment.

# High-Frequency Jet Ventilator Circuits

1. Two main types

a. Subglottic catheters

i. Most commonly used in planned endotracheal/laryngeal procedures

ii. Various diameters and materials

iii. Rigid (ventilating) bronchoscope can also be included in this category

iv. These are usually placed using direct laryngoscopy after induction of anesthesia (can also be placed after topicalization of the airway with local anesthesia).

b. Invasive catheters

i. Most commonly placed through the cricothyroid membrane

ii. Often placed in emergent situations (cannot ventilate, cannot intubate patient); can be set up using basic supplies on hand in most operating rooms

iii. More complications with this technique

iv. Displacement of the catheter can result in significant subcutaneous emphysema, making it more difficult to replace the cannula or perform a definitive surgical airway.

v. Delivery of high pressure for extended periods of time can result in tension pneumothorax and/or cardiovascular collapse.

vi. If the patient does not have a patent glottic or supraglottic area (i.e., patients with obstructing airway tumors or redundant pharyngeal tissue), this technique is of limited utility and results in air trapping and hyper-expansion of the lungs.

vii. Insertion technique

(1) Identify the cricothyroid membrane by palpation.

(2) Attach a 10 mL or 20 mL syringe partially filled with saline to a large-bore angiocatheter.

(3) Insert through the cricothyroid membrane at a 30-degree angle, pointing the needle caudally (down the trachea).

(4) Aspirate while inserting; air will bubble up through the syringe.

(5) Thread the angiocatheter off the needle into the trachea; once the angiocatheter is inserted completely, the position should be reconfirmed by withdrawing air.

(6) Attach the jet ventilation source to the angiocatheter.

viii. Complications (in order of incidence)

(1) Subcutaneous emphysema (most common)

(2) Bleeding

(a) Often this is minor.

(b) If an anterior jugular vein, thyroid isthmus, or innominate artery is encountered, the bleeding can be significant.

(3) Barotrauma

(4) Pneumothorax

(5) Esophageal injury

(6) Arterial laceration

(7) Cardiovascular compromise from air trapping

# Jet Ventilator Parameters

1. Frequency

2. Percent inspiratory time

a. Recommended initial setting is 40%.

3. Inspiratory oxygen content

4. Driving pressure

a. Driving pressure is the residual oxygen pressure in the ventilator that is available to deliver a breath to the patient.

b. Maximum recommended driving pressure is 50 psi.

5. Peak inspiratory pressure (PIP)

a. Measured from the pressure line

b. Detects high pressures in the system

   c.   The alarm will disable breath delivery until elevated PIP is corrected.

   d.   Recommended initial pressure settings for the PIP is 28 cm $H_2O$ in adults and 12 cm $H_2O$ in children.

6.   Pause pressure (PP)

   a.   Measured in the jet line 10 milliseconds prior to the delivery of each breath

   b.   The purpose of the PP is to prevent breath stacking and barotraumas.

   c.   Recommended pressure limit is 24 cm $H_2O$.

7.   Humidification level

## Ventilation Technique, General Recommendations

1.   Adults will require a pressure of at least 30 psi for ventilation to be effective (flow through common gas outlet is approx. 50–55 psi).

2.   For children, the recommendation is 0.4 psi/kg.

3.   Inspiration should be less than 1 second followed by 2–3 seconds of expiration time.

4.   Keep in mind that in cases of severe airway obstruction the only outlet for expiration may be the angiocatheter, and this is not a large enough orifice to allow for exhalation of the delivered volume.

   a.   Establishing a patent proximal airway or placement of a larger diameter catheter may be required to allow for adequate exhalation.

   b.   There are multi-lumen (two-, three-, or four-lumen) endotracheal tubes designed specifically for jet ventilation. These provide a dedicated lumen for gas inflow, outflow, pressure measurement, and cuff inflation.

   c.   Monitoring airway pressures is important to prevent complications; however, in an emergency situation this is not always possible or available.

   d.   Intermittent disconnection may be needed to allow exhalation and to avoid barotrauma.

5.   $CO_2$ monitoring should be performed.

   a.   Side-channel sampling of $CO_2$ is often unreliable.

   b.   Arterial blood gas sampling may be needed.

## KO Treatment Plan

### Pre-operative

1.   Complete history and physical examination

2.   If HFJV is the anesthetic plan, discuss the goals for the patient's ventilation and your plan if these goals are not met.

   a.   Intubation

   b.   Aborting the procedure

### Intra-operative

1.   Apply standard ASA monitors.

   a.   Oxygenation during jet ventilation can usually be adequately monitored using pulse oximetry.

   b.   The absence of tidal volume precludes the use of standard ventilator disconnect monitoring intra-operatively.

   c.   Insist on $CO_2$ monitoring with side-channel sampling.

2.   Consider the placement of an arterial line for frequent $CO_2$ sampling.

3.   Intravenous induction using lidocaine, fentanyl, propofol, and rocuronium

4.   Maintenance anesthesia: propofol and remifentanil infusion

   a.   Good for rapid onset and termination

   b.   Volatile anesthetics cannot be used with the HFJV technique.

5.   The HFJV catheter should be placed beyond the vocal cords using direct laryngoscopy.

6.   Use the HFJV technique that you are the most comfortable with.

   a.   Microcomputer-controlled jet ventilator

   b.   Subglottic catheter

## Bibliography

Barash PG, Cullen BF, Stoelting RK, et al. *Clinical Anesthesia*, 8th ed. Philadelphia: Lippincott Williams & Wilkins, 2017, p. 1062.

Butterworth JF, Mackey DC, Wasnick JD. *Morgan & Mikhail's Clinical Anesthesiology*, 6th ed. New York: McGraw-Hill Education, 2018, p. 1345.

Gropper MA. *Miller's Anesthesia*, 9th ed. Philadelphia: Elsevier, 2020, p. 1332.

Yao FSF, Fontes ML, Malhotra V. *Yao & Artusio's Anesthesiology: Problem-Oriented Patient Management*, 6th ed. Philadelphia: Lippincott Williams & Wilkins, 2008, pp. 77–80.

# Chapter 23

# One-Lung Ventilation

Elliott Chiartas

## Sample Case

A 60-year-old, 120 kg male is scheduled for a right middle lobectomy for carcinoma of the lung. He has a 50-pack-per-year smoking history. He suffers from chronic obstructive pulmonary disease (COPD) and asthma. His pulse is 70 bpm and blood pressure is 145/90 mm Hg. What are your concerns? How will you secure this patient's airway? What are your intra-operative concerns? If the intubation was difficult, how would you change the double-lumen tube (DLT) to a single-lumen tube?

## Clinical Issues

### Indications for Separation of the Two Lungs/One-Lung Ventilation

1. Absolute

    a. Isolation to prevent spillage or contamination

        i. Infection
        ii. Massive hemorrhage

    b. Control of ventilation

        i. Bronchopleural fistula
        ii. Bronchopleural cutaneous fistula
        iii. Surgical opening of a major conducting airway
        iv. Giant unilateral lung cyst or bulla
        v. Tracheobronchial tree disruption
        vi. Life-threatening hypoxemia from unilateral lung disease

    c. Unilateral bronchopulmonary lavage

        i. Pulmonary alveolar proteinosis

2. Relative

    a. Surgical exposure

        i. Thoracic aortic aneurysm
        ii. Pneumonectomy
        iii. Upper lobectomy
        iv. Mediastinal exposure
        v. Thoracoscopy
        vi. Middle and lower lobectomies
        vii. Esophageal resection
        viii. Thoracic spine surgery
        ix. Tracheoesophageal fistula repair

    b. Severe hypoxemia from unilateral lung disease

### Contraindications for One-Lung Ventilation

1. Relative

    a. Dependence on two-lung ventilation
    b. Prior pulmonary resection
    c. Intraluminal mass in bronchus that may be dislodged

### Techniques for Lung Separation

1. Bronchial blocker

    a. Physiologically the same effect as that produced by clamping one lumen of a DLT
    b. Clinical indications

        i. Critically ill patients in whom it may not be feasible to place a DLT
        ii. Intubated patients
        iii. Patients with a known difficult airway
        iv. Need for post-operative ventilation

            (1) May avoid a risky post-operative change from a DLT to a single-lumen tube

    c. Limitations

        i. Slow lung deflation time
        ii. Slow lung reinflation time
        iii. Difficult suctioning of the operative lung

2. Endobronchial placement of a regular endotracheal tube (ETT)

    a. Clinical indications

        i. Rapid, easy way of effectively separating two lungs, especially in cases of massive hemoptysis
        ii. In most situations, the tube will guide to the right mainstem.

            (1) A fiber-optic bronchoscope is used to guide the tube into place.
            (2) If the left mainstem must be intubated, the patient's head is turned to the right, and the tube is rotated 180 degrees.

    b. Limitations

        i. If entering the right mainstem bronchus, there is a high probability that the right upper lobe (secondary) bronchus may be blocked off, leading to serious hypoxemia.

    ii.   Unable to suction the operative lung

3.   DLT (Fig. 23.1)

    a.   Placement of a DLT (Fig. 23.2)

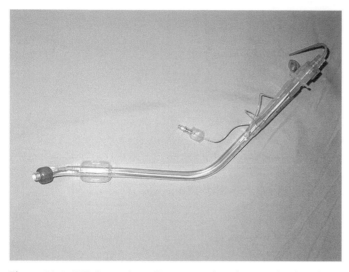

**Figure 23.1** DLT. Source: https://commons.wikimedia.org/wiki/File:Carlens .jpg (photo credit: bigomar2 (May 23, 2007)).

    b.   Verification of DLT placement by auscultation (Fig. 23.3 and Table 23.1)

    c.   Verification of DLT placement by fiber-optic bronchoscopy

       i.   In a left-sided DLT, placing the fiber-optic scope through the tracheal lumen will reveal a view of the tracheal carina, with the upper surface of the blue left endobronchial balloon just visible below the tracheal carina, off to the left.

      ii.   The cuff should not be herniated over the carina.

**TKO:** Major malpositions are frequently tested! Know the signs of malposition both by auscultation and fiber-optic bronchoscopy! Fiber-optic bronchoscopy will reveal a mispositioning incidence as high as 78%. Therefore, even after appropriate auscultation, verification of precise placement with a fiber-optic scope is critical.

## KO Treatment Plan

### Pre-operative

1.   Patients presenting for thoracic surgeries often have an associated history of COPD and a history of cigarette smoking.

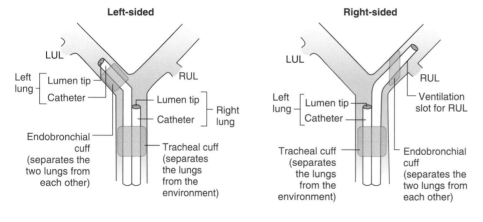

**Figure 23.2** Placement of a DLT. Source: This figure was published in *Anesthesia*, 6th edition, RD Miller, LA Fleisher, RA Johns, et al., Page 1874, Copyright Elsevier (2005). Reprinted with permission.

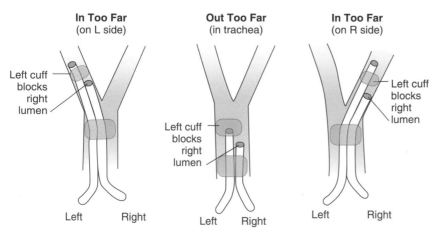

**Figure 23.3** Verification of DLT placement by auscultation. Source: This figure was published in *Anesthesia*, 6th edition, RD Miller, LA Fleisher, RA Johns, et al., Page 1879, Copyright Elsevier (2005). Reprinted with permission.

**Table 23.1** Procedure and breath sounds heard

| Procedure | Breath sounds heard | | |
|---|---|---|---|
| | In too far left | Out too far | In too far right |
| Clamp tracheal lumen, both cuffs inflated | Left | Left and right | Right |
| Clamp bronchial lumen, both cuffs inflated | None or very decreased | None or very decreased | None or very decreased |
| Clamp tracheal lumen, deflate bronchial cuff | Left | Left and right | Right |

Adapted from Miller RD, ed. *Miller's Anesthesia*, 6th ed. Philadelphia: Churchill Livingstone, 2005, p. 1879.

    a. Evaluate the respiratory and cardiovascular functions of these patients appropriately.

       i. Pre-operative pulmonary function tests may be indicated to establish a baseline and identify patients unable to tolerate the planned procedure.

         (1) Tests also indicate if improvement in respiratory function occurs following bronchodilator therapy.

      ii. EKG and other studies may be indicated from the patient's history and physical examination.

        (1) This is considered an intermediate-risk surgery per the ACC/AHA guidelines, with cardiac risk generally reported as <5%.

      iii. Evaluate for hematologic abnormalities and follow baseline blood counts with hematocrit and coagulation studies.

        (1) Coagulation studies are especially important if thoracic epidural anesthesia is planned for post-operative pain relief.

2. Evaluate for appropriate post-operative pain control.

    a. Regional anesthesia techniques ensure optimal patient comfort and minimize pulmonary complications. Options include thoracic epidural analgesia and paravertebral and erector spinae plane blocks. Choice of regional technique is dependent on patient risk factors, surgery performed, and physician preference.

## Intra-operative

1. Assuming the patient has a normal airway, place a DLT after the induction of general anesthesia.

    a. Verify the correct placement immediately and in the lateral position using auscultation and direct visualization with the fiber-optic scope.

2. Maintain two-lung ventilation as long as possible.
3. Use 100% FiO$_2$.

4. Begin one-lung ventilation without changing tidal volumes, unless peak pressures are prohibitive of this maneuver.

    a. Keep the plateau airway pressures <25 cm H$_2$O. In order to achieve this, permissive hypercapnia may be required.

    b. Low tidal volumes (4–6 mL/kg) and moderate positive end-expiratory pressure (PEEP) (5–10 cm H$_2$O) are used to theoretically prevent barotrauma.

    c. Be vigilant of air trapping or auto-PEEP in patients who may require a prolonged expiratory phase of respiration, for example those with COPD or asthma.

5. Treatment of hypoxemia

    a. If severe, switch to two-lung ventilation immediately!

    b. Check the position of the DLT with fiber-optic bronchoscopy.

    c. Eliminate nonpulmonary causes of hypoxemia – that is, CHF, right-sided heart failure, hypotension.

    d. Utilize alveolar recruitment maneuvers to the dependent lung to increase tidal volumes and improve oxygenation.

    e. Apply PEEP, 5–10 cm H$_2$O to the dependent lung.

    f. Apply continuous positive airway pressure (CPAP), 5–10 cm H$_2$O to the nondependent lung. This overcomes the atelectasis in the nonventilated lung, decreasing the shunt fraction.

    g. Apneic oxygenation insufflation to the nondependent lung

    h. Adjust the CPAP and PEEP in an attempt to find the optimal end-expiratory pressure for each lung.

    i. Intermittently ventilate both lungs.

    j. In an emergency, have the surgeon clamp the pulmonary artery. This increases perfusion to the dependent lung.

    k. Use veno-venous ECMO (extracorporeal membrane oxygenation) if one-lung ventilation is critical and no other options are available.

## Post-operative

1. The post-operative course should be guided by the patient's pre-operative cardiopulmonary condition and intra-operative course.
2. If the trachea is to be extubated, the patient must meet extubation criteria as defined in this review book.
3. If the patient is to remain on mechanical ventilation, the DLT must be changed to a single-lumen tube and the position of the tube should be verified with end-tidal $CO_2$ monitoring and auscultation.
   a. In the setting of a difficult initial intubation, the problem of maintaining adequate post-operative ventilation exists. There are a number of possible solutions, all of which may be appropriate in a given set of circumstances.
      i. Leaving the DLT *in situ* and withdrawing the bronchial lumen into the trachea
         (1) This avoids any further manipulation of the airway but is bulky and should not be used if there is a suspicion that post-operative ventilation will last for an extended period of time.
         (2) In addition, few intensive care units are comfortable with caring for a DLT, and as a member of the patient care team, it is important to maintain such consideration.
      ii. Exchange of DLT for single-lumen tube via an extended tube changer
         (1) This would be the author's method of choice.
         (2) It requires an assistant to remove the DLT over a tube changer while direct laryngoscopy is maintained by the anesthesiologist. The single-lumen tube is then threaded over the tube changer by the assistant.
      iii. In the setting of a known pre-operative difficult airway, the DLT may be avoided, and a bronchial blocker placed instead.
         (1) This avoids the post-operative problems of changing the tube, and allows for maintenance of mechanical ventilation.
         (2) This is also a successful option in patients who are intubated pre-operatively, as the change from a single-lumen tube to a DLT may lead to loss of airway control.
4. If the patient remains mechanically ventilated, an aggressive respiratory care regimen is necessary to remove secretions, diagnose/prevent/treat infections, and dilate the airways.

## Bibliography

Campos JH, Feilder A. Hypoxia during one-lung ventilation: a review and update. *J Cardiothorac Vasc Anesth* 2018;32(5):2330–8

Colquhoun DA, Leis AM, Shanks AM, et al. A lower tidal volume regimen during one-lung ventilation for lung resection surgery is not associated with reduced postoperative pulmonary complications. *Anesthesiology* 2021;134 (4):562–76

Gropper MA. *Miller's Anesthesia*, 9th ed. Philadelphia: Elsevier, 2020, pp. 1663–73.

Jaffe RA, Samuels SI, eds. *Anesthesiologist's Manual of Surgical Procedures*, 3rd ed. Philadelphia: Lippincott Williams & Wilkins, 2004, pp. 206–17.

Lohser J. Evidence-based management of one-lung ventilation. *Anesthesiol Clin* 2008;26(2):241–72.

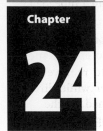

**Chapter**

# 24

# Hypotension

Winston Singleton, Robert C. Lee, and Jessica A. Lovich-Sapola

## Sample Case

A 58-year-old female sustained a right femur fracture. She had a prior right total hip arthroplasty and will need a revision. Her past medical history includes hypertension, mild obstructive sleep apnea, hiatal hernia, and obesity. The patient is terrified of needles and states she had a bad experience with a prior cesarean section after multiple attempts at a spinal anesthetic. She is taken to the operating room and general anesthesia is induced with IV esmolol, lidocaine, fentanyl, propofol, and rocuronium. The tracheal intubation is uneventful. The femoral prosthesis with bone cement is placed. Two minutes later, you notice the end-tidal $CO_2$ decrease to 25 mm Hg when it had been 35–40 mm Hg during the entire case. The minute ventilation has remained the same and you cycle the blood pressure cuff. The blood pressure is 78/45 mm Hg. A repeat blood pressure is 67/38 mm Hg and the end-tidal $CO_2$ is now 12 mm Hg. What would you do next? What is your differential diagnosis?

## Clinical Issues

### Definition of Hypotension

1. The blood pressure is low enough to cause signs and symptoms of inadequate blood flow to the vital organs.
2. A blood pressure less than 90/60 mm Hg is sometimes considered the cutoff for hypotension, but this may be a perfectly acceptable value in some people.

### Signs and Symptoms of Hypotension

1. An alert and awake patient may start complaining of lightheadedness, dizziness, nausea, fatigue, shortness of breath, chest pain, lack of concentration, and blurred vision.
2. The patient may have a syncopal episode and/or have cold, clammy, and pale skin.
3. A patient under general anesthesia will have a drop in blood pressure greater than 20% of his or her normal baseline.
4. You may see changes in the EKG (ischemic; such as ST segment depressions or elevations), pulse oximeter (hypoxia), heart rate (reflex tachycardia), and end-tidal $CO_2$ (decreased secondary to a decreased cardiac output state).

## Differential Diagnosis of Hypotension

**TKO:** This list is extremely important for the oral board exam. In almost every exam, at some point, the patient will become hypotensive. You should have this list memorized so that you can easily determine the possible causes of the patient's hypotension and be able to quickly treat the problem.

1. Pulmonary: hypoxia, hypercarbia, and tension pneumothorax
2. Hypovolemia: fluid deficit and acute blood loss
3. Cardiac: rate/rhythm abnormality, inotropic failure, myocardial ischemia, contusion, tamponade, rupture, congestive heart failure, cardiomyopathy, and valvular injury or lesion
4. Shock: hypovolemic, cardiogenic, and septic
5. Surgical compression of the heart, aorta, inferior vena cava, or abdominal contents
6. Embolus: pulmonary, air, fat, and amniotic
7. Electrolyte and hormonal abnormalities: hypoglycemia, hypocalcemia, adrenal insufficiency, antidiuretic hormone suppression, and hypermagnesemia
8. Anaphylaxis: latex; transfusion; drugs such as antibiotics (penicillin, cephalosporin, sulfa, vancomycin), local anesthetic (usually an ester), muscle relaxants (rocuronium, atracurium, mivacurium, d-tubocurarine, succinylcholine), and opioids (morphine, meperidine), protamine, colloids, iodine, and IV contrast dye
9. Deep anesthesia, drug overdose, and medications such as angiotensin converting enzyme inhibitors and angiotensin receptor blockers
10. Hypothermia
11. Sympathetic blockade and neuraxial block
12. Vasodilation
13. Laparoscopy
    a. Hypercarbia
    b. Dysrhythmia
    c. Increased vagal tone from excessive stretching of the peritoneum
    d. Compression of the inferior vena cava causing a decrease in cardiac output
    e. Venous gas embolism

# KO Treatment Plan

## Pre-operative

1. Validate the blood pressure by re-checking it. Make sure the cuff is the appropriate size and/or that the arterial line transducer is at the correct level.
2. Evaluate the patient and inquire about specific symptoms such as lightheadedness, dizziness, nausea, blurred vision, and chest pain.
3. Perform a physical exam.

   a. Auscultate the heart and lungs.
   b. Palpate for a carotid or femoral pulse.
   c. Check the mucous membranes and extremities to help assist in a rough estimate of the patient's volume status.
   d. Assess the airway, breathing, and circulation.
   e. Check the patient's temperature.
   f. Look for signs of bleeding.

4. Provide supplemental oxygen.
5. Increase IV fluid administration until the cause of the hypotension is determined.
6. Review the patient's medical history.
7. Review the patient's medication list. Determine when her medications were last given.
8. Attempt to determine the patient's baseline blood pressure.
9. Consider getting a 12-lead EKG to evaluate the patient's cardiac rate and rhythm.
10. Order an arterial blood gas, check electrolytes, and get a chest radiograph.
11. Initiate therapy directed at the etiology of the hypotension, if indicated, and re-confirm the diagnosis.
12. Consider postponement of an elective procedure, especially if the patient is experiencing symptoms from the hypotension, unless the cause of the hypotension can be treated surgically.

## Intra-operative

1. Confirm the blood pressure measurement. Check the transducer and/or blood pressure cuff.
2. Evaluate the airway, breathing, circulation, vital signs, temperature, and end-tidal $CO_2$. Pay particular attention to the patient's cardiac rate and rhythm.
3. Place the patient on 100% oxygen.
4. Decrease the volatile inhalational agent, if tolerated.
5. Increase IV fluid administration until the etiology is determined with consideration for colloid solution, such as albumin, and/or blood products.
6. Evaluate the surgical field and consult with the surgeon to evaluate bleeding and inferior vena cava compression.
7. Review the history and physical exam.
8. Consider placement of invasive hemodynamic monitors and transesophageal echocardiography, if available.

9. Stop infusions that may cause vasodilation.

   a. Stop any antihypertensive agents such as β-blockers, calcium channel blockers, nitroglycerin, nitroprusside, isoproterenol, and fenoldopam.

10. Start ionotropic therapy (bolus and/or infusion).

    a. Phenylephrine

       i. Selective $\alpha_1$ receptor agonist
       ii. Noncatecholamine
       iii. Peripheral vasoconstriction

          (1) Increase in systemic vascular resistance
          (2) Increase in arterial blood pressure
          (3) Reflex decrease in the heart rate mediated by the vagus nerve
          (4) Reduced cardiac output

       iv. Can be given either as a bolus or an infusion
       v. Short duration of action: 15 minutes after a single dose
       vi. Tachyphylaxis can occur with infusions

    b. Ephedrine

       i. Noncatecholamine sympathomimetic
       ii. Indirect $\alpha_1$ and $\beta_1$ agonist, and direct $\beta_2$ receptor agonist
       iii. Increases the blood pressure, heart rate, contractility, and cardiac output
       iv. Bronchodilator
       v. Usually used as a bolus agent
       vi. Can also be given intramuscularly
       vii. Longer duration of action than epinephrine

    c. Epinephrine

       i. Endogenous catecholamine
       ii. $\alpha_1$, $\alpha_2$, $\beta_1$, and $\beta_2$ receptor agonist
       iii. Direct stimulation of $\beta_1$ receptors of the myocardium

          (1) Increase in blood pressure
          (2) Increase in cardiac output
          (3) Increase in myocardial oxygen demand secondary to increase in the heart rate and contractility

       iv. $\alpha_1$ stimulation

          (1) Decreases splanchnic and renal blood flow
          (2) Increases coronary perfusion pressure secondary to increasing aortic diastolic pressure
          (3) Increase in systolic blood pressure

       v. $\beta_2$ stimulation

          (1) Vasodilation in the skeletal muscles
          (2) Relaxes bronchial smooth muscle

vi. Used to treat

    (1) Anaphylaxis

    (2) Ventricular fibrillation

vii. Used as a bolus and infusion

d. Norepinephrine

    i. Direct $\alpha$ and $\beta_1$ and limited $\beta_2$ receptor agonist

    ii. Causes an increase in systemic vascular resistance with intense vasoconstriction of the arterial and venous vessels

    iii. Increased myocardial contractility from the $\beta_1$ effects

    iv. Increase in systolic and diastolic pressures

    v. Reflex decrease in heart rate and increased afterload may prevent the increase in cardiac output

    vi. Decreased renal and splanchnic blood flow

    vii. Increased myocardial oxygen requirements

    viii. Used as bolus and infusion

    ix. Agent of choice for management of shock

e. Dopamine

    i. Endogenous nonselective direct and indirect adrenergic and dopaminergic agonist

    ii. Clinical effects vary by dose

        (1) Low dose (0.5–3 μg/kg/min): primarily activates dopaminergic receptors

            (a) Vasodilates renal vasculature

            (b) Promotes diuresis and natriuresis

            (c) Has no beneficial effect on kidney function

        (2) Moderate doses (3–10 μg/kg/min): activates both $\beta_1$ and $\alpha_1$ receptors

            (a) $\beta_1$ stimulation increases myocardial contractility, heart rate, systolic blood pressure, and cardiac output.

            (b) Myocardial oxygen demand increases more than supply.

        (3) Higher doses (>10 μg/kg/min) cause a more prominent $\alpha_1$ receptor effect.

            (a) Increase in peripheral vascular resistance

            (b) Fall in renal blood flow

    iii. Used as an infusion

f. Dobutamine

    i. $\beta_1$ and $\beta_2$ agonist

    ii. Increased cardiac output secondary to the increase in myocardial contractility

    iii. The $\beta_2$-caused decrease in peripheral vascular resistance usually prevents much of an increase in blood pressure.

    iv. Increase in myocardial oxygen consumption

    v. Used in pharmacological stress testing

g. Milrinone

    i. Phosphodiesterase inhibitor

    ii. Leads to an increase in cyclic AMP

    iii. This results in an increase in myocardial contractility and cardiac output.

    iv. There is a decrease in systemic vascular resistance by blocking cyclic GMP metabolism.

11. Placing the patient in a head-down tilt or Trendelenburg position is controversial. It does increase the central blood volume and transiently increases the cardiac output, but ultimately activates baroreceptors and can worsen peripheral vasodilation.

**TKO:** Intra-operative hypotension (MAP $\leq$ 75 mmHg) may be associated with adverse clinical outcomes.

1. Increased 30-day major adverse cardiac events

    a. Myocardial infarction

    b. Death

2. Increased 30-day major adverse cerebrovascular events

    a. Stroke

    b. Delirium

3. Intra-operative hypotension is potentially avoidable.

## Post-operative

1. Confirm the blood pressure measurement. Check the transducer and/or blood pressure cuff.
2. Evaluate the patient, perform a physical exam, and check airway, breathing, and circulation.
3. Provide supplemental oxygen.
4. Increase IV fluid administration as hypovolemia is the most common etiology of hypotension in the post-operative period.
5. Consider a 12-lead EKG to check the cardiac rate and rhythm.
6. Investigate any recent drug administration and the anesthesia record.
7. Stop any infusion that may cause vasodilation.
8. Consider arterial blood gas, complete blood count, and chest radiograph.
9. Aim therapy at the etiology. Perform any maneuver that may help with venous return or help alleviate symptoms if present.
10. If crystalloid solution is not sufficient, consider plasma expanders, such as albumin, or blood products.
11. Ionotropic therapy
12. If fluid administration does not improve the blood pressure, myocardial dysfunction may be a possibility. Monitor for myocardial ischemia and end-organ damage.

## Case Discussion

The case presented is classic for an embolism from the cement used for the femoral prosthesis. The patient also may have suffered from a fat embolism secondary to the femur fracture. The treatment for this patient would be supportive care. The first mode of action should be to immediately call for help. Inform the surgeon of the likely diagnosis. The blood pressure in this scenario had been re-checked. Provide 100% oxygen. Decrease or stop all volatile anesthetics. Palpate for a carotid pulse. If there is no palpable pulse, call for the crash cart and begin the Advanced Cardiovascular Life Support protocol. Intravenous fluids should be given "wide open." Place an arterial line and obtain an arterial blood gas. If the arterial line is difficult, the arterial blood gas should be drawn first. Consider placing a central line to monitor the central venous pressure. The patient should be taken to the intensive care unit immediately post-operatively with continued mechanical ventilation.

## Bibliography

Barash PG, Cullen BF, Stoelting RK. *Clinical Anesthesia*, 8th ed. Philadelphia: Lippincott Williams & Wilkins, 2017, pp. 301–32.

Butterworth JF, Mackey DC, Wasnick JD. *Morgan & Mikhail's Clinical Anesthesiology*, 6th ed. New York: McGraw-Hill Education, 2018, pp. 239–48.

Gregory A, Stapelfeldt WH, Khanna AK, et al. Intraoperative hypotension is associated with adverse clinical outcomes after noncardiac surgery. *Anesth Analg* 2021 **132**(6): 1654–65.

# Hypertension

Winston Singleton, Robert C. Lee, and Jessica A. Lovich-Sapola

## Sample Case

A 48-year-old female is scheduled for a laparoscopic cholecys-tectomy. She has a history of hypertension, diabetes mellitus type II, and hyperlipidemia. She is taking lisinopril, metopro-lol, metformin, and atorvastatin. She states that she did not take any of her medications this morning. Her pre-operative blood pressure is 181/112 mm Hg. A repeat blood pressure is 184/117 mm Hg. She states she is a little nervous and denies any other symptoms. General endotracheal anesthesia is per-formed uneventfully using propofol, fentanyl, and vecuro-nium. An arterial line is placed. Shortly after skin incision, her blood pressure increases from 130/80 mm Hg to 170/100 mm Hg. What is your differential diagnosis? What steps would you take to determine the cause of the intra-operative hypertension? Would you be concerned with the patient's pre-operative blood pressure? Is there a specific blood pressure reading that would cause you to postpone the surgery?

## Clinical Issues

### Definition of Hypertension

1. An adult whose systemic blood pressure is greater than 130/80 mm Hg on at least two different occasions is considered to be hypertensive.
2. Hypertension can be further broken down into stages
   a. Normal: <120/<80 mm Hg
   b. Elevated: 120–129/<80 mm Hg
   c. Stage 1: 130–139/80–89 mm Hg
   d. Stage 2: ≥140/≥90 mm Hg
3. A hypertensive crisis occurs when the systolic blood pressure rises to greater than 180 and/or the diastolic blood pressure rises to greater than 120 mm Hg.
4. Hypertensive urgency: the patient is not showing evidence of target end-organ damage.
5. Hypertensive emergency: the patient develops signs or symptoms of target end-organ damage.

### Types of Target End-Organ Damage

The highest risk of death is seen in patients with systolic arterial pressures greater than 180 mm Hg.
1. Ischemic heart disease
2. Congestive heart failure
3. Cerebrovascular accident

4. Arterial aneurysm
5. End-stage renal disease

## Differential Diagnosis

**TKO:** This list is extremely important for the oral board exam. In almost every exam, at some point, the patient will become hypertensive. You should have this list memorized so that you can easily determine the possible causes of the patient's hyper-tension and be able to quickly treat the problem.

1. Pre-existing hypertension and end-organ dysfunction of the brain, heart, and kidneys
2. "White coat" hypertension
3. Pulmonary: hypoxia, hypercarbia, pulmonary edema, and obstructive sleep apnea
4. Renal: renovascular disease, renal parenchymal disease, renin-secreting tumor, and polycystic kidney disease
5. Neurologic: elevated intracranial pressure, spinal cord injury, Guillain–Barré syndrome, and dysautonomia
6. Cardiac: ischemia, stiff vessels, aortic coarctation, and fluid overload
7. Endocrine: Cushing's syndrome, pheochromocytoma, thyrotoxicosis, hyperaldosteronism, and hyperparathyroidism
8. Vascular: coarctation of the aorta, vasculitis, and collagen vascular disease
9. Drugs: vasopressors, cocaine, monoamine oxidase inhibitors interaction, such as with tyramine, tricyclic antidepressants, naloxone, glucocorticoids, mineralocorticoids, oral contraceptives, withdrawal from antihypertensive therapy, and withdrawal from drugs of abuse
10. Pain, anxiety, inadequate anesthesia
11. Bladder distension
12. Malignant hyperthermia
13. Hypothermia
14. Electrolyte abnormalities: hypercalcemia, hypoglycemia
15. Autonomic instability

## Risk Factors for Hypertension

1. Black or African American
2. Hypertension in either parent
3. Excess alcohol intake
4. Excess sodium intake

5. Overweight and obesity
6. Physical inactivity

## KO Treatment Plan

### Pre-operative

1. Confirm the blood pressure measurement. Check the blood pressure cuff to ensure it is the appropriate size.
2. Evaluate the patient, assess airway, breathing, and circulation; and look for evidence of end-organ damage.
3. Review the history and pharmacology of the drugs that the patient is on for blood pressure control. Check to see what drugs the patient has been taking during the peri-operative period, including the day of surgery.

   a. If a patient has been on chronic β-blocker therapy, it should be continued.

4. The decision of whether to cancel a case is highly debatable. Delaying the surgery for the purpose of blood pressure control may not be necessary, especially in patients with mild to moderate hypertension. It is recommended that an elective case should be postponed if the hypertensive patient exhibits signs of target end-organ damage that can be improved with a delay, or if the damage requires further evaluation prior to the surgery. Strict care should be taken to ensure peri-operative hemodynamic stability because labile hemodynamics, rather than pre-operative hypertension, appear to be more closely related with adverse cardiovascular complications.

   a. Review blood pressure readings over the past few weeks and look for a trend.
   b. Is the patient compliant with her medications?
   c. Is her blood pressure elevated today only because she is nervous and/or did not take her medications?
   d. Counsel the patient on the importance of good blood pressure control with respect to the risks of anesthesia, including heart attack, stroke, arrhythmias, and death.
   e. Many patients will choose to delay the surgery to establish better blood pressure control.
   f. If the case is an emergency, consider the placement of a pre-induction arterial line to help titrate in antihypertensive agents.
   g. There is no consensus on the upper limit of the systemic blood pressure for case delay or postponement.
   h. According to the American College of Cardiology/ American Heart Association, if the patient's systolic blood pressure is ≥180 mm Hg and/or the diastolic blood pressure is ≥110 mm Hg then consideration of the potential benefits of delaying the surgery to optimize the effects of the antihypertensive medications should be weighed against the risk of delaying the surgical procedure. With rapid-acting intravenous agents, the blood pressure can be controlled within hours. An attempt should be made to treat these blood pressures with antihypertensive medications prior to going into the operating room.

      i. The intra-operative arterial blood pressure should be maintained within 20% of the best estimate of the pre-operative arterial pressure, especially in patients with markedly elevated pre-operative pressures. This recommended intra-operative pressure may still be in the hypertensive range.

### Induction

1. Expect an exaggerated blood pressure (both hypo- and hypertensive) response to the anesthetic drugs and increased cardiovascular lability.

   a. A patient with chronic hypertension will have an associated increase in systemic vascular resistance and a relative hypovolemia.
   b. The anesthetics will cause systemic vasodilation and associated hypotension.
   c. Patients with chronic hypertension also have a more vigorous response to laryngoscopy and intubation than normotensive or controlled hypertensive patients.

2. Consider maneuvers to suppress tracheal reflexes and blunt the sympathetic responses to tracheal intubation by using lidocaine, opioids, β-blockers, or vasodilators.
3. Attempt to limit the duration of tracheal manipulation.
4. Consider pre-induction invasive hemodynamic monitors, such as an arterial line.

### Intra-operative

1. Confirm the blood pressure measurement. Check the transducer and/or blood pressure cuff.
2. Evaluate airway, breathing, circulation, and end-tidal $CO_2$. Check all the vital signs.
3. Verify adequate oxygenation and ventilation. Place the patient on 100% oxygen.
4. Review the history and physical exam to guide your differential diagnosis.
5. Consider placement of invasive hemodynamic monitors, such as an arterial line.
6. Antihypertensive agents:

   a. β-blockers

      i. Decrease heart rate, myocardial contractility, and peripheral vascular resistance
      ii. Avoid if heart rate is <60 bpm
      iii. Use with caution in asthmatics
         (1) They can induce bronchospasm in severe asthmatics.
         (2) They are usually safe for mild to moderate asthmatics.
      iv. Examples:

(1) Esmolol

    (a) Ultrashort-acting selective $\beta_1$-antagonist

    (b) Reduces heart rate more than blood pressure

    (c) Used to treat tachycardia and hypertensive response to perioperative stimuli (i.e., intubation, surgical incision, and emergence)

    (d) Used to treat ventricular rate of patients with atrial fibrillation

    (e) Short duration of action secondary to rapid redistribution and hydrolysis by red blood cell esterase

    (f) Avoid in patients with: sinus bradycardia, heart block greater than first degree, cardiogenic shock, and low ejection fraction heart failure.

    (g) Bolus or infusion administration

(2) Metoprolol

    (a) Selective $\beta_1$-antagonist

    (b) No intrinsic sympathomimetic activity

    (c) Available for oral and intravenous use

(3) Propranolol

    (a) Nonselectively blocks $\beta_1$ and $\beta_2$ receptors

    (b) Lowers arterial blood pressure by decreasing myocardial contractility, lowered heart rate, and diminished renin release

    (c) Cardiac output and myocardial oxygen demand are reduced.

    (d) Slows atrioventricular conduction and the ventricular response to supraventricular tachycardia

    (e) Side effects: bronchospasm ($\beta_2$), heart failure, bradycardia, and atrioventricular block ($\beta_1$)

    (f) Long half-life compared to esmolol

(4) Nebivolol

    (a) Newer generation $\beta$-blocker

    (b) High affinity for $\beta_1$ receptors

    (c) Causes direct vasodilation via its stimulatory effect on endothelial nitric oxide synthase

b. Mixed antagonists

  i. Labetalol

    (1) Blocks $\alpha_1$, $\beta_1$, and $\beta_2$ receptors: ratio of $\alpha$ to $\beta$ blockade is 1:7

    (2) Heart rate and cardiac output are only slightly depressed or unchanged

    (3) Decreases peripheral vascular resistance and blood pressure

    (4) Lowers blood pressure without reflex tachycardia

    (5) Beneficial in patients with coronary artery disease

    (6) IV dose: peak effect at 5 minutes

    (7) Side effects: left ventricular heart failure, paradoxical hypertension, and bronchospasm

  ii. Carvedilol

    (1) Mixed $\beta$- and $\alpha$-blocker

    (2) Used to treat heart failure secondary to cardiomyopathy, left ventricular dysfunction after an acute myocardial infarction, and hypertension

c. $\alpha$-blocker

  i. Phentolamine

    (1) Competitive (reversible) blockade of $\alpha_1$ and $\alpha_2$ receptors

    (2) Peripheral vasodilation

    (3) Decreases arterial blood pressure

    (4) Reflex tachycardia and postural hypotension

    (5) Used to treat pheochromocytoma, clonidine withdrawal, and used prior to circulatory arrest in children undergoing repair of cardiac lesions

    (6) Bolus or infusion administration

  ii. Prazosin

  iii. Phenoxybenzamine

d. $\alpha_2$ receptor agonists:

  i. Decreases systemic vascular resistance and heart rate

  ii. Sedative properties

  iii. Examples:

    (1) Clonidine

      (a) Used as an antihypertensive: long-term use can lead to super-sensitization and upregulation of receptors; abrupt discontinuation can lead to withdrawal syndrome and hypertensive crisis.

      (b) Decreases anesthetic and analgesic requirements

      (c) Decreases minimum alveolar concentration

      (d) Provides sedation and anxiolysis

      (e) Prolongs duration of nerve blocks

      (f) Decreased post-operative shivering

      (g) Inhibition of opioid-induced muscle rigidity

      (h) Attenuation of opioid withdrawal symptoms

      (i) Treats acute post-operative pain and some chronic pain syndromes

(j) Side effects: bradycardia, hypotension, respiratory depression, sedation, and dry mouth

(2) Dexmedetomidine

(a) Used for sedative properties

(b) Higher affinity for the $\alpha_2$ receptor than clonidine

(c) Shorter half-life than clonidine

(d) Sedative

(e) Analgesic

(f) Sympatholytic: blunts peri-operative cardiovascular responses

(g) Decreases anesthetic requirements

(h) Rapid administration may elevate the blood pressure

(i) Hypotension and bradycardia can occur with ongoing therapy

e. Calcium channel antagonists

i. Dose-related arteriolar selective vasodilators

ii. Examples:

(1) Nicardipine

(2) Clevidipine

(a) Ultra-short acting with a plasma half-life of 1 minute secondary to rapid metabolism by blood esterases

(b) Lipid emulsion

f. Vasodilators

i. Sodium nitroprusside

(1) Balanced arteriolar and venous dilator that results in decreased systemic vascular resistance

(2) Reflex tachycardia and coronary steal syndrome are both possible

(3) Potent and reliable antihypertensive

(4) Rapid onset of action (1–2 minutes)

(5) Short duration

(6) Frequent blood pressure monitoring is required with an arterial line recommended

(7) Risk: acute cyanide toxicity

(a) Treatment: ventilation with 100% oxygen and sodium thiosulfate or 3% sodium nitrite or cyanocobalamin

ii. Nitroglycerin

(1) Direct vasodilator that acts on the venous system more than the arterial system

(2) Reduces preload, myocardial oxygen demand, and platelet aggregation

(3) Increases myocardial oxygen supply

(4) Dilates pulmonary vasculature and relaxes bronchial smooth muscle

(5) Uterine relaxant

(6) Used to treat myocardial ischemia, hypertension, and ventricular failure

(7) Can be administered intravenously, sublingually, and transdermally

(8) Side effects: headache

iii. Hydralazine

(1) Relaxes arterial smooth muscle

(2) Used to treat hypertension

(3) Hydralazine has a slower onset (10–20 minutes) and longer duration (2–4 hours) compared to β-blockers.

(4) The associated baroreceptor reflex may increase heart rate, myocardial contractility, and cardiac output.

(5) Potent cerebral vasodilator

iv. Fenoldopam

(1) Selective dopamine D1 receptor agonist

(2) Hypotensive agent

(3) Decreases peripheral vascular resistance

(4) Increases renal blood flow, diuresis, and natriuresis

(5) Indicated for patients with severe hypertension with renal impairment

(6) Rapid onset of action

(7) Easily titratable

(8) Short elimination half-life

(9) Increases heart rate (slow titration results in less reflex tachycardia)

(10) Can lead to a rise in intraocular pressure (avoid in glaucoma patients)

(11) Increases kidney blood flow

(12) Side effects: headache, flushing, nausea, tachycardia, hypokalemia, and hypotension

7. Monitor for myocardial ischemia.

a. Pay close attention to the electrocardiogram and look for ST segment changes.

b. Transesophageal echocardiography is helpful to evaluate for intra-operative wall motion abnormalities.

## Post-operative

1. Confirm the blood pressure measurement. Check the transducer and/or blood pressure cuff.

2. Evaluate airway, breathing, and circulation.

3. Review the history and physical exam.

4. Rule out the most common etiologies such as pain, hypercapnia, hypoxemia, urinary retention, or excessive intravascular fluid volume.

5. Antihypertensive therapy should be given with the goal to gradually resume the patient's regimen of oral antihypertensive drugs.

6. Monitor for signs of end-organ damage.

# Bibliography

Barash PG, Cullen BF, Stoelting RK, et al. *Clinical Anesthesia*, 8th ed. Philadelphia: Lippincott Williams & Wilkins, 2017, pp. 592–3.

Butterworth JF, Mackey DC, Wasnick JD. *Morgan & Mikhail's Clinical Anesthesiology*, 6th ed. New York: McGraw-Hill Education, 2018, pp. 248–60.

Gropper MA. *Miller's Anesthesia*, 9th ed. Philadelphia: Elsevier, 2020, pp. 918–98.

Hanada S, Kawakami H, Goto T, et al. Hypertension and anesthesia. *Curr Opin Anaesthesiol* 2006;**19**(3):315–19.

Hines, M. *Stoelting's Anesthesia and Co-existing Disease*, 7th ed. Philadelphia: Churchill Livingstone, 2018, pp. 183–98.

Howell SJ, Sear JW, Foex P. Hypertension, hypertensive heart disease, and perioperative cardiac risk. *Br J Anaesth*, 2004;**92**(4):570–83.

Whelton PK, Carey RM, Aronow WS, et al. ACC/AHA/AAPA/ABC/ACPM/AGS/APhA/ASH/ASPC/NMA/PCNA Guideline for the prevention, detection, evaluation, and management of high blood pressure in adults: a report of the American College of Cardiology/American Heart Association Task Force on Clinical Practice Guidelines. *Hypertension*. 2018;**71**:e13–e115.

**Chapter**

# 26 Arrhythmias

Saima Karim and Jessica A. Lovich-Sapola

## Sample Case

An 80-year-old male just woke up after an emergency pinning of his left hip. You are called to the recovery room because the patient's heart rate suddenly increased from 80 to 160 beats/min. How would you evaluate? What would you do if his blood pressure was 120/80 mm Hg? What if his blood pressure was 60/30 mm Hg?

## Clinical Issues

### Diagnosis of Arrhythmias

1.  Classified by heart rate (HR)

    a.  Bradyarrhythmia (HR <60 beats/min)
    b.  Tachyarrhythmia (HR >100 beats/min)
    c.  Conduction blocks (HR at any rate)

2.  Classified by the anatomic origin within the heart

    a.  Ventricular
    b.  Supraventricular
    c.  Junctional
    d.  Elsewhere

### Intra-operative Factors Contributing to Arrhythmias

1.  General anesthetics

    a.  Volatile anesthetics can produce an arrhythmia through a re-entrant mechanism.
    b.  Halothane sensitizes the myocardium to endogenous catecholamines.
    c.  Cocaine and ketamine block the reuptake of norepinephrine and can facilitate the development of epinephrine-induced arrhythmias.

2.  Local anesthetics

    a.  Pharmacological sympathectomy leading to a parasympathetic dominance and bradycardia

3.  Abnormal arterial blood gases and electrolytes

    a.  Abnormalities in pH
    b.  Hypoxia/hypercarbia

4.  Sympathetic response to endotracheal intubation
5.  Reflexes

    a.  Vagal: sinus bradycardia, atrioventricular block, or asystole
    b.  Carotid sinus stimulation: bradycardia
    c.  Oculocardiac reflex: bradycardia or asystole

6.  Central nervous system stimulation
7.  Dysfunction of the autonomic nervous system
8.  Pre-existing cardiac disease

    a.  Myocardial ischemia/infarction
    b.  Congestive heart failure (CHF)
    c.  Cardiomyopathy
    d.  Valvular disease
    e.  Conduction system abnormalities

9.  Central venous cannulation

    a.  Insertion of the wire or catheter into central circulation

10. Surgical manipulation of the cardiac structures

    a.  Atrial sutures
    b.  Venous bypass cannulas

11. Location of the surgery

    a.  Dental

        i.   Profound stimulation of the sympathetic and parasympathetic nervous system
        ii.  Trigeminal (fifth cranial) nerve stimulation leading to stimulation of the autonomic nervous system

12. Pain
13. Hypovolemia
14. Hypotension
15. Anemia
16. Endocrine abnormalities

    a.  Hyperthyroidism
    b.  Pheochromocytoma

17. Temperature abnormalities

    a.  Hyperthermia
    b.  Hypothermia

# KO Treatment Plan

## Continued Assessment of an Arrhythmia

1. What is the arrhythmia?
   a. Usually best evaluated in limb lead II because it will show the largest P wave.
   b. What is the HR?
   c. Is the rhythm regular?
   d. Is there one P wave for each QRS complex?
   e. What is the relationship between the P and QRS complex?
   f. Is the QRS complex normal?
   g. Is the rhythm dangerous?
2. Does it produce a hemodynamic disturbance?
3. What treatment is required?
4. How urgently does it need to be treated?
   a. Treatment should be initiated immediately if the arrhythmia is associated with marked hemodynamic impairment.
   b. Treatment should be started promptly if the arrhythmia is a precursor to a more severe arrhythmia.
   c. Treatment should also be initiated if the arrhythmia is detrimental to the patient's underlying cardiac disease.
      i. Tachycardia in a patient with mitral stenosis

# Asystole and Pulseless Electrical Activity (PEA)

## Clinical Issues

### Definitions

1. Asystole (Fig. 26.1)
   a. No discernible electrical activity on the EKG

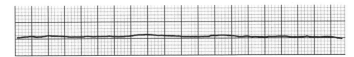

**Figure 26.1** Asystole. Drawing credit: J. Lovich-Sapola, MD, MBA, FASA.

b. Always confirm by checking the monitor for loose leads, no power, too low a signal gain, or operator error (Figs. 26.2–26.3).
   c. Usually there is a poor prognosis
   d. Asystole can be the endpoint rhythm for patients initially in ventricular fibrillation or ventricular tachycardia.
2. PEA
   a. Heterogeneous group of rhythms that are organized or semi-organized but lack a palpable pulse
   b. It is any organized rhythm without a pulse except for ventricular fibrillation, ventricular tachycardia, or asystole.
   c. A poor outcome is likely unless diagnosed and treated quickly and aggressively.
   d. This arrhythmia can often be perpetrated by noncardiac causes.

### Causes

1. Asystole and PEA
   a. Hypovolemia
   b. Hypoxia
   c. Hydrogen ion (acidosis)
   d. Hyper- and hypokalemia
   e. Hypoglycemia
   f. Hypothermia
   g. Toxins/tablets
   h. Tamponade (cardiac)
   i. Tension pneumothorax
   j. Thrombosis (pulmonary, coronary)
   k. Trauma

## KO Treatment Plan

1. Call for help.
2. Cardiopulmonary resuscitation (CPR)
3. Oxygen
4. Attach the monitor/defibrillator.
5. Early epinephrine 1 mg intravenous or intraosseous (IV/IO)
6. Resume CPR.
7. Epinephrine 1 mg IV/IO (may repeat every 3–5 minutes)

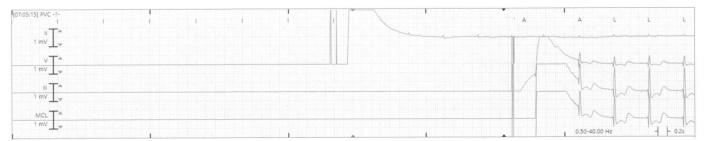

**Figure 26.2** Example of pseudo-pause due to lead disconnection. Credit: Saima Karim, DO.

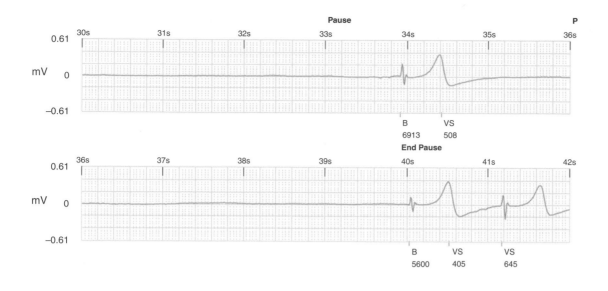

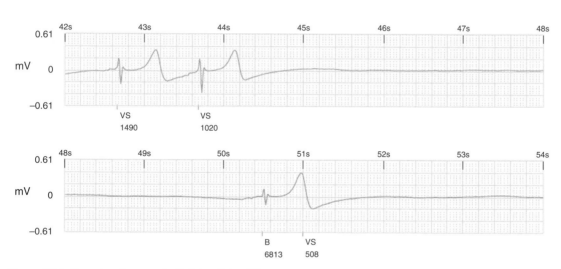

**Figure 26.3** Examples of pauses. Credit: Saima Karim, DO.

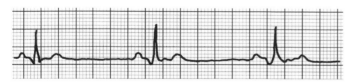

**Figure 26.4** Sinus bradycardia. Drawing credit: J. Lovich-Sapola, MD, MBA, FASA.

8. Look for and treat the underlying cause.
9. There is no evidence that attempting to defibrillate or transcutaneous pace asystole or PEA is helpful.

# Sinus Bradycardia (Fig. 26.4)

## Clinical Issues

### Definition

1. HR <60 beats/min

2. HR <50 beats/min in patients with chronic β-blocker therapy
3. Regular rhythm
4. Normal QRS complex unless there is underlying intraventricular conduction delay, bundle branch block, or paced ventricular rhythm

### Side Effects of Bradycardia

1. Decreased cardiac output
2. Decreased blood pressure
3. Syncope, vertigo, lightheadedness, and dizziness

### Causes

1. Hypoxia/hypercarbia
2. Drug effects

   a. Opioids

b. β-blockers

c. Calcium channel blockers

d. Antiarrhythmic medications such as amiodarone and sotalol

e. Succinylcholine

f. Anticholinesterase inhibitors

g. Anesthetic overdose

3. Acute inferior myocardial infarct

4. Vagal stimulation

   a. Oculo-cardiac reflex

   b. Visceral stimulation

5. High sympathetic blockade

   a. High spinal

   b. Spinal shock

6. Acidosis

7. Allergic reaction

8. Hypertension

9. Increased intracranial pressure (ICP): Cushing's response

10. Baseline slow HR: well-trained athletes may have large stroke volumes and large cardiac output reserve that allow for normal resting bradycardia.

## KO Treatment Plan

1. Check all vital signs.

2. Check the baseline HR.

3. Ensure a secure airway with adequate oxygenation and ventilation.

4. Obtain a 12-lead EKG.

5. HR <40 beats/min is often poorly tolerated even in healthy patients.

6. Treatment is recommended if hypotension, ventricular arrhythmias, or signs of poor peripheral perfusion are observed.

7. Atropine 0.5 mg IV bolus repeated every 3–5 minutes, up to 3 mg

8. Ephedrine 5–10 mg IV bolus

9. Dopamine 2–20 μg/kg/min IV infusion

10. Epinephrine 2–10 μg/min IV infusion

11. Temporary transcutaneous pacing or transvenous pacemaker: this should be done immediately if the patient is symptomatic with significant bradycardia.

# Sinus Tachycardia (Fig. 26.5)

## Clinical Issues

### Definition

1. Most commonly occurring arrhythmia in the perioperative period

2. HR 100–160 beats/min

3. Regular rhythm

4. Normal QRS complex unless there is underlying intraventricular conduction delay, bundle branch block, or paced ventricular rhythm

5. Normal sinus P wave

### Causes

1. Hypoxia/hypercapnia

2. Pain/anxiety

3. Inadequate anesthesia

4. Hypovolemia/anemia

5. Fever/malignant hyperthermia/sepsis

6. Congestive heart failure

7. Drug effect

   a. Catecholamines

   b. Pancuronium

   c. Anticholinergics

   d. Vasodilators

8. Endocrine abnormalities

   a. Hyperthyroidism

   b. Thyrotoxicosis

   c. Pheochromocytoma

9. Electrolyte abnormalities

   a. Hypoglycemia

10. Surgery

11. Pulmonary embolism

12. Pneumothorax

13. Pacemaker malfunction

14. Drug withdrawal

15. Bladder distension

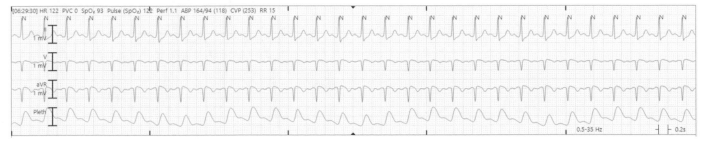

**Figure 26.5** Sinus tachycardia. Credit: Saima Karim, DO.

## KO Treatment Plan

### Stable Tachycardia

1. Check all vital signs.
2. Check an EKG.
3. Check the baseline HR.
4. Check the oxygenation and ventilation.
5. Prolonged tachycardia can precipitate congestive heart failure.
6. Tachycardia decreases coronary perfusion time.
7. Treat the underlying disorder.
8. β-blockers in patients with underlying ischemic heart disease

### Unstable Tachycardia with a Pulse

1. A patient has unstable tachycardia if he or she
   a. Is hypotensive
   b. Shows signs of shock
   c. Has an altered mental status
   d. Has ongoing chest discomfort
   e. Has shortness of breath
   f. Has syncope
2. Support the airway, breathing, and circulation.
3. Give oxygen.
4. Check all vital signs.
5. Establish IV access.
6. Persistent tachyarrhythmia: synchronized cardioversion
   a. Narrow regular: 50–100 J
   b. Narrow irregular: 120–200 J biphasic or 200 J monophasic
   c. Wide regular: 100 J
   d. Wide irregular: defibrillation (not synchronized)

## Premature Atrial Contractions (PAC; Fig. 26.6)

### Clinical Issues

#### Definition

1. An ectopic pacemaker site in the left or right atrium initiates the atrial premature beat.
2. The P wave will generally have a different shape from the usual sinus beat.
3. The PR interval will vary depending on the site of the ectopic focus.

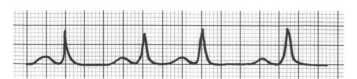

**Figure 26.6** Exaamples of PAC couplet. Drawing credit: J. Lovich-Sapola, MD.

4. It has a normal sinus cycle with no compensatory pause.
5. The HR is variable, but usually less than 100 beats/min.
6. The rhythm is irregular.

## KO Treatment Plan

1. Rarely needed
2. Digitalis, β-blockers, or verapamil may be considered if hemodynamic function is impaired.

## Paroxysmal Supraventricular Tachycardia (PSVT; Figs. 26.7–26.8)

### Clinical Issues

#### Definition

1. Rapid, regular rhythm
2. Narrow QRS complex unless there is aberrancy during supraventricular tachycardia or intraventricular conduction delay or bundle branch block at baseline
3. Typically lacks the normal sinus P wave, but can still be positive in inferior lead and negative in V1 if focal atrial origin is close to the sinus node. Sometimes P waves can be difficult to visualize.
4. Usually abrupt in onset and termination
5. HR is 130–270 beats/min.

#### Associated with the Following

1. Seen in 5% of normal adults and in patients with Wolff–Parkinson–White syndrome
2. Intrinsic heart disease
3. Systemic illness
4. Thyrotoxicosis
5. Digitalis toxicity
6. Pulmonary embolism
7. Pregnancy
8. Changes in the autonomic nervous system
9. Drug effect
10. Intravascular volume shifts

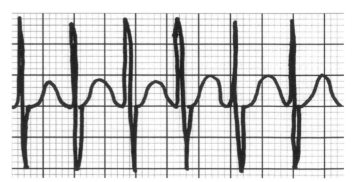

**Figure 26.7** PSVT. Drawing credit: J. Lovich-Sapola, MD, MBA, FASA.

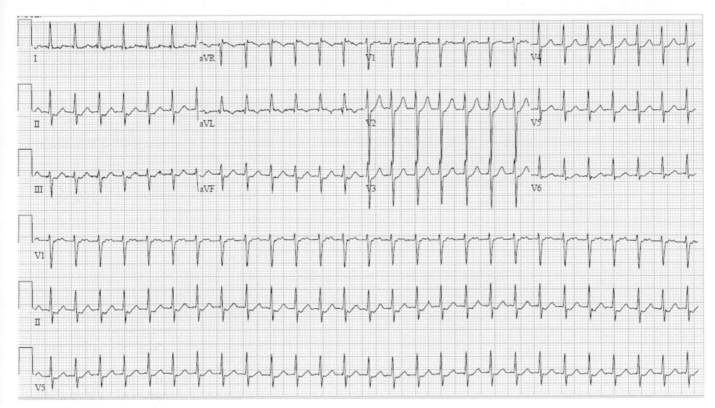

**Figure 26.8** PSVT Credit: Saima Karim, DO.

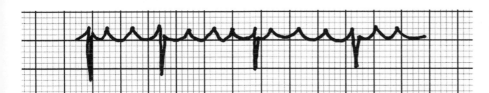

**Figure 26.9** Atrial flutter. Drawing credit: J. Lovich-Sapola, MD, MBA, FASA.

## KO Treatment Plan

1. Often must be treated because of its rapid rate and associated poor hemodynamic function
2. Vagal maneuvers
3. Give adenosine 6 mg rapid IV bolus, followed by a second and third dose, if necessary, at 12–18 mg per bolus.
4. Verapamil 2.5–10 mg IV
5. Amiodarone 150 mg IV infusion over 10 minutes
6. Esmolol 1 mg/kg bolus IV and 50–200 mg/kg/minute infusion
7. Edrophonium 5–10 mg IV bolus
8. Give phenylephrine 100 μg IV if the patient is hypotensive.
9. Digoxin 0.5–1.0 mg IV
10. Rapid overt pacing in an attempt to capture the ectopic focus
11. Synchronized cardioversion in incremental doses of 50, 100, 200, 300, and 360 J: this should be done immediately if the patient is hemodynamically unstable.

## Atrial Flutter (Figs. 26.9–26.10)

### Clinical Issues

**Definition**

1. Classic sawtooth flutter waves in typical flutter, but sometimes typical sawtooth pattern is absent
2. Atrial rate is generally 250–350 beats/min.
3. Ventricular rate varies
4. Rhythm is regular
5. The QRS complex is the same as it is during sinus unless there is aberrancy.
6. Macro re-entrant arrhythmia

**Causes**

1. Severe heart disease
2. Coronary artery disease
3. Mitral valve disease
4. Pulmonary embolism
5. Hyperthyroidism

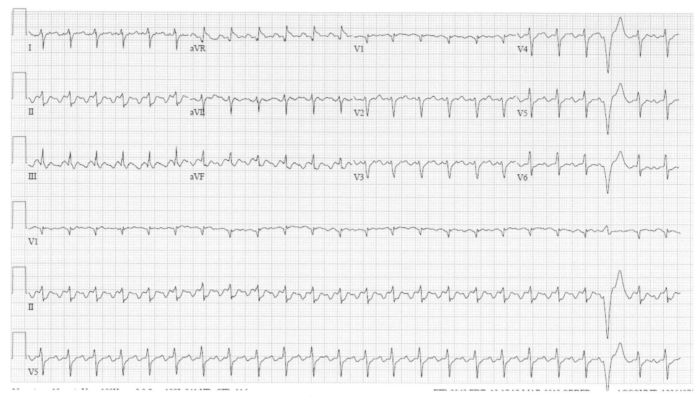

**Figure 26.10** Atrial flutter with PVC. Credit: Saima Karim, DO.

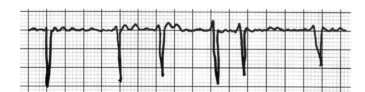

**Figure 26.11** Atrial fibrillation. Drawing credit: J. Lovich-Sapola, MD, MBA, FASA.

6. Cardiac trauma
7. Cancers of the heart
8. Myocarditis

## KO Treatment Plan

### Hemodynamically Stable

1. Consider pharmacologic or synchronized cardioversion after ruling out the risk of a thromboembolic event.
2. Control the ventricular response rate by slowing the conduction through the atrioventricular node with β-blockers such as esmolol and metoprolol or calcium channel blockers such as diltiazem.

### Hemodynamically Unstable

1. Start synchronized DC cardioversion with 100 J, gradually increasing to 360 J if needed.

2. Procainamide 5–10 mg/kg IV loading dose with a 0.5 mg/kg/minute infusion
3. Rapid atrial pacing from within the atrium can help maintain sinus rhythm.

## Atrial Fibrillation (Figs. 26.11–26.13)

### Clinical Issues

#### Definition

1. Irregular atrial focus with variable ventricular conduction with no P waves or no consistent P wave-appearing morphology on the EKG
2. Irregularly irregular rhythm
3. Atrial rate 350–500 beats/min
4. Ventricular rate varies significantly.
5. P waves are absent or there can be coarse atrial fibrillation with no recognizable P wave pattern or consistent morphology.
6. QRS complex is the same as it is during sinus unless there is aberrancy.

#### Causes

1. Cardiac disease
2. Other causes are similar to those associated with atrial flutter.

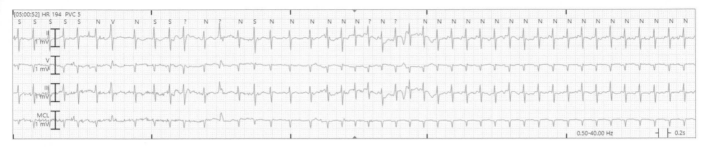

**Figure 26.12** Atrial fibrillation example. Credit: Saima Karim, DO.

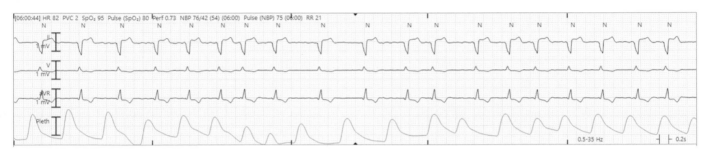

**Figure 26.13** Atrial fibrillation example. Credit: Saima Karim, DO.

## Clinical Significance

1. Loss of atrial "kick" may reduce the ventricular filling and significantly compromise cardiac output by 10–20%.
2. Atrial fibrillation may be associated with atrial thrombi after 24 hours, which can result in pulmonary and systemic embolization.

## KO Treatment Plan

### Acute Atrial Fibrillation

1. IV diltiazem or esmolol
2. Consider synchronized cardioversion in patients with pronounced hemodynamic instability. Start with 100–200 J, then 300 J, then 360 J.
3. If atrial fibrillation has been present for over 48 hours without anticoagulation, there is an increased risk of thromboembolism.
   a. Consider a transesophageal echocardiogram (TEE) to rule out an atrial thrombus.
   b. Adequate anticoagulation for 4 weeks should be considered prior to cardioversion if a thrombus is present.

### Long-Term Therapy

1. Employ anticoagulation therapy with warfarin or direct-acting oral anticoagulants, depending on the risk of thromboembolic events, but even without significant risk of thromboembolic events if rhythm control has to be undertaken
2. β-blockers, calcium channel blockers, and digitalis can be used to control the HR if it is >100 beats/min.

3. Initiate antiarrhythmic therapy with consideration of the patient's renal function, hepatic function, and presence of coronary artery disease or structural heart disease.
4. Atrial fibrillation ablation
5. Electrode catheter ablation of the atrioventricular junction and permanent pacemaker insertion

### Antiarrhythmic Agents for Prevention of Recurrence

1. Propafenone
2. Flecainide
3. Sotalol
4. Amiodarone
5. Dofetilide
6. Dronedarone
7. Quinidine

## Junctional Rhythms (Fig. 26.14)

### Clinical Issues

#### Definition

1. Cells in the sinus node are not able to act as pacemakers.
2. The ectopic activity is initiated at the site of the AV junction.
3. P waves are abnormal.
4. Variable HR of 40–180 beats/min.
5. Regular rhythm
6. QRS complex is normal unless there is underlying intraventricular conduction delay, bundle branch block, or paced ventricular rhythm.

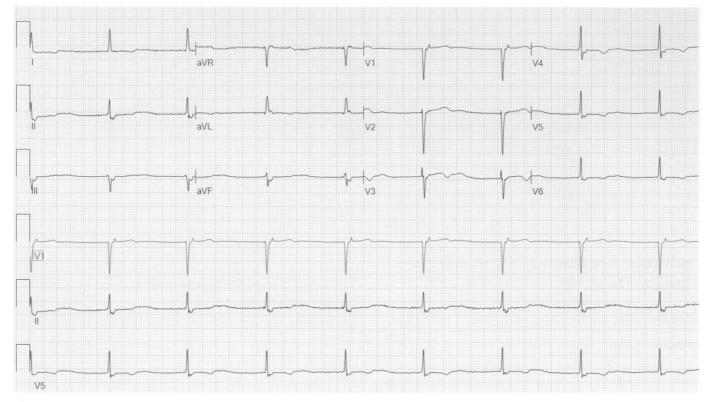

**Figure 26.14** Junctional rhythm. Credit: Saima Karim, DO.

## Causes

1. Junctional rhythms are common under general anesthesia, especially with halogenated anesthetic agents. Isoproterenol use can also induce junctional rhythm. Some antiarrhythmics that suppress sinus activity may also result in junctional rhythm.

## Significance

1. Junctional rhythms frequently decrease blood pressure and cardiac output by about 15%.

## KO Treatment Plan

1. Usually requires no treatment
2. If the patient becomes hypotensive and has poor perfusion, treatment is indicated.
3. IV atropine, ephedrine, or isoproterenol can be used in an effort to increase the activity of the sinoatrial (SA) node.
4. A small 10 mg dose of succinylcholine while under general anesthesia may revert a nodal rhythm to a sinus rhythm.
5. Temporary pacing is rarely needed.
6. Permanent dual chamber or atrial pacing is rarely needed.

# Premature Ventricular Contractions (PVC; Figs. 26.15–26.16)

## Clinical Issues

### Definition

1. Ectopic pacemaker activity arising inferior to the AV junction
2. Wide QRS complex (>0.12 seconds)
3. No P wave or retrograde P wave
4. Rhythm is irregular or bradysphygmia may occur.

### Causes

1. Common during anesthesia, especially in patients with pre-existing cardiac disease
2. Electrolyte and blood gas abnormalities
3. Drug interactions
4. Brainstem stimulation
5. Trauma to the heart
6. Pre-existing structural heart disease
7. Cardiac ischemia

### Significance

1. May be a life-threatening event
2. The arrhythmia may progress to ventricular tachycardia or fibrillation.

## KO Treatment Plan

1. Correct the underlying abnormality, such as decreased serum potassium or low arterial oxygen tension.

    a. Check arterial blood gas, electrolytes, EKG, and chest X-ray.

2. If very frequent or symptomatic PVCs occur, may treat with a lidocaine 1.5 mg/kg or amiodarone 150 mg IV bolus – but it is rarely needed unless this is a new recurrence without a correctable underlying cause.

3. Recurrent ventricular premature beats can be treated with an IV infusion of lidocaine at 1–4 mg/min or amiodarone at 1 mg/min, esmolol, propranolol, procainamide, quinidine, atropine, verapamil, or overdrive pacing.

## Ventricular Tachycardia (VT) with a Pulse (Figs. 26.17–26.19)

### Clinical Issues

#### Definition

1. The presence of three or more PVCs is known as nonsustained VT. If the ventricular arrhythmia lasts for more than 30 seconds, then it is known as sustained VT.

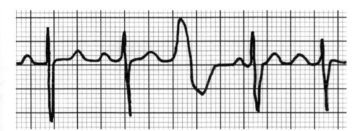

**Figure 26.15**  PVC. Drawing credit: J. Lovich-Sapola, MD, MBA, FASA.

2. The presence of a fusion beat, capture beat, and atrioventricular dissociation
3. HR of 100–250 beats/min
4. Usually a regular rhythm but can be irregular
5. Wide QRS complex greater than 0.12 seconds. There are usually more ventricular complexes than atrial complexes.

#### Significance

1. Acute onset is life-threatening and requires immediate treatment.

### KO Treatment Plan

1. Amiodarone 150 mg IV infusion over 10 minutes
2. Synchronized cardioversion: start with 100–200 J, then 300 J, then 360 J.

## Ventricular Fibrillation (VF; Figs. 26.20–26.21)

### Clinical Issues

#### Definition

1. Irregular rhythm
2. Erratic ventricular contractions
3. The EKG has a bizarre ventricular pattern of various sizes.
4. P waves are not visible.
5. Rapid, grossly disorganized rhythm
6. QRS is not seen.

#### Causes

1. Myocardial ischemia
2. Hypoxia
3. Hypothermia

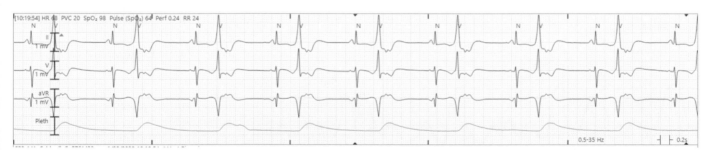

**Figure 26.16**  Frequent monomorphic PVCs in bigeminal pattern.

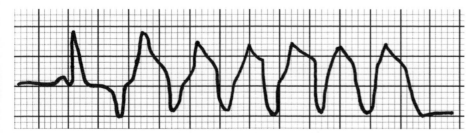

**Figure 26.17**  Non-sustained ventricular tachycardia. Drawing credit: J. Lovich-Sapola, MD, MBA, FASA.

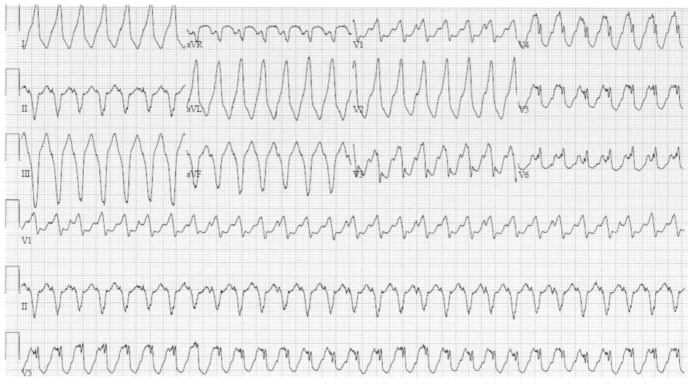

**Figure 26.18** Sustained VT. Credit: Saima Karim, DO.

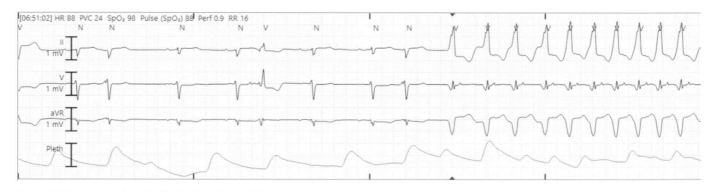

**Figure 26.19** Nonsustained VT. Credit: Saima Karim, DO.

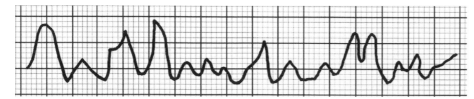

**Figure 26.20** Ventricular fibrillation. Drawing credit: J. Lovich-Sapola, MD, MBA, FASA.

4. Electric shock
5. Electrolyte imbalance
6. Drug effect
7. Prolonged QT interval

**Significance**

1. No effective cardiac output
2. Can be fatal unless treated immediately and aggressively.

## KO Treatment Plan for VF and Pulseless VT

1. CPR
2. Oxygen
3. Attach the monitors/defibrillator.
4. Asynchronous defibrillation (one shock with 120–200 J for biphasic defibrillator or 360 J for a monophasic defibrillator)

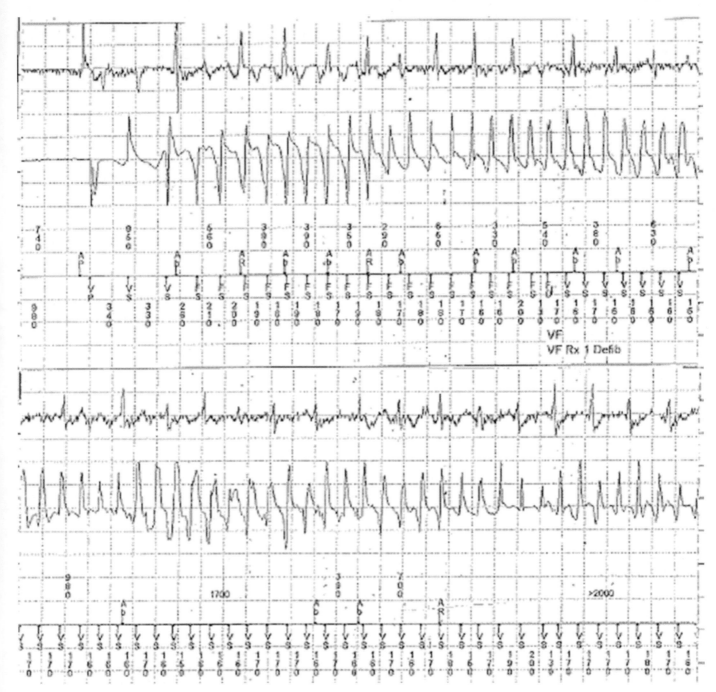

**Figure 26.21** VF during a code. Credit: Saima Karim, DO.

5. Resume CPR for 2 minutes.
6. Continue to alternate one shock and CPR as long as the patient maintains a shockable rhythm.
7. Once the patient has an IV, give epinephrine 1 mg IV/IO (may repeat every 3–5 minutes).
8. Consider an antiarrhythmic such as:
   a. Amiodarone 300 mg IV/IO once, then consider an additional dose of 150 mg IV/IO.
   b. Lidocaine 1–1.5 mg/kg first dose, then 0.5–0.75 mg/kg IV/IO, with a maximum of three doses or 3 mg/kg.
   c. Magnesium 1–2 g IV/IO for torsades de pointes.
9. After five cycles or CPR/shock, reevaluate the rhythm.

# Torsades de Pointes (Fig. 26.22)

## Clinical Issues

### Definition

1. VT with a prolonged QT
2. Rapid, polymorphic VT with a characteristic twist of the QRS complex around the isoelectric baseline

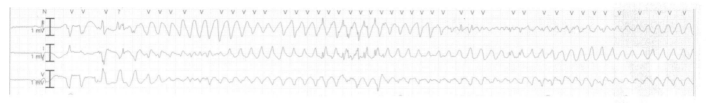

**Figure 26.22** Torsades de pointes. Credit: Saima Karim, DO.

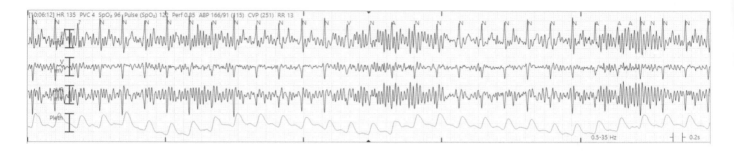

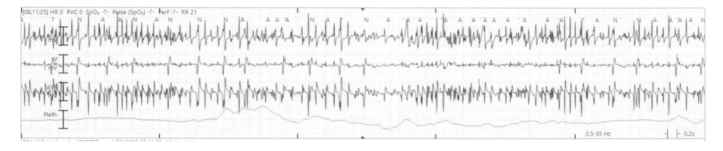

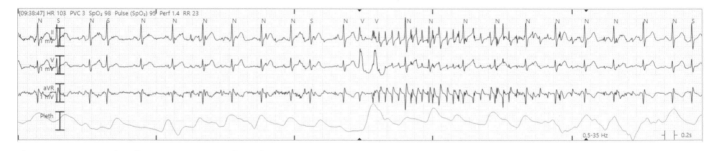

**Figure 26.23** Examples of noise that can be confused for an arrythmia. Credit: Saima Karim, DO.

3. May mimic VF
4. It is a life-threatening arrhythmia.
5. Rate is usually 150–250 beats/min.
6. No atrial component
7. P wave is buried in the QRS.
8. Ventricular rhythm is regular or irregular.

### Causes

1. Occurs in the presence of disturbed repolarization: prolonged QT

2. Seen also with electrolyte disturbances such as hypokalemia, hypocalcemia, and hypomagnesemia

## KO Treatment Plan

1. Discontinue the drugs that led to the prolonged QT and correct any electrolyte abnormality.
2. Asynchronous defibrillation
3. 1–2 g IV magnesium sulfate, IV amiodarone, and/or IV isoproterenol
4. Overdrive pacing

## Bibliography

American Heart Association. *American Heart Association 2020 Guidelines for* *Advanced Cardiovascular Life Support.* Dallas: AHA, 2020.

Barash PG, Cullen BF, Stoelting RK, et al. *Clinical Anesthesia*, 8th ed. Philadelphia: Lippincott Williams & Wilkins, 2017, pp. 1661–82.

Gropper MA. *Miller's Anesthesia*, 9th ed. Philadelphia: Elsevier, 2020, pp. 2713–42.

# Chapter 27

# Cardiac Conduction Blocks

Cristian M. Prada

## Sample Case

A 15-year-old female is scheduled for a mastoidectomy. Her mother reports that she was 8 weeks premature and has significant developmental delays. She is followed closely at an outside hospital for her primary care. Her mother also tells you that she was recently diagnosed with a second-degree heart block (Mobitz type II). She hands you a copy of the cardiologist's note. He recommends a follow-up appointment and EKG in 3 months, but no medications or pacemaker. The patient is currently asymptomatic. Are you concerned? How will you treat this patient? Would you place external pacemaker pads? Would you like another cardiology consult?

## Clinical Issues

### Definitions

1. Conduction systems of the heart
   a. Sinoatrial (SA) node
   b. Atrioventricular (AV) node
   c. His–Purkinje system (AV bundle [of His], Purkinje fibers of the right and left bundle branches)
2. Heart block above the AV node is transient and benign; below the AV node is more progressive and permanent.
3. Elderly patients
   a. Increase in the incidence of bradydysrhythmias and conduction abnormalities
      i. Caused by a progressive fibrosis in both the SA and the AV conduction system
      ii. For the SA node: fat accumulation, which separates it from the atria musculature
   b. SA pacemaker cells decrease progressively from 60 years of age: at 75 years old, approximately 10% of the original numbers of cells are present.
   c. Bradydysrhythmias may be present pre-operatively but can have an unexpected onset as heart block under general anesthesia, mainly in the elderly population.

## Sinus Node Block

1. Failure of the normal pacemaker of the SA node
2. This rarely causes symptoms, because if the patient has a complete block at the SA node, the secondary pacemaker

of the heart would be the AV node, which depolarizes at 40–60 beats/min.

a. Sinus node arrest
   i. Absence of spontaneous depolarization
   ii. Prolonged sinus pauses caused by failure of sinus impulse formation

b. Sinus node exit block
   i. No electrical propagation
   ii. Block of conduction of sinus impulses from the SA node to the surrounding atrial tissue

c. Atrial tissue failure
   i. Depolarization does not reach the AV node.

d. Sick sinus syndrome
   i. A combination of symptoms caused by SA node dysfunction and manifested by marked bradycardia, sinoatrial block, or sinus arrest
   ii. Can have associated episodes of supraventricular tachycardia; often called bradycardia–tachycardia syndrome
      (1) Dizziness
      (2) Confusion
      (3) Fatigue
      (4) Syncope
      (5) Congestive heart failure (CHF)
   iii. Treatment
      (1) Atrial or dual-chamber pacemaker
      (2) These patients are at a high risk of developing a pulmonary embolism and should be started on anticoagulation therapy.

## Atrioventricular Node Block

1. Presence of P waves without ventricular activation
2. Temporary or permanent; anatomic or functional impairment of conduction
3. Classification: first-, second-, or third- (complete) degree block and high-grade AV block (Fig. 27.1)
   a. First-degree block

First degree AV block

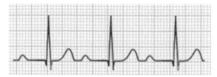

Second degree AV block (Mobitz I or Wenckebach)

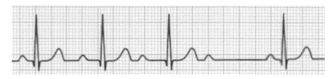

Second degree AV block (Mobitz II)

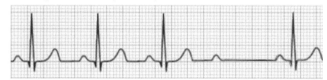

Second degree AV block (2:1 block)

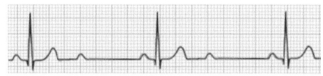

Third degree AV block with junctional escape

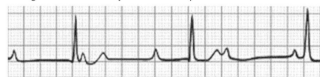

**Figure 27.1** Heart blocks. Source: Dr. Nicholas Patchett (https://commons .wikimedia.org/wiki/File:Heart_block.png).

i. Prolonged PR interval >200 msec on a 12-lead EKG

ii. Benign

   (1) Sometimes significant bradycardia can occur during spinal anesthesia.

   (2) Rare progression to higher degrees of block; reported only with spinal or general anesthesia

   (3) If the PR interval is >400 msec, then an apparent AV dyssynchrony and higher-grade AV block can develop if the atrial rate increases (exercise, trauma, anemia), because not all of the atrial impulses are conducted to the ventricles.

iii. Causes

   (1) AV nodal disease

   (2) Enhanced vagal tone (athlete)

   (3) Myocarditis

   (4) Acute myocardial infarction

   (5) Electrolyte disturbances

   (6) Medication

      (a) Calcium channel blockers

      (b) β-blockers

      (c) Cardiac glycosides

      (d) Cholinesterase inhibitors

      (e) Digitalis

iv. Treatment depends on symptomatology, but can include:

   (1) Correction of any electrolyte imbalances

   (2) Withholding of any offending medications

   (3) Admission of the patient to the coronary care unit if it is associated with a myocardial infarction, or otherwise continuing with outpatient follow-up.

b. Second-degree block

i. Some impulses are blocked.

   (1) Mobitz I (Wenckebach): the PR interval progressively lengthens until the ventricles fail to activate (P wave not followed by QRS).

      (a) Disease of the AV node

      (b) If the patient is hemodynamically stable, the treatment is observation only.

      (c) This is usually a benign condition.

   (2) Mobitz II: intermittently nonconducted P waves are not preceded by PR prolongation.

      (a) Disease along the His–Purkinje system

      (b) May progress rapidly to a complete heart block

         (i) Cardiac arrest and sudden death

      (c) May occur with an antero-septal infarct

      (d) Treatment: pacemaker

      (e) Some recommend prophylactic pacemaker implanted pre-operatively in patients with 2:1 AV block even without symptoms.

c. Third-degree block

i. No atrial impulses are conducted to the ventricles.

ii. Complete heart block

iii. P wave without relation to the QRS complexes

iv. Causes

   (1) Coronary ischemia

   (2) Congenital: lupus

   (3) Fibrosis and/or sclerosis (Lenègre disease), calcification (Lev disease)

(4) Cardiomyopathy (sarcoidosis, amyloidosis, hemochromatosis, malignancy, infectious, idiopathic)

(5) Hyperkalemia, hypo- or hyperthyroidism, trauma, degenerative neuromuscular disease

(6) Drugs: beta-blockers, calcium channel blockers, digoxin, adenosine, antiarrhythmics

(7) Post-valvular surgery or correction of congenital heart disease

(8) Transcatheter aortic valve implantation, ablation of arrhythmias, transcatheter closure of ventricular septal defect, alcohol septal ablation for hypertrophic cardiomyopathy

(9) Risk factors for AV block: increased systolic blood pressure and high values of fasting glucose levels

v. Treatment

(1) Dual-chamber pacemaker

vi. Treatment if the patient has acutely hemodynamically unstable heart block

(1) Pharmacologic: continuous infusion of isoproterenol; possibly atropine, ephedrine, epinephrine, dopamine, dobutamine (if heart failure with reduced ejection fraction)

(a) Glycopyrrolate is indicated only for vagally induced bradycardia.

(b) These treatments can sometimes cause uncontrolled sinus tachycardia.

(2) Pacing: transcutaneous, transvenous, transthoracic, or transesophageal

vii. Treatment of hemodynamically stable heart block

(1) Transcutaneous pacing

(2) Evaluate for causes

d. High-grade AV block: intermittent atrial conduction to the ventricle with two or more consecutive blocked P waves but without complete AV block.

## Bundle Branch Blocks (Fascicular Blocks)

1. Left bundle branch block (Fig. 27.2)

a. Activation of the left ventricle is delayed, which results in the left ventricle contracting later than the right.

i. Usually indicates an underlying cardiac pathology

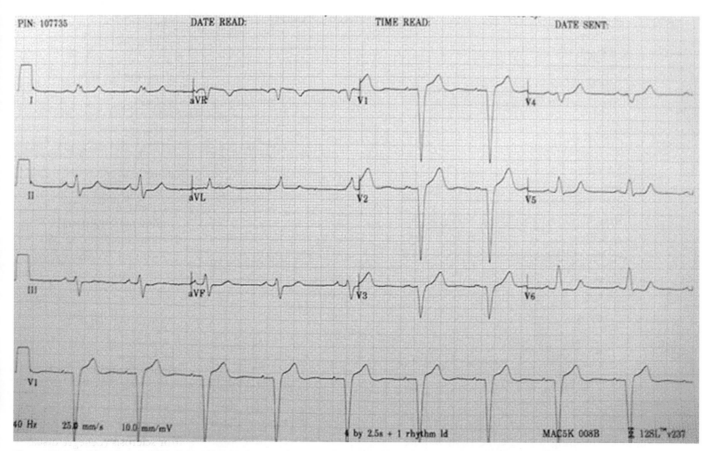

**Figure 27.2** Left bundle branch block: EKG. Source: James Heilman, MD (https://commons.wikimedia.org/wiki/File:LBBB2009.JPG).

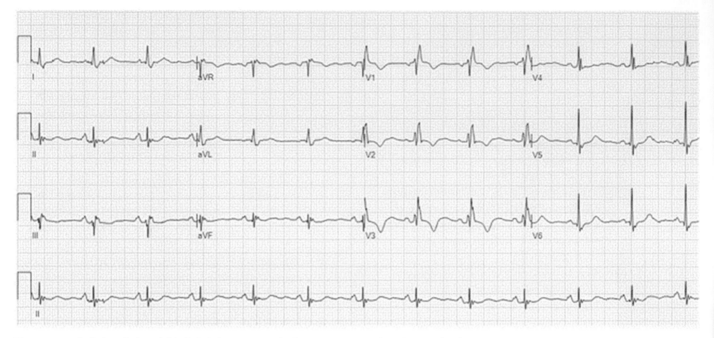

**Figure 27.3** Right bundle branch block: EKG. Source: Ewingdo (https://commons.wikimedia.org/wiki/File:ECG_NSR_with_RBBB_74_bpm.jpg).

(1) Dilated or hypertrophic cardiomyopathy
(2) Hypertension
(3) Aortic valve disease
(4) Coronary artery disease: myocardial infarction

b. Causes

  i. Hypertension
  ii. Myocardial infarction
  iii. Excessive coronary artery disease
  iv. Primary conduction defect

c. Diagnosis

  i. Heart rhythm must be supraventricular in origin.
  ii. The QRS duration must be ≥120 msec.
  iii. There should be a QS or RS complex in lead V1.
  iv. There should be a monophasic R wave in leads I and V6.

    (1) R, R′ in the left chest leads (V5 or V6)

  v. The T wave should be deflected opposite the terminal deflection of the QRS complex.

d. Treatment

  i. Requires a complete cardiac evaluation
  ii. Patients with syncope, CHF, and prolonged QRS may require a pacemaker.

2. Right bundle branch block (Fig. 27.3)

a. The right ventricle is not directly activated by impulses traveling through the right bundle branch.

  i. First, the left ventricle receives the electrical impulse, followed by the right ventricle.
  ii. The left ventricle is normally activated by the left bundle branch.
  iii. These impulses travel through the myocardium of the left ventricle and activate the right ventricle.
  iv. New onset with symptoms

    (1) Screen for pulmonary embolism, chronic lung disease, cardiomyopathy, CHF, atrial and ventricular septal defects, Ebstein anomaly, blunt chest trauma, and polymyositis.

b. Causes

  i. Central line placement (right side)
  ii. Increased prevalence with increased age

    (1) It is usually a marker in slow progressive degenerative disease.

  iii. Can be a normal variant in healthy patients

c. Diagnosis

  i. The heart rhythm must be supraventricular in origin.
  ii. The QRS duration must be ≥120 msec.
  iii. There should be a terminal R wave in lead V1.

    (1) R, R′ in the right chest leads (V1 or V2)

  iv. There should be a slurred S wave in leads I and V6.
  v. The T wave should be deflected opposite the terminal deflection of the QRS complex.

d. Treatment

    i. Generally asymptomatic and does not require treatment.

    ii. Pacemaker if syncope occurs

## KO Treatment Plan

### Pre-operative

1. The patient was diagnosed with Mobitz II second-degree heart block.

    a. May progress to complete heart block

    b. Usually treated with a pacemaker

2. Since the surgery is elective, I would postpone the surgery to get a second opinion cardiology consult.

3. If the surgery suddenly became an emergency:

    a. Place external pacer pads.

    b. Have the pacer/defibrillator in the operating room.

### Intra-operative

1. Standard ASA monitoring

2. Begin general anesthesia with an endotracheal tube so that the patient already has a secure airway if she goes into complete heart block and requires cardiac pacing.

### Post-operative

1. Maintain the pacer pads in the post-anesthesia care unit.

2. Close observation on a telemetry or coronary care unit floor

3. Order a cardiology consult for close follow-up management.

## Bibliography

American Heart Association. CPR & first aid, emergency cardiovascular care. https://cpr.heart.org/en/resuscitation-science/cpr-and-ecc-guidelines/algorithms (accessed 2 January 2023).

*Circulation.* Management of symptomatic bradycardia and tachycardia. *Circulation* 2005;**112**:67–77.

Dubin D. *Rapid Interpretation of EKGs*, 6th ed. Tampa: Cover, 2000, pp. 174–94.

Gropper MA. *Miller's Anesthesia*, 9th ed. Philadelphia: Elsevier, 2020, pp. 1815–25.

Kerola T, Eranti A, Aro AL, et al. Risk factors associated with atrioventricular block. *JAMA Netw Open* 2019;**2**(5):e194176.

Lobato EB, Gravenstein N, Kirby RR. *Complications in Anesthesiology*, 3rd ed. Philadelphia: Lippincott Williams & Wilkins, 2008, pp. 256–9.

Longnecker DE, Brown D, Newman M, et al. *Anesthesiology*. New York: McGraw Hill. 2008, p. 349.

Sauer WH. Third degree (complete) atrioventricular block. In: Ganz LI, Yeon, SB, eds. *UpToDate* (accessed 2 January 2023).

Shigematsu-Locatelli M, Kawana T, Nishigaki A, et al. General anesthesia in a patient with asymptomatic second-degree two-to-one atrioventricular block. *JA Clin Rep* 2017;**3**:27.

Suzuki M, Sakaue T, Tanaka M, et al. Association between right bundle branch block and impaired myocardial tissue-level reperfusion in patients with acute myocardial infarction. *J Am Coll Cardiol* 2006;**47**:2122–4.

Yao FSF, Hemmings HC, Malhotra V, Fong J. *Yao & Artusio's Anesthesiology: Problem-Oriented Patient Management*, 9th ed. Alphen aan den Rijn: Wolters Kluwer. 2021, pp. 182–4.

# Acute Coronary Syndrome

Cristian M. Prada and Jessica A. Lovich-Sapola

**Chapter 28**

## Sample Case

A 68-year-old female, 231 lb. and 5'1″ tall, with a history of hypertension, diabetes mellitus, and large joint chronic arthritis, is scheduled for a laparoscopic cholecystectomy. The patient is noncompliant with her medication: atenolol and glyburide. On the morning of the surgery, the patient's blood pressure was 145/86 mm Hg, heart rate (HR) 88, respiratory rate (RR) 20, oxygen saturation 97% on room air, and temperature 36.8 °C. Her blood glucose was 186 mg/dL. Physical examination revealed no abnormalities, and the airway was assessed as a Mallampati class II. After a smooth induction of general anesthesia with midazolam, fentanyl, propofol, and rocuronium, a #7.0 endotracheal tube was placed atraumatically. Anesthesia was maintained with mechanical ventilation, isoflurane, oxygen, air, fentanyl boluses, and rocuronium. About 30 minutes after the incision, the patient's HR increased to 112 beats/min and her blood pressure became 184/99 mm Hg. The anesthesiologist also noticed a depression of the ST segment in the monitored V5 cardiac lead.

What would you do? What treatment would you give? Could this event have been prevented? Would you extubate this patient? What is your plan for the post-operative care of this patient?

## Clinical Issues

### Definitions

1.  Acute coronary syndrome (ACS)

    a.  Patient with coronary atherosclerosis

    b.  Spectrum of clinical syndromes

        i.   Unstable angina
        ii.  Non-ST-segment elevation myocardial infarction (NSTEMI)
        iii. ST-segment elevation myocardial infarction (STEMI)
        iv.  Sudden cardiac death

    c.  Varying degree of coronary occlusion

    d.  Symptoms

        i.   Acute chest discomfort: pain, pressure, tightness, burning
        ii.  Dyspnea
        iii. Epigastric pain
        iv.  Pain in one or both arms, jaw, neck, or back
        v.   Nausea
        vi.  Sweating
        vii. Dizzy or lightheadedness

2.  Two groups of patients, based on electrocardiogram (ECG):

    a.  Acute chest pain and persistent (>20 min) ST-segment elevation

        i.   Named: ST-segment elevation ACS
        ii.  Total or subtotal coronary occlusion: development of STEMI
        iii. Treatment: immediate reperfusion by primary percutaneous coronary intervention (PCI), or fibrinolytic therapy

    b.  Acute chest pain but *no persistent* ST elevation (NSTEMI)

        i.   Transient ST-segment elevation: persistent or transient ST-segment depression, T wave inversion, flat T waves, pseudo-normalization of T waves, or even normal ECG.
        ii.  Cardiomyocyte necrosis (NSTEMI) or, less frequently, myocardial ischemia without cell damage (unstable angina)
        iii. Immediate coronary angiography and, if appropriate, revascularization for:

            (1) Ongoing chest pain
            (2) ST-segment depression
            (3) Heart failure
            (4) Hemodynamic instability
            (5) Electrical instability

3.  Acute myocardial infarction (AMI): cardiomyocytes necrosis in a clinical setting of acute myocardial ischemia.

    a.  Criteria for diagnosis:

        i.   Increase or decrease of a cardiac biomarker: high-sensitivity cardiac troponin (hs-cTn) T or I, with at least one value above 99%.
        ii.  At least one of the following:

            (1) Symptoms of myocardial ischemia
            (2) New ischemic ECG changes
            (3) Pathological Q waves on ECG
            (4) Imaging evidence of loss of viable myocardium or new regional wall abnormality

(5) Intracoronary thrombus: angiography or autopsy

4. Types of myocardial infarction:

a. Type 1: atherosclerotic plaque: rupture, ulceration, fissure, erosion – resulting in intraluminal thrombus

b. Type 2: other than plaque: hypotension, hypertension, tachyarrhythmias, bradyarrhythmia, anemia, hypoxemia, coronary spasm, spontaneous coronary artery dissection, coronary embolism, coronary microvascular dysfunction

c. Type 3: death without biomarkers available

d. Type 4: related to PCI

e. Type 5: related to coronary artery bypass grafting (CABG)

5. Chronic stable angina

a. Anginal pain: substernal, exertional, radiating

b. Pain is relieved by rest or nitroglycerin

c. Can be asymptomatic: silent ischemia

i. More common with diabetics

ii. Occurs with an extensive collateral blood supply

d. Symptoms occur when atherosclerotic lesions cause 50–75% occlusion

6. Unstable angina

a. Abrupt increase in severity, frequency, or duration of angina attacks

b. Angina at rest

c. New onset of angina with severe or frequent episodes

d. Partially occluding thrombus that produces symptoms of ischemia

e. Treatment: antiplatelet agents

i. Aspirin

ii. Clopidogrel (Plavix)

iii. Glycoprotein IIb/IIIa receptor inhibitors

(1) Fibrinolytic therapy is not effective.

f. Additional treatment

i. Oxygen

ii. Nitroglycerine (sublingual or intravenous)

iii. β-blockers

iv. Heparin

## Mechanism of Cardiac Ischemia

1. Imbalance between the supply and demand of oxygen to the myocardium

a. Supply of oxygen to the myocardium: determined by coronary perfusion pressure and the duration of the diastole

i. Coronary perfusion pressure is maintained by:

(1) Normal to high diastolic arterial pressure

(2) Normal to low left ventricular end-diastolic pressure (LVEDP)

ii. Increased length of diastole increases the supply of oxygen.

b. Demand of oxygen by the myocardium is determined by:

i. HR

(1) Decreasing HR

(a) Increases oxygen supply by prolonging diastole

(b) Decreases oxygen demand as the heart is doing less work

(c) Avoid severe bradycardia which causes decreased diastolic arterial pressure and increased LVEDP.

(d) Use β-blockers.

ii. Contractility

(1) Difficult to measure; even by cardiac output or left ventricular ejection fraction

(a) Decreased contractility may be beneficial in coronary artery disease (CAD) as long as coronary perfusion pressure is maintained.

(b) Potent volatile anesthetic agents: isoflurane and halothane

(c) Myocardial depressants are useful for patients with CAD as long as the coronary perfusion pressure is maintained.

iii. Myocardial wall tension

(1) Increased during systole against high after-loads, resulting in higher oxygen demand, despite the increase in coronary perfusion pressure.

## Factors That Influence Peri-operative Myocardial Ischemia and Infarction

1. Increased myocardial oxygen demand

a. HR

i. Maintain a normal rate and rhythm.

b. Blood pressure

i. Maintain a normal blood pressure within 20% of the peri-operative mean.

c. Surgical stress and post-operative pain can lead to a hyperadrenergic state that can result in tachycardia and increased oxygen demand.

2. Decreased myocardial oxygen supply occurs with improper ventilation of the patient.

3. Coronary artery spasm
4. Anesthetic effects: see below
5. Rupture of atherosclerotic plaque: coronary thrombosis
6. Coagulation abnormalities: surgically induced

   a. Prothrombotic state secondary to the stress response and direct activation of the coagulation cascade by the surgical injury
   b. Platelet activation

## Cardiac Cascade

1. Progressive sequence of pathophysiologic events triggered by myocardial ischemia: coronary artery occlusion
2. Diastolic abnormalities: increase in LVEDP
3. Systolic abnormalities: regional wall motion abnormalities
4. Hemodynamic abnormalities
5. EKG changes
6. Angina: symptoms may not occur (silent myocardial infarction)

## Take-Home Message for the Evaluation and Diagnosis of Chest Pain

1. Chest pain means more than pain. It can present as pain, pressure, tightness, or discomfort in the chest, shoulders, arms, back, and jaw.

   a. Can also present as shortness of breath and fatigue
   b. Women are more likely to present with nausea and shortness of breath.

2. Highly sensitive cardiac troponins are the preferred standard for diagnosis of an AMI.
3. Early care for acute symptoms is key to survival.
4. Routine testing is not needed for low-risk patients.
5. Rule out other causes of chest pain:

   a. Pulmonary

      i. Embolism
      ii. Pneumonia
      iii. Pneumothorax

   b. Aortic dissection
   c. Esophageal/gastrointestinal

      i. Rupture
      ii. Esophagitis
      iii. Peptic ulcer
      iv. Gall bladder

   d. Herpes zoster
   e. Noncoronary cardiac

      i. Aortic stenosis
      ii. Pericarditis
      iii. Myocarditis

**TKO:** Reversal of the ischemia signs is not in the same temporal order: the stunned myocardium may have wall motion abnormalities despite EKG signs of resolution.

1. High likelihood of myocardial ischemia if the patient has any of the findings below:

   a. History

      i. Chest or left arm pain or discomfort plus:

         (1) Current pain is similar to prior angina
         (2) Known CAD, myocardial infarction

   b. Physical exam

      i. Transient mitral regurgitation
      ii. Hypotension
      iii. Diaphoresis
      iv. Pulmonary edema or rales

   c. EKG

      i. New transient ST deviation ($\geq$0.5 mm)
      ii. T wave inversion ($\geq$2 mm) with symptoms

   d. Cardiac markers

      i. Elevated troponin I or T – if available: hs-cTn test at 0 and 2 hours
      ii. Elevated CK-MB – not routinely recommended if hs-cTn available
      iii. Determine BNP (B-type natriuretic peptide) for prognostic

2. Intermediate likelihood: if the patient has no high likelihood findings and has any of the findings below

   a. History

      i. Chest or left arm pain or discomfort plus

         (1) Age >70 years
         (2) Male sex
         (3) Diabetes mellitus

   b. Physical exam

      i. Extracardiac vascular disease

   c. EKG

      i. Fixed Q waves
      ii. Abnormal ST segments or T waves that are not new

   d. Cardiac markers

      i. Any finding in the intermediate likelihood category plus normal cardiac enzymes

3. Low likelihood: if the patient has no high or intermediate risk findings and has any of the findings below

   a. History

      i. Probable ischemic symptoms
      ii. Recent cocaine use

   b. Physical exam

i. Chest discomfort can be reproduced by palpitation (15% of patients with musculoskeletal pain will have a myocardial infarction).

c. EKG

i. Normal EKG

ii. T wave flattening

iii. T wave inversion in leads with dominant R waves

d. Normal cardiac markers

## Clinical Tools to Detect Ischemia

1. EKG

a. Most useful

b. Noninvasive

c. Continuous monitor

i. Lead changes and the associated artery and area of damage

(1) V1–V2

(a) Left coronary artery

(i) Left anterior descending artery (LAD) and septal branch

(b) Septum, atrioventricular (AV) bundle, and bundle branches

(c) Complications: infranodal block and bundle branch blocks (BBB)

(2) V3–V4

(a) Left coronary artery

(i) LAD and diagonal branch

(b) Anterior wall of the left ventricle (LV)

(c) Complications: LV dysfunction, congestive heart failure (CHF), BBB, complete heart block, and premature ventricular complex (PVC)

(d) Associated with a poor prognosis and sudden death

(3) V5–V6 plus I and aVL

(a) Left coronary artery

(i) Circumflex branch

(b) High lateral wall LV

(c) Complications: LV dysfunction and AV nodal block

(4) II, III, aVF

(a) Right coronary artery

(i) Posterior descending branch

(b) Inferior wall LV and posterior wall LV

(c) Complications: hypotension and sensitivity to nitroglycerine and morphine sulfate

(5) V4 R

(a) Right coronary artery

(i) Proximal branches

(b) Right ventricle (RV), inferior wall LV, and posterior wall LV

(c) Complications: hypotension, supranodal and AV-nodal blocks, atrial fibrillation/flutter, premature atrial complex (PAC), and adverse medical reactions

(6) V1–V4 (marked depression)

(a) Either left coronary artery (circumflex) or right coronary artery (posterior descending branch)

(b) Posterior wall LV

(c) Complication: LV dysfunction

2. Transesophageal echocardiography (TEE)

a. Most sensitive

i. Reduction of the normal degree of thickening across the ventricular wall during systole (systolic wall thickening): the most sensitive marker of ischemia

b. Most recognizable sign: reduction in movement of the ventricular wall toward the center of the ventricle (endocardial excursion)

c. Wall motion abnormalities: not always specific – e.g., hypovolemic or hypervolemic states

3. Coronary angiogram

4. Coronary computed tomographic angiography – recommended as an alternative to invasive angiography

5. Myocardial perfusion imaging

6. Stress test

7. Pulmonary artery (PA) catheterization

a. Information about systolic dysfunction, diastolic dysfunction, and mitral regurgitation

b. Questionable sensitivity and safety of catheterization

## Initial Management of an Acute Coronary Syndrome

Immediate treatment goal: relieve pain, improve blood flow, and restore heart function

1. Immediate assessment

a. Vital signs

b. Oxygen saturation

c. Obtain intravenous (IV) access.

d. 12-lead EKG

e. Brief targeted history

f. Fibrinolytic checklist
g. Cardiac markers
h. Electrolytes and coagulation studies
i. Portable chest X-ray
j. Assess for the following:

    i. HR ≥100
    ii. Systolic blood pressure (SBP) ≤100 mm Hg
    iii. Pulmonary edema (rales)
    iv. Signs of shock

2. Immediate treatment

a. Oxygen

    i. May limit ischemic myocardial injury, reducing the amount of ST-segment elevation

b. Nitroglycerin

    i. Dilates the coronary arteries and vascular smooth muscle in veins, arteries, and arterioles
    ii. Reduces ischemic pain
      (1) Routes
        (a) Sublingual (SL) tablet: 0.4 mg, may repeat two times every 3–5 minutes
        (b) Sublingual spray: 1 or 2 sprays repeated two times at 3–5 minute intervals
        (c) Intravenous (IV): 12.5–25 µg bolus, 0.5–10 µg/kg/min infusion
      (2) Treatment goals
        (a) Relief of ischemic discomfort
        (b) Limit the blood pressure drop
      (3) Contraindications/cautions
        (a) SBP <90 mm Hg
        (b) Severe bradycardia (HR <50)
        (c) Tachycardia (HR >100)
        (d) RV infarction
        (e) Recent use (within 24–48 hours) of phosphodiesterase inhibitor for erectile dysfunction

c. Aspirin

    i. Inhibits thromboxane $A_2$ platelet aggregation to reduce coronary reocclusion and recurrent events after fibrinolytic therapy
    ii. Effective for unstable angina
    iii. Recommendations
      (1) For all patients with acute coronary syndrome unless they have a true aspirin allergy
        (a) Aspirin allergy: consider clopidogrel.
      (2) 160–325 mg of nonenteric coated aspirin orally: crushed or chewed
        (a) Rectal suppository if the patient has nausea/vomiting or peptic ulcer disease

    iv. Cautions
      (1) Active peptic ulcer disease
      (2) True allergy
      (3) Bleeding disorders
      (4) Severe hepatic disease

d. Morphine

    i. Dilates the arteries and veins
      (1) Redistributes blood volume
      (2) Reduces ventricular preload and afterload
      (3) May reduce pulmonary edema

    ii. The analgesic effects reduce chest pain.
    iii. It decreases oxygen requirements.
    iv. Recommendations
      (1) 2–4 mg IV
      (2) May give an additional dose of 2–8 mg IV at 5–15-minute intervals

    v. Indicated for patients with ischemic pain not relieved by nitroglycerin and acute coronary syndrome without hypotension
    vi. May be useful to redistribute blood volume in patients with pulmonary edema
    vii. Cautions
      (1) Do not use in patients with hypotension or suspected hypovolemia.
      (2) If hypotension develops without pulmonary edema, elevate the patient's legs and give a 250–500 mL bolus of IV normal saline.

# Triage

1. ST-segment elevation or a new left BBB (LBBB)
a. High specificity for an evolving STEMI
b. Treat with β-blockers, clopidogrel, and heparin.
c. Evaluate for reperfusion candidacy if ≤12 hours from the onset of symptoms.
d. During PCI: bivalirudin (0.75 mg/kg IV bolus, followed by 1.75 mg/kg/h for up to 4 h after the procedure), as an alternative to unfractionated heparin plus GP IIb/IIIa inhibitors.
e. Admit to a monitored bed, assess risk status, and consider cardiac catheterization if it has been >12 hours from the onset of symptoms.

    i. Start statin and ACE inhibitor/ARB therapy.

2. ST-segment depression or dynamic T wave inversion
a. Strongly suggestive of ischemia
b. High-risk subset of patients with unstable angina/NSTEMI
c. Start treatment with nitroglycerin, β-blockers, clopidogrel, heparin, and glycoprotein IIb/IIIa receptor inhibitor.
d. Admit to a monitored bed.

e. Assess risk status.

   i. Consider cardiac catheterization.
   ii. Start statin and ACE inhibitor/ARB therapy.

3. Nondiagnostic or normal EKG

   a. If the patient continues to have chest pain

      i. Repeat the EKG.
      ii. Order serial cardiac markers.
      iii. Myocardial imaging/2D echocardiography
      iv. Continue medical observation.

## Fibrinolytic Therapy

1. Goals

   a. Limit infarct size
   b. Preserve LV function
   c. Reduce mortality
   d. Door-to-drug time ≤30 minutes

2. Most effective in the following patients:

   a. ST-segment elevation or a new LBBB
   b. Early presentation
   c. Larger infarction
   d. Younger patients with a lower risk of intracerebral hemorrhage

3. Can be harmful

   a. ST-segment depression
   b. Patients >24 hours after the onset of pain
   c. Presence of high blood pressure (SBP >175 mm Hg) on presentation denotes an increased risk of stroke after fibrinolytic therapy.

4. Absolute contraindications

   a. Any prior intracranial hemorrhage
   b. Known structural cerebral vascular lesion
   c. Known malignant intracranial neoplasm
   d. Ischemic stroke within 3 months (unless it is acute, within 3 hours)
   e. Suspected aortic dissection
   f. Active bleeding
   g. Significant closed head trauma within 3 months

5. Relative contraindications

   a. History of chronic, severe, poorly controlled hypertension
   b. Traumatic or prolonged CPR (>10 minutes)
   c. Recent internal bleeding (2–4 weeks)
   d. Noncompressible vascular puncture
   e. Pregnancy
   f. Active peptic ulcer disease
   g. Current anticoagulant use

## KO Treatment Plan

### Pre-operative

1. Complete history and physical

   a. Functional capacity

2. Cardiac history

   a. Chest pain
   b. Shortness of breath
   c. Peripheral edema

3. ACC/AHA guidelines for the sample case

   a. Intermediate risk surgery
   b. Minor clinical risk secondary to her uncontrolled hypertension

      i. These guidelines require no further cardiac workup unless the patient had symptoms of cardiac ischemia (i.e., chest pain).

4. Pre-operative medications

   a. β-blockade

      i. Clinical evidence shows that patients who are appropriately β-blocked before the surgery have less ischemia than those who are not or who receive only calcium channel blockers; this appears to be related to less tachycardia in β-blocked patients.

   b. Short-acting calcium channel blockers

      i. Patients who are on short-acting calcium channel blockers in the pre-operative period have resulted in worse outcomes after cardiac ischemia.

         (1) Possibly due to the resulting negative inotropic effect
         (2) However, they may be beneficial in preventing stunned myocardium.

   c. Nitrates

      i. There are no good data available for the use of pre-operative nitrate treatment in the prevention of myocardial ischemia.

         (1) Rarely used, except in patients with high risk, such as patients with acute unstable angina requiring noncardiac surgery

### Intra-operative

1. Rapid assessment of which determinants of the myocardial $O_2$ balance have been compromised

   a. Tachycardia (in most instances)
   b. This patient became tachycardic and hypertensive.

2. Improve the patient's hemodynamics.

a. This may require deepening of the patient's anesthesia. Light anesthesia could lead to hypertension, tachycardia, and cardiac ischemia.

3. Evaluate her IV access.
4. 100% oxygen
5. Medications
   a. Nitroglycerin
   b. Morphine
   c. β-blockers
      i. Initially, give short-acting esmolol.
      ii. Decreases HR

6. 12-lead EKG
7. Labs
   a. Cardiac markers
   b. Complete blood count
   c. Electrolytes
   d. Coagulation panel

8. Chest X-ray
9. Inform the surgeon. Cancel or finish the case ASAP.
10. Look for resolution or worsening of the ST-depression.
11. Consult cardiology.
12. If the patient becomes hemodynamically unstable, consider TEE for further cardiac evaluation.
13. This situation may have been prevented with better hemodynamic maintenance during the surgery. According to the ACC/AHA guidelines, the patient did not require any further pre-operative workup.

## Preferred Anesthetic Technique for a High-Cardiac Risk Patient

1. There is no evidence that a specific anesthetic technique is associated with a better cardiac outcome.
2. Regional versus general anesthesia for the at-risk (myocardial ischemia) patients in the noncardiac surgical setting:
   a. Regional anesthesia
      i. Advantages
         (1) Stress response is attenuated or blocked.
            (a) Thoracic epidurals may suppress the stress response to surgery and reduce myocardial oxygen demand better than lumbar epidural anesthesia.
         (2) Vasodilation
            (a) During vascular surgery, the vasodilation can facilitate surgical anastomoses and graft perfusion.
         (3) Decreased risk of deep vein thrombosis

      ii. Disadvantages
         (1) Spontaneous ventilation during lengthy surgery in a compromised patient
         (2) Hypotension and bradycardia from a high sympathectomy

   b. Inhalational anesthetic effects
      i. Common potent volatile anesthetic effects:
         (1) Dose-related decrease in arterial blood pressure
         (2) Decreased oxygen consumption
         (3) Increase in coronary blood flow
         (4) Studies have shown the volatile anesthetics to all be essentially similar in terms of myocardial ischemia and adverse cardiac outcomes, assuming the patients received opioids during the anesthetic.

      ii. Isoflurane
         (1) Maintains cardiac output
         (2) Increase in HR by 10–20% at 1 MAC
         (3) Less negative inotropic effects than halothane, except in the elderly
         (4) Potent peripheral and coronary vasodilator
         (5) No effect on cardiac conduction system
         (6) Theoretical concerns about "coronary steal syndrome"

      iii. Desflurane
         (1) Maintains cardiac output
         (2) Increased HR
            (a) Increase of 10–20% at greater than 1 MAC
            (b) The increase in HR is specifically associated with rapid increases in the inspired concentration.
            (c) The associated tachycardia can be lessened by pretreatment with narcotics or clonidine.
         (3) Rapid increase in inhaled concentration also results in hypertension.
            (a) During induction, a 1.0–1.5 MAC (end-tidal 7.5–10.9%) can lead to sympathetic hyperactivity and myocardial ischemia in patients with CAD.
            (b) Lower concentrations, such as 0.55–0.83 MAC (end-tidal 4–6%) often result in no clinically significant sympathetic stimulation.
            (c) If the sympathetic stimulation is decreased with opioids, propofol, esmolol, or clonidine, then desflurane can be used in patients at risk for myocardial ischemia.

iv. Sevoflurane

    (1) Maintains cardiac output and HR

    (2) Does not increase HR, blood pressure, or plasma norepinephrine concentrations at 1.5–2.7 MAC

    (3) Same cardiac contractility effects as isoflurane and desflurane

    (4) Same incidence of myocardial ischemia in patients with or at high risk for CAD as isoflurane

    (5) No sympathetic stimulation: some prefer it for patients with hypertension and normal left ventricular function.

v. Nitrous oxide

    (1) Increases sympathetic nervous system activity

    (2) Increases vascular resistance at 40% concentration

c. Narcotics

    i. Lack of intrinsic myocardial depression

    ii. Vagotonic effects

    iii. Minor decrease in blood pressure

    iv. Dose–response relationship between plasma levels of opioid and suppression of adrenergic responses is extremely variable, and there is risk of breakthrough hypertension and tachycardia.

d. Benzodiazepines: significant hypotension because of peripheral vasodilation.

## Post-operative

1. If hemodynamically stable:

    a. Resolution of patient's ST-depression

    b. Extubate

        i. Closely monitor the patient and treat any hypertension and tachycardia.

        ii. Be prepared to abort the extubation if the patient develops ST changes.

    c. Maintain hemodynamics.

    d. Send the patient to a cardiac-monitored floor.

    e. Cardiology consult

2. If hemodynamically unstable:

    a. Keep intubated.

    b. Coronary care unit (CCU)

    c. Cardiology consult

# Bibliography

American Heart Association. *American Heart Association 2020 Guidelines for Advanced Cardiovascular Life Support.* Dallas: AHA, 2020.

Barash PG, Cullen BF, Stoelting RK, et al. *Clinical Anesthesia*, 8th ed. Philadelphia: Lippincott Williams & Wilkins, 2017, pp.1661–83.

Butterworth JF, Mackey DC, Wasnick JD. *Morgan & Mikhail's Clinical Anesthesiology*, 6th ed. New York: McGraw-Hill Education, 2018, pp. 395–6.

Circulation. Stabilization of the patient with acute coronary syndromes. *Circulation*, 2005;**112**:IV89–IV110.

Collet J-P, Thiele H, Barbato E, et al. 2020 ESC Guidelines for the management of acute coronary syndromes in patients presenting without persistent ST-segment elevation. *Eur Heart J* 2021;**42** (14):1289–367.

Field JM, American Heart Association. *Advanced Cardiac Life Support Guidelines. Handbook of Emergency Cardiovascular Care for Healthcare Providers.* Dallas: AHA, 2006, pp. 22–42.

Gulati M, Levy P, Mukherejee D, et al. 2021 AHA/ACC/ASE CHEST/SAEM/SCCT/ SCMR guideline for the evaluation and diagnosis of chest pain: a report of the American College of Cardiology/American Heart Association Joint Committee on Clinical Practice Guidelines. *Circulation* 2021;**144**(22):e368–e454.

Kirby RR, Gravenstein N, Lobato E, et al. *Clinical Anesthesia Practice*, 2nd ed. New York: Elsevier, 2002, pp. 810–26.

Reed AP, Yudkowitz FS. *Clinical Cases in Anesthesia*, 3rd ed. New York: Churchill Livingstone, 2005, pp. 11–20.

# Embolism

Cristian M. Prada

## Sample Case

A 73-year-old female underwent a repair of an abdominal aortic aneurysm. She has a history of heavy smoking, severe chronic obstructive pulmonary disease (COPD), hypertension (HTN), diabetes mellitus, and is noncompliant with her insulin treatment. Toward the end of the surgery, the patient was transferred to another anesthesia provider, who took her to the post-anesthesia care unit (PACU) intubated, sedated, and with the arterial line and central venous pressure (CVP) monitors in place. Approximately 15 minutes after the patient's arrival in the PACU, the anesthesiologist was called emergently to see the patient. The patient had become severely hypotensive. After a quick examination, the anesthesiologist noticed that one of the peripheral infusions was placed on an inflated pressure bag and there was no fluid in the bag or in the intravenous (IV) line. What do you think happened? How would you further assess the patient? What is your treatment?

## Venous Thromboembolism

### Clinical Issues

#### Definition of Pulmonary Embolism (PE)

1. A thrombotic embolism that originates in the deep veins of the legs or pelvis and embolizes to the pulmonary artery.
2. Presents as asymptomatic to fulminate cardiovascular collapse depending on the amount of clot and the patient's physiologic reserve.
3. A large clot can obstruct the pulmonary artery (PA), causing right heart strain/failure, severe V/Q mismatch, and release of thromboxane and serotonin, which also increase the PA pressure.
4. Unusual to occur intra-operatively: more frequent in the post-operative period

#### Physiologic Causes of Venous Thromboembolism

1. Venous stasis, vessel wall damage, and hypercoagulability (Virchow's triad)
2. During general anesthesia
   a. Vasodilatory effects of the anesthetic drugs
   b. Immobility of the lower extremities
   c. Hypercoagulability
   d. Stress response to surgery

e. Direct damage to the venous endothelium during surgery

#### Signs and Symptoms of PE

1. Dyspnea
2. Chest pain
3. Cough
4. Blood-tinged sputum
5. Fever
6. Tachycardia
7. Tachypnea
8. Coarse breath sounds
9. Mild hypoxemia
10. New S4 heart sound
11. Accentuation of the pulmonic component of the S2 heart sound
12. Abrupt increase in the gradient between $PaCO_2$ (high) and end-tidal $CO_2$ (low)

#### Diagnosis of PE

1. Gold standard is the pulmonary angiogram
2. Laboratory
   a. Not typically used (including arterial blood gas [ABG]) for diagnosing or ruling out PE
   b. Even patients with a normal $PaO_2$ can still have a PE.
   c. A low $PaO_2/FiO_2$ ratio (less than 200) or D-dimer presence are nonspecific.

3. Imaging studies
   a. Ventilation–perfusion (V/Q) scan for patients with renal failure (avoids the IV contrast used in a pulmonary angiogram)
      i. Algorithm elaborated by PIOPED (Prospective Investigation of Pulmonary Embolism Diagnosis) study, followed by PIOPED-2 funded by the NIH (National Institute of Health)
      ii. First, use clinical signs and symptoms to give the probability of PE (low, medium, high).
      iii. Then, factor the symptoms with the results of the V/Q scan (low to high probability of PE).
   b. Computerized tomography (CT): spiral (helical) CT often replaces the V/Q scans secondary to the speed of

the study and the ability to evaluate other potential embolic sources (i.e., legs, pelvis).

    i. The sensitivities can be up to 90% with a single detector scan.

c. CT pulmonary angiogram (CTPA) combined with CT venography has a higher sensitivity for venous thromboembolism (VTE).

    i. A negative CT angiogram does not rule out a subsegmental PE.

    ii. According to the PIOPED-2 study, the pretest clinical probability of all post-surgical patients is considered to be an intermediate risk at minimum.

    iii. Only patients with a high pretest (clinical) probability and a negative CT scan should undergo compression ultrasonography of the extremities to rule out VTE.

## Diagnosis Pathways

### Excluding PE

1. Clinical probability assessment

    a. Low: normal D-dimer

    b. Moderate:

        i. Negative high-quality CTPA

        ii. Negative V/Q single-photon emission CT (SPECT)

        iii. Normal V/Q

        iv. Negative pulmonary angiogram

        v. Negative CTPA combined with negative lower extremity Doppler ultrasound (LE DUS) or non-high-probability V/Q combined with negative LE DUS

    c. High:

        i. Negative high-quality CTPA

        ii. Negative V/Q SPECT

        iii. Normal V/Q or negative pulmonary angiogram

### Confirming PE

1. Clinical probability assessment

    a. Low:

        i. Positive CTPA

        ii. Positive V/Q SPECT

        iii. High-probability V/Q or positive pulmonary angiogram

    b. Moderate:

        i. Positive CTPA

        ii. Positive V/Q SPECT

        iii. High-probability V/Q

        iv. Positive pulmonary angiogram or nondiagnostic V/Q combined with positive LE DUS

    c. High:

        i. Positive CTPA

        ii. Positive V/Q SPECT

        iii. High probability of V/Q

        iv. Positive pulmonary angiogram

        v. Nondiagnostic V/Q combined with positive LE DUS or positive LE DUS

## Etiology

1. Upper extremity deep venous thrombosis (DVT)

    a. There is a 9% incidence of symptomatic PE arising from the upper extremities.

    b. This type of DVT results from

        i. Central venous catheters

        ii. Patients with cancer

        iii. Paget–Schroetter syndrome

    c. Rarely spontaneous

    d. It presents clinically with swelling, erythema, and arm pain.

2. Pulmonary emboli

    a. There is a 90% incidence of a PE arising from extremities (lower or upper) and 10% from pelvic veins, renal veins, inferior vena cava (IVC), or heart.

3. Surgical procedures related to the risk of VTE

    a. Highest for (in order) total hip arthroplasty, excision/destruction/biopsy of the brain, total knee arthroplasty, abdominal aortic surgery, splenectomy, and coronary artery bypass graft (CABG) surgery.

## Risk Factors for DVT

1. Patient-related

    a. Elderly

    b. Obesity

    c. Bedridden patients

    d. Limb paralysis

    e. Prolonged immobilization (including long-distance travel by plane or car)

    f. Pregnancy

    g. Varicose veins

    h. Congenital venous malformations

    i. Sickle-cell disease

2. Hypercoagulable and inflammatory states

    a. Factor V Leiden deficiency

    b. Activated protein C resistance

    c. Antiphospholipid syndrome

    d. Dyslipoproteinemia

    e. Nephrotic syndrome

    f. Inflammatory bowel disease

    g. Infection

    h. Bechet's syndrome

i. Myeloproliferative diseases

j. Neoplasms

3. Predisposing factors

a. Previous VTE

b. Trauma

c. Respiratory failure

d. Paroxysmal nocturnal hemoglobinuria

e. Superficial vein thrombosis

f. Central venous catheter

g. Vena cava filter

h. Intravenous drug abuse

4. Medications

a. Oral contraceptives

b. Hormone replacement therapy

c. Heparin-induced thrombocytopenia

d. Chemotherapy

e. Tamoxifen

f. Thalidomide

g. Antipsychotics

## KO Treatment Plan

1. Prevent formation of the DVT

a. Low molecular weight heparin (LMWH)

b. Intermittent pneumatic compression (IPC) devices

c. Elastic stockings

d. Regional anesthesia

i. Only surgical anesthesia from an epidural, but not post-operative analgesia from an epidural, lowers the peri-operative risk of VTE.

ii. Evaluate the patient's coagulation status before neuraxial anesthesia.

e. IVC filters

i. DVTs of the proximal (above the knee) lower extremities have a high likelihood of pulmonary embolization.

(1) These patients usually require therapeutic anticoagulation.

(2) If anticoagulation is contraindicated (recent surgery, continued bleeding), consider the insertion of an IVC filter.

ii. Also, prophylactic insertion is recommended in morbidly obese or high-risk trauma patients.

2. Treatment of an acute PE

a. Therapeutic anticoagulation

b. IVC filter

c. Clot thrombolysis with tissue plasminogen activator (TPA) or streptokinase/urokinase

d. Surgical embolectomy

### Preventive Therapy Related to the Risk of Developing DVT

1. Low risk

a. Minor surgery

b. Age <40 years old

c. No risk factors

i. Prevention = early mobilization

2. Moderate risk

a. Minor surgery (patient with risk factors)

b. Age 40–60 years (patient with no risk factors)

c. Major surgery (age <40 years old, no risk factors)

i. Prevention = unfractionated heparin (UFH) every 12 hours, LMWH, or IPC

3. High risk

a. Minor surgery (age >60 years old or with risk factors)

b. Major surgery (age >40 or with risk factors)

i. Prevention = UFH every 8 hours, LMWH, or IPC

4. Highest risk

a. Major surgery (age >40 years old and with major risk factors = prior VTE, malignancy, hip or knee replacement, major trauma, hip fracture surgery, spinal cord injury, or thrombophilia)

i. Prevention = LMWH or adjusted heparin dose

## Venous Air Embolism

### Clinical Issues

#### Definition

1. Occurs when air enters venous circulation through an incised or cannulated vein

2. Frequent IV introduction of small amounts of air during injections or infusions of medications

a. 100 mL air per second can flow into a 14-gauge IV catheter with a 5 cm $H_2O$ pressure gradient.

b. The amount of air needed to cause a problem can be as low as 20 mL and is relative to the rate of air infusion.

#### Surgeries and Procedures at Increased Risk of Venous Air Embolism (VAE)

1. TURP (transurethral resection of prostate) or radical prostatectomy

a. Less in robotic-assisted laparoscopic radical prostatectomies than in radical retropubic ones

2. Sitting craniotomy: 76% risk of VAE

3. Spinal surgery: including laminectomy; scoliosis surgery in children

4. Laparoscopic surgery: carbon dioxide embolism (insufflation directly into a vein)
5. Endoscopic bowel procedures
6. Hip replacement
7. Arthroscopic joint procedures
8. VATS: video-assisted thoracoscopic surgeries
9. Chest trauma
10. Any procedure with human- or pump-delivered infusions (e.g., angiography)

## Physiology of the VAE

1. Slow entrainment of a large volume of air is well tolerated in a dog model.
2. Small amounts of air are well tolerated in healthy patients if the air is isolated to the right heart and pulmonary circulation.
   a. Even a small amount of air, if it goes into the coronary or cerebral circulation, can cause an embolic event.
3. Large amounts of air (>50 mL) entering rapidly can cause increased pulmonary pressures, hypotension, and eventual cardiac collapse.
4. In an awake and spontaneously ventilating patient, an air embolus will present with the following:
   a. Dyspnea
   b. Cyanosis
   c. Arrhythmias
   d. Hypotension
   e. Increased central venous and pulmonary artery pressures
   f. Decreased cardiac output
   g. "Mill wheel" murmur
   h. Cardiac collapse

## Diagnosis

1. Signs of cardiac ischemia
2. Look for signs of increased pulmonary artery pressure (PAP).
3. Hypotension
4. Acute decrease in end-tidal $CO_2$ and increase in $PaCO_2$
   a. Increase in alveolar dead space and decrease of cardiac output, increased PVR
5. Increased $ETN_2$ (end-tidal nitrogen)
6. Precordial (right atrium) Doppler ultrasound: detection of "mill wheel" murmur
7. Air with aspiration of a right atrium multi-orifice catheter
8. TEE: right ventricular dilation or hypokinesis
   a. Sometimes presents as PA hypertension: but this symptom is nonspecific since it is also present in patients with chronic obstructive lung disease.
9. Air embolism is more severe than a carbon dioxide (less dramatic) embolization

## Monitoring for Patients at High Risk for VAE

1. Observation (surgical field)
   a. Noninvasive
   b. Not sensitive
2. $ETCO_2$
   a. Noninvasive
   b. Sensitive
   c. Nonspecific
   d. Widely used
3. Precordial Doppler ultrasound
   a. Sensitive
   b. Easy signal detection
   c. Difficult placement in the prone position, obese patient, or the patient with a chest deformity
   d. Nonquantitative
4. End-tidal nitrogen
   a. Specific
   b. Hypotension lowers sensitivity
5. Multi-orifice right atrial catheter (used only in sitting position craniotomies)
   a. Quantitative
   b. Not good for continuous screening
6. TEE (transesophageal echocardiography)
   a. Sensitive
   b. Expensive
   c. Not widely available
7. Arterial line: in prone or sitting position craniotomies, place the transducer at the level of the circle of Willis.

# Patient Outcome with a VAE

1. The outcome depends on the volume of air that enters the pulmonary circulation and, when present, the amount of air that crosses into the systemic arterial circulation and enters the brain.
2. Large amounts of venous air create an airlock, increase right heart pressures, and may open a patent foramen ovale.
3. Usually resolves if detected and treated early
   a. If this occurs in the operating room, surgery can almost always resume once the patient is stable.
4. Undetected and prolonged VAE results in cardiac arrest.
   a. In that situation: emergently change the patient to supine position and start CPR.
   b. Always have a cart outside the operating room for surgeries in prone position.

## Complications of the VAE

1. Pulmonary
   a. Hypoxemia
   b. Pulmonary hypertension
   c. Pulmonary edema
   d. Hypercarbia
   e. V/Q mismatch

2. Cardiovascular
   a. Hypotension
   b. Arrhythmias
   c. Myocardial ischemia
   d. Right heart failure
   e. Cardiac arrest

3. Central nervous system
   a. Stroke
   b. Brain edema

## Prevention of VAE

1. When cannulating veins, keep vein elevation below the level of the heart.
   a. Position the patient in the Trendelenburg position for the placement of central catheters in the internal jugular or subclavian veins.
   b. Removal of large-bore catheters
      i. Should be done with the patient supine
      ii. Apply compression to the vein.

2. Monitor the stopcock position and IV-line connection to prevent entry of air into lines.
3. Modern IV pumps should have air detection and alarm systems.
4. Patients who are at a high risk for VAE should have precordial Doppler monitoring during the anesthetic.
5. Minimize the elevation of the surgical site from the heart.
6. Keep the patient euvolemic.
7. Avoid medications that increase venous capacitance: nitroglycerin.

## KO Treatment Plan

1. Lower the site of air entry to below the heart.
2. Notify the surgeon.
3. Secure the airway and ensure adequate oxygenation and ventilation.
4. Stop the nitrous oxide and place the patient on 100% $O_2$.
5. Flood the surgical field with saline.
6. Compression of the proximal vein: internal jugular vein in sitting cases
7. Aspiration of right atrial catheter, if present
8. IV saline bolus

9. Support the circulation by starting a vasopressor, if needed.
   a. Inotropic support may help clear the air bubble.

10. Position the patient in the left lateral decubitus position in an attempt to keep the intraventricular air from entering the PA.
    a. Air rises to the nondependent portion of the ventricle.
       i. This may help, but you may not be able to maintain this position because of the need to perform chest compressions.

11. Positive end-expiratory pressure (PEEP) does not decrease the incidence of VAE.

**TKO:** The presented sample case is likely an example of a VAE, due to the injection of air into a venous line under pressure.

1. IV bolus with saline
2. Support the patient's hemodynamics.
3. Aspirate from her CVP catheter.
4. Consider placing her in the left lateral decubitus position if she is stable.
5. If she is hemodynamically unstable:
   a. Patient intubated already: change to 100% $O_2$.
   b. Pressors
   c. Chest compression (CPR)
   d. Advanced cardiac life support (ACLS)

# Fat Venous Embolism/Fat Embolism Syndrome (FES)

## Clinical Issues

### Definition

1. Fat embolism to the venous and pulmonary circulation is common during orthopedic surgeries and in trauma patients.
2. The presence of fat globules that obstruct circulation, usually the result of fractures of a long bone, burns, parturition, or the fatty degeneration of the liver
3. Mechanism
   a. Disruption of the venous system at the surgical or injury site allows fat from the bone marrow or adipose tissue to enter the venous system.
   b. Increased intraosseous pressure (which occurs during the placement of rods or nails in bones) pushes the fat into the venous system.

4. Most commonly occurs in hip replacement, knee replacement, and intramedullary nailing of the diaphysis (bone shaft)
5. The course can vary from benign to fulminate pulmonary failure with cardiovascular collapse.

6. The current theory about the mechanism is that it is not a mechanical obstruction of the pulmonary arterial circulation but rather an immune reaction caused by the breakdown of the embolic fat into free fatty acids causing an inflammatory cascade in the pulmonary and systemic circulation.

   a. There is some degree of fat embolism in up to 90% of all long bone fractures and orthopedic procedures that instrument into bone marrow.

## Fat Embolism Syndrome

1. Described more than 100 years ago
2. Lack of a gold standard for diagnosis
3. FES occurs in 0.5–2.0% of long bone fractures and 10% of multiple long bone fractures or concomitant pelvic fractures.
4. The mortality in FES is 1–20%, with variability depending on the patient's pre-existing comorbid conditions.

### Diagnosis of FES

1. FES is not clinically recognized in most patients because only a few develop the traditional signs and symptoms.
2. Triad
   a. Hypoxemia
   b. Neurological abnormalities: altered mental status
   c. Petechiae: occur 12–72 hours after initial trauma or instrumentation

### Signs and Symptoms of FES

1. Hypoxia-associated tachypnea
2. Dyspnea
3. Central nervous system (CNS) depression, including lethargy, confusion, seizures, focal deficits (in paradoxical fat embolism)
4. Petechial rash: head, neck, torso, and axilla
5. Fever
6. Tachycardia
7. Retinal fat emboli
8. Decreased end-tidal $CO_2$
9. Increased PAP
10. Bronchospasm
11. Hypotension
12. Acute respiratory distress syndrome (ARDS)
13. Disseminated intravascular coagulation (DIC)

### Laboratory Findings of FES

1. Lipiduria
2. Fat in the alveoli: bronchio-alveolar lavage
3. Fat in the blood: aspirate of pulmonary blood or systemic blood
4. Fat in the right ventricle: TEE
5. Ground glass opacity: high-resolution computer tomography

## KO Treatment Plan

1. Early fracture fixation may prevent FES.
2. Therapy: supportive
3. 50% of patients will require intubation and mechanical ventilation secondary to severe hypoxemia.
4. ARDS: "low stretch protocol" to minimize alveoli trauma
   a. Goal: keep the $PaO_2$ >60 mm Hg, without excessive $O_2$ or volutrauma.
   b. Tidal volume less than 6 mL/kg and plateau pressures less than 30 cm $H_2O$
5. The patient will be at an increased risk for anemia and thrombocytopenia, so monitor for DIC.
6. Epinephrine or milrinone can be given to improve right ventricular function.

# Amniotic Fluid Embolism Syndrome (AFES)
## Clinical Issues
### Definition

1. Amniotic fluid (including fetal squamous cells, lanugo hair, and mucin) enters the venous system and eventually the pulmonary circulation. Incidence is 1 in 40,000 deliveries, or 1.7–7.7 per 100,000 deliveries.
2. The pathogenesis is unclear. It is not a mechanical outflow obstruction but is postulated to be secondary to an immune response to the amniotic fluid contents, or an immune reaction triggered by leukotrienes or arachidonic acid within the fluid. Abnormal activation of the maternal proinflammatory mediators occurs in response to fetal tissue exposure.
3. Profound multi-organ failure can occur.
   a. Respiratory failure: intubation and mechanical ventilation
   b. Cardiogenic shock: vasopressors
   c. DIC: 83%
   d. Similar to the systemic inflammatory response syndrome from severe sepsis and anaphylaxis
4. AFES can occur as early as 20 weeks' gestation, but is more likely to occur during labor and delivery or in the 48 hours postpartum.
5. AFES can occur after abortions and amniocentesis.
6. Pulmonary and systemic hypertension can occur during the initial phase of AFES.
   a. Pulmonary hypertension can worsen right ventricular failure and contribute to low cardiac output, which may resolve quickly, only to be followed by hypotension due to left ventricular failure.
7. The incidence in the United States is 1 in 20,000 to 1 in 30,000 deliveries.
8. The mortality is 16–80%, and is a leading cause of perinatal maternal mortality.

a. Survivors have a high morbidity due to cerebral hypoxia.

## Risk Factors for AFES

1. Tumultuous labor
2. Trauma
3. Multiparity
4. Advanced maternal age
5. Cesarean section
6. Increased gestational age
7. Induction of labor
8. Abruption
9. Placenta previa
10. Cervical laceration
11. Uterine rupture

### Signs and Symptoms of AFES

1. Usually presents with an abrupt onset and rapid clinical deterioration
2. Restlessness or confusion leading to decorticate posturing
   a. Altered mental status and seizures
   b. Headache
   c. Nausea and vomiting
3. Cardiovascular
   a. Hypotension and cardiogenic shock
   b. Arrythmia
      i. PEA (25%)
      ii. Bradycardia (20%)
      iii. Asystole
      iv. Ventricular fibrillation
4. Pulmonary
   a. Hypoxia
   b. Bronchospasm
   c. ARDS
   d. Pulmonary edema: capillary leak from embolism, left heart failure, and cardiogenic shock
   e. Increased PAP
   f. Increased end-tidal $CO_2$
5. Consumptive coagulopathy (DIC)
   a. Low fibrinogen
   b. Low platelets
   c. Abnormal PT and PTT
6. Uterine atony

7. Fetal distress and death
8. Fever

### Differential Diagnosis

1. Pulmonary thromboembolism
2. VAE
3. Hemorrhage
4. Anaphylaxis
5. Transfusion reaction
6. Myocardial infarction

### Laboratory Diagnosis

1. Fetal squamous cells in the patient's blood are thought to be pathognomonic for AFES but have been found in women without the syndrome.

## KO Treatment Plan

1. There are no known strategies to prevent AFES.
2. The management is supportive.
3. A high percentage of patients require intubation and mechanical ventilation for hypoxia, secondary to the associated pulmonary edema.
   a. Pulmonary edema tends to clear up more rapidly than in patients with typical ARDS.
4. Severe hemodynamic instability of the patient requires invasive monitoring and vasopressors.
5. Laboratory studies for coagulopathies/DIC are required to determine the need for blood, plasma, or platelet transfusion.
6. Parturients who have not delivered will require immediate delivery of the fetus to prevent further hypoxic damage to the fetus and facilitate cardiopulmonary resuscitation of the mother.
7. Medication treatment to consider:
   a. A-OK is mnemonic for medications that have been proposed to be helpful in the treatment of AFE in case studies.
      i. Atropine (1 mg): vagal response
      ii. Ondansetron (8 mg): serotonin
      iii. Ketorolac (30 mg): thromboxane $A_2$
8. There are a few case reports of using hemofiltration, exchange transfusion, cardiopulmonary bypass, and extracorporeal membrane oxygenation. These are not available in all birthing centers.

## Bibliography

Broaddus VC, Ernst JD, King TE, et al. *Murray and Nadel's Textbook of Respiratory Medicine,* 7th ed. Philadelphia: Elsevier, 2021, pp. 1101–22.

Free Dictionary. Fat embolism. http://medical-dictionary.thefreedictionary.com/fat+embolism (accessed January 3, 2023).

Gropper MA. *Miller's Anesthesia,* 9th ed. Philadelphia: Elsevier, 2020, p. 2035.

Lobato EB, Gravenstein N, Kirby RR. *Complications in Anesthesiology,* 3rd ed.

Philadelphia: Lippincott Williams & Wilkins, 2008, pp. 193–203.

Richard C, Ricome JL, Rimailho A, et al. Fatal pulmonary embolism with a normal PaO2. *Ann Med Interne (Paris)* 1983;**134** (6):559–62.

Talbot M, Schemitsch EH. Fat embolism syndrome: history, definition, epidemiology. *Injury* 2006;**37**(Suppl. 4):S3–S7.

Yao F-SF, Hemmings HC, Malhotra V, et al. *Yao and Artusio's Anesthesiology: Problem-Oriented Patient Management*, 9th ed. Alphen aan den Rijn: Wolters Kluwer, 2021, pp. 401–2, 410, 575–7, 605–6.

**Chapter**

# 30

# Cardiac Tamponade

Cristian M. Prada

## Sample Case

A 65-year-old female, morbidly obese, smoker (one pack per day for 35 years), with a history of hypertension (HTN), coronary artery disease (CAD), and diabetes mellitus treated with insulin, underwent an uneventful coronary artery bypass graft (CABG). The patient was taken, sedated and intubated, to the intensive care unit (ICU), with dopamine at 5 μg/kg/min and insulin 2 IU/h as continuous infusions. After 3 hours in the ICU, the patient suddenly became tachycardic, and her blood pressure decreased dramatically. She had no response to a higher dose of dopamine and norepinephrine infusion. The surgical fellow on call in the ICU performed an emergent needle pericardial aspiration, which removed 100 cc of fresh blood. The patient was taken emergently to the operating room (OR) on a wide-opened epinephrine drip. After a thoracotomy and pericardiocentesis, the patient's hemodynamic status improved significantly. How would you have prepared this patient for surgery? What would be your choice of induction drugs, and why?

## Clinical Issues

### Etiology of Cardiac Tamponade

1. Most often: malignancies and post-cardiocentesis
2. Other
   a. Idiopathic pericarditis
   b. Uremic pericarditis
   c. Hemorrhagic
      i. Post-cardiopulmonary bypass
      ii. Any cardiac surgery
      iii. Dissecting aortic aneurysm
   d. Autoimmune disease
      i. Systemic lupus erythematosus (SLE)
      ii. Collagen vascular disease
      iii. Rheumatoid arthritis (autoimmune disease)
   e. Hypothyroidism
   f. Radiation
   g. Air
   h. Infection: viral or bacterial
   i. Inflammation after myocardial ischemia
   j. Trauma

3. Acute: occurs within minutes, hours, or less than five days post-cardiac surgery.
4. Delayed: occurs 5–7 days post-cardiac surgery.

## Presenting Symptoms of Cardiac Tamponade

1. Chest pain
2. Shortness of breath
3. Tachypnea
4. Tachycardia
5. Enlarged neck veins
6. Syncope
7. Edema
8. Nausea
9. Fever
10. Hypotension

## Physiology

1. Tamponade: fluid in the pericardial sac limits filling of the heart.
   a. Acute setting: small amounts of pericardiac fluid can cause tamponade (100–150 mL).
   b. Chronic setting: as much as 1–2 L of fluid may accumulate before tamponade.

2. Hemodynamic manifestations: mainly due to atrial rather than ventricular compression.
3. Initially, diastolic filling is limited, causing a reduced stroke volume that stimulates sympathetic reflexes resulting in increased heart rate and contractility to maintain the cardiac output.
4. Rising right atrial (RA) pressure stimulates reflex tachycardia and peripheral vasoconstriction.
5. Blood pressure is maintained by vasoconstriction, but cardiac output begins to fall as the pericardial fluid increases.
6. The jugular venous pulse has a small Y-descent but a prominent X-descent because the diastolic filling is decreasing.
7. The pericardial pressure–volume curve approaches vertical because any additional fluid greatly restricts cardiac filling and reduces diastolic compliance.

8. RA pressure, pulmonary artery (PA) diastolic pressure, and pulmonary capillary wedge pressure (PCWP) equilibrate to within 5 mm Hg of each other.

9. A precipitous blood pressure drop leads to reduced coronary artery blood flow and subendocardial ischemia.

## Diagnostic

1. Triad of acute tamponade

   a. Decreasing arterial pressure and tachycardia

   b. Increasing venous pressure (elevated jugular venous pressure)

   c. Small, quiet heart (muted heart sounds); pulsus paradoxus (and pericardial rub when pericarditis)

2. CVP = PAD = PAOP (CVP = central venous pressure; PAD = pulmonary artery diastolic pressure; PAOP = pulmonary artery occlusion pressure)

   a. This is rarely observed in the post-operative CABG patient because the transected pericardium is left open.

3. Pulsus paradoxus

   a. May be seen with cardiac tamponade

   b. Defined as a fall in systolic pressure >12 mm Hg during inspiration

   c. It is caused by a reduced left ventricular (LV) stroke volume produced by increased filling of the right heart during inspiration.

      i. Pulsus paradoxus may also be present with:

         (1) Obstructive pulmonary disease

         (2) Right ventricular (RV) infarction

         (3) Constrictive pericarditis

         (4) Pulmonary embolism

      ii. Pulsus paradoxus is absent with:

         (1) LV dysfunction

         (2) Positive pressure ventilation

         (3) Atrial septal defect (ASD)

         (4) Severe aortic regurgitation

4. The inspiratory venous pressure remains steady or increases (Kussmaul's sign) rather than decreases.

5. The EKG can show the following:

   a. Low-voltage QRS

   b. Electrical alternans

   c. T wave abnormalities

   d. Sinus rhythm

6. Echocardiography is the most reliable noninvasive method for the diagnosis of cardiac tamponade.

   a. Exaggerated motion of the heart within the pericardial sac

   b. Diminished LV dimensions and mitral valve excursions during inspiration

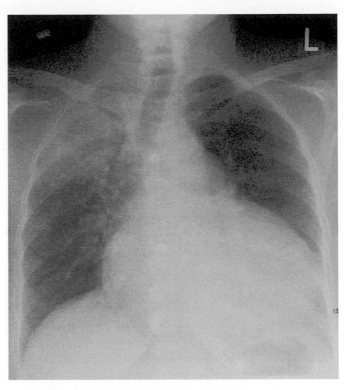

**Figure 30.1** Cardiac tamponade X-ray: pericardial effusion due to malignancy. Source: James Heilman (https://commons.wikimedia.org/wiki/File: Tamponade.PNG).

   c. Shifting of the interventricular septum toward the left ventricle

   d. RA (at end-diastole) and ventricular (in early diastole) collapse

   e. Left atrial collapse: 25% of hemodynamic compromised patients and very specific; less left ventricle collapse: more muscular

   f. Respiratory variations in volumes and flows – pulsus paradoxus

   g. Inferior vena cava (IVC) plethora: dilation and less than 50% IVC diameter reduction during inspiration

   h. Echocardiography can also be used to guide the needle or catheter for aspiration.

7. Chest X-ray (anterior–posterior view; Fig. 30.1)

   a. Normal or extremely enlarged heart, depending on the acuity and chronicity of the tamponade process

   b. A lateral view may also show an enlarged heart.

8. Normal pericardial fluid: 15–25 mL

   a. Tamponade physiology: 150 mL (acute) to 1000 mL (chronic)

9. After cardiac surgery, tamponade due to hemorrhage requires immediate mediastinal exploration.

   a. It is often difficult to diagnose cardiac tamponade after cardiac surgery because the classic signs are often missing.

b. If the patient has a persistently poor cardiac output with increased and equalized RA and LA pressures, strongly consider the possibility of cardiac tamponade.

c. An echocardiogram should be performed whenever a patient is not progressing as expected in the post-operative period and has signs of end-organ dysfunction (decrease in urine output, increased blood urea nitrogen [BUN] and creatinine).

## KO Treatment Plan

TKO: Emergency treatment

1. Pericardiocentesis: quick removal of the pericardial fluid from the pericardial sac that surrounds the myocardium using a needle or long, thin tube (catheter)

    a. Technique

        i. Blind (in emergent situations)
        ii. Using transthoracic echocardiography or fluoroscopy
        iii. Bedside, catheterization lab, or OR

    b. Relative contraindications of pericardiocentesis:

        i. Severe pulmonary hypertension
        ii. Bleeding diathesis (low platelets)/uncorrected coagulopathy
        iii. Avoid the subcostal approach if there is a risk of fatal liver injury.

    c. Indication for pericardiocentesis

        i. Blunt or penetrating trauma injury causing accumulation of blood in the pericardial sac with hemodynamic instability or cardiac arrest
        ii. Acute or chronic pericardial effusion without evidence of tamponade to aid in diagnosis of the effusion
        iii. Palliation of symptoms: dyspnea, edema, or prevention of effusion progressing to an emergent situation
        iv. Cardiac tamponade

2. Pericardial window, surgical pericardiectomy, or thoracotomy

3. Supportive therapy

    a. Antibiotics
    b. Serial monitoring of echocardiograms
    c. Treatment of pain
    d. Anti-inflammatory medication
    e. Blood transfusion

## Pre-operative Preparation

1. Complete history, physical examination, and labs
2. Key areas of concern identified and addressed

    a. Respiratory distress: give supplemental $O_2$, review the chest X-ray, and order blood gas labs.

    b. Positive pressure ventilation: avoid (can further impair cardiac filling) unless the clinical picture suggests that the patient will develop cardiac arrest.

    c. Oliguria: reflects prerenal or renal (acute tubular necrosis) processes secondary to decreased cardiac output and vasoconstriction.

        i. Optimize hemodynamics – dobutamine preferred agent
        ii. Do not give diuretics.
        iii. The most effective treatment is pericardiocentesis.

    d. Elevated prothrombin time (PT) and partial thromboplastin time (PTT)

        i. Treat the coagulopathy.
        ii. Check a complete blood count (CBC).
        iii. Have 4–6 units of packed red blood cells (PRBCs) in the OR before starting surgery.

    e. Premedication

        i. Do not give an anxiolytic.
        ii. The most effective and safest technique in this situation to decrease the patient's anxiety is to communicate with the patient.

    f. Sympathoadrenal activation is supporting perfusion of vital organs through selective vasoconstriction and tachycardia.

        i. Do not give any medications to decrease the patient's tachycardia pre-operatively.

3. Communication with the surgical team is very important so that you will be able to follow the surgeon's findings in the operating field and be ready to treat the dramatic hypotension that usually occurs upon opening of the pericardium.

## Intra-operative

1. Transport the patient to the OR.

    a. Monitors

        i. Standard ASA monitors
        ii. Pre-induction arterial line

    b. Oxygen by face mask

        i. Increase the $FiO_2$ as needed.

    c. Have all equipment for intubation immediately available.
    d. Have a cardioversion unit available.
    e. Have all emergency drugs available, including:

        i. Phenylephrine (0.1–0.5 mg boluses, 25–125 µg/min infusion)
        ii. Epinephrine (0.01–0.1 µg/kg/min)
        iii. Calcium chloride (2–4 mg/kg)

iv. Lidocaine (1–2 mg/kg)

v. Atropine (0.01 mg/kg)

2. Anesthetic medications

a. Ketamine: first choice for induction agent in pericardial tamponade

   i. Induction dose: 1 mg/kg IV

   ii. Rapid onset

   iii. Peak plasma concentration is achieved in less than 1 minute.

   iv. The patient's unconsciousness will last for 10–15 minutes, but the analgesic effect (somatic > visceral) will last for an additional 30 minutes or longer.

   v. Effects: small increases in blood pressure, heart rate, cardiac output, and myocardial oxygen demand

   vi. Direct central sympathetic stimulation and inhibition of norepinephrine uptake into the sympathetic nerve endings

   vii. Intrinsic myocardial depressant

b. Etomidate: second choice for induction agent in pericardial tamponade

   i. Preferred when cardiovascular collapse is anticipated

   ii. Induction dose: 0.2–0.3 mg/kg IV

   iii. No myocardial depression

   iv. Limiting factors: pain at the injection site, involuntary muscle movements, reduction of the seizure threshold, and enhanced duration of the seizure limit its use.

c. Propofol: not indicated for induction in pericardial tamponade

   i. May cause up to a 30% reduction in systemic blood pressure or even cardiovascular arrest

   ii. Antiarrhythmic effect on the atrioventricular (AV) node

     (1) Therefore, use with caution in combination with calcium channel blockers, β-blockers, or digoxin.

d. Fentanyl

   i. Not a depressant on myocardial contractility

   ii. Causes a vagotonic decrease in heart rate and mild sympatholytic (central outflow) effects. The resulting decrease in blood pressure may be more profound in shock or pre-shock and when in combination with benzodiazepines, or propofol.

   iii. Give with caution.

e. Midazolam: do not give to the patient pre-operatively.

   i. Mild to moderate systemic vasodilation, especially when used in combination with narcotics

3. Induction

a. Standard ASA monitors and arterial line

b. Surgical team ready (gowned), with the patient sterilely prepared and draped

c. Induction with IV ketamine or etomidate and a muscle relaxant (depolarizing or nondepolarizing)

   i. Keep the patient breathing spontaneously prior to induction.

d. Be prepared to treat circulatory collapse.

e. Management of hypotension

   i. Vasoactive drugs

   ii. Cardioactive drugs

   iii. Fluid challenge

   iv. Reduce inspiratory positive pressure (decrease tidal volume or change to hand-ventilation) to facilitate cardiac filling.

   v. Surgical relief of the tamponade is the definitive treatment.

f. Hemodynamic changes upon chest opening

   i. Normalizes the pressure relationship between the pericardium and the heart chambers

   ii. Relieves the tamponade and its hemodynamic effects

   iii. Dramatic improvements in blood pressure and stroke volume, unless the myocardium is injured or stunned

   iv. The patient can usually wean quickly from most vasoactive and cardioactive drugs.

   v. Expect to see improvements in the oxygenation, acid–base status, and urine output.

## Complications

1. Myocardial injury
2. Hemorrhage into the pericardium
3. Pneumothorax
4. Great vessel injury
5. Liver injury
6. Abdominal viscera injury
7. Arrhythmia
8. Infection

## Post-operative

1. Extubation criteria

a. Clinically stable with no significant inotropic or vasoactive support

b. Neurologically intact: the patient is alert and follows simple commands.

c. Adequate pulmonary function: acceptable acid–base status and weaning parameters should be fulfilled (tidal volume, respiratory rate, vital capacity, inspiratory effort)

---

d. Normal body temperature
e. Intact neuromuscular function (reverse paralysis if needed)
f. Normal coagulation factor studies

2. Hypertension in the ICU after the surgical treatment of cardiac tamponade
   a. Primary: exclude hypoxia, hypercarbia, acid–base derangements, and pain.
   b. First few hours in the ICU: hypertension
      i. Uncertain etiology
      ii. Possible sympathoadrenal activation including pain, vasoconstriction, or local stress mediators
   c. Treat with:
      i. IV sodium nitroprusside
      ii. β-blockers (labetalol, metoprolol, atenolol, esmolol, or propranolol): theoretical concerns of myocardial depression and bradycardia are not justified in practice.

# Bibliography

Abdullah RS. Restoration of circulation after cessation of positive pressure ventilation in a case of "Lazarus Syndrome." *Anesth Analg* 2001;**93**:241.

American Heart Association. *American Heart Association 2020 Guidelines for Advanced Cardiovascular Life Support.* Dallas: American Heart Association, 2020.

Ben-David B, Stonebraker VC, Hershman R, et al. Survival after failed intraoperative resuscitation: a case of "Lazarus Syndrome." *Anesth Analg* 2001;**92**:690–2.

Gropper MA. *Miller's Anesthesia,* 9th ed. Philadelphia: Elsevier, 2020, pp. 2713–42.

Hoit BD. Cardiac tamponade. In Yeon SB, ed., *UpToDate.* www.uptodate.com/contents/cardiac-tamponade (accessed January 3, 2023).

Kaplan JA, Augoustides JGT, Manecke JR, et al. *Kaplan's Cardiac Anesthesia,* 7th ed. Philadelphia: Elsevier, 2017, pp. 945–8.

Wilner DA, Grossman SA. Pericardiocentesis. In: *StatPearls.* Treasure Island: StatPearls Publishing, 2022.

Yao FSF, Hemmings Jr HC, Malhotra V, Fong J. *Yao & Artusio's Anesthesiology: Problem-Oriented Patient Management,* 9th ed. Alphen aan den Rijn: Wolters Kluwer, 2021, pp. 279–302.

# Chapter 31

# Current ACC/AHA Guidelines for Peri-operative Cardiac Evaluation for a Noncardiac Surgery

Saima Karim and Jessica A. Lovich-Sapola

## Sample Case

A 46-year-old male presents for gastric bypass surgery. He weighs 160 kg. He has obstructive sleep apnea and a functional capacity of less than 4 METs. He denies chest pain. He reports shortness of breath with walking, even a short distance. What further tests would you like to order? Does he need further cardiac workup? EKG? Cardiac stress test?

## Clinical Issues

### Risk Predictors

1. Clinical risk factors (patient-specific risk factors)

   a. Revised Cardiac Risk Index (RCRI)

      i. Unstable coronary artery disease; ischemic heart disease

         (1) History of myocardial infarction (MI)
         (2) History of a positive treadmill test
         (3) Use of nitroglycerine
         (4) Current complaints of chest pain are thought to be secondary to coronary ischemia.
         (5) EKG with abnormal Q waves or concerning ST changes

      ii. History of congestive heart failure (CHF)

         (1) Pulmonary edema
         (2) Paroxysmal nocturnal dyspnea
         (3) Peripheral edema
         (4) Bilateral rales
         (5) S3 heart sound
         (6) Chest radiograph with pulmonary vascular redistribution

      iii. Cerebrovascular disease

         (1) History of transient ischemic attack (TIA)
         (2) History of stroke

      iv. Diabetes mellitus (on insulin)
      v. Chronic renal failure (CR >2.0 mg/dL)

## Cardiac Risk Stratification for Noncardiac Surgical Procedures

1. Vascular (high risk): reported cardiac risk is often more than 5%.

   a. Aortic and other major vascular surgery
   b. Emergency surgery
   c. Anticipated long procedures with associated fluid shifts and large estimated blood loss

2. Intermediate-risk surgery: reported cardiac risk is generally 1–5%.

   a. Intraperitoneal and intrathoracic surgery
   b. Carotid endarterectomy
   c. Head and neck surgery
   d. Orthopedic surgery
   e. Prostate surgery

3. Low-risk surgery: reported cardiac risk is generally less than 1%.

   a. Endoscopic procedures
   b. Superficial procedures
   c. Cataract surgery
   d. Breast surgery
   e. Ambulatory surgery

## Peri-operative Risk Based on Combined Clinical and Surgical Risk

1. RCRI ≥2

   a. Surgical risk ≥1% (intermediate- or high-risk surgery)

      i. METs ≥4: no further testing
      ii. METs <4: pharmacologic stress test if it will impact patient care

2. Acute coronary syndrome

   a. Evaluate and treat

3. Low-risk surgery (<1% risk)

   a. Requires no further testing

## Application of Recommendations

1.  Class I: benefit ≫ risk. Procedure/treatment should be performed/administered.
2.  Class IIa: benefit ≫ risk. Additional studies with focused objectives are needed. It is reasonable to perform/ administer treatment.
3.  Class IIb: benefit ≥ risk. Additional studies with broad objectives are needed. The procedure/treatment may be considered.
4.  Class III: benefit ≤ risk. No additional studies are needed. Procedure/treatment should not be performed/ administered since it is not helpful and may be harmful.

# Recommendations

## Recommendations of Pre-operative Resting 12-Lead ECG

1.  Class IIa:
    a.  Persons with known coronary artery disease, significant arrythmia, peripheral arterial disease, cerebrovascular disease, or other structural heart disease, except those undergoing low-risk surgery
    b.  EKG is recommended for all patients undergoing high- and intermediate-risk surgery if they have the following:
        i.  Known coronary artery disease
        ii.  Significant arrythmia
        iii.  Peripheral arterial disease
        iv.  Cerebrovascular disease
        v.  Structural heart disease
    c.  Low-risk surgery: do not require an EKG independent of age or medical history unless they have a recent change in medical condition (i.e., chest pain or acute shortness of breath).
2.  Class IIb:
    a.  Asymptomatic patients without known coronary artery disease, except those undergoing low-risk surgery
3.  Class III: no benefit
    a.  Not indicated in asymptomatic persons undergoing low-risk surgical procedures

## Recommendation for Noninvasive Exercise Stress Testing Before Noncardiac Surgery

1.  Class IIa:
    a.  For patients with elevated risk and excellent functional capacity (>10 METs), forgo further exercise testing and proceed to surgery.

2.  Class IIb:
    a.  Elevated risk and unknown functional capacity, perform exercise testing to assess for functional capacity if it will change management.
    b.  Elevated risk and moderate to good functional capacity (≥4–10 METs), forgo further cardiac testing and proceed to surgery.
    c.  Elevated risk and poor functional capacity (<4 METs), perform exercise testing with cardiac imaging to check for myocardial ischemia if it will change management.
3.  Class III:
    a.  Not useful for patients undergoing low-risk noncardiac surgery

## Recommendation for Pharmacologic Stress Testing before Noncardiac Surgery

1.  Class IIa:
    a.  Elevated risk for noncardiac surgery and poor functional capacity (<4 METs) to undergo noninvasive pharmacologic stress testing if it will change management
2.  Class III: no benefit
    a.  Not useful in patients undergoing low-risk noncardiac surgery

## Pre-operative Coronary Angiography

1.  Class III
    a.  Routine pre-operative coronary angiography is not recommended.

## Recommendations for Pre-operative Coronary Revascularization with Coronary Artery Bypass Grafting (CABG) or Percutaneous Coronary Intervention (PCI)

1.  Class I:
    a.  Recommended in circumstances in which revascularization is indicated
2.  Class III:
    a.  Not recommended that routine coronary artery revascularization be performed before noncardiac surgery exclusively to reduce peri-operative cardiac events

## Timing of Elective Noncardiac Surgery in Patients with Previous PCI

1.  Class I:

a. Elective noncardiac surgery should be delayed 14 days after balloon angioplasty and 30 days after bare metal stent (BMS) implantation.

b. Elective noncardiac surgery should be delayed 365 days after drug eluting stent (DES) implantation.

2. Class IIa:

a. In patients for whom noncardiac surgery is required, there should be a consensus among the treating physicians as to the relative risks of surgery and discontinuation or continuation of antiplatelet therapy.

3. Class IIb:

a. Elective noncardiac surgery may be considered after DES implantation after 180 days if the risk of further delay is greater than the expected risk of ischemia and stent thrombosis.

4. Class III: Harm

a. Elective noncardiac surgery should not be performed within 30 days after BMS or within 12 months after DES in patients for whom dual antiplatelet therapy will need to be discontinued peri-operatively.

b. Elective noncardiac surgery should not be performed within 14 days of balloon angioplasty in patients for whom aspirin therapy will need to be discontinued peri-operatively.

# Recommendations for β-Blocker Medical Therapy

1. Class I:

a. Continued in patients undergoing surgery who are already receiving β-blockers chronically

2. Class IIa:

a. It is reasonable for β-blockers after surgery to be guided by clinical circumstances, independent of when the agent was started.

3. Class IIb:

a. If intermediate- or high-risk myocardial ischemia is noted in the pre-operative risk stratification tests, it may be reasonable to begin peri-operative β-blockers.

b. With patients having three or more RCRI risk factors, it may be reasonable to begin β-blockers before surgery.

c. Compelling long-term indication for β-blocker therapy but no other RCRI risk factors: initiating β-blockers in the peri-operative setting as an approach to reduce peri-operative risk is of uncertain benefit.

d. For patients in whom β-blocker therapy has been initiated, it may be reasonable to begin peri-operative β-blocker therapy long enough in advance to assess safety and tolerability more than 1 day before surgery.

4. Class III:

a. Should not be given to patients undergoing surgery who have an absolute contraindication to β-blockade.

b. Should not be started on the day of surgery.

# Recommendations for Statin Therapy

1. Class I:

a. Continue if currently taking statins.

2. Class IIa:

a. Statin use is reasonable for patients undergoing vascular surgery with or without clinical risk factors.

3. Class IIb:

a. May be considered in patients with clinical indications who are undergoing elevated-risk procedures

# Recommendations for Angiotensin-Converting Enzyme Inhibitors (ACEI)

1. Class IIa

a. Continuing ACEIs peri-operatively is reasonable.

b. If ACEI is held, restart as soon as clinically possible post-operatively.

# Recommendations for Management of Implantable Cardioverter-Defibrillators (ICDs)

1. Class I

a. Patients with ICDs who have pre-operative reprogramming to inactivate tachytherapy should be on continuous cardiac monitoring during the entire time it is inactivated.

b. External defibrillation equipment should be immediately available.

c. Reprogram the ICD before leaving the peri-operative area.

2. Generic guidelines

a. Pacemaker: must be interrogated within 12 months of the surgery, with a report in the medical records.

b. ICD: must be interrogated within 6 months of the surgery, with a report in the medical records.

# Recommendations for Use of Pulmonary Artery (PA) Catheters

1. Class IIb:

a. Pre-operative admission to the ICU for PA catheter monitoring is rarely required and should be restricted to a very small number of highly selected patients whose presentation is unstable and who have multiple comorbid conditions.

i. When the underlying medical condition significantly affects hemodynamics (heart failure, severe valvular disease, combined shock states) and cannot be corrected before surgery

2. Class III:

   a. Routine use of a PA catheter in patients, even those with elevated risk, is not recommended.

## Recommendation for Use of Transesophageal Echocardiography (TEE)

1. Class IIa:

   a. Emergency use of TEE is reasonable in patients with hemodynamic instability undergoing noncardiac surgery to determine the cause of the instability when it persists despite corrective therapy.

2. Class III: no benefit

   a. Routine use of TEE to screen for cardiac abnormalities or monitor myocardial ischemia is not recommended in patients without risk factors or procedural risks for significant hemodynamic, pulmonary, or neurological compromise.

## Recommendation for Maintenance of Body Temperature

1. Class IIb:

   a. Maintenance of normothermia is recommended for most procedures other than during periods in which mild hypothermia is intended to provide organ protection (e.g., during high aortic cross-clamping).
   b. Normothermia may be reasonable to reduce peri-operative cardiac events.

## Recommendations for Surveillance for Peri-operative MI

1. Class I

   a. Post-operative serum troponin measurement is recommended in patients with EKG changes or chest pain typical of acute coronary syndrome (signs or symptoms suggestive of myocardial ischemia).
   b. Obtaining an EKG is recommended in setting or signs of myocardial ischemia or arrythmia.

2. Class IIb

   a. Usefulness of post-operative screening with troponin levels in patients at high risk for peri-operative myocardial ischemia but without signs of ischemia is uncertain.
   b. Usefulness of post-operative EKG in patients at high risk but without symptoms is uncertain.

3. Class III

   a. Routine post-operative screening with troponin levels without signs or symptoms of ischemia is not useful for guiding peri-operative management.

## KO Treatment Plan

### Pre-operative

1. Assuming the patient has no diabetes or diagnosed cardiovascular risk, he does not require any further cardiac workup.
2. The patient has no RCRI clinical predictors and is having an intermediate-risk surgery.
3. According to the ACC/AHA guidelines, he can proceed to the operating room.
4. No further cardiac testing is required.

**TKO:** Remember that you can always order any test that you want within reason; you just have to be able to explain why you are ordering it and be prepared to respond to the results.

## Bibliography

Fleisher LA, Fleischmann KE, Auerbach AD, et al. 2014 ACC/AHA guideline on perioperative cardiovascular evaluation and management of patients undergoing noncardiac surgery. *Circulation* 2014;**130**: e278–e333.

# Pacemaker/Implantable Cardioverter-Defibrillators (ICDs): Considerations for Anesthesiologists

Donald M. Voltz and Jessica A. Lovich-Sapola

## Sample Case

A 71-year-old man presents for a right hemicolectomy after a suspicious polyp was found during a routine colonoscopy. He has a past medical history of hypertension and sick-sinus syndrome for which he had a pacemaker placed 8 years ago. He is currently active, has no known drug allergies, and has been NPO for 16 hours except for a bowel prep. He last saw his cardiologist 1 year ago and was without any limitations according to the patient. What are your concerns? Does this patient need to be seen by his cardiologist prior to his surgery? What do you need to know about his pacemaker? Will the pacemaker affect your anesthetic?

## Clinical Issues

### Incidence of Pacemakers and ICDs

1. There are roughly 200,000 pacemakers and 60,000 ICDs implanted each year.
2. With recent recalls on some of the leads and/or devices, the number of devices needing to be replaced also adds to these figures.

### Indications for Pacemaker/ICD Placement

1. Pacemaker
   a. Sinus node dysfunction
      i. Symptomatic bradycardia
      ii. Syncopal episodes
      iii. Sick-sinus syndrome
   b. Atrioventricular (AV) node dysfunction
      i. Third-degree or high-grade second-degree AV block
   c. Bi-fascicular block
   d. Second- or third-degree AV block after an ST elevation myocardial infarction
   e. Hypersensitive carotid sinus syndrome and neurocardiogenic syncope
   f. Cardiac transplantation patients that develop persistent bradycardia
   g. Other conditions
      i. Neuromuscular disease
      ii. Cardiac sarcoidosis
      iii. Central obstructive sleep apnea
   h. Prevention and termination of supraventricular tachycardia
   i. Hemodynamic indications
      i. Cardiac resynchronization therapy
      ii. Hypertrophic cardiomyopathy with sinus node or AV node dysfunction
   j. Congenital heart disease
2. ICDs
   a. Secondary prevention of sudden cardiac death in patients with a previous VT/VF cardiac arrest
   b. Primary prevention of a sudden cardiac death

## Pacemaker Nomenclature

The North American Society for Pacing and Electrophysiology (NASPE) and the British Pacing and Electrophysiology Group (BPEG) devised a standardized nomenclature for all implantable pacemakers and defibrillators. This nomenclature consists of a five-letter code to describe the functionality of these devices. This standardized code was last updated in 2002.

### Position 1: Chamber Being Paced

O – No chamber paced

A – Atria

V – Ventricle

D – Dual – atria and ventricle

### Position 2: Chamber Being Sensed

O – No chamber sensed

A – Atria

V – Ventricle

D – Dual – atria and ventricle

### Position 3: Response of Device to a Sensed Event

O – No response to sensed event

T – Trigger device when event sensed

I – Inhibit device when event sensed

D – Dual – triggered and inhibited

### Position 4: Programmability and Rate Modulation

O – No programmability

R – Rate modulation activated

### Position 5: Multi-site Pacing

O – No chamber paced

A – Atria

V – Ventricle

D – Dual – atria and ventricle

## How Magnets Affect Pacemakers and ICDs

1. Most of the pacemakers that have been developed and are clinically in use contain an electronic component (Reed switch) which is affected by the application of a magnetic field to the device.
2. When the Reed switch comes in contact with a magnetic field, it can either close a circuit or disrupt electrical flow.
3. In many pacemakers, placement of a magnet over the generator will result in the pacemaker being converted to a continuous asynchronous mode.
   a. This is not the case for all pacemakers.
   b. Those in anesthesiology sometimes get the sense that the addition of a Reed switch was placed for anesthesiologists to quickly set a pacemaker to an asynchronous mode and prevent interference from electrocautery.
   c. Magnets were not initially intended to change pacemaker modes in the operating room, but instead were incorporated to test certain functions of these devices, such as battery life.
   d. Not all pacemakers are switched to an asynchronous mode with the application of a magnet and some pacemakers may not revert back to their baseline settings once the magnet is removed.
4. Some pacemakers will be completely deactivated with the placement of a magnet.
5. In order to be clear about what will happen with the placement of a magnet, one needs to ascertain the brand and model of the implanted device.
6. This can sometimes be uncovered with a chest X-ray; however, most need to be interrogated by specialized devices typically found in the cardiology department.
7. ICDs and pacemakers respond differently to the placement of a magnet.
   a. The algorithms for detection of fatal ventricular arrhythmias lead these devices to respond to electromagnetic interference differently from standard pacemakers.
   b. In light of this, ICDs need to be deactivated prior to surgical procedures where electrocautery or other electromagnetic interference may occur.

c. Deactivating the device renders these patients without protection from ventricular arrhythmias, so one will need to be prepared to apply external cardiac defibrillation should a life-threatening arrhythmia develop when the patient is in the operating room.
d. Many ICDs also contain protection against bradycardia, thereby functioning as pacemakers in addition to their antiarrhythmic functionality.
e. Inactivation or disabling an implantable device:
   i. Not straightforward
   ii. Demands vigilance and investigation prior to proceeding to the operating room

f. Application of a magnet to an ICD will most commonly disable the defibrillation option. This is not an absolute, however, since different models exist with a wide variety of default configurations in the presence of a magnet. Another important point to realize is that combined pacemakers and ICDs do not uniformly respond to the application of a magnet. Many of the current pacemakers revert to an asynchronous state when a magnet is placed over the device. Combined ICD-pacemakers do not all revert to an asynchronous pacing mode in the presence of a magnetic field.

**TKO:** Due to inconsistencies between the many pacemakers and ICD devices on the market, it is advisable to interrogate each device to know what a patient's underlying rhythm is, what the device defaults to in the presence of a magnet, and the state of the device (battery charge, lead integrity, overall device health). Following a case, the device should be re-interrogated to determine whether any changes are required to restore it to its pre-operative status.

## Electromagnetic Interference Problems with Implanted Devices

1. Inhibition of the pacemaker
2. Inappropriate delivery of anti-tachycardia therapy by the ICD
3. Changes in lead parameters
4. Runaway pacemaker
5. Pacemaker failure
6. Conversion from VOO back to backup mode (reprogramming)
7. Loss of capture
8. Dislodgement of leads
9. Rate-adaptive pacing
10. Oversensing and inhibition with lithotripsy
11. Noise reversal mode
12. Myocardial burns

# Pre-operative Evaluation of Pacemakers and ICDs

1. Retrospective investigation into the failure rates of implantable pacemakers and ICDs showed an outright failure in 1.4 pacemakers and 36.4 ICDs per 1000 implants.
2. In light of this failure rate, the large variation in how the devices respond to electromagnetic interference, and often unclear reason for device placement, it is important to investigate these devices prior to elective and semi-emergent surgical procedures.
3. Depending upon how long the device has been in place as well as the number and types of leads that have been placed, a pre-operative chest X-ray might help to determine which vessels contain the pacemaker/ICD leads.
4. If a central line is planned for a given procedure, understanding the path of the leads might influence which vessel is cannulated, since lead disruption or central line entanglement has been reported.
5. All implantable devices should be interrogated by someone who is competent to interrogate these devices and make peri-operative setting changes for the safety of the patient.
   a. Pacemaker should have been interrogated within 12 months
   b. ICDs should have been interrogated within 6 months
6. A copy of the interrogation and settings should be kept with the patient's chart so any changes can be undone after the procedure is completed.
7. The interrogation will provide valuable information about the device.
   a. Remaining battery life
   b. Integrity of the leads
   c. Patient's underlying cardiac rhythm
   d. Current settings and recent discharges of the device (ICDs)
8. Understanding the patient's underlying rhythm is important.
   a. Determines the mode and rate at which to set the backup pacing
   b. Gives an understanding of what the device will default to when a magnet is placed over the generator
9. Some pacemakers have modes that respond to minute ventilation in order to increase the pacing rate with exercise.
   a. During a surgical procedure, this minute ventilation rate responsiveness and other programmed rate responsive functions should be disabled.
10. Any anti-tachycardic functionality should be disabled since electrocautery interference with the device can lead to inappropriate discharge.

## TKO: Risk Mitigation Strategies

1. Use bipolar when possible.
2. Use short bursts of monopolar cautery: 5 seconds or less.
3. Place the return current pad in such a way as to avoid crossing the generator.
4. Have rescue equipment.
5. Avoid activating the electrocautery in the area of the generator.

# Peri-operative Pacemaker Settings

1. Intrinsic pacemaker functions are often disrupted by the electromagnetic interference that occurs during surgery.
   a. Pacemakers need to be reprogrammed prior to the procedure if the device is within 15 cm of the planned surgical field.
   b. The patient's baseline settings should be restored following the conclusion of the procedure.
2. Reprogramming a pacemaker to an asynchronous mode at a rate greater than the patient's underlying basal rate ensures that over- and under-sensing by the device does not occur.
   a. An asynchronous mode is not completely protective and can result in a malignant arrhythmia.
      i. Most patients who undergo pacemaker placement have coexisting disease of the myocardium.
      ii. This places them at a higher risk for arrhythmias.
3. In a device that contains anti-tachycardia protection (ICDs), this feature should be turned off.
   a. One needs to be prepared for external cardiac defibrillation in the event of a malignant ventricular arrhythmia occurring while the device is inactive.
   b. External defibrillation pads or external paddles should be available.

# Peri-operative Pacemaker Failure

1. Pacemakers are mechanical devices with the potential to fail at any time. Pacemaker failure can result from the following:
   a. Inability to capture
   b. Lead disruption
   c. Generator failure
      i. Peri-operative lead or generator failure occurs at a much lower level than failure to capture.
      ii. Proper pre-operative interrogation should confirm the integrity of the device and leads.
2. Pacemaker wires are placed so that contact between the wire and the myocardium occurs.
   a. Over time, the pacemaker lead often becomes densely adherent to the myocardium due to a fibrotic reaction between the leads and the myocardium.

3. Certain situations that occur in the operating room can inhibit the conduction of an electrical impulse from the pacemaker generator to the myocardium and therefore impede conduction and capture of the signal resulting in a failure to capture.

    a. Ischemia
    b. Acidosis
    c. Antiarrhythmic medications
    d. Electrolyte disturbances

4. In the event of a noncapturing pacemaker in a patient who is dependent on the device for cardiac function, emergency external pacing might be required.

## Post-operative Pacemaker Management

1. Any changes that were made to a pacemaker or ICD prior to surgery should be restored to the patient's baseline settings to ensure the best outcome for the patient.
2. Many of these devices are adjusted on an individual basis to ensure device longevity as well as to optimize a patient's cardiac function.
3. Leaving them in a peri-operative default setting can:

    a. Greatly impact the patient's performance.
    b. Increase the drain on the battery leading to a more rapid deterioration of the device and necessitate a replacement.

4. If an ICD has been deactivated, this should be restored as quickly as possible following the procedure.

    a. Until ICD function has been restored, an external pacer/defibrillator should be immediately available.

5. Most pacemaker manufacturers recommend a complete re-interrogation of the devices following surgery to ensure that:

    a. Electrocautery did not inflict any damage to the device.
    b. Electrocautery did not prematurely drain the battery.

## KO Treatment Plan

### Pre-operative

1. This patient has had a pacemaker for a number of years and his underlying rate, rhythm, and dependence on the device are unclear.
2. The patient may or may not know if he also has ICD functionality in the device.
3. If there is no record of recent interrogation, the device should be studied prior to proceeding with surgery.
4. Assuming the device and leads are intact and adequate battery life remains, we can safely proceed with the procedure after the device is reprogrammed.
5. If on interrogation it was discovered that the pacemaker battery did not have sufficient charge, the leads had an unsafe level of resistance, or the device revealed some

other problem, the case should be postponed until a new device and/or leads can be implanted.

6. Given that this patient has an underlying bradycardic rhythm of 60 beats/min, the device should be reprogrammed to an asynchronous mode with a rate of 70 beats/min.
7. In addition, if the device had anti-tachycardic features, these should be disabled.

### Intra-operative

1. No special monitoring or techniques need to be employed in the operating room.
2. Be careful about the placement of the electrocautery grounding pad so that it does not cause damage to the pacemaker generator.
3. Be vigilant for any failure in pacemaker capture that could occur.
4. Correct any acid–base or electrolyte disturbances should they occur, as these can affect the pacemaker response.
5. If this case was a true emergency:

    a. Place the electrocautery grounding pad away from the pacemaker.
    b. Place external pacer pads on the patient and have a defibrillator/pacer connected in monitoring mode.
    c. Place a magnet on the pacemaker/ICD once external pads are in place and a continuous EKG tracing is present. Observe what happens to the pacemaker rhythm with the application of the magnet.
    d. Obtain a stat chest X-ray intra-operatively; some devices have a series of codes that can be determined with a chest X-ray.
    e. Consult cardiology to evaluate the patient intra-operatively. If this is not possible, the device needs to be interrogated immediately following the procedure.

        i. Until the device is re-interrogated, you cannot be certain that the pre-operative pacemaker settings have been restored or that the ICD is indeed functional.
        ii. Continuation of external pacing/defibrillation pads and monitoring should continue until the device is interrogated and reset by the cardiology team.

### Post-operative

1. Following the conclusion of the procedure, re-interrogate the device to reset it to the pre-operative settings.
2. If an ICD was deactivated, it should be reactivated.
3. Finally, document the device integrity and battery life. Forward this information to the physician who is managing the device.

## Bibliography

Barash PG, Cullen BF, Stoelting RK, et al. *Clinical Anesthesia*, 8th ed.Philadelphia: Lippincott Williams & Wilkins, 2017, pp. 1724–31.

Maisel WH, Moynahan M, Zuckerman BD, et al. Pacemaker and ICD generator malfunctions: analysis of Food and Drug Administration annual reports. *JAMA* 2006;**295**:1901–6.

Miller R. *Miller's Anesthesia*. Philadelphia: Elsevier, 2005, pp. 1416–18.

**Chapter**

# 33 Cardiac Valvular Abnormalities

Donald M. Voltz and Jessica A. Lovich-Sapola

## Sample Case

A 71-year-old female was scheduled to undergo an elective total hip arthroplasty. Her activity level is minimal due to arthritic changes of her hips. She has a history of hypertension and hypothyroidism, both under good control with medication. Prior to her surgery, a systolic murmur was appreciated, prompting a full cardiac workup. A transthoracic echocardiogram revealed aortic stenosis with a peak gradient across the aortic valve of 48 mm Hg and a left ventricular ejection fraction of 35% with concentric hypertrophy. No evidence of stress-induced ischemia was appreciated on a dobutamine stress test.

## Clinical Issues

### Importance of Understanding Cardiac Valvular Lesions

1. Myocardial optimization depends on a balance between oxygen utilization and its supply.

    a. Optimization of myocardial performance is greatly impacted both by oxygen imbalance and the loading conditions on the ventricles.

    b. Due to a high incidence and severity of complications that occur in patients with hemodynamically significant lesions, it is important to understand how to optimize these patients.

2. Important hemodynamic variables in patients with valvular disease include the following:

    a. Rhythm

    b. Heart rate (HR)

    c. Preload (PL)

    d. Contractility

    e. Afterload (AL)

    f. Systemic vascular resistance (SVR)

        i. Control of these factors and understanding how they are altered in valvular pathologic situations is important to safely get these patients through surgery and optimize them both pre-operatively and in the peri-operative period.

3. Important variables

    a. Systemic blood pressure is directly related to the product of cardiac output and SVR.

    b. Cardiac output is the product of stroke volume (SV) (ventricular end diastolic volume − ventricular end systolic volume) and HR.

    c. Ventricular end diastolic volume is impacted by preload conditions and the compliance of the ventricle during diastole.

    d. Ventricular end systolic volume is impacted by afterload conditions and the contractile state of the ventricle.

        i. All of these variables are impacted by hemodynamically significant valvular disease and all play a role in the myocardial oxygen balance at both a baseline state and during surgical and anesthetic stresses.

        ii. Understanding the impact of these factors on myocardial performance and oxygen balance is different for each of the major valvular disorders.

4. Principles of normal and pathologic flow states across a valve orifice

    a. Flow across any orifice is positively correlated to:

        i. Cross-sectional valve area.

        ii. The square root of the pressure gradient across the valve.

        iii. The amount of time a given volume of blood transits the valve orifice.

            (1) Since flow across any of the cardiac valves impacts overall cardiac output and the perfusion pressure of the body, optimizing flow across diseased valves while limiting oxygen debt situations is important for improving patient outcomes.

    b. Flow conditions are responsive to loading conditions in some pathologic states (i.e., regurgitant lesions) while in others they are fixed (i.e., stenotic lesions).

        i. Transvalvular flow depends on the point of the cardiac cycle and the type of valvular pathology.

        ii. Valvular disease presents mainly as two types of lesions: stenosis or regurgitation.

            (1) In stenotic valvular lesions there is a pressure overload state on the preceding cardiac chamber (i.e., the left ventricle in aortic stenosis).

146

(a) For stenotic lesions, the ratio of transvalvular flow/duration of the cardiac cycle where flow occurs (i.e., systole for aortic stenosis) is important for cardiac function.

(b) In the case of aortic stenosis, when the flow increases or the duration of the systole shortens, this ratio increases leading to more pressure strain on the left ventricle.

(c) Minimizing any increases in flow or increasing the systolic period will help to reduce the pressure stress on the heart.

(2) In regurgitant lesions, there is a volume overload state placed on the preceding chamber (i.e., the left atrium in mitral regurgitation).

(a) Management of all cardiac lesions depends on minimizing either the pressure or volume overload state while maintaining or enhancing systemic cardiac output.

5. Understanding how changes in HR can affect the duration of systole and diastole is also important when it comes to valvular lesions and their optimization.

a. A rapid HR leads to a proportionately greater decrease in filling time during diastole than systole.

b. Slowing the heart increases both the diastolic filling time as well as the duration of systole.

c. This is important to understand for both stenotic and regurgitant lesions.

6. Systemic and pulmonic vascular resistance (afterload on the left and right ventricles, respectively) is also important to understand.

a. Increasing the afterload can lead to a greater degree of regurgitation while a significant drop in afterload can be poorly tolerated in stenotic lesions.

b. When afterload is reduced, the resulting blood pressure drop triggers the cardiac system to increase its output, either by an increase in HR, increase in SV, or often an increase in both.

c. For regurgitant lesions, a decreased afterload makes forward cardiac flow easier, leading to a physiologic improvement and less regurgitation.

d. This is not the case for stenotic lesions, however.

i. During a reduction in afterload, the cardiac response is an elevation in HR leading to more blood that must traverse a stenotic valve.

ii. To increase blood flow, velocity must increase, which occurs by increasing the pressure behind the stenosis.

iii. As the stenosis becomes worse, a patient's ability to increase cardiac output during a reduction in afterload becomes limited; patients often will not be able to maintain their blood pressure.

iv. With a decrease in blood pressure, there is a reduction in cardiac perfusion (that occurs during diastole when the heart is relaxing) leading to myocardial ischemia that further limits cardiac output.

v. In patients with significant aortic stenosis, a drop in afterload can result in cardiac arrest.

vi. Slow induction of anesthesia is important to maintain some afterload pressure in the aorta to ensure that coronary vessels are perfused.

## Pathophysiology of Aortic Stenosis

1. The main etiology for aortic stenosis is senile fibrocalcific degeneration leading to aortic sclerosis and stenosis.
2. The main etiology used to be rheumatic heart disease, although this has been decreasing in frequency.
3. In a subset of patients, a congenital bicuspid aortic valve leads to an acceleration of fibrocalcific deposits and these patients tend to present with significant aortic stenosis at an earlier age.
4. In about 50% of the patients who present with aortic stenosis, significant coronary artery disease is also present, leading to a combined aortic valve replacement as well as a bypass operation.

## Symptoms of Aortic Stenosis

1. Patients are often asymptomatic as the disease begins.

a. As the degree of stenosis impacts the myocardial reserve, symptoms begin to develop.

b. The presence and severity of symptoms are related to the prognosis of this disease.

c. Ideally, intervention is best during the early stages to avoid irreversible myocardial damage and to allow the myocardium to remodel itself.

d. Patients with worsening aortic stenosis often present with SAD: syncope, angina, and dyspnea.

2. Syncope

a. In the presence of a normal cardiovascular system, as systemic oxygen requirements increase during exercise or other physiologic stress, both the HR and SV increase to produce a higher cardiac output, thereby increasing the delivery of oxygen and removal of waste generated by the tissues.

b. In the presence of aortic stenosis, a fixed defect limiting the amount of blood that can be ejected from the heart, there is a limit on increasing cardiac output to meet peripheral oxygen demands.

c. When tissues increase their metabolism, such as during times of exertion or other physiologic stresses, vasodilatation of the capillary beds occurs to increase tissue perfusion and prevent an oxygen debt.

    i. In patients who have severe aortic stenosis, higher oxygen requirements by tissues during times of exertion lead to vasodilatation; however, a concomitant increase in cardiac output to overcome this drop in SVR cannot occur, resulting in hypotension and a decreased perfusion of the brain.

    ii. If the drop in cerebral perfusion is severe enough, syncope can result.

    iii. This problem occurs when the aortic valve becomes severely narrowed, limiting an increase in cardiac output.

  d. When patients with aortic stenosis present with syncope, their 3-year mortality without aortic valve replacement approaches 50%.

3. Angina

  a. Aortic stenosis leads to progressive myocardial hypertrophy to generate high compensatory left ventricular (LV) pressures and maintain cardiac output.

  b. Both myocardial oxygen demand and supply are altered in the presence of aortic stenosis.

  c. Myocardial hypertrophy necessitates a higher oxygen requirement while aortic stenosis leads to a decrease in aortic root pressure, the driving force behind myocardial perfusion pressure during diastole.

  d. When the oxygen demand is not met by the supply, an oxygen debt results in the development of angina.

  e. Patients with critical aortic stenosis cannot increase their cardiac output to any great extent without developing ischemia and angina.

  f. This becomes a vicious spiral since ischemia leads to myocardial dysfunction, which further impacts LV function, a drop in cardiac output, and further drops in myocardial perfusion.

  g. For patients who develop angina in the presence of aortic stenosis, their 5-year mortality approaches 50%.

4. Dyspnea

  a. Dyspnea in the presence of aortic stenosis arises from the increased LV pressures required to pump blood across the stenotic aortic valve.

  b. As the valve area decreases, the LV pressure must increase to maintain a normal cardiac output.

  c. If the LV pressure becomes too great, the pressure backs up blood flow and affects the pulmonary system.

  d. In the initial phases of aortic stenosis, the myocardium hypertrophies to generate these higher pressures; but with increasing degrees of stenosis, the myocardium is not able to keep up, leading to

progressive systolic and diastolic dysfunction culminating in congestive heart failure (CHF).

  e. When patients progress to CHF, their prognosis becomes poor without an aortic valve replacement.

    i. Two-year mortality as high as 50% has been reported in patients who develop CHF in the presence of aortic stenosis.

5. Summary

  a. Patients who present with syncope, angina, or dyspnea and have severe or critical aortic stenosis have a much-increased risk of dying without surgical aortic valve replacement.

  b. To preserve cardiac function, the goal is to delay the progression of this disease or intervene surgically before irreversible myocardial damage has resulted.

  c. With replacement of the diseased aortic valve, a fair amount of myocardial remodeling can occur, allowing for increased longevity in these patients.

## Assessment of the Severity of Aortic Stenosis

1. The normal aortic valve area is 2.5–3.5 $cm^2$.

  a. As stenosis progresses, this valve area decreases with a concomitant increase in LV pressures to move the same amount of blood across the valve.

  b. In a normal situation, the pressure gradient between the left ventricle and the aorta is only a few mm Hg; but as the stenosis progresses, this pressure gradient can become quite elevated.

  c. The degree of aortic stenosis as measured by the pressure gradient across the valve correlates to the degree of reduced aortic valve area.

2. Mild aortic stenosis

  a. The valve area falls to below 2.5 and 1.5 $cm^2$, resulting in a minimal elevation in peak gradient to less than 20 mm Hg.

3. Moderate aortic stenosis

  a. Valve area of 1.0–1.5 $cm^2$ and a peak gradient of greater than 50 mm Hg

4. Severe aortic stenosis

  a. Valve areas <1.0 $cm^2$ and peak gradients greater than 50 mm Hg; can be as high as 100 mm Hg

5. Critical aortic stenosis

  a. Aortic valve orifice is reduced to <0.5 $cm^2$

## Management of Cardiac Valvular Disease

1. To safely manage patients who present with cardiac valvular disease, you must understand the following five factors and how changes in these physiologic parameters can improve or impede the clinical situation of patients with valve disease.

a. Cardiac rhythm
b. HR
c. Preload
d. Contractility
e. Afterload

2. Optimal management of patients who present with any cardiac valvular lesion will depend on these parameters and is addressed below for each pathologic condition.

# Knock Out Management Strategies

## Aortic Stenosis

1. Rhythm: maintain normal sinus rhythm

    a. Patients with aortic stenosis often develop both systolic and diastolic dysfunction as a result of this disease.
    b. Myocardial hypertrophy leads to a decrease in the compliance of the LV and thereby a decrease in the passive filling of the LV during diastole.
    c. In a normal situation, atrial systole provides 20–30% of the LV filling volume.
    d. Due to a decreased compliance, the importance of the left atrial systole is exaggerated in patients with aortic stenosis if they are to maintain their cardiac output.
    e. Maintenance of a normal sinus rhythm is important; atrial fibrillation is poorly tolerated in this patient population.
    f. If these patients develop an unstable or rapid arrhythmia, immediate cardioversion should be performed.

2. HR: avoid bradycardia (decreases cardiac output) and tachycardia (ischemia).

    a. Patients with severe aortic stenosis have a narrow window regarding HR.
    b. In all situations, maintenance of their baseline, resting HR should be maintained.
    c. As mentioned above, these patients have a poorly compliant ventricle and therefore require a longer time and higher left atrial pressures to adequately fill the LV.
    d. This filling comes during diastole, the period of the cardiac cycle most affected by increases in HR.
    e. A rapid HR increases oxygen requirements while at the same time limiting supply, placing these patients at an increased risk for ischemia, leading to further myocardial dysfunction.
    f. Based on this information, one would assume bradycardia would be best for patients with aortic stenosis; however, due to the fixed lesion at the aortic valve limiting the amount of blood ejected during each cardiac cycle (i.e., a fixed SV), a drop in HR can significantly limit cardiac output, leading to hypotension and peripheral perfusion problems.

    g. Maintenance of HR at the patient's baseline level, usually 70–90 beats/min, allows for an adequate cardiac output while at the same time maintaining a balanced oxygen delivery and consumption.

3. Preload: maintain or increase

    a. With a decrease in LV compliance and therefore a higher requirement on left-sided filling pressures to ensure an adequate cardiac output, adequate preload is important in these patients.
    b. A loss of intravascular volume resulting from dehydration or blood loss is poorly tolerated since this leads to underfilling of the LV and a resulting decrease in cardiac output.
    c. Overzealous fluid administration can also lead to complications since the left atrial pressures and pulmonary capillary pressures are elevated to overcome the poorly compliant LV and allow for adequate filling.
    d. Too much intravascular volume can tip the balance and place these patients in pulmonary edema.
    e. Careful monitoring and management of preload status is important in the optimization of patients with aortic stenosis.

4. Contractility

    a. As with all valvular lesions, the ventricular and atrial chambers become modified to deal with the abnormal fluid and pressure dynamics.
    b. As a result of ventricular hypertrophy to overcome the narrowing of the aortic valve, ventricular performance decreases.
    c. Individual myocytes are forced to work harder and their contractile force for unit of energy burned is lessened, resulting in an overall decrease in contractility.
    d. Further decreases in contractility that result from ischemia or other myocardial insults must be avoided to maintain adequate cardiac output and systemic pressures.

5. Afterload: maintain or increase

    a. Like many of the other cardiac parameters, maintenance of SVR and afterload is important so that coronary perfusion is not impacted.
    b. As mentioned in the case above, peripheral vasodilatation is normally offset by a compensatory increase in cardiac output.
    c. With aortic stenosis and a relatively fixed stroke volume, a drop in SVR leads to a precipitous fall in blood pressure and a significant drop in coronary perfusion pressure.
    d. It is important to maintain the afterload at baseline levels since hypotension leads to a decrease in coronary perfusion, further dropping cardiac output, perpetuating the problem.

## Aortic Insufficiency

1. Rhythm: sinus

   a. Patients with aortic insufficiency maintain the best forward cardiac output with a slightly tachycardic state.

   b. Uncontrolled tachycardia leads to a decrease in performance and an increase in oxygen requirements.

   c. Typically patients with aortic insufficiency are best optimized with HRs of 90–110 beats/min.

2. HR: increase

   a. The hemodynamic goals in aortic insufficiency are to maintain an adequate forward cardiac output.

   b. In any regurgitant valvular lesion there is a balance between forward blood flow and the regurgitant flow that results through the incompetent valve.

   c. It is only the forward flow that allows for end-organ perfusion; the regurgitant flow is lost at the expense of extra-myocardial work.

   d. In aortic insufficiency, regurgitation occurs during diastole, so limiting this period of the cardiac cycle will limit the amount of backward flow.

   e. A slightly tachycardic rate allows for both an overall increase in cardiac output as well as a decrease in the amount of regurgitation.

      i. This comes at the expense of an increased oxygen requirement from increasing HR.

   f. Bradycardia results in a lower oxygen requirement for each beat of the heart but allows for a longer diastolic time and therefore a reduction in forward cardiac output.

      i. This inefficient cardiac output leads to more myocardial work without a resulting benefit in systemic perfusion.

   g. Patients tolerate a mild increase in HR to promote forward flow and to compensate for the regurgitant flow.

   h. Aortic insufficiency also leads to a precipitous drop in aortic root pressure during diastole, which reduces coronary perfusion pressure and flow.

      i. An increased HR and limitation of diastole corrects some of this problem.

3. Preload: slightly increased

   a. The LV in patients with aortic insufficiency tends to dilate to make room for the extra volumes that occur in diastole.

   b. These patients have normal filling during diastole from the left atrium; however, they also have a fraction of the forward cardiac output entering the LV through an incompetent aortic valve.

   c. This results in a situation in which the LV has an exaggerated preload for the next cardiac cycle.

   d. Remodeling of the ventricle to accommodate this extra volume is accomplished by dilation.

   e. In the event of significant intravascular depletion, the LV can become under-filled and have a detrimental effect on cardiac output.

   f. Patients with aortic insufficiency must not be overzealously fluid resuscitated leading to acute decompensation of the LV and concomitant pulmonary edema.

4. Contractility

   a. With dilation of the LV to accommodate the extra volume from aortic regurgitation, the myocytes become stretched and could result in a decrease in contractility, and ultimately myocardial failure.

5. Afterload: decreased

   a. With an increase in systemic pressure and elevations in afterload, the forward cardiac output decreases, leading to a higher fraction of regurgitant blood.

   b. A slight, controlled drop in SVR promotes forward cardiac flow and a decrease in regurgitation.

   c. Uncontrolled drops in SVR or exaggerated increases in blood pressure/afterload can lead to cardiovascular collapse and therefore need to be eliminated.

## Mitral Stenosis

1. Rhythm: maintain normal sinus rhythm

   a. Maintaining these patients in a sinus rhythm at their baseline HR is ideal; however, due to a chronic increase in left atrial pressures and a resulting left atrial dilation to accommodate these pressures, many patients present with atrial fibrillation.

   b. Atrial fibrillation leads to a decrease in late diastolic filling and can reduce end diastolic volumes by up to 30%.

      i. This is overcome by the increased left atrial pressures and higher than normal early and late diastolic fillings that result from these increased pressures.

   c. Given that many of these patients present in atrial fibrillation, and most are unlikely to be successfully converted to a normal sinus rhythm due to atrial dilation, control of their HR at 70–90 beats/min is important.

      i. Rapid ventricular response is not well tolerated in these patients since an increase in ventricular rate impacts diastolic filling times and decreases cardiac output.

2. HR: maintain at the low end of normal; avoid tachycardia.

   a. As with aortic stenosis, ventricular filling occurs during diastole.

b. Given this situation, maintaining a baseline HR at 70–90 beats/min provides adequate diastolic filling time while preserving an HR-dependent cardiac output.

c. Both uncontrolled increases and precipitous decreases in HR can lead to an uncompensated situation and an overall reduction in cardiac output.

   i. If the HR falls too low, the fixed nature of aortic stenosis limits the amount of LV filling and therefore results in a fall in cardiac output.

   ii. Increasing the HR normally leads to an increase in cardiac output; however, in patients with flow-limiting mitral stenosis, every elevation in HR decreases filling of the LV due to a shortening of the diastolic time as well as the flow limitation imposed by the stenosis.

3. Preload: maintain, avoid hypovolemia

   a. A fixed, reduced mitral valve area in patients with flow-limiting mitral stenosis necessitates maintenance of adequate preload.

   b. Ventricular filling both during early and late diastole is limited by the reduction in cross-sectional area of the stenotic mitral valve.

   c. A drop in preload results in a drop in left atrial pressure resulting in a decrease in LV filling.

   d. With a fall in LV end diastolic volume, a concomitant fall in cardiac output occurs.

   e. Patients with mitral stenosis compensate by maintaining a greatly elevated left atrial pressure that ultimately leads to atrial dilatation, and a vast majority of patients present with atrial fibrillation.

4. Contractility

   a. In the early stages of mitral stenosis, the LV contractility is not impacted.

   b. With progression of the disease or the presence of multiple valvular lesions such as combined mitral and aortic stenosis that occurs in rheumatic heart disease, the LV function may be impacted.

5. Afterload

   a. Mitral stenosis results in a fixed lesion and therefore a fixed SV due to limitations on getting blood into the LV during diastole.

   b. In a normal situation, a fall in afterload would be compensated by an increase in cardiac output.

   c. Patients with mitral stenosis are not able to increase their cardiac output by a modification of SV.

   d. In addition, an increase in HR would normally lead to an increased cardiac output, but in these patients it further limits diastolic filling and is detrimental to LV filling.

   e. Given this, patients with mitral stenosis do not respond well to precipitous drops in afterload, requiring an increase in their cardiac output.

# Mitral Insufficiency

1. Rhythm

   a. Maintenance of a mild degree of tachycardia is best to promote adequate LV filling while limiting the amount of time in diastole.

   b. With significant regurgitation, the left atrium can become enlarged and dilated to accommodate the regurgitant volumes which increases likelihood of atrial fibrillation.

   c. Uncontrolled tachycardia from a rapid ventricular response should be avoided.

2. HR: avoid bradycardia and maintain a mild tachycardia.

   a. In a manner similar to aortic insufficiency, patients with mitral insufficiency are attempting to optimize the amount of forward cardiac output.

   b. A slight increase in HR leads to a decrease in the diastolic time and therefore limits the amount of regurgitation that can occur.

   c. Excessive elevations in HR are not good since these ultimately impact coronary oxygen supply and demand.

   d. A mild tachycardia of 90–110 beats/min is usually optimal for these patients.

   e. Profound bradycardia is not well tolerated since this can lead to acute LV fluid overload when a significant amount of the cardiac output flows through the incompetent mitral valve.

3. Preload: increase slightly

   a. Patients with mitral insufficiency often maintain adequate levels of preload and the LV is presented with higher than normal volumes during diastole as a result of the mitral insufficiency.

4. Contractility

   a. Many patients who present with mitral insufficiency also have ventricular dysfunction.

   b. A poorly functioning ventricle leads to hypertrophy and dilation of the mitral annulus, resulting in chronic mitral insufficiency.

   c. In these patients, the ventricular function is depressed, and further myocardial depressants can lead to decompensation.

   d. It is important to understand the etiology of valvular dysfunction and how the inciting disease processes can be worsened, leading to cardiac decompensation.

5. Afterload: mild decrease in afterload

   a. The balance between afterload and left atrial pressures determines the fraction of regurgitant flow and forward cardiac output.

   b. A slight reduction in SVR leads to an increase in forward cardiac output and is well tolerated by patients with mitral insufficiency.

c. Precipitous increases in afterload decrease forward cardiac output and cause an increase in left atrial and pulmonary capillary pressure.

d. If this increase is too great, pulmonary edema can result.

e. In patients with severely depressed left ventricular function leading to a significant amount of mitral regurgitation, surgical repair of the valve can lead to LV decompensation.

f. This occurs because in the diseased state any increase in afterload does not present as a further strain on the LV.

g. The lower-pressured left atrium would serve as a "pop-off" mechanism thereby limiting the strain on the LV.

h. Once the mitral valve is replaced or repaired, restoring competence, any increase in afterload strain is directly transferred to the LV.

i. If the increase in afterload is too great, LV failure can develop in the peri-operative period.

## KO Treatment Plan

### Pre-operative

1. The patient presented above is at an increased risk of developing complications in the peri-operative period.

2. Although her pre-operative stress echocardiogram did not reveal any areas of ischemia, she has moderate to severe aortic stenosis with a decrease in her LV function (LVEF 35%).

3. Since this is an elective case, it is prudent to evaluate this patient for an aortic valve replacement prior to repairing her hip.

4. If this patient presented for an emergency operation, the luxury of repairing her valve would not be present.

   a. In an emergent situation, pre-operative optimization would be required.

      i. In the setting of an emergency case, a pre-induction arterial line is required to be able to closely monitor and respond to any fluctuations in blood pressure.

      ii. Ideally, maintaining this patient at her baseline HR and blood pressure is best.

      iii. Avoidance of profound drops in blood pressure is important since this drop greatly effects myocardial perfusion pressure and can result in ischemia followed by cardiac arrest.

         (1) Due to the limitation in aortic valve area, CPR is often not effective in patients with severe AS and therefore any drops in blood pressure should be managed aggressively.

      iv. In choosing an anesthetic technique, medications that maintain blood pressure without significantly impacting HR should be chosen.

         (1) Many people avoid the use of spinal anesthetics due to the technique's potential for a profound and unpredictable drop in blood pressure.

         (2) However, patients have successfully been managed with regional anesthesia provided they are dosed correctly and slowly.

      v. A gentle induction with etomidate and fentanyl will likely provide hemodynamic stability from a blood pressure and HR standpoint.

### Intra-operative

1. During this case, the patient's HR and blood pressure need to be continually observed and addressed to reduce peri-operative complications.

2. Despite not having any areas of ischemia on her pre-operative stress echocardiogram, she is at an increased risk to develop ischemia because of the higher oxygen requirements of her myocardium.

3. Her history of hypertension as well as aortic stenosis have likely led to hypertrophy of her myocardium, bringing about these increased oxygen requirements.

4. During the procedure, with swings in blood loss or fluid administration, we would see episodes of hyper- or hypotension.

5. In addition, she may also develop tachycardia, further adding to her oxygen requirements.

6. Any deviation from her baseline hemodynamic status should be addressed, albeit slowly and carefully, to avoid large swings in blood pressure or profound decreases in HR.

7. Since these patients do not tolerate atrial fibrillation, you must be prepared to cardiovert them to restore them to sinus rhythm.

### Post-operative

1. Close monitoring of her blood pressure, HR, and end-organ perfusion should continue.

2. The stress response to surgery and shifts in fluids can occur for many days post-operatively.

3. Restoration of her baseline medications and maintenance of her blood pressure and HR to her pre-surgical baseline are best for this patient.

## Bibliography

Barash PG, Cullen BF, Stoelting RK, et al. *Clinical Anesthesia*, 8th ed. Philadelphia: Lippincott Williams & Wilkins, 2017, pp. 1082–9.

Butterworth JF, Mackey DC, Wasnick JD. *Morgan & Mikhail's Clinical Anesthesiology*, 6th ed. New York: McGraw-Hill Education, 2018, pp. 415–25.

Kurup V, Haddadin AS. Valvular heart diseases. *Anesthesiol Clin* 2006;**24**:487–508.

Otto CM. Valvular aortic stenosis: disease severity and timing of intervention. *J Am Coll Cardiol* 2006;**47**:2141–51.

Rapaport E. Natural history of aortic and mitral valve disease. *Am J Cardiol* 1975;**35**:221.

# Transcatheter Aortic Valve Replacement

Maninder Singh and Zaid H. Jumaily

## Sample Case

An 83-year-old patient with hypertension, diabetes, chronic kidney disease, and coronary artery disease requiring multiple stents presents to the emergency department with worsening dyspnea and syncope. Physical exam reveals a systolic murmur and bedside echocardiogram is consistent with severe aortic stenosis. He is referred to cardiology and cardiothoracic surgery for treatment. What aortic valve interventions are options? When would a transcatheter aortic valve replacement (TAVR) procedure be indicated? What are the anesthetic considerations?

## Clinical Issues

### Indications for Aortic Valve Intervention

1. Severe aortic stenosis

    a. Symptomatic (dyspnea on exertion, syncope, exertional angina)

    b. Aortic jet velocity >4.0 m/s or mean pressure gradient >40 mm Hg

    c. Aortic valve area <1.0 cm$^2$

2. Aortic valve replacement (AVR) is recommended for the following patients:

    a. Symptomatic with high-gradient severe aortic stenosis

    b. Asymptomatic severe high-gradient aortic stenosis with left ventricular ejection fraction (LVEF) <50%

    c. Asymptomatic severe high-gradient aortic stenosis undergoing other cardiac surgery

    d. Asymptomatic, very severe high-gradient aortic stenosis and low surgical/TAVR risk

    e. Asymptomatic, very severe aortic stenosis with decreased exercise tolerance or hypotension with exercise

3. Choice of TAVR over the surgical AVR option

    a. The TAVR has become an approved therapy for the replacement of a stenotic aortic valve in patients at extreme and high risk for an open, surgical valve replacement.

    b. Requires a focused risk assessment by an experienced multidisciplinary team based on the patient's comorbidities

    c. Currently, TAVR is approved for moderate- and high-risk patient populations, and is undergoing trials for low-risk patients.

    d. Absolute contraindications to TAVR

        i. Life expectancy <12 months due to noncardiac reasons or comorbidities disallowing improvement in quality of life

        ii. Other valvular lesions with major contribution to patient's symptoms that would otherwise be treatable with surgery

        iii. Inadequate aortic annulus size, bicuspid valve

        iv. Endocarditis

        v. High risk of coronary ostia obstruction

    d. Relative contraindications to TAVR

        i. Acute myocardial infarction (MI) within 30 days

        ii. Coronary artery disease; untreated and amenable to bypass graft

        iii. Hemodynamic instability requiring inotropic support

        iv. Hypertrophic cardiomyopathy

        v. Severe pulmonary hypertension and right ventricular dysfunction

        vi Elevated risk of annular rupture

        vii Issues related to retrograde arterial access

4. Valve types

    a. Two types of valves approved in the United States

        i. SAPIEN 3 (balloon expandable)

        ii. EVOLUT (self-expanding)

## KO Treatment Plan for TAVR

### Pre-operative

1. Assess the patient's concurrent comorbidities and optimize the patient for cardiac surgery.

2. Institutional variation regarding location (catheterization lab versus hybrid operating room)

3. Multidisciplinary discussion regarding the following:

    a. Primary access site (cut-down access requires general anesthesia)

        i. Femoral artery (percutaneous, most common)

        ii. Axillary/subclavian artery (cut-down)

iii. Transapical/aortic (thoracotomy/sternotomy)
iv. Transcaval
v. Transcarotid

b. Secondary access site (femoral artery vs. radial)
c. Arterial access for blood pressure monitoring (left side is usually preferred)
d. Peripheral access and central access

4. Trained multidisciplinary team

a. Interventional cardiologist
b. Cardiothoracic surgeon
c. Perfusionist (with a cardiopulmonary bypass [CPB] machine available)
d. Anesthesiologist
e. Nursing teams
f. Echocardiogram sonographer (if the transesophageal echocardiogram [TEE] cannot be done by the cardiac anesthesiologist)

5. Type and cross for at least 4 units of PRBCs

## Intra-operative

1. Type of anesthetic:

a. MAC with sedation: most common for primary percutaneous femoral access
b. General anesthesia when cut-down or thoracotomy/ sternotomy is required, or patient factors disallow sedation (back pain, orthopnea, severe sleep apnea, etc.)

2. Hemodynamic goals

a. Sinus rhythm

i. Avoid supraventricular tachycardia (SVT) and atrial fibrillation.
ii. Avoid loss of atrioventricular (AV) synchrony.
iii. Avoid tachycardia or severe bradycardia (heart rate goal of 60–80 beats/min).

b. Maintain afterload.

i. Avoid hypotension. Treat with a vasoconstrictor (phenylephrine preferred, or norepinephrine if inotropy is also required).
ii. Pre-emptive treatment of hypotension with phenylephrine if induction of general anesthesia is required
iii. Avoid hypertension. Treat with β-blocker if the heart rate is elevated.

c. Maintain contractility

i. Myocardial depression after induction of general anesthesia is common. This can be managed with norepinephrine.

3. The steps of the procedure

a. Apply standard ASA monitors, defibrillator/pacing pads, and cerebral oximetry.
b. Peripheral IV access and arterial invasive blood pressure monitoring
c. Induction if general anesthesia
d. TEE if general anesthesia
e. Primary access (e.g., femoral artery)
f. Secondary access (e.g., contralateral femoral artery or radial artery)
g. Central venous access (for transvenous pacing and resuscitation)
h. Balloon valvuloplasty (often done at time of deployment)
i. Upsize the primary access to fit the device introducer.
j. Anti-coagulate the patient (heparin), goal ACT >250.
k. Advance the valve to the annulus. Assess position on TEE if applicable.
l. Deploy the valve with rapid transvenous pacing (180 beats/min). Avoid treating expected hypotension at this stage.
m. Monitor and manage resultant arrhythmia (pacing), ischemia (valve covering ostium), and hemodynamic instability.
n. Transthoracic echocardiogram (TTE)/TEE to assess for valve positioning, perivalvular leak, pericardial effusion, etc.
o. Closure and reversal of heparinization
p. Emergence from anesthesia; transfer to ICU setting for monitoring.

## Complications

1. Vascular complications of access site

a. Dissection, perforation, hemorrhage
b. Have blood available for resuscitation.

2. Pacing malfunction during deployment and arrhythmias
3. Aortic insufficiency following balloon valvuloplasty

a. May need inotropic support
b. Prolonged time to deployment can cause improper deployment and may require valve-in-valve transcatheter aortic valve implantation (TAVI).

4. Device embolization
5. Coronary occlusion

a. Prior coronary artery bypass graft (CABG) surgery is protective.
b. High-risk patients may have a coronary wire in place.

6. Conversion to open surgery and CPB
7. Stroke

a. If sedation technique is used, you may obtain a neurologic exam.
b. If under general anesthesia, precipitous drop in cerebral oximetry

c. Most commonly due to embolization of aortic plaque

## Post-operative

1. Plan for post-operative monitoring.

   a. Monitor for conduction abnormalities.

2. Echocardiogram and ECG post-procedure

   a. Repeat at 30 days and then annually.

b. Assess valve function.

c. Assess left ventricle size and function.

d. Pulmonary artery systolic pressure

e. Cardiac rhythm

3. Pain management

4. Early mobilization

5. Long-term antithrombotic therapy and endocarditis prophylaxis

## Bibliography

Brecker SJD, Aldea GS. Choice of intervention for severe calcific aortic stenosis. In *UpToDate* (accessed October 30, 2021).

Fontes ML. Intraoperative hemodynamic management of aortic and mitral valve disease in adults. In *UpToDate* (accessed October 30, 2021).

Miller RD, Fleisher LA, Johns RA, et al. *Anesthesia*, 9th ed. New York: Churchill Livingstone, 2020, pp 1790–1, 2307–8).

# Point of Care Ultrasound

**Chapter 35**

Daniel Guay and Augusto Torres

## Clinical Issues

### Point of Care Ultrasound (POCUS)

#### Definitions

1.  Narrowed ultrasound examination performed at the bedside meant to answer a clinical question or assist in a diagnosis.

    a.  POCUS can be used to assist in many clinical scenarios.

    b.  It is commonly used in the emergency department in the setting of abdominal trauma for a focused assessment of abdominal trauma (FAST).

2.  Anesthesiologists utilize POCUS in three typical domains: cardiac, thoracic, and gastric.

### Characteristics

1.  Adjunct to physical exam
2.  Designed to help answer binary yes/no questions (i.e., presence of pericardial effusion or not, as opposed to quantitative measurement of effusion)
3.  Not comprehensive: focuses on explaining an abnormality
4.  May not necessarily make a definitive diagnosis
5.  Helps physician at the bedside gather crucial information to assess the patient's physiologic status, refine a differential diagnosis, and decide on future interventions

### Cardiac POCUS

#### Definition

1.  A focused examination of the cardiovascular system performed by a physician using ultrasound as an adjunct to the physical examination to recognize specific ultrasonic signs that represent a narrow list of potential diagnoses in specific clinical settings (American Society of Echocardiography).
2.  Focused cardiac ultrasound (FoCUS) is a standardized but restricted scanning protocol used as an extension of the clinical examination.

#### Indications

1.  Hemodynamic instability or undifferentiated shock
2.  Cardiac arrest
3.  Pericardial effusion/tamponade
4.  Heart failure
5.  High cardiac risk patients
6.  Adjunct to physical examination

#### Image Acquisition

1.  Phased array transducer (2–7.5 MHz)
2.  With limited diagnostic targets, only a select number of views are required:

    a.  Parasternal long axis (PLAX)

        i.  Used to assess, in order of importance:

            (1)  Left ventricle (LV) size and function
            (2)  Right ventricle (RV) size
            (3)  Mitral valve
            (4)  Aortic valve
            (5)  Left pleural effusion
            (6)  Pericardial effusion
            (7)  Aortic root dilatation, which may indicate a dissection

    b.  Parasternal short-axis (PSAX)

        i.  Used to assess, in order of importance:

            (1)  LV size and function
            (2)  RV size and function
            (3)  Pericardial effusion

        ii.  Limited look at regional wall motion abnormalities

            (1)  LV filling (dilation)
            (2)  RV:LV pressure
            (3)  Interventricular septal kinetics
            (4)  Volume status

    c.  Apical 4-chamber:

        i.  Used to assess, in order of importance:

            (1)  LV size and function
            (2)  RV size and function
            (3)  Mitral valve
            (4)  Tricuspid valve
            (5)  Right atrium (RA) and left atrium (LA) size
            (6)  Pericardial effusion

    d.  Subcostal 4-chamber:

        i.  Used to assess, in order of importance:

156

(1) LV size and function

(2) RV size and function (best look at the RV and RV wall thickness)

(3) Mitral valve

(4) Tricuspid valve

(5) RA and LA size

(6) Pericardial effusion

(7) Cardiac motion during cardiac arrest

(8) Subcostal inferior vena cava (IVC): assess volume status with a view of the IVC, by calculating the IVC collapsibility index.

(9) Abdominal aorta

## Advantages of FoCUS

1. Results are in "real time."
2. Less invasive than transesophageal ultrasound or pulmonary artery catheters
3. Can be performed comfortably in an awake patient

## Disadvantages/Challenges of FoCUS

1. Experience of physician; if acquired images are poor, limited information is obtained.
2. Qualitative assessment; therefore it is not meant to grade disease severity.
3. Variable quality of ultrasound equipment
4. Effect of mechanical ventilation on image equality
5. Inaccessibility (i.e., wound dressing, surgical draping over thorax)
6. Patient positioning (i.e., prone, arm draped over chest, etc.)
7. Obesity

## Clinical Scenarios for FoCUS

1. Poor cardiac function

   a. Patients with poor functional capacity without access to or without prior cardiovascular workup present for emergent or urgent surgery.

   b. Focused evaluation of patients may reveal poor LV function and allow clinicians to adjust peri-operative management.

2. Cardiac arrest

   a. May be difficult to perform

   b. Look for reversible causes: hypovolemia, myocardial infarction, RV failure, LV failure, cardiac tamponade, or pulmonary embolism.

3. Pulmonary embolism

   a. Images seen on ultrasound

      i. Normally the RV is two-thirds the size of the LV; with a massive pulmonary embolism, the RV may appear larger than the LV.

      ii. Parasternal short-axis view may show flattening of the interventricular septum and a small LV.

iii. Subcostal view: the IVC will be plethoric with minimal respiratory variation.

4. Cardiac tamponade

   a. Images on ultrasound

      i. Presence of pericardial effusion

      ii. Dilated IVC

      iii. Late diastolic inversion of the RA free wall and RV diastolic collapse

      iv. Swinging heart surrounded by pericardial effusion

5. Valvular pathology

   a. Visual inspection of the aortic valve with restriction of extent of aortic cusps can alert to significant aortic stenosis.

6. Volume status assessment

   a. During spontaneous ventilation, IVC diameter <2.1 cm with inspiratory collapse of >50% during a sniff correlates with right atrial pressure of 0–5 mm Hg.

   b. Generally, IVC diameter <1 cm is considered an indicator of hypovolemia, although very low systemic vascular resistance (SVR) can produce similar findings.

# Thoracic POCUS

## Definitions

1. Lung sliding: characteristic shimmering/sparkling along the pleural line synchronous with respiration is due to normal sliding of the parietal and visceral pleurae.

2. A-lines: horizontal lines equidistant from one another.

   a. Reverberation artifact generated by the pleural line

   b. Normal lung surface finding

3. B-lines ("comet tail"): vertical lines that extend from the pleura to through the image

   a. Focal B-lines may suggest pneumonia.

   b. Diffuse B-lines on both sides of the chest suggests a diffuse alveolar interstitial process such as pulmonary edema or ARDS.

   c. B-lines decrease with aeration (emphysema and hyperinflation).

4. Acoustic shadow: black cones of shadow due to reflection of ultrasound beams by bone/ribs

5. M-Mode: time/motion display of ultrasound line

   a. Allows depiction of pleural line over time to increase sensitivity for detecting sliding

6. Lung-point: pathognomonic for pneumothorax

   a. Portion of pleura with lung sliding and portion with fixed pleura

## Indications

1. Symptoms include: shortness of breath, acute dyspnea, hypoxia, pleuritic chest pain, congestive heart failure, or chest trauma.
2. Evaluation for pneumothorax
3. Evaluation for pleural effusion, lung edema, and consolidation
4. Verify placement of the endotracheal tube.
5. Lung ultrasound has been shown to have increased sensitivity and specificity when compared to both chest X-ray and physical examination in detecting pleural effusions and pneumothorax, as well as determination of bilateral ventilation.

## Image Acquisition

1. A high-frequency (5.0–10.0 MHz) linear transducer is used, though a curvilinear probe may be needed in some cases.
2. The patient is positioned supine, assessing anterior segments of the chest, where air would rise in the presence of pneumothorax.
3. Absence of lung sliding is not definitive for pneumothorax; it may represent apnea, bronchial intubation, pleural adhesion, or large infiltrates; therefore clinical context is important.
4. Similarly, presence of bilateral lung sliding does not rule out pneumothorax, only that there was no pneumothorax at the area assessed. It is therefore important to investigate as many regions as clinically necessary.
5. Can utilize M-mode to increase detection of lung sliding
   a. A characteristic "sandy beach" sign indicates pleural sliding.
   b. A "barcode" sign indicates lack of sliding, typically due to lack of opposition of visceral and parietal pleura (i.e., pneumothorax).
6. Observation of the lung-point is pathognomonic for pneumothorax.
7. Assessing for bilateral lung sliding following endotracheal intubation has shown to have increased sensitivity and specificity (99% and 100%) when compared to auscultation for bilateral breath sounds.
8. Pleural effusion is best assessed in the sitting position, placing the transducer on dependent regions of the posterior/lateral chest wall.
   a. Loculated effusions may be seen in superior portions of lung.

# Gastric POCUS

## Definition

1. Ultrasound examination of the stomach
2. Pulmonary aspiration of gastric contents in the perioperative period has been associated with severe morbidity and death.

a. Fasting for 6–10 hours does not guarantee an empty stomach, irrespective of comorbidities.
b. Noninvasive measurement of the gastric contents by qualitative and quantitative measures can be used to risk-stratify and mitigate this risk.

## Risk Factors for Aspiration

1. Emergency procedure
2. Gastrointestinal obstruction
3. Morbid obesity
4. Gastroesophageal reflux disease
5. Diabetes mellitus
6. Recent oral intake
7. Recent opioid administration
8. Major trauma
9. Previous gastric bypass surgery
10. Pregnancy

## Indication

1. Uncertain prandial status
   a. Unclear history
   b. Cognitive dysfunction
   c. Language barriers
   d. Pediatric patients
2. Known/suspected delayed gastric transit
   a. Diabetes mellites
   b. Chronic kidney disease
   c. Pregnancy
   d. Obesity
   e. Systemic medications (e.g., opioids)

## Image Acquisition

1. Low-frequency (1–5 MHz) curvilinear probe
2. Patient in supine and right lateral decubitus positions (possible semi-recumbent if unable to tolerate lateral)
3. Probe in sagittal plan over epigastrium
4. Sonographic landmarks include liver, pancreas, aorta, superior mesenteric artery, and vertebral bodies. Gastric antrum will be the only visible gastric structure.

## Interpretation

The risk of aspiration correlates with the quantity of gastric contents. The most accepted upper limit for gastric secretions is 1.5 mL/kg of body weight (~100–130 mL), which accounts for roughly 95% of fasted surgical patients. A volume of >1.5 mL/kg is rarely seen in the fasting state and either suggests delayed emptying or recently ingested fluids.

1. Empty
   a. Grade 0 antrum: "bulls-eye" appearance with thick muscularis propria layer.
      i. Low aspiration risk
2. Clear fluid

a. Grade 1 antrum: hypoechoic, distended antrum. Fluid is only visible in right lateral position.

   i. Low aspiration risk; <1.5 mL/kg of gastric fluid

b. Grade 2 antrum: fluid is visible in both supine and right lateral positions.

   i. High aspiration risk; >1.5 mL/kg gastric fluid

c. Presence of thick fluids is associated with high risk of pulmonary aspiration.

3. Solid

   a. Distended antrum

   b. Recently digested food is associated with a "frosted glass" appearance.

   c. Later stages are associated with hyperechoic, heterogeneous consistency.

   d. High aspiration risk

### Clinical Implications

1. Gastric ultrasound should not be used as a sole mechanism for assessing gastric status and does not replace a thorough history and physical exam.

2. It is important to consider the urgency of the surgery, prandial history, and other risk factors for pulmonary aspiration (i.e., altered mentation, stroke, swallowing disorders).

3. These considerations with additional insight from gastric ultrasound may allow one to make improved informed medical decisions.

4. Changes in patient care may be related to the timing of anesthesia (i.e., proceed, delay, or cancel), anesthetic technique (i.e., general anesthesia with a protected airway vs. regional vs. sedation), and need for aspiration precautions including tracheal intubation, need for rapid sequence intubation, or placement of a gastric tube.

# Bibliography

Chowdhury AR, Punj J, Pandey R, et al. Ultrasound is a reliable and faster tool for confirmation of endotracheal intubation compared to chest auscultation and capnography when performed by novice anaesthesia residents: a prospective controlled clinical trial. *Saudi J Anaesth* 2020;14(1):15–21.

Coker BJ, Zimmerman JM. Why anesthesiologists must incorporate focused cardiac ultrasound into daily practice. *Anesth Analg* 2017;124(3):761–5.

El-Boghdadly K, Wojcikiewicz T, Perlas A. Perioperative point-of-care gastric ultrasound. *BJA Educ*. 2019;19(7):219–26.

Engelhardt T, Webster NR. Pulmonary aspiration of gastric contents in anaesthesia. *Br J Anaesth*. 1999;83(3):453–60.

Porter TR, Shillcutt SK, Adams MS, et al. Guidelines for the use of echocardiography as a monitor for therapeutic intervention in adults: a report from the American Society of Echocardiography. *J Am Soc Echocardiogr* 2015;28(1):40e56

Sharma G, Jacob R, Mahankali S, Ravindra MN. Preoperative assessment of gastric contents and volume using bedside ultrasound in adult patients: a prospective, observational, correlation study. *Indian J Anaesth* 2018;62(10):753–8.

Virtual Transthoracic Echocardiography. Focused cardiac ultrasound (FOCUS). http://pie.med.utoronto.ca/tte/TTE_con tent/focus.html#intructions (accessed January 3, 2023).

# Intra-operative Transesophageal Echocardiography

Maninder Singh, Elvera L. Baron, and Varun Dixit

**Chapter 36**

## Sample Case

A 63-year-old female is at the end of her atrial fibrillation ablation. The procedure was completed uneventfully. While you are preparing to extubate the patient, she becomes hypotensive. While you are supporting her blood pressure and managing her hemodynamically, what other tests would you like to do to make a diagnosis?

## Clinical Issues

### Intra-operative Transesophageal Echocardiography (TEE)

1. Uses sound waves to create an image of underlying tissues
2. Provides valuable information about cardiac anatomy and myocardial function during surgery
3. Can be used intraoperatively to detect regional and global ventricular abnormalities, chamber dimensions, valvular anatomy, and the presence of intracardiac air
4. May assist in guiding the placement of intracardiac and intravascular catheters and devices. These may include guidewires for central line or intra-aortic balloon pump placement, or confirming cannulation sites, such as coronary sinus and/or bicaval cannulation.
5. Regional wall motion abnormalities from myocardial ischemia often appear before EKG changes occur.
6. Regional wall motion abnormalities can be classified into three categories: hypokinesis (reduced wall motion), akinesis (no wall motion), and dyskinesis (paradoxical wall motion).

### Indications

1. Intra-operative evaluation of acute, persistent, and life-threatening hemodynamics in which patients have not responded to treatment; this use is not limited to cardiac surgeries.
2. Intra-operative use in coronary reperfusion, valve repair or replacement, congenital repair, hypertrophic obstructive cardiomyopathy, placement of durable devices (left and right assist devices [LVADs, RVADs]), pericardial window procedures, use in aortic dissections with possible valve involvement, and for endocarditis when pre-operative testing was inadequate or extension of infection to perivalvular tissue is suspected.

3. Peri-operative use in trauma patients with possible injuries to major vessels, tamponade, and increased risk of myocardial ischemia or infarction

### Contraindications

1. Absolute
   a. Patient refusal
   b. Previous full esophagectomy
   c. Severe esophageal obstruction
      i. Stricture, webs, rings, masses
   d. Esophageal perforation
   e. Ongoing esophageal hemorrhage

2. Relative
   a. Esophageal diverticulum, varices, fistula, and previous esophageal surgery including partial esophagectomy
   b. History of gastric surgery, mediastinal irradiation, or unexplained swallowing difficulties
   c. Other esophageal or gastric diseases that may be worsened by placement and manipulation of the TEE probe (Mallory–Weiss tear, scleroderma, etc.)

### Complications

1. Sore throat
2. Dental trauma
3. Submucosal hematoma
4. Jaw subluxation
5. Tonsillar bleeding
6. Esophageal or gastric perforation
7. Endotracheal tube migration or extubation

### TEE Probe Insertion

1. Inserted into an anesthetized patient like an orogastric tube, well-lubricated
2. The stomach should be emptied of gastric contents and air for best imaging prior to TEE probe placement.
3. Force should be avoided if resistance is encountered.
4. This is a semi-invasive procedure.

There are at least 28 basic views recommended for the comprehensive multiplane TEE examination. However, 11

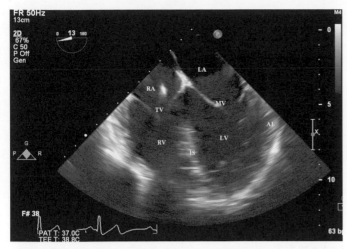

**Figure 36.1** Mid-esophageal 4-chamber view. Image credit: M. Singh.

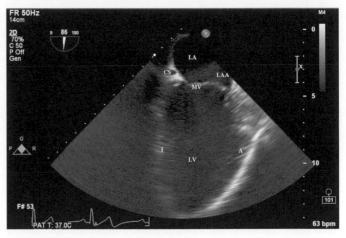

**Figure 36.2** Mid-esophageal 2-chamber view. Image credit: M. Singh.

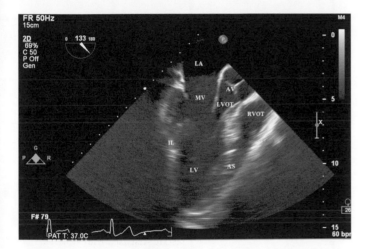

**Figure 36.3** Mid-esophageal long-axis view. Image credit: M. Singh.

basic views can provide diagnosis for most unstable surgical patients.

1. All of these views can be obtained by the placement of the TEE probe in three positions in the gastrointestinal tract: upper esophageal, mid-esophageal, and transgastric positions.
2. There can be significant individual variability and each suspected pathology should be verified in multiple views.

## Mid-esophageal 4-Chamber View (Fig. 36.1)

1. Commonly referred to as the "home base" view, it is one of the most comprehensive views available to evaluate cardiac anatomy and function.
2. Using the omniplane function, the probe should be adjusted until all of the following structures are identified: left atrium (LA), right atrium (RA), left ventricle (LV), right ventricle (RV), mitral valve (MV), tricuspid valve (TV), anterolateral wall of the LV (AL), and inferoseptal wall of the LV (IS). This is typically found at 0–10 degrees.
3. The mid-esophageal 4-chamber view is used to evaluate:

   a. LA, RA, RV, and LV size and function
   b. TV and MV anatomy and function
   c. Diastolic function
   d. The presence of atrial or ventricular septal defects
   e. Pericardial effusion
   f. Volume status and wall motion abnormalities
   g. Ejection fraction of the LV

## Mid-esophageal 2-Chamber View (ME 2Ch) (Fig. 36.2)

1. Using the omniplane function, the probe should be adjusted until all of the following structures are identified: LA, left atrial appendage (LAA), MV, LV, anterior wall of the LV, and inferior wall of the LV, and coronary sinus (CS). This is typically found at around 90 degrees.
2. The mid-esophageal 2-chamber view is used to evaluate:

   a. LV anterior and inferior wall size and function
   b. LV apex and presence or absence of apical thrombus
   c. MV disease and annular measurements
   d. Left atrial appendage mass, thrombus, or flow velocities

## Mid-esophageal Long-Axis View (ME LAX) (Fig. 36.3)

1. Using the omniplane function, the probe should be adjusted until all of the following structures are identified: LV, anteroseptal wall of the LV, inferolateral wall of the LV, left ventricular outflow tract (LVOT), right ventricular outflow tract (RVOT), aortic valve (AV), and MV. This is typically found at around 120 degrees.
2. The mid-esophageal long-axis view is used to evaluate:

   a. LV anteroseptal and posterior wall function
   b. LVOT diameter and pathology
   c. MV anatomy and function

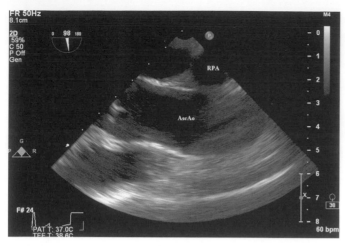

**Figure 36.4** Mid-esophageal ascending aortic long-axis view. Image credit: M. Singh.

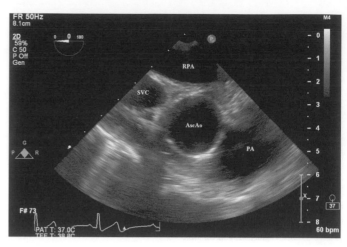

**Figure 36.5** Mid-esophageal ascending aortic short-axis view. Image credit: M. Singh.

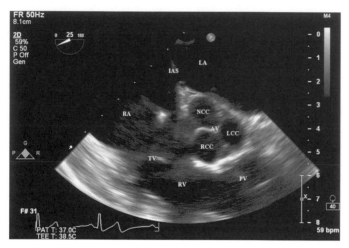

**Figure 36.6** Mid-esophageal aortic valve short-axis view. Image credit: M. Singh.

d. AV anatomy and function (only two AV cusps are visualized)

e. Interventricular septum pathology

## Mid-esophageal Ascending Aortic Long-Axis View (ME Asc Ao LAX)(Fig. 36.4)

1. Using the omniplane function and slight withdrawal of the probe, the probe should be adjusted until all of the following structures are identified: ascending aorta (Asc Ao) in the long-axis view and the right pulmonary artery (RPA) in the short-axis view.

2. The mid-esophageal ascending aortic long-axis view is used to evaluate:

   a. Ascending aorta in the long axis (atheroma, dissection, diameter)

   b. Pulmonary artery (PA) in the short axis

      i. Pulmonary embolus via visualization of the main and right pulmonary artery

   c. Pericardial effusion

## Mid-esophageal Ascending Aortic Short-Axis View (ME Asc Ao SAX)(Fig. 36.5)

1. "Great vessel view"

2. The probe should be adjusted until all of the following structures are identified: main PA in the long-axis, RPA in the long-axis, the proximal ascending aorta (Asc Ao) in the short-axis, and superior vena cava (SVC) in the short-axis.

3. The mid-esophageal ascending aortic short-axis view is used to evaluate:

   a. The ascending aorta dimensions and the presence of any dissection flaps

   b. The PA (pathology, diameter, thrombosis) and position of the tip of the PA catheter

   c. Central line catheter placement in the SVC

## Mid-esophageal Aortic Valve Short-Axis View (ME AV SAX) (Fig. 36.6)

1. The probe should be adjusted until all of the following structures are identified: AV, right (RCC), left (LCC), and noncoronary cusp (NCC), inter-atrial septum (IAS), LA, RA, TV, RV, and PV.

2. "Mercedes Benz" sign

3. The mid-esophageal aortic valve short-axis view is used to evaluate:

   a. The size, number, appearance, and motion of AV cusps

   b. The area of the AV orifice

   c. The presence of aortic insufficiency and/or aortic stenosis

   d. The integrity of the IAS, including patent foramen ovale (PFO) or other atrial septal defect (ASD)

   e. LA size

   f. Coronary artery pathology

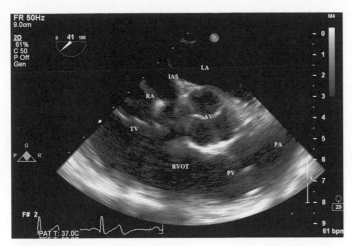

**Figure 36.7** Mid-esophageal right ventricular inflow–outflow view. Image credit: M. Singh.

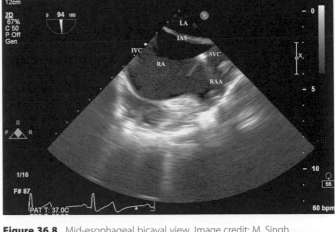

**Figure 36.8** Mid-esophageal bicaval view. Image credit: M. Singh.

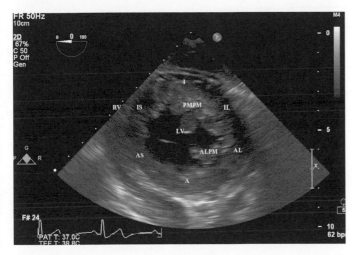

**Figure 36.9** Transgastric midpapillary short-axis view. Image credit: M. Singh.

## Mid-esophageal Right Ventricular Inflow–Outflow View (ME RV inflow-outflow) Fig. 36.7)

1. The probe should be adjusted until all of the following structures are identified: AV, TV, PV, PA, RVOT, LA, RA, and IAS.

2. The mid-esophageal right ventricular inflow–outflow is used to evaluate:

   a. PV anatomy and function (pulmonic insufficiency)
   b. RV and RVOT structure and function
   c. TV anatomy and function
   d. Passage of a PAC across the RV to the PA
   e. PA pathology
   f. Ventricular septal defect (VSD)

## Mid-esophageal Bicaval View (ME bicaval) (Fig. 36.8)

1. The probe should be adjusted until all of the following structures are identified: RA, SVC on the right, IAS, LA, and inferior vena cava (IVC) on the left of the screen.

2. The mid-esophageal bicaval view is used to evaluate:

   a. The integrity of the IAS to detect a PFO or ASD
   b. Real-time placement of catheters, wires, and venous cannula in both the SVC and IVC
   c. For the presence of thrombus or tumors

## Transgastric Midpapillary Short-Axis View (TG SAX) (Fig. 36.9)

1. To obtain this view, begin with the mid-esophageal 4-chamber view. With the LV in the center of the image, advance the probe into the stomach. Gently anteflex the probe and optimize the view so that both papillary muscles are imaged.

2. The probe should be adjusted until all of the following structures are identified: LV walls: (starting at noon and moving clockwise) inferior (I), inferolateral (IL), anterolateral (AL), anterior (A), anteroseptal (AS), inferoseptal (IS), papillary muscles: anterolateral (ALPM), posteromedial (PMPM), and RV.

3. The trans-gastric midpapillary ventricular short-axis view is used to evaluate:

   a. LV size, function, and cavity volume
   b. Interventricular septal motion, VSD
   c. Pericardial effusion
   d. Global ventricular systolic function and regional wall motion
   e. Volume status in the hemodynamically unstable patient
   f. Any wall motion abnormality. Each LV wall segment is supplied by a branch of coronary artery, such that territories of all three coronary arteries are seen simultaneously. Any new wall motion abnormality can signify potential ischemia.

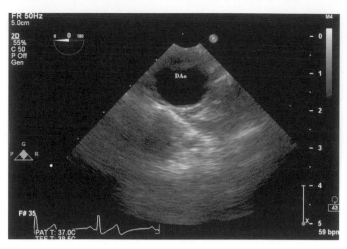

**Figure 36.10** Mid-esophageal descending aortic short-axis view. Image credit: M. Singh.

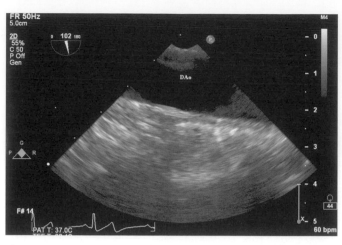

**Figure 36.11** Mid-esophageal descending aortic long-axis view. Image credit: M. Singh.

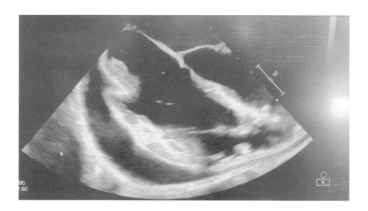

**Fig 36.12** Pericardial effusion TEE. Image credit: V. Dixit.

## Descending Aortic Short- and Long-Axis View (Desc Ao SAX, Desc Ao LAX) (Figs. 36.10–36.11)

1. To obtain this view, insert the probe to the mid-esophagus. Turn the probe to the left to find the aorta.
2. The probe should be adjusted until the descending aorta is identified.
3. The mid-esophageal descending aortic views are used to evaluate:
   a. Aortic pathology, atherosclerosis, aortic dissection, aortic insufficiency, intra-aortic balloon pump tip position, and left pleural effusion
   b. Right pleural effusion
   c. Placement of guidewires and cannula

## KO Treatment Plan

Since the patient is still under general anesthesia, a TEE can provide valuable information to rule in or out reasons for sudden deterioration. TEE is a relatively low-risk procedure and gives valuable information. In this patient, a TEE examination was performed and it showed pericardial effusion (Fig. 36.12). The pericardial effusion was drained by the cardiologist in the procedure room and a drain was left in place to avoid re-collection of fluid. The most likely cause of fluid collection was from perforation while performing the procedure. After drainage, the patient was stabilized and extubated with no complications.

# Extra Scenario TEE Images (Figs 36.13–36.16)

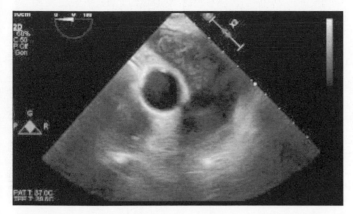

**Fig 36.13** Pulmonary emboli. Image credit: V. Dixit

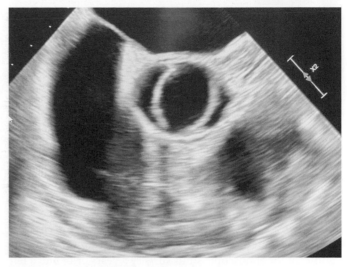

**Fig 36.14** Bicuspid aortic valve. Image credit: V. Dixit

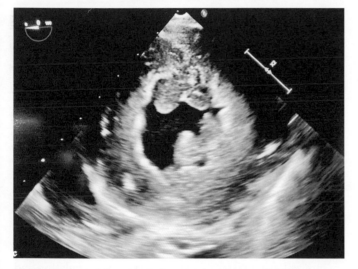

**Fig 36.15** Severe left ventricular hypertrophy. Image credit: V. Dixit

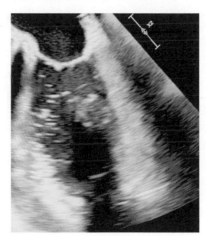

**Fig 36.16** Air in Ventricle. Image credit: V. Dixit.

# Bibliography

Barash PG, Cullen BF, Stoelting RK, et al. *Clinical Anesthesia*, 8th ed. Philadelphia: Lippincott Williams & Wilkins, 2017, pp. 735–41.

Butterworth JF, Mackey DC, Wasnick JD. *Morgan & Mikhail's Clinical Anesthesiology*, 6th ed. New York: McGraw-Hill Education, 2018, pp. 108–15.

Gropper MA. *Miller's Anesthesia*, 9th ed. Philadelphia: Elsevier, 2020, pp 1194–227.

Hahn RT, Abraham T, Adams MS, et al. Guidelines for performing a comprehensive transesophageal echocardiographic examination: recommendations from the American society of echocardiography and the society of cardiovascular anesthesiologists. *J Am Soc Echocardiography* 2013;26(9):921–64.

Reeves S, Finley A, Skubas N, et al. Basic perioperative transesophageal echocardiography examination: a consensus statement of the American Society of Echocardiography and the Society of Cardiovascular Anesthesiologists. *J Am Soc Echocardiography* 2012;26:443–56.

Toronto General Hospital Department of Anesthesia. Virtual transesophageal echocardiography standard and alternative views modules. Perioperative Interactive Education. http://pie.med.utoronto.ca/TEE (accessed January 3, 2023).

Varon AJ, Smith CE. *Essentials of Trauma Anesthesia*. New York: Cambridge University Press, 2012, pp. 138–153.

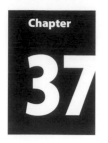

# Cardiopulmonary Bypass (CPB) and Associated Anticoagulation

Donald M. Voltz and Jessica A. Lovich-Sapola

## Sample Case

A 69-year-old female is scheduled to undergo a coronary revascularization, as well as an aortic valve replacement for severe aortic stenosis. Her past medical history is significant for a non-ST segment myocardial infarction (MI), hypertension, progressive aortic stenosis with mildly depressed left ventricular function, and diabetes mellitus. Her past surgical history is significant for endoscopic sinus surgery 3 years prior and a left femoral-distal bypass graft 2 years ago. She does not report any adverse anesthetic complications but does report a fall in her platelet count when she was hospitalized for lower extremity ischemia. What are your concerns? What pre-operative workup would you like? How does her medical history affect your intra-operative plans?

## Clinical Issues

### Basics of Cardiopulmonary Bypass (CPB)

1. CPB diverts venous blood (usually from the right atrium [RA]) away from the heart, adds oxygen, removes $CO_2$, and returns the blood through a cannula in a large artery (usually the ascending aorta or femoral artery).
2. Blood bypasses the heart and lungs.
3. CPB provides artificial ventilation and perfusion via the systemic circulation.
4. Nonphysiologic conditions
    a. Mean arterial pressure is less than normal.
    b. Nonpulsatile blood flow
5. To minimize damage
    a. Systemic hypothermia
    b. Topical hypothermia
    c. Cardioplegia

### Basic Circuit

1. Reservoir: receives the blood from the patient via venous cannulas in the RA, superior or inferior vena cava (SVC, IVC), or the femoral vein
2. Oxygenator: blood–gas interface
    a. Oxygenation of venous blood: one of the primary functions of the lungs
        i. During cardiac surgery and CPB, the surgeon places one or two cannula into the vena cava in order to drain venous blood into the CPB circuit's venous reservoir.
        ii. This blood is then passed through either a membrane or bubble oxygenator.
3. Heat exchanger: cooled or warmed by conduction
4. Main pump
    a. Roller pumps
    b. Centrifugal pumps
    c. Pulsatile pumps
5. Arterial filter: helps reduce systemic embolism by filtering particulate matter (thrombi, fat, tissue debris)
6. Accessory pumps and devices
    a. Cardiotomy suction: aspirates blood from the surgical field
    b. Left ventricular vent
    c. Cardioplegia pump
    d. Ultrafiltration: used to increase the patient's hematocrit during CPB without giving a transfusion

### Evaluation of Adequacy of Anticoagulation for CPB

1. Anticoagulation must be established before CPB to prevent acute disseminated intravascular coagulation and formation of clots in the CPB pump.
2. Heparin is often utilized for the following reasons:
    a. Consistent in its dose and the achievement of adequate anticoagulation
    b. Rapid onset time
    c. Easy to monitor in the operating room setting
    d. Adequate therapeutic window
    e. Specific means of reversing its effects to restore coagulation back to baseline
3. Adequacy of coagulation is usually confirmed by measuring the activated clotting time (ACT).
    a. ACT longer than 400–480 seconds is adequate.
    b. Heparin 300–400 units/kg is usually given before aortic cannulation (measure ACT 3–5 minutes after the heparin is given).
    c. If ACT is less than 400 seconds, give another 100 units/kg of heparin.
    d. Resistance to heparin can be seen in patients with antithrombin III deficiency; these patients require an

infusion of antithrombin III or fresh frozen plasma (FFP).

## Contraindications to Heparin Use

1. The only contraindication to the use of heparin for cardiac surgery is a history of heparin-induced thrombocytopenia (HIT).

   a. This is not entirely clear since some patients who have experienced HIT have been safely anticoagulated with a heparin for cardiac surgery.

## Potential Coagulation Problems that Occur with CPB

1. HIT: these patients produce heparin-dependent antibodies that agglutinate platelets and produce thrombocytopenia and occasionally thromboembolism.

   a. Develops in 5–28% of patients who receive heparin.

   b. There are two commonly agreed upon subtypes of this syndrome.

      i. HIT type I

         (1) Results in a mild decrease in the number and/or function of platelets following the administration of heparin

         (2) This drop in platelet levels is thought to be due to an enhanced aggregation of platelets.

         (3) Heparin binds to the surface of platelets and to platelet factor 4.

         (4) This binding facilitates platelets clumping together and these aggregates are removed from circulation by the reticulo-endothelial system.

      ii. HIT type II

         (1) More severe syndrome

         (2) Shares some similarity with type I

         (3) Patients who present with HIT type II tend to have received heparin for a longer time period (5–10 days).

         (4) There is a decrease in platelet levels due to aggregation and removal from circulation; however, there is an additional antibody-mediated effect.

            (a) Antibodies are generated and bind to the heparin-platelet factor 4 complex.

            (b) This leads to activation of the inflammatory system as well as activation of the complement cascade.

            (c) These reactions and activations lead to endothelial cell damage and additional activation and clumping of platelets at these areas of endothelial damage.

         (5) Thrombotic complications in patients with HIT have been reported to be as high as 20%, and if these clots occur in the heart, lungs, or brain, a mortality rate as high as 40% has been reported in patients.

   c. A final understanding of HIT has not yet been achieved.

      i. Measurement of antibody levels in patients who survive an HIT type II reaction become undetectable several weeks after cessation of heparin.

      ii. In addition, repeated exposure to heparin does not always reproduce the HIT type II reaction.

      iii. It is unclear what to do with these patients who are in need of cardiac surgery and anticoagulation.

      iv. There have been reports of patients who were removed from heparin for a number of weeks resulting in a disappearance of antibodies and then a safe, brief administration of heparin for CPB and surgery.

## Alternatives for Anticoagulation during CPB

There are a few experimental alternatives to heparin for anti-coagulation during cardiac surgery. None of these compounds have been FDA-approved for clinical use in CPB at this point; however, they have interesting properties and may at some point be used for clinical anticoagulation.

1. Bivalirudin

   a. Small peptide with a short half-life of 24 minutes

   b. It was synthesized from hirudin and acts by binding to the active site on thrombin, preventing its ability to cleave fibrinogen into fibrin.

   c. It is cleaved by thrombin itself, leading to elimination in the plasma, and is not dependent on an organ for its removal.

      i. There is no specific reversal agent for bivalirudin; one must wait for it to be cleaved by thrombin for restoration of normal clotting activity.

   d. In order to be used for cardiac surgery, a bolus is delivered followed by an infusion to maintain anticoagulation for the duration of the CPB.

   e. This peptide has been used for some interventional cardiology procedures; however, monitoring its activity is not as easy as for heparin.

   f. The anticoagulation effects of bivalirudin are not accurately measured with ACT and it is recommended that an ecarin clotting time (ECT) be utilized to guide therapeutic levels.

      i. The ECT is not a standard assay as of yet, making this difficult to use in surgery.

2. Hirudin
3. Anacrod
4. Argatroban

## Role of Antifibrinolytic Medications in CPB

1. The coagulation system tends to favor anticoagulation until endothelial damage occurs.
2. In a normal setting, the endothelial cells play a role in the prevention of platelet activation and aggregation, and the generation of fibrin clotting.
   a. Endothelial cell membranes contain heparin sulfate, which inhibits clotting factors.
   b. Endothelial cells are also responsible for releasing prostacyclin, which causes vasodilation and stabilizes platelet cells, preventing their activation and the formation of a platelet plug.
   c. Endothelial cells, except those present in the cerebral circulation, synthesize and display thrombomodulin on their cell surface.
      i. Thrombomodulin greatly decreases activation of the clotting cascade.
   d. When endothelial cells are damaged, these factors are no longer present and the balance is switched to a prothrombotic state in the local area where the endothelial cells are absent.
3. When endothelial cells become damaged, the subendothelial matrix becomes exposed and there is an activation of the clotting pathway.
4. Thrombosis occurs when both platelets and fibrin become intertwined, filling the area of endothelial damage.
   a. The first phase of clotting occurs (after endothelial damage) with a decrease in prostacyclin and an increase in thromboxane.
      i. This results in vasoconstriction.
   b. A platelet plug forms at the area of endothelial damage and this, coupled with the vasoconstriction, limits bleeding and provides a scaffolding upon which a clot can form.
5. Tissue factor becomes exposed when the endothelial cells are damaged, and is the primary initiator of the clotting cascade.
6. Thrombin appears to be the main initiator of clotting; however, it has a central role in turning off the clotting system once it has been inactivated when most of it is bound up into the clot by fibrin.
7. The final phase of coagulation is a remodeling of the clot and a direct repair of the endothelial cell injury by the fibrinolytic system.
8. CPB stimulates the coagulation system as well as the fibrinolytic system.

   a. Specific drugs are available to decrease the activation of the fibrinolytic system, decrease the destruction of clots, and decrease the amount of bleeding.
   b. During cardiac surgery, as well as other major surgeries where there is a supra-physiologic increase in the fibrinolytic system, the use of these agents can significantly decrease the amount of blood loss and thereby decrease the transfusion requirements.
   c. One must be cautious with their use, however, because complete inhibition of the fibrinolytic system can lead to an increased risk of thrombosis.
   d. Three main antifibrinolytic drugs are used to decrease peri-operative blood loss and decrease the number of blood transfusions.
      i. Epsilon-amino caproic acid (Amicar)
      ii. Tranexamic acid
      iii. Bovine pancreatic trypsin inhibitor (aprotinin)
      iv. Tranexamic acid and epsilon-amino caproic acid are lysine analogs that reversibly bind to plasminogen, preventing it from being activated.
      v. Aprotinin, a serine protease, decreases activation of fibrinolysis. This action is similar to that of epsilon-amino caproic acid and tranexamic acid; however, it also binds to kallikrein, an initiator of the clotting cascade, thereby limiting activation of the intrinsic clotting pathway.
         (1) Recently, aprotinin has not been used in cardiac surgery due to increases in renal dysfunction and higher cardiac mortality. Prolonged CPB has been implicated in peri-operative renal dysfunction and some authors argue that complex surgeries requiring prolonged CPB are more likely to receive aprotinin over the other antifibrinolytic agents.

## Additional Medications This Patient Might Have Been Exposed to That Can Lead to Coagulopathies during CPB

1. Patients often present to the operating room following an unsuccessful intervention in the cardiac catheterization lab.
   a. Antiplatelet medications
      i. A class of medications that are great for minimally invasive interventions such as balloon angioplasty or stenting.
      ii. Peri-operative period risk: increased blood loss
      iii. The most commonly used antiplatelet medication, especially in patients who are admitted to the hospital with an acute MI, is aspirin.
         (1) Aspirin irreversibly inhibits the enzyme cyclooxygenase, which is in the

prostaglandin synthesis pathway and leads to the production of thromboxane, a potent platelet activating molecule.

    (2) Aspirin, due to its irreversible inhibition of cyclooxygenase, causes platelet dysfunction for the life of the platelet: 10 days.

iv. In addition to aspirin, potent antiplatelet medications are used by cardiologists to decrease the risk of thrombosis in coronary arteries following interventions to restore their patency.

    (1) Glycoprotein IIb/IIIa receptor

    (2) This receptor is inhibited by a number of agents used in the cardiology suite.

        (a) Abciximab (Reopro)

        (b) Eptifibatide (Integrelin)

        (c) Tirofiban (Aggrastat)

            (i) All work by binding to this receptor and greatly decreasing the activation and aggregation potential of platelets.

            (ii) This is a great benefit when thrombogenic stents or the exposure of atherosclerotic plaques occur in angioplasty; however, when the patient proceeds to surgery, the lack of platelet function greatly limits the initial phase of clot formation.

v. A third class of antiplatelet medications acts by binding to and inhibiting platelet ADP receptors.

    (1) ADP is a potent molecular stimulant of platelet aggregation.

    (2) Ticlopidine (Ticlid) and clipidogrel (Plavix) are two medications in this class.

    (3) All of these medications have been shown to cause an increase in operative blood loss, leading to a higher incidence of peri-operative blood transfusions and/or a higher requirement for re-exploration due to bleeding or a bleeding complication such as cardiac tamponade.

2. Since none of these medications have specific reversal agents, the only treatment is to administer platelets to patients who have received these medications prior to cardiac surgery.

    a. One consideration we must be aware of with these medications is that they can have an effect on the platelets that are transfused as well as the patient's native platelets.

    b. Transfusion of platelets will interact with these medications until the free serum level of the antiplatelet medications is zero.

    c. To reduce the indiscriminate transfusion of platelets in these patients, specific platelet function testing may

be useful, although it can take time to perform in the operating room.

    d. The use of a thromboelastograph has shown some utility in the operating room to diagnose and monitor the treatment of platelet dysfunctions as well as other coagulopathies.

        i. Routine use of these devices has not yet occurred and some skill is required to interpret the results.

## Weaning from CPB

1. Assess systemic arterial pressure, ventricular volumes and filling pressures, and cardiac function on transesophageal echocardiogram (TEE).
2. Progressive clamping of the venous return line tubing
3. As the beating heart fills, ventricular ejection resumes.
4. Pump flow is gradually decreased.
5. Once the venous line is completely occluded and the systolic blood pressure is >80–90 mm Hg, the pump flow is stopped.

## Mode for the Reversal of Heparin after Separation from CPB

1. Heparin is the anticoagulant of choice for cardiac surgery.

    a. Quick onset

    b. Adequate therapeutic window

    c. Quick and effective reversal with protamine

2. The *in vivo* half-life of heparin is 90 minutes; however, this is far too long to allow for its natural removal for restoration of the coagulation system; therefore, IV protamine is used.
3. ACT returns to pre-anticoagulation levels within a few minutes from IV protamine due to the strong electrostatic interaction between heparin (negatively charged) and protamine (positively charged).

    a. Keep in mind that protamine itself can be a weak anticoagulant if an excessive amount is administered.

    b. Each milligram of protamine effectively neutralizes 100 U of heparin.

    c. In a standard cardiac case, the initial 300–400 U/kg administration of heparin is reversed, even though additional heparin may be used by the perfusionist during the course of CPB.

        i. The initial heparin dose is used for the reversal calculation to account for metabolism and removal of heparin from the system.

## Adverse Effects of Protamine

1. Protamine is a highly positively charged protein that binds effectively and inactivates heparin.
2. Adverse hemodynamic effects of protamine:

    a. Vasodilation

    b. Myocardial depression

c. Pulmonary hypertension
d. Anaphylaxis

  i. Patients who have been exposed to protamine or similar antigens in the past have the potential, albeit a rare adverse reaction, to develop an anaphylactic reaction resulting in profound vasodilatation and cardiovascular collapse.

    (1) Previous exposure
    (2) Fish allergies
    (3) Diabetics using insulin (NPH): since protamine is used to prolong insulin effects
    (4) Men who have undergone vasectomies or episodes of orchitis are also at risk for exposure to antigens leading to immunologic sensitization.

      (a) Treatment of this reaction is the same as any other anaphylactic reaction.

        (i) Support of the cardiovascular system
        (ii) Administration of diphenhydramine and epinephrine to block histamines effects as well as halt the degranulation of leukocytes

## Post-Bypass Period

1. Bleeding controlled
2. Bypass cannulas removed
3. Anticoagulation reversed
4. Chest closed
5. Goal: systolic blood pressure <140 mm Hg
6. Blood, colloids, and crystalloids are guided by the observation of the left ventricle on TEE, filling pressures, and post-bypass hematocrit

   a. Goal hematocrit is 25–30%.

## Post-Bypass Persistent Bleeding Differential Diagnosis

1. Inadequate surgical control
2. Incomplete reversal of heparin
3. Thrombocytopenia
4. Platelet dysfunction
5. Hypothermia-induced coagulation defects
6. Undiagnosed pre-operative hemostatic defects
7. Newly acquired factor deficiency or hypofibrinogenemia

## KO Treatment Plan

### Pre-operative

1. The anticoagulation in this patient can present some challenges.

a. The history of a fall in platelet count following her revascularization surgery is of note.
b. In patients who have had a drop in platelet count following the administration of heparin, one must be concerned about HIT.
c. An evaluation of her current platelet count should be done as well as a determination of the presence of antiheparin antibodies.

  i. This is a specialized test necessitating the involvement of a hematologist for administration and interpretation of the result.

d. Currently, there is no good clinical substitute in the United States for heparin.
e. Heparin has been used safely in CPB in patients who have a history of HIT; however, consultation with a hematologist would be warranted.

### Intra-operative

1. The presence of aortic stenosis along with coronary artery disease warrants a combined aortic valve replacement as well as coronary revascularization.

   a. This will prolong CPB and therefore place this patient at a higher risk for coagulopathies.

     i. Knowing this, as well as her history of thrombocytopenia, she will likely require the administration of platelets and possibly coagulation factors once she is weaned from CPB.

   b. Her prior history of vascular surgery suggests that she has been exposed not only to heparin, but also likely was reversed with protamine.

     i. Keeping this in mind will be important during reversal of her heparin.
     ii. Prior exposure to protamine places her at a small increased risk of undergoing an anaphylactic reaction to repeat exposure.
     iii. Test-dosing the protamine and closely monitoring for any adverse reaction will be important.

### Post-operative

1. Following the separation from CPB and the reversal of her heparinization with protamine, close monitoring of her coagulation system and blood count will determine whether additional platelets or clotting factors will be required.
2. With her prior history of thrombocytopenia, daily monitoring of her platelet level and potentially the measurement of antiheparin antibodies will be important to ensure she does not become profoundly coagulopathic.

# Bibliography

Barash PG, Cullen BF, Stoelting RK, et al. *Clinical Anesthesia*, 8th ed. Philadelphia: Lippincott Williams & Wilkins, 2017, pp. 1090–104.

Butterworth JF, Mackey DC, Wasnick JD. *Morgan & Mikhail's Clinical Anesthesiology*, 6th ed. New York: McGraw-Hill Education, 2018, pp. 443–94.

Castelli R, Casserino E, Cappellini MD, et al. Heparin induced thrombocytopenia: pathogenetic, clinical, diagnostic and therapeutic aspects. *Cardiovasc Hematol Disord Drug Targets* 2007;7(3):153–62.

Despotis GJ, Joist JH. Anticoagulation and anticoagulation reversal with cardiac surgery involving cardiopulmonary bypass: an update. *J Cardiothorac Vasc Anesth* 1999;13 (4 Suppl. 1):18–29.

Despotis GJ, Levine V, Hoist JH, et al. Antithrombin III during cardiac surgery: effect on response of activated clotting time to heparin and relationship to markers of hemostatic activation. *Anesth Analg* 1997;85 (3):498–506.

Gropper MA. *Miller's Anesthesia*, 9th ed. Philadelphia: Elsevier, 2020, pp. 1735–73.

Hartmann M, Sucker C, Boehm O, et al. Effects of cardiac surgery on hemostasis. *Transfus Med Rev* 2006;20 (3):230–41.

Kam PC. Anaesthetic management of a patient with thrombocytopenia. *Curr Opin Anesthesia* 2008;21(3):369–74.

Maslow AD, Chaudrey A, Bert A, et al. Perioperative renal outcome in cardiac surgical patients with preoperative renal dysfunction: aprotinin versus epsilon aminocaproic acid. *J Cardiothorac Vasc Anesth* 2008;22(1):6–15.

Miller, RD. *Miller's Anesthesia*, 6th ed. Philadelphia: Churchill Livingston, 2005.

Ngaage DL, Cale A, Cowen A, et al. Aprotinin in primary cardiac surgery: operative outcome of propensity score-matched study. *Ann Thorac Surg* 2008;86(4):1195–202.

Taneja R, Fernandes P, Marwaha G, et al. Perioperative coagulation management and blood conservation in cardiac surgery: a Canadian survey. *J Cardiothorac Vasc Anesth* 2008;22(5):662–9.

Warkentin, TES. Heparin-induced thrombocytopenia and the anesthesiologists. *Can J Anaesth* 2002;49:S36–S49.

Young, JA, Kisker CT, Doty, DB. Adequate anticoagulation during cardiopulmonary bypass determined by activated clotting time and the appearance of fibrin monomers. *Ann Thorac Surg* 1978;26:231.

**Chapter**

# 38

# Carotid Surgery

Adrienne Gomez and Matthew A. Joy

## Sample Case

An 80-year-old male with a past medical history of moderate left carotid artery stenosis presents for a left carotid endarterectomy (CEA). How would you monitor the patient's central nervous system (CNS) during the procedure? Would you use a regional or general anesthetic? Why?

## Clinical Issues

### Introduction

1. One of the more challenging cases facing anesthesiologists is the management of the patient presenting for a CEA.

   a. The patient population presenting with carotid atherosclerotic stenosis (CAS) typically possesses multiple medical problems.

      i. Coronary artery disease (CAD): may predispose the patient to significant hemodynamic changes in the operating room.

         (1) Accordingly, cardiac complications arising peri-operatively during CEA still remain a major source of morbidity and mortality.

      ii. Hypertension
      iii. Diabetes
      iv. Tobacco abuse and its associated pulmonary consequences
      v. Angina and previous myocardial infarction

2. The current ACC/AHA guidelines for cardiac risk stratification for noncardiac surgical procedures list carotid surgery as an intermediate-risk procedure.

   a. Reported risk: 1–5%
   b. The anesthesiologist managing these patients with cardiovascular disease is encouraged to read these guidelines closely.

### Definition of CEA

1. CEA is a surgical procedure that attempts to revascularize the carotid artery via the removal of an atherosclerotic plaque.
2. CEA is one of the more commonly performed vascular procedures in the United States, with approximately 130,000 performed annually.
3. Locations

   a. Bifurcation of the common carotid artery into the internal and external carotid arteries
   b. Proximal internal carotid artery

4. Enlargement of luminal plaques results in narrowing and ulceration, thus CEA surgery is done to reduce the potential risk of transient ischemic attacks (TIA) and stroke in selected patients.
5. Plaques tend to form at arterial branches due to turbulent blood flow.

### Pre-operative Assessment

1. The patient presenting for CEA surgery poses numerous issues for the surgeon and anesthesiologist.
2. Patient selection is critical for successful outcomes, and although operative candidates are primarily determined by the vascular or neurosurgeon performing the procedure, the anesthesiologist should be familiar with the published guidelines for appropriate patient choice and identification of risk factors and predictors of morbidity and mortality, which may have an impact on outcome.

   a. The general indications are that symptomatic patients with angiographic evidence of 70–99% carotid stenosis are candidates for a CEA.
   b. Individuals should not be considered for surgery if the stenosis is less than 50%.
   c. For asymptomatic disease with stenosis of 60–99%, CEA can be considered.
   d. Stratification of symptomatic versus asymptomatic disease is only one part of the criterion for selection of patients for surgery.
   e. Other clinical data should be ascertained prior to a CEA (see the following).

3. Critical information obtained should include the following:

   a. Overall pre-operative health status

      i. Presence of clinical markers

         (1) Major, intermediate, and minor clinical predictors
         (2) Functional capacity
         (3) Cardiac risk of the noncardiac procedure: as mentioned, CEA is typically regarded as an intermediate-risk procedure.

b. Comprehensive cardiac evaluation is indicated in selected patients.

   i. Typically those patients with major clinical predictors of increased cardiac risk have the following:

     (1) Unstable coronary syndromes

     (2) Decompensated heart failure

     (3) Significant arrhythmias

       (a) High-grade atrioventricular block

       (b) Symptomatic ventricular arrhythmias in the presence of underlying heart disease

       (c) Supraventricular arrhythmias with an uncontrolled ventricular rate

     (4) Severe valvular disease

4. The ultimate goal is to identify patients who are at significant risk for adverse myocardial outcomes and reduce the risk by either peri-operative management (e.g., aggressive β-blockade, blood pressure control, smoking cessation) or pre-operative cardiac intervention, as might be the case in the very small subset of patients with highly symptomatic coronary disease and carotid stenosis.

## Surgical Considerations

1. The degree of carotid stenosis of the ipsilateral artery as well as the degree of contralateral carotid disease is critical for collateral perfusion during cross-clamping.

2. Clearly define whether the patient is presenting for asymptomatic versus symptomatic revascularization.

  a. This has direct ramifications on surgical indication, risk stratification, and post-operative neurologic outcome.

   i. Categorization of patients into symptomatic versus asymptomatic is derived from the combined results of multiple prospective trials, from which these evidence-based recommendations are derived.

   ii. The type of symptoms, if present, should also be clearly delineated as part of the patient's risk profile, as these variables are also factored in patient selection, prognostication, and timing of surgery.

     (1) TIA

     (2) Reversible ischemic neurologic deficit (RIND)

     (3) Cerebral vascular accident (CVA)

     (4) Neurologically symptomatic patients

       (a) Active pre-operative TIAs are typically in need of more urgent carotid revascularization than the patient with a recent CVA.

3. As previously mentioned, the angiographic anatomy has a direct bearing on patient selection and outcome predictions.

  a. Additionally, the native carotid anatomy influences the selection of:

   i. Neuromonitoring: EEG, BIS, carotid stump pressure, cerebral oximetry

   ii. Surgical approach: shunting, patch angioplasty

   iii. Anesthetic choice: regional, local, and general anesthesia

## Anesthetic Approaches

1. Regional technique (awake)

  a. Several different approaches have been described for performing regional anesthesia for a CEA.

   i. Adequate blockade of the C2–C4 dermatomes via a cervical plexus block (CPB) either deep, intermediate, and/or superficial block or an intermediate CPB provides adequate anesthesia for CEA. Deep and superficial CPBs are more commonly utilized. Both blocks have advantages and disadvantages, but both are considered to be equally efficacious.

     (1) Deep CPB

       (a) Frequently utilized because of its reliability

       (b) Most commonly employed regional technique for CEA

       (c) Disadvantages

        (i) Diaphragmatic dysfunction: due to inadvertent phrenic nerve block

        (ii) Greater risk of epidural, subarachnoid, and vertebral artery injection

        (iii) Horner's syndrome

        (iv) Unintentional blockade of the recurrent laryngeal and vagus nerves

     (2) Superficial CPB

       (a) Lower reported complication rate and easier to perform than the technically challenging deep CPB, the superficial CPB may be the preferred technique for regional CEA anesthesia in selected patients.

   ii. Cervical epidural block (CEB)

     (1) Utilized by a few experienced regional anesthesiologists via a catheter placed in the epidural space

     (2) This technique has not gained widespread use due to the potential of associated

blockade of the thoracic nerve roots which could result in hypotension, bradycardia, and possible respiratory failure due to changes in pulmonary function.

(3) This block has not been reported to be more efficacious than both deep and superficial CPB, and carries more risk potential; therefore, it is typically not recommended.

iii. Local anesthetic infiltration block

(1) Straight local anesthetic infiltration performed by either the surgeon or anesthesiologist

(2) This technique is rarely performed due to inefficacy, resulting commonly in significant patient discomfort.

b. Despite regional modalities being utilized much less frequently than general anesthesia for CEA, the CPB remains a useful technique in selected patients undergoing this procedure, especially when there is concern of severe carotid disease and possible plaque embolization during the surgery, which might not be discernible in an unconscious patient under general anesthesia regardless of the neuromonitoring techniques employed.

c. Regional techniques can be supplemented with intravenous sedation; however, the anesthesiologist must always be cognizant of the level of sedation to facilitate neurologic assessment throughout the surgery.

d. Unlike cerebral monitors, which lack sensitivity and specificity (see the following), an awake patient provides a very specific and sensitive indicator of cerebral function.

e. Before one embarks upon a regional technique, it is imperative that this approach be acceptable to both the surgeon and patient; hence a lengthy discussion regarding the anesthetic plan and expectations should be held with both the patient and surgeon pre-operatively.

**TKO:** It is beyond the scope of this chapter to review the detailed techniques involved in performing the previously mentioned blocks. However, anesthesiologists should be familiar with the CPB, and an ABA candidate should be able to accurately describe the technique employed, regional anatomy, landmarks, distribution of anesthesia, block dynamics, choice of local anesthetic, and possible complications involved. Additional reading can be obtained from any standard regional anesthesia textbook and the informative website www.nysora.com.

2. General anesthesia

a. The majority of CEA cases in North America are still performed with a general anesthetic technique.

b. Although an awake patient is considered the gold standard for cerebral monitoring for a CEA, there is

no conclusive evidence that this procedure is best performed under a regional technique.

c. In addition to maintaining hemodynamic stability, a general anesthetic poses additional challenges compared to regional techniques.

i. Unlike regional anesthesia, additional neuromonitoring techniques may need to be employed for assessment of cerebral perfusion, since an awake responsive patient is no longer an option (see below for neuromonitoring techniques).

d. Several different techniques for general anesthesia have been proposed, each with purportedly superior advantages.

i. Total intravenous anesthesia techniques (TIVA)

(1) Induction and maintenance with propofol and remifentanil

(2) Advocates cite superior hemodynamic stability and rapid emergence as justification for this particular technique.

ii. Inhalational technique

(1) Takes advantage of the theoretical improved cerebral protection with agents such as isoflurane as the basis of their selection

(2) It is recommended that if used as part of a general anesthetic technique, nitrous oxide should be discontinued prior to carotid artery cross-clamping in order to minimize the risk of air embolism that may occur during this phase of the procedure.

e. Regardless of the general anesthetic technique employed, the overall goal should remain the same.

i. Blunting of noxious stimuli: intubation, incision, surgical pain and the associated stress response

ii. Protection of vital organs from ischemic injury, including the heart and brain

iii. Peri-operative hemodynamic stability, including heart rate and blood pressure control

iv. Maintaining cardiovascular stability (especially in this patient population)

v. Expeditious emergence from the anesthetic, allowing for rapid neurologic assessment

vi. An anesthetic that does not negatively impact the neuromonitoring technique employed (see below) for the surgery

## Monitoring Techniques

1. Standard ASA monitors
2. Continuous ST monitoring of leads II and V5
3. Direct invasive intra-arterial blood pressure monitoring

4. Rarely is pulmonary artery catheter (PAC) monitoring indicated for this surgery. The routine use of this catheter for CEA procedures is unsupported.
5. Cerebral monitors
   a. A regional anesthetic technique with an awake and responsive patient likely provides the gold standard neurologic monitor for CEA procedures.
   b. General anesthetics require other modalities of monitoring cerebral ischemia, and anesthesiologists should be aware of the advantages and disadvantages of the various techniques employed.
      i. A 16-channel electroencephalogram (EEG)
         (1) Considered by some sources as the gold standard of neuromonitoring under general anesthesia
            (a) Monitors cortical surface cells electrical activity
            (b) During occlusion of the carotid artery, EEG changes occur in 20% of patients.
            (c) Post-operative neurologic changes are associated with EEG changes lasting over 10 minutes.
            (d) Ischemia is noted on EEG as decreased frequency and amplitude, with isoelectric readings being associated with severe ischemia.
         (2) Advantages
            (a) Readily available
            (b) Reliability
            (c) Correlation with cerebral ischemia
         (3) Disadvantages
            (a) Possible need for a trained technician for interpretation
            (b) High false positive rate
            (c) Possible anesthetic agent influences
            (d) Inability to detect subcortical ischemia
            (e) Focal embolic events may be missed
      ii. Processed EEG: BIS monitoring techniques
         (1) Advantages
            (a) Availability
            (b) Ability to identify severe cerebral ischemia
            (c) Ease of use
         (2) Limitations
            (a) Reliability
            (b) Inability to detect focal ischemia
      iii. Somatosensory evoked potentials (SSEP)
         (1) Advantages

            (a) Equivalent efficacy to EEG
            (b) Detects deep brain structure injury
         (2) Disadvantages
            (a) Complexity
            (b) Need for a trained technician
            (c) Limitations of inhalational anesthetic use due to effects on interpretation
      iv. Transcranial Doppler (TCD)
         (1) Advantages
            (a) Ability to monitor cross-clamp hypoperfusion and shunt malfunction
            (b) Ability to assess cerebral blood flow and embolic phenomena
         (2) Limitations
            (a) Technical complexity involving monitor placement and interpretation of TCD data
            (b) May require additional trained personnel
      v. Cerebral oximetry devices (i.e., near-infrared spectrophotometry [NIRS])
         (1) Advantages
            (a) Simplicity of use
         (2) Disadvantages
            (a) Low sensitivity and specificity
      vi. Carotid stump pressure (CSP)
         (1) This is a simple technique in which the surgeon measures the mean arterial carotid pressure distal to the cross-clamp.
         (2) Presently, clinicians utilize 50 mm Hg as a cutoff for shunting.
         (3) Advantages
            (a) Simplicity
            (b) Lack of expense
         (4) Disadvantages
            (a) Lack of validation
            (b) Lack of a critical CSP value in assessing collateral flow, below which a shunt should be placed
6. The importance of such monitoring
   a. There is a subsequent clinical response if signs of altered cerebral perfusion are noted during carotid cross-clamping, which in most centers is the placement of a carotid shunt (selective shunting).
   b. The anesthesiologist managing these patients along with the candidate preparing for a clinical scenario of

CEA should be aware of the signs and indexes of altered perfusion of these devices, especially the CSP, its clinical significance, and implication for intra-operative management.

# KO Treatment Plan

## Pre-operative

1. Complete history and physical

   a. Patients often have multiple associated medical problems.

      i. CAD: angina and myocardial ischemia
      ii. Hypertension
      iii. Diabetes
      iv. History of CVA
         (1) Ask about residual symptoms.
         (2) This is especially relevant if a regional technique is planned (i.e., the patient must be able to follow commands).
      v. Smoking history and related lung pathology

2. Labs

   a. This patient population is frequently on anticoagulant therapy.

      i. Check with the prescribing physician before discontinuation, bridging therapy if needed, and timing of therapy resumption.
         (1) Especially in the case of clopidogrel and warfarin
      ii. These patients and others at risk for coagulation defects should have at minimum the following labs:
         (1) Coagulation panel (PT, INR, PTT)
         (2) A complete blood count (CBC) and electrolyte panel for baseline values for all patients
         (3) For anemic patients, a blood type and screen is probably not unreasonable.

3. Cardiac workup

   a. EKG
   b. A comprehensive cardiac evaluation should be done in any patient who is considered to have major clinical predictors of increased cardiac risk.

4. Pulmonary workup

   a. Chest X-ray in select patients

      i. Chronic obstructive pulmonary disease (COPD)
      ii. Cardiopulmonary pathology

## Intra-operative

1. The anesthetic technique chosen should be the best suited for the anesthesiologist, the patient, and the surgeon.

   a. Regardless of whether regional or general techniques are implemented, the goals are the same.

      i. Avoid ischemic injury to the brain.
      ii. Maintain adequate cerebral perfusion.
      iii. Maintain cardiovascular stability.
      iv. Provide a rapid anesthetic recovery allowing for a neurologic exam.

   b. Select one patient-specific anesthetic plan and defend it.
   c. For this particular case, a general anesthetic was chosen. After consultation with the surgeon it was deemed that a general anesthetic would allow for better surgical exposure in this patient with complex carotid anatomy. The patient also preferred a general anesthetic due to a previous unpleasant experience with regional anesthesia.
   d. For other cases of CEA, a regional technique might be a preferred method, and the ABA candidate should be prepared to discuss it.

2. Pre-induction arterial catheter for continuous blood pressure monitoring
3. Pre-medication with judicious amounts of intravenous fentanyl and lidocaine to blunt the sympathetic response to direct laryngoscopy
4. Application of the standard ASA monitors
5. Intravenous induction with etomidate for hemodynamic stability
6. Placement of the endotracheal tube

   a. Monitor the patient closely during laryngoscopy.
   b. Treat elevations of heart rate or blood pressure with short-acting medications such as esmolol and judicious amounts of opioid.
   c. Be prepared to treat sudden hypotension on induction with bolus dosing of phenylephrine.

7. Maintenance of anesthesia would include isoflurane, based upon its purported cerebral protective effects, and a remifentanil infusion, based on its short half-life, which allows for a rapid anesthetic emergence.

   a. Phenylephrine and nitroglycerin infusions should be prepared and available in advance for administration in the event of significant hemodynamic changes as needed.

8. Cerebral monitoring

   a. CSP

      i. Simple technique
      ii. Inexpensive
      iii. Commonly used

b. Processed EEG (BIS): especially if an EEG is not available or practical

    i. Ease of use

    ii. Readily available

    iii. Interpret cautiously, as it is not validated for this particular indication and may not reliably detect cerebral ischemia.

**TKO:** Be prepared to discuss all of the techniques of cerebral monitoring for CEA.

## Post-operative

1. The patient should be monitored closely in either the intensive care unit or on a telemetry floor.

    a. CEA surgery is associated with significant hemodynamic lability for the first 24 hours.

# Bibliography

Allain R, Marone LK, Meltzer J, Jeyabalan G. Carotid endarterectomy. *Int Anesthesiol Clin* 2005;**43**(1):15–38.

Augoustides J, Gutsche J. Anesthesia for carotid endarterectomy and carotid stenting. In Nussmeler N, ed., *UpToDate*, 2020. www.uptodate.com/contents/anesthesia-for-carotid-endarterectomy-and-carotid-stenting (accessed March 8, 2022).

Barrett J, Harmon D, Loughnane F, Finucane B, Shorten G. *Peripheral Nerve Blocks and Peri-operative Pain Relief.* London: Saunders Elsevier, 2004, pp. 51–4.

Chaturvedi S, Bruno A, Feasby T, et al. Carotid endarterectomy: an evidence-based review: report of the Therapeutics and Technology Assessment Subcommittee of the American Academy of Neurology. *Neurology* 2005;**65**(6):794–801.

Chelly JE, *Peripheral Nerve Blocks: A Color Atlas*, 3rd ed. Philadelphia: Lippincott Williams & Wilkins, 2009, pp. 162–8.

Erickson KM, Cole DJ. Review of developments in anesthesia for carotid endarterectomy. *Curr Opin Anesthesiol* 2005;**18**:466–7.

European Carotid Surgery Trialists Collaborative Group. Endarterectomy for moderate symptomatic carotid stenosis: interim results from the MRC European Carotid Surgery Trial. *Lancet* 1996;**347**:1591–3.

Farhoomand L, Berger J, Lehfeldt S. Controversies in anesthesia for carotid endarterectomy: general versus regional anesthesia. *Semin Anesth Periop Med Pain* 2004;**23**(30):244–7.

Ferguson GG, Eliasziw M, Barr HW, et al. The North American Symptomatic Carotid Endarterectomy Trial: surgical results in 1415 patients. *Stroke* 1999;**30**:1751–8.

Fleisher LA, Beckman JA, Brown KA, et al. ACC/AHA 2014 Guidelines on perioperative cardiovascular evaluation and care for noncardiac surgery: a report of the American College of Cardiology/American Heart Association Task Force on Practice Guidelines (Writing Committee to Revise the 2002 Guidelines on Perioperative Cardiovascular Evaluation for Noncardiac Surgery). *Circulation* 2014;**130**:e278–e333.

Hadzic A. *Textbook of Regional Anesthesia and Acute Pain Management.* New York: McGraw-Hill Medical, 2007.

Hobson RW, Weiss DG, Fields WS, et al. Efficacy of carotid endarterectomy for asymptomatic carotid stenosis: the Veterans Affairs Cooperative Study Group. *N Engl J Med* 1993;**328**(4):221–7.

Huncke T, Bekker A. Carotid endarterectomy: anesthetic choices and cerebral monitoring. *Curr Rev Clin Anesth* 2008;**28**:239.

Ivanec Z, Mazul-Sunkol B, Lovricević I, et al. Superficial versus combined (deep and superficial) cervical plexus block for carotid endarterectomy. *Acta Clin Croat* 2008;**47**(2):81–6.

Kaplan JA, Lake CL, Murray MJ. *Vascular Anesthesia*, 2nd ed. Philadelphia: Elsevier, Churchill Livingston, 2004, pp. 93–105.

Kaplan JA, Lake CL, Murray MJ. *Vascular Anesthesia*, 2nd ed. Philadelphia: Elsevier, Churchill Livingston, 2004, pp 187–98.

Maharaj R. A review of recent developments in the management of carotid artery stenosis. *J Cardiothorac Vasc Anesth* 2008;**22**(2):277.

Miller RD, Fleisher LA, Johns RA, et al. *Anesthesia*, 9th ed. New York: Churchill Livingstone, 2005, pp. 1855–64

OpenAnesthesia. Carotid endarterectomy: CNS monitoring. www.openanesthesia.org/carotid_endarterectomy_cns_monitoring (accessed April 19, 2022).

Pandit JJ, Satya-Krishna R, Gration P. Superficial or deep cervical plexus block for carotid endarterectomy: a systematic review of complications. *Br J Anaesth* 2007;**99**(2):159–69.

Rerkasem K, Rothwell PM. Local versus general anaesthesia for carotid endarterectomy. Cochrane Database Syst Rev 2008;**4**:CD000126.

Schwartz AJ, Matjasko MJ, Otto CW, et al. *Refresher Courses in Anesthesiology*, vol. **31**. Philadelphia: Lippincott Williams & Wilkins, 2003, pp. 91–103.

Yastrebov K. Intraoperative management: carotid endarterectomies. *Anesthesiol Clin N Am* 2004;**22**(2):265–87.

# Mediastinal Mass

Maureen S. Harders

## Sample Case

A 28-year-old male presents to his primary care doctor with weight loss and a nonproductive cough. He is diagnosed with a mediastinal mass. He presents to the operating room for a diagnostic mediastinoscopy. What are your concerns? How will you induce anesthesia?

## Clinical Issues

### Definition

1. The mediastinum contains all of the organs in the chest except for the lungs.

   a. Heart
   b. Aorta
   c. Thymus
   d. Trachea
   e. Esophagus
   f. Nerves
   g. Lymph nodes
   h. Superior and inferior vena cava

2. The mediastinum is divided into three parts.

   a. The anterior portion is bordered by the sternum anteriorly and the pericardium posteriorly.
   b. The middle mediastinum is defined as the pericardium and all of its contents.
   c. The posterior mediastinum is defined as the area posterior to the pericardial wall and anterior to the thoracic vertebral bodies.

3. Masses in the anterior mediastinum are more likely to be malignant.

4. The four most common masses are the thymoma, (terrible) lymphoma, teratoma, and the ectopic thyroid (the 4 Ts).

5. Myasthenia gravis is present in 25% of patients diagnosed with a mediastinal mass. Consider this in your anesthetic plan.

### Mediastinoscopy

1. Indications

   a. Visualization of the contents of the mediastinum
   b. To assess the spread of bronchial carcinoma
   c. Staging of lymph nodes

   d. Diagnosis of sarcoidosis
   e. Diagnosis of lymphoma

2. Contraindications (relative)

   a. Previous mediastinoscopy (because of scarring)
   b. Superior vena cava (SVC) syndrome
   c. Thoracic aortic aneurysm
   d. Cerebrovascular disease: occlusion of the innominate artery can cause cerebral ischemia in patients with already compromised cerebral blood flow.
   e. Tracheal deviation

3. Complications

   a. Hemorrhage
   b. Pneumothorax
   c. Infection
   d. Recurrent laryngeal nerve injury
   e. Pressure on the right innominate (brachiocephalic) artery can cause decreased cerebral perfusion as well as decreased blood flow to the right upper extremity.
   f. Chylothorax
   g. Hemothorax
   h. Venous air embolism

## Differential Diagnosis of Increased Airway Resistance

1. Bronchospasm
2. Foreign body
3. Tension pneumothorax
4. Endobronchial intubation
5. Poor compliance secondary to lung disease
6. Mediastinal mass

## KO Treatment Plan

### Pre-operative

1. Review the patient's symptoms.

   a. Dyspnea with positional changes

      i. Shortness of breath in the supine position

   b. Hoarse voice or noisy breathing
   c. Dysphagia
   d. Signs of SVC obstruction

   i. Cerebral edema

     (1) Headache

     (2) Mental status change

     (3) Confusion

     (4) Coma

   ii. Facial cyanosis and flushing

  iii. Venous distension in the neck

   iv. Venous distension of the upper arms and chest

    v. Upper limb edema

   vi. Lightheadedness

  vii. Upper airway edema

     (1) Cough

     (2) Dyspnea

     (3) Dysphagia

     (4) Stridor

2. Review the pertinent studies.

  a. CT scan: look for tracheal or main stem bronchial compression.

  b. Flow volume loops: collapse during expiration is a sign of intrathoracic compression.

  c. Echocardiogram: look for right ventricular (RV) outflow obstruction and/or right heart dysfunction.

3. If there is severe obstruction of the airway or right ventricular outflow tract (RVOT), discuss with the surgeon the possibility of performing the mediastinoscopy under local anesthesia. This will help avoid the possibility of further compression on the RVOT, which could lead to cardiovascular collapse.

4. Remember that respiratory complications in the peri-operative period may occur even though pre-operative studies would not have predicted difficulties.

# Intra-operative

1. Monitors and intravenous (IV) access

  a. A large-bore IV is needed. Consider a lower extremity IV if there is significant compression on the SVC.

  b. A right radial arterial line is very sensitive and will dampen with pressure of the mediastinoscope on the innominate artery.

  c. The pulse oximeter waveform can also be used to help alert the anesthesiologist to pressure being placed on the innominate artery, but is not quite as sensitive or as reliable as the arterial line.

  d. Consider bilateral femoral lines if there is a possibility of complete airway obstruction and the need to start cardiopulmonary bypass or femorofemoral ECMO (extracorporeal membrane oxygenation). May consider placing

these under local anesthesia prior to induction if the mass is large.

  e. Have two units of cross-matched blood available. Remember that the mediastinum is full of large blood vessels.

2. Airway management

  a. The goal is to not give up the airway.

  b. Keep the patient breathing spontaneously. Spontaneous respirations help maintain a normal transpulmonary pressure gradient and help distend the airway.

  c. Avoid muscle relaxation since it can diminish airway tone. This may be critical to the patient for maintaining his airway.

  d. Awake fiber-optic intubation with a reinforced endotracheal tube should be the first option for a patient who has an obstruction.

  e. An inhalational induction with sevoflurane in the sitting position is also a consideration. Remember that you may lose the airway as the induction proceeds, and you must be prepared to deal with that complication.

3. Lost-airway maneuvers

  a. Change the patient's position to lateral or prone.

  b. Reverse the muscle relaxant.

  c. Try to get the patient breathing spontaneously.

  d. Use a rigid bronchoscope to push past the obstruction.

4. Maintaining spontaneous respirations will not only aid in maintaining the airway but it is also important in patients with RVOT obstruction, since compression of the RVOT can lead to cardiovascular collapse.

  a. Intermittent positive pressure ventilation (IPPV) may decrease the cardiac output.

  b. The supine position also may aggravate the RV outflow obstruction.

  c. Pressure from the mass may also cause arrythmias

# Post-operative

1. Extubation

  a. The patient needs to be watched closely. He may develop a complication that requires reintubation due to increased airway obstruction from swelling or impaired respiratory muscle function.

  b. Respiratory complications including airway obstruction occur with a higher incidence in patients with greater than 50% compression of the trachea in pre-operative exams.

2. Patients who remain intubated may need pressure control ventilation to maintain an open airway.

# Bibliography

Barash PG, Cullen BF, Stoelting RK, et al. *Clinical Anesthesia*, 8th ed. Philadelphia: Lippincott Williams & Wilkins, 2017, pp. 1059–61.

Bechard P, Letourneau L, Laacasse Y, et al. Perioperative cardio-respiratory complications in adults with mediastinal mass: incidence and risk factors. *Anesthesiology* 2004; **100**(4): 826–34.

Brodsky JB. *Thoracic Anesthesia: Problems in Anesthesia*, vol. **4**. Philadelphia: Lippincott, 1990, pp. 334–8.

Erdos, G, Tzanova, I. Perioperative anesthetic management of mediastinal masses in adults. *Eur J Anesthesiol* 2009;**26**(8):627–32.

Gropper MA. *Miller's Anesthesia*, 9th ed. Philadelphia: Elsevier, 2020, pp. 1688, 1705–7.

# Treatment of Elevated Intracranial Pressure

Adrienne Gomez and Jessica A. Lovich-Sapola

## Sample Case

A 19-year-old male presents to the emergency room after falling two stories from a balcony. He is confused and agitated. His blood pressure is 198/99 mm Hg and his heart rate is 110 beats/min. The emergency medical services reports that the patient had one episode of emesis during his transport to the hospital. On examination his pupils are dilated. How do you determine whether the patient's intracranial pressure (ICP) is increased? Why is it important to know? If elevated, what steps would you take to reduce ICP?

The neurosurgeon determines that the patient requires an emergent surgery. Immediately after opening the skull, the surgeon says that the dura is taut. How will you treat this? The surgeon says the brain is bulging. What are your next steps in management?

## Clinical Issues

### ICP

1. The normal ICP wave is pulsatile and varies with spontaneous respiration.
2. The mean ICP should remain below 15 mm Hg.
   a. Sustained ICPs over 20 mm Hg leads to worsened outcomes.
   b. With ICP >30 mm Hg, cerebral blood flow (CBF) progressively decreases. The resulting ischemia leads to edema which leads to increased ICP and more ischemia. If left untreated, this cycle will continue until the patient dies from progressive neurologic damage and herniation.
3. Treatment of elevated ICP should begin once it reaches values of greater than 20–25 mm Hg. Higher values may be tolerated if the cerebral perfusion pressure (CPP) is adequate.
4. CPP = mean arterial pressure (MAP) – ICP or central venous pressure (CVP) (whichever is greater).
   a. Goal CPP in the range of 60–70 mm Hg
   b. CPP <60 mm Hg adversely affects brain tissue oxygenation and metabolism.

### Signs and Symptoms of Elevated ICP

1. Altered and/or loss of consciousness
2. Dilated or nonreactive pupils

3. Flexor or extensor posturing
4. Nausea and vomiting
5. Headache
6. Papilledema
7. Focal neurologic deficits

### Causes of Elevated ICP

1. Expanding tissue or fluid mass
2. Injury
   a. Depressed skull fracture
3. Excess CBF
4. Increase in cerebral spinal fluid (CSF) volume secondary to obstruction of circulation or impaired absorption
5. Increase in blood volume from vasodilation or a hematoma
6. Increased brain tissue volume secondary to a tumor or edema
7. Anxiety
8. Painful stimulation
9. Induction of anesthesia

### Complications Associated with an Elevated ICP

1. Reduced blood flow to the brain
2. Brain herniation across the meninges, down the spinal canal, or through an opening in the skull
   a. Herniation can lead to neurologic deterioration and death.

### Anesthetic Effects on Brain Physiology

1. Volatile anesthetics result in:
   a. Increase in CBF secondary to direct cerebral vasodilation, leading to an increased ICP under conditions of abnormal intracranial elastance
   b. Decreased cerebral metabolic rate (CMR)
2. Intravenous anesthetics
   a. Propofol
      i. Preferred over volatile anesthetics because it does not have a direct vasodilatory effect; therefore, it does not increase ICP.
      ii. Decreases CMR

iii. Decreases CBF

iv. Decreases ICP

v. Can decrease the MAP, leading to a decrease in CPP. Doses must be titrated carefully.

b. Etomidate

i. Decreases CMR

ii. Decreases CBF

iii. Direct vasoconstrictor

iv. It does not produce clinically significant cardiovascular depression.

v. Likely decreases ICP

vi. Considered the induction agent of choice

c. Benzodiazepines (midazolam)

i. Decrease CMR

ii. Decrease CBF

iii. May decrease the ICP

d. Opioids (fentanyl and remifentanil)

i. Minor reduction or no effect on CBF and CMR

e. Barbiturates

i. Decrease CMR

ii. Decrease CBF

iii. Decrease ICP

iv. Can decrease the MAP, leading to a decrease in CPP. Doses must be titrated carefully.

v. Decrease seizure activity

## Drugs to Avoid

1. Etomidate

a. There are theoretical concerns as the standard propylene glycol formulation may induce cerebral tissue hypoxia, tissue acidosis, and neurological deficits. Currently, it is still considered the induction agent of choice.

2. Nitrous oxide

a. NMDA receptor antagonist

b. Possible direct neurotoxic effects
When administered alone nitrous oxide has the following neurologic effects:

i. Increases CMR

ii. Increases CBF

iii. Increases ICP

iv. Disturbs CBF/CMR coupling in humans receiving sevoflurane

v. The increased CBF and ICP can be blunted by administering barbiturates, benzodiazepines, and morphine.

3. Flumazenil

a. Benzodiazepine antagonist

b. Give with caution, if at all, in patients with elevated ICP secondary to the reversal of the CMR, CBF, and ICP lowering effects of benzodiazepines.

4. Ketamine

a. Increases CBF and CMR

# KO Treatment Plan

## Pre-operative

### Indications for ICP monitoring

1. Severe head injury defined by the Glasgow coma scale (GCS) as less than 8

2. Abnormal head CT findings including hematoma, contusions, edema, or compressed basal cisterns

3. Severe traumatic brain injury, even with a normal head CT, if the patient has any of the following conditions:

a. Age greater than 40 years

b. Motor posturing

c. Systolic blood pressure less than 90 mm Hg

### Ventriculostomy

1. Compared to intraparenchymal monitoring, a ventriculostomy is considered safer, more accurate, and a more cost-effective method to monitor ICP.

2. A ventriculostomy also has diagnostic and therapeutic capabilities.

3. Complications such as infection and hemorrhage are relatively infrequent.

## Plan for Treatment of Elevated ICP

1. Positional therapy

a. Optimal venous drainage and the movement of CSF from the cranium to the spinal canal is achieved with head-up positioning.

i. The patient's head should be about 30 degrees above heart level.

ii. Ensure that objects around the neck are not restrictive, including cervical collars, tracheostomy ties, and endotracheal tube ties.

iii. Reduce extremes of neck positioning, for example flexion and extension.

b. This sitting position also allows for improved ventilation–perfusion matching and therefore improved cerebral oxygen delivery.

2. Support hemodynamics

a. Arterial blood pressure should be maintained within 10% of awake values.

b. The CPP should be kept at values >60 mm Hg.

c. The blood pressure should be maintained until direct ICP monitoring can be instituted and the CPP directly targeted.

3. Analgesia and sedation

   a. Adequate sedation and pain control are important secondary to the resulting increase in ICP from agitation.

   b. Intravenous esmolol, narcotics, and lidocaine can be used to blunt the sympathetic response to direct laryngoscopy and other painful stimuli.

   c. Be aware that oversedation in the post-operative period may impede sequential neurologic assessments.

   d. A short-acting agent such as propofol may be preferable.

      i. The use of propofol usually requires the subsequent use of a vasoactive drug to maintain the MAP and, in turn, the CPP.

   e. Intravenous barbiturates and benzodiazepines can also be used.

4. Avoid hypoxemia ($PaO_2$ <60 mm Hg).

   a. Maintain adequate oxygenation and ventilation.

      i. Goal $PaO_2$ >100 mm Hg
      ii. Goal $PaCO_2$ 30–35 mm Hg

   b. Positive end-expiratory pressure (PEEP) was once believed to increase the ICP, but it may actually decrease the ICP by improving cerebral oxygenation.

   c. Use the lowest possible airway pressure settings.

5. Hyperventilation

   a. Appropriate treatment for urgent situations that require a rapid reduction in ICP, for example brain herniation

   b. The current guidelines recommend maintenance of $PaCO_2$ at about 30–35 mm Hg. For rapid reduction in urgent situations, patients can be hyperventilated to a $PaO_2$ of 26–30 mm Hg.

   c. Recent studies have shown that the hyperventilation-induced vasoconstriction leads to an acute decrease in ICP. However, long-term use may result in hypoxic injury and possible stroke.

6. The goal hematocrit should be greater than 30%.

7. Patients should be normothermic.

   a. Hypothermia: if the patient presents to the hospital in a hypothermic state, active and aggressive rewarming should be avoided secondary to an increase in observed mortality. Special care should be used to avoid shivering.

      i. There are no data that show hypothermia improves outcome.

   b. Hyperthermia: hyperthermia should be treated aggressively, since the increase in CMR has been shown to worsen the neurologic exam.

8. Drainage of cerebrospinal fluid (CSF) per the surgeon

   a. This decreases the intracranial volume and the ICP.

   b. Drainage of CSF is obtained from the lateral cerebral ventricles or the lumbar subarachnoid space.

   c. Lumbar drainage of CSF is usually not recommended secondary to the risk of cerebellar herniation.

9. Osmotic therapy

   a. Mannitol

      i. Osmotic diuretic and cerebral arteriolar vasoconstrictor

      ii. Helps move excess interstitial fluid into the vascular space, therefore lowering the ICP.

      iii. The dose is 0.25–1.0 g/kg IV over 10–15 minutes. This dose usually results in a 100 mL removal of water from the patient's brain and a decrease in the ICP within 30 minutes. The maximum effect is seen within 1–2 hours.

         a. Boluses are preferred over continuous infusions.
         b. Boluses lower ICP and improve CBF.

      iv. Urine output can exceed 1–2 L within an hour. Infusion of a crystalloid solution is necessary to replace the intravascular fluid loss.

      v. Rapid administration can lead to paradoxical vasodilation of the cerebral vasculature, ultimately leading to excessive fluid in the brain and intracranial hypertension.

      vi. It is contraindicated in patients who are not adequately volume resuscitated.

   b. Furosemide

      i. Useful in a patient with increased vascular fluid and pulmonary edema
      ii. May be used in conjunction with mannitol to maintain osmotic gradient
      iii. Dose: 1 mg/kg IV
      iv. May lead to hypovolemia and electrolyte disturbances

   c. Hypertonic saline (NaCl 3–5%)

      i. May be beneficial in patients refractory to mannitol therapy

10. Decrease intravenous fluids.

11. Barbiturate coma

   a. This is used in patients with intractable elevations in ICP.

   b. Lowers the CMR and results in a decrease in excitatory neurotransmitter release

   c. Consider only when CPP cannot be maintained with previously described therapies. It usually requires pulmonary artery catheterization and vasoactive agents.

d. High-dose barbiturates are especially effective for treating elevated ICP after an acute head injury, but studies have shown that it is not associated with any improvement in outcome.

12. Neuromuscular blockade: these drugs may be necessary for a temporary treatment of an elevated ICP, but they are not recommended for long-term use secondary to their interference with the neurologic exam.

13. Corticosteroids

a. Effective for patients with elevated ICP secondary to localized cerebral edema around a brain tumor, particularly metastatic tumors and glioblastomas

14. Decompressive craniectomy: a surgical procedure that is used to control severely elevated ICP and prevent herniation and stroke.

15. Decompressive laparotomy: indicated in patients with coexisting injuries or after a vigorous volume infusion in which the patient develops increased intra-abdominal pressure to greater than 20 mm Hg. This increase in abdominal pressure worsens the pulmonary mechanics and therefore requires a higher MAP to maintain arterial oxygen saturation. The increase in ventilating pressure leads to an increase in intra-thoracic pressure and impaired venous drainage from the head, therefore leading to an increased ICP if not treated.

16. Avoid ketamine, nitrous oxide, hypotonic crystalloid solutions, and glucose-containing solutions.

## Intra-operative

1. Transport of the patient should be kept to a minimum.

2. Surgical interventions should be for life- or limb-threatening procedures only.

3. Urgent surgeries – for example, the fixation of a long bone – should only be performed once the CPP is being successfully managed.

4. Continue all of the above therapies during the surgery, including positional therapy, when possible; aggressive hemodynamic monitoring and resuscitation, administration of osmotic agents, and deep levels of anesthesia and sedation.

5. Induction of anesthesia is usually performed with a rapid sequence intubation (RSI).

a. Blunt the sympathetic response to laryngoscopy with intravenous fentanyl (3 μg/kg) and/or intravenous lidocaine (1.5 mg/kg).

b. Pretreatment with 0.01 mg/kg of vecuronium 3 minutes prior to giving succinylcholine helps to prevent the associated increase in ICP.

c. Etomidate is the induction agent of choice secondary to its hemodynamic stability and decreasing effect on ICP.

6. Maintenance of anesthesia should include narcotics and low concentrations of volatile anesthetics. Avoid nitrous oxide.

7. Treat a taut dura or a bulging brain with IV boluses of propofol, barbiturates, benzodiazepines, and/or mannitol/furosemide. Also consider positional therapy, hyperventilation, increased neuromuscular blockade, and drainage of the CSF. Verify normothermia and proper oxygenation. Continued communication with the surgeon is extremely important in this situation.

## Bibliography

Barash PG, Cullen BF, Stoelting RK, et al. *Clinical Anesthesia*, 8th ed. Philadelphia: Lippincott Williams & Wilkins, 2017, pp. 1008–9, 1303.

Butterworth JF, Mackey DC, Wasnick JD. *Morgan & Mikhail's Clinical Anesthesiology*, 6th ed. New York: McGraw-Hill Education, 2018, pp. 601–3.

Gropper MA. *Miller's Anesthesia*, 9th ed. Philadelphia: Elsevier, 2020, pp. 2675–8.

Rakel RE, Bope ET. *Conn's Current Therapy*. Philadelphia: Saunders, 2008, chapter 240.

Smith ER, Hanjani-Amin S. Evaluation and management of elevated intracranial pressure in adults. In *UpToDate* (accessed October 20, 2021).

Stoelting RK, Dierdorf SF. *Anesthesia and Co-Existing Disease*, 4th ed. Philadelphia: Churchill Livingstone, 2002, pp. 236–8.

# 41 Somatosensory-Evoked Potentials (SSEPs) and Motor-Evoked Potentials (MEPs)

Jessica A. Lovich-Sapola and Samuel DeJoy

## Sample Case

A 47-year-old male is scheduled for a surgical repair of his cervical spine. He was in a high-speed motor vehicle accident 1 week ago and has been in a cervical collar since. Does this patient require SSEP and/or MEP monitoring? Why? If SSEP/MEP monitoring is used, how will this affect your anesthesia? Would a wake-up test be better than SSEP/MEP monitoring?

## Clinical Issues

### Evoked Potentials

1. Used intra-operatively to monitor the integrity of a specific sensory or motor pathway

### General Treatment Issues

1. Communication between the anesthesia team, neuromonitoring clinician, and surgeon is critical. The neuromonitoring clinician should be informed prior to any significant changes in the administration of anesthesia during the case (i.e., any bolus of medication or nitrous oxide [$N_2O$]/volatile anesthetic change). The goal should be to make no major anesthetic changes after the induction of anesthesia and the baseline neuromonitoring measurements.
2. Changes in levels of inhaled anesthetics, temperature, $CO_2$, and blood pressure affect interpretations of SSEP/MEP monitoring. Therefore, these levels should be kept as constant as possible during the case. In the management of patient hemodynamics, it is preferred that boluses of medications are avoided. Adjusting the infusion rates of the intravenous medications is preferred. Boluses of β-blockers, hydralazine, phenylephrine, and ephedrine are preferred if a bolus is required.
3. Compatibility of a given anesthetic protocol with SSEP or MEP monitoring is not all-or-nothing; it is a continuum. It depends on multiple factors, and the same anesthetic protocol will not work with all patients.
4. Each patient should have baseline SSEP/MEP measurements once anesthesia is induced and the patient is positioned.
5. The anesthesia and surgical teams must provide full disclosure of the risks and benefits of the neuromonitoring and anesthesia, including but not limited to the possibility of awareness and intra-operative movement, tongue or lip injury, and vision changes.

## SSEP

### Clinical Issues

#### Definition

1. SSEPs evaluate the functional integrity of the ascending sensory pathways.
2. SSEPs are recorded after electrical stimulation of a peripheral mixed nerve.
3. The stimulation is usually with a surface electrode or a fine-needle electrode.
4. Nerves commonly stimulated include the median nerve at the wrist, the common peroneal nerve at the knee, and the posterior tibial nerve at the ankle.
5. Compromise or injury to the pathway manifests as an increase in the latency and/or a decrease in the amplitude of the evoked potential waveform.
6. A 50% reduction in amplitude is considered to be significant and warrants a change in action, either by anesthesia or the surgeon.
7. It is important to limit outside factors that can also affect the waveform.
   a. Maintain a constant level of the anesthetic drug.
   b. Avoid boluses of anesthetics and significant changes in the inhaled anesthetic.

#### Indications

1. Intramedullary/extramedullary spinal cord tumors or cysts
2. Vascular lesions in the spine
   a. Arterial-venous malformations
   b. Arterial-venous fistulas
3. Cervical or thoracic spine herniated discs that cause spinal cord compression
4. Spinal cord decompression and stabilization after an acute spinal cord injury
5. Spinal fusion
6. Cervical spondylosis
7. Ossification of the posterior longitudinal ligament
8. Scoliosis correction
9. Brachial plexus exploration after injury
10. Resection of a fourth ventricular cyst
11. Release of a tethered spinal cord
12. Clipping of an intracranial aneurysm

13. Carotid endarterectomy
14. Resection of a thalamic tumor
15. Abdominal and thoracic aneurysm repair
16. Repair of coarctation of the aorta

## KO Treatment Plan SSEP

### Intra-operative

1. Benzodiazepines produce minimal changes on the SSEP waveform when given in low doses.

    a. 1–2 mg of midazolam IV can safely be given in the pre-operative period.

    b. At high doses, diazepam can cause an increase in latency and a decrease in amplitude.

    c. Midazolam causes a decrease in amplitude, with no change in latency, at escalating doses.

2. IV induction doses of propofol, ketamine, or etomidate do not tend to affect the SSEP waveform recordings.

    a. Propofol can have an effect when given at high doses.

    b. It is notable that etomidate actually causes an increase in the wave amplitude, but also increases latency.

    c. Continuous propofol infusion (50–100 µg/kg/min) can be added as a supplement if needed.

3. A muscle relaxant (i.e., rocuronium or vecuronium) can be used for induction and as needed throughout the case.

4. High concentrations of volatile agents essentially eliminate the evoked potential. They cause a dose-dependent increase in latency and a decrease in amplitude.

    a. Up to 0.5 MAC of isoflurane, sevoflurane, or desflurane is acceptable.

5. $N_2O$ produces a profound depressant effect on the SSEPs, especially when used in combination with volatile anesthetics. It causes a decrease in amplitude with minimal effects on the latency.

    a. It is recommended to use no $N_2O$.

6. Opioids produce minimal changes in the SSEP waveform even in high doses.

    a. Continuous infusion of fentanyl or remifentanil is recommended.

    b. Boluses of opioids should still be avoided during critical times when neurologic injury may occur.

7. Clonidine and dexmedetomidine are $\alpha_2$-receptor agonists that can be used to decrease anesthetic requirements. Both agents can be used without compromising SSEP monitoring.

    a. Recommended dexmedetomidine infusion rate: 0.2–0.4 µg/kg/h

8. Ketamine increases the cortical SSEP amplitude.

    a. Recommended infusion rate: 0.25–2 mg/kg/h

9. Physiologic factors such as temperature, blood pressure, $PaO_2$, and $PaCO_2$ can alter the SSEPs. The goal is to maintain a fairly constant value without any major fluctuations.

    a. Maintain normothermia. Hypo- and hyperthermia both can affect the SSEP monitoring.

    b. Hypotension less than the cerebral autoregulation set point produces a progressive decrease in amplitude on the SSEPs.

    c. Hypoxia produces SSEP changes including a decrease in amplitude.

    d. Anemia results in increased latency of the SSEP waveform.

10. Mean arterial pressure (MAP) should be maintained at 90–110 mm Hg for cervical spine procedures (modify based on the patient's medical history and surgical input).

11. The anesthesia team should frequently communicate with neuromonitoring regarding bolus medications given and the adequacy of the monitoring waveforms, and participate in the differential diagnosis of nonreassuring waveforms.

12. The neuromonitoring technologist must communicate with the anesthesia team and surgeon regarding concerning trends in neuromonitoring. EEG evaluation and interpretation regarding the patient's adequacy of anesthetic depth and amnestic state must be communicated with the anesthesia team. If further clarification is needed, the anesthesiologist can contact the monitoring neurologist.

## MEP

## Clinical Issues

### Definition

1. MEPs test the integrity of the descending motor pathway.
2. Eliminate the need for a "wake-up test"

    a. A "wake-up test" is when you lighten the anesthesia of a patient during the surgery and ask him or her to move the extremities to evaluate for any spinal cord damage. This can be dangerous, especially if the patient is in the prone position. It also carries a higher risk of intra-operative awareness, which can be very disturbing for many patients.

3. MEPs should universally be combined with SSEP monitoring.

### Indications

1. Intramedullary spinal cord tumors
2. Vascular lesions in the spine

    a. Arterial-venous malformations

    b. Arterial-venous fistulas

3. Cervical or thoracic spine herniated discs that cause spinal cord compression
4. Scoliosis surgery
5. Removal of cerebral tumors involving the motor cortex or subcortical motor pathways
6. Aortic reconstruction

### Contraindications to Transcranial MEP

1. Patients with a history of seizure
2. Skull fracture
3. Implanted metal devices
   a. Cardiac pacemakers
   b. Central venous or pulmonary artery catheters

## KO Treatment Plan SSEP Plus MEP

### Intra-operative

1. Small 1–2 mg IV boluses of midazolam can be safely given in the pre-operative period.
2. Induction with IV propofol, etomidate, or ketamine can be done safely.
3. A single dose of muscle relaxant can be used for the intubation but should not be repeated.
   a. Some sources say that a low-dose infusion of IV muscle relaxants, maintaining one or two twitches in a train of four, can produce a reliable MEP waveform. This is very department-specific since there is no set protocol in the literature.

4. A bite block must be in place prior to turning the patient prone to decrease the risk of tongue and lip laceration.
   a. Use a reinforced endotracheal tube.
5. Volatile anesthetics have significant depressant effects on the MEP waveform. No volatile anesthetic agents should be used (i.e., isoflurane, sevoflurane, or desflurane).
6. $N_2O$ causes less suppression of the MEP waveforms than volatile anesthetics.
   a. It is still recommend to use no $N_2O$.
7. Continuous infusion of propofol (50–150 µg/kg/min)
8. Continuous infusion of fentanyl or remifentanil
9. Ketamine infusion can be used at a recommended rate of 0.25–2 mg/kg/h.
   a. Be mindful that up to 35% of patients with ketamine infusions after spine surgery report hallucinations and delirium.
   b. If the surgery is long, the ketamine infusion should be limited to critical times and not the entire surgery.
10. Avoid hypothermia, hypoxia, and hypotension.
    a. MAP should be maintained at 90–110 mm Hg for cervical spine procedures, but modified based on the patient's medical history and surgical input.

## Bibliography

Bal E, Sessler DI, Nair DR, et al. Motor and sensory evoked potentials are well maintained in patients given dexmedetomidine during spine surgery. *Anesthesiology* 2008;**109**:417–25.

Banoub M, Tetzlaff JE, Schubert A. Phamacologic and physiological influences affecting sensory evoked potentials. *Anesthesiology* 2003;**99**:716–37.

Barash PG, Cullen BF, Stoelting RK. *Clinical Anesthesia*, 5th ed. Philadelphia: Lippincott Williams & Wilkins, 2006, pp 760–3.

Calancie B, Harris W, Broton JG et al. "Threshold-level" multipulse transcranial electrical stimulation of motor cortex for intraoperative monitoring of spinal motor tracts: description of method and comparison to SSEP monitoring. *J Neurosurg* 1999;**90**:376.

Clapcich AJ, Emmerson, RG, Roye DP. Propofol/remifentanil is superior to nitrous oxide/isoflurane/remifentanil for cortical somatosensory evoked potentials assessment

in children undergoing spinal surgery. *Anesthesiology* 2002;**96**:A306.

Clapcich AJ, Emmerson, RG, Roye DP, et al. The effects of propofol, small-dose isoflurane, and nitrous oxide on cortical somatosensory evoked potential and bispectral index monitoring in adolescents undergoing spinal fusion. *Anesth Analg* 2004;**99**(5):1334–40.

Fletcher JE, Hinn AR, Heard CM, et al. The effects of isoflurane and desflurane titrated to a bispectral index of 60 on the cortical somatosensory evoked potential during pediatric scoliosis surgery. *Anesth Analg* 2005;**100**(6):1797–803.

Gropper MA. *Miller's Anesthesia*, 9th ed. Philadelphia: Elsevier, 2020, pp. 1252–6.

Gulur P, Der T, Nelli A, Murray S. ASA presentation: ketamine infusions for pain control in acute care – prevalence and side effects. Chapel Hill: Duke University, October 21, 2019

Haghighi SS. Influence of isoflurane anesthesia on motor evoked potentials

elicited by transcortical, brainstem, and spinal root stimulation. *Neurol Res* 1998;**20**(6):555–8.

Lovich-Sapola JA, DeJoy S. NeuroMonitoring Anesthesia Protocol. Cleveland: MetroHealth Medical Center, 2020.

Lyon R, Feiner J, Lieberman J. Progressive suppression of motor evoked potentials during general anesthesia: the phenomenon of "anesthetic fade." *J Neurosurg Anesthesiol* 2005;**17**:13–19.

Miller RD, Cucchiara RF, Millere E, et al. *Anesthesia*, 5th ed. Philadelphia: Churchill Livingstone, 2000, pp. 1335–45.

Strahm C, Min K, Boos N, et al. Reliability of perioperative SSEP recordings in spine surgery. *Spinal Cord* 2003;**41**(9):483–9.

van Dongen EP, ter Beek HT, Schepens MA, et al. Within-patient variability of myogenic MEPs to multipulse transcranial electrical stimulation during two levels of partial neuromuscular blockade in aortic surgery. *Anesth Analg* 1999;**88**:22–7.

# 42 Posterior Fossa Craniotomy

Brian M. Osman

## Sample Case

A 5-year-old boy presents with a 1-week history of headaches, visual changes, and ataxia. A large infratentorial mass is discovered on MRI. He is scheduled for craniotomy and resection of the tumor. What are your specific concerns: pre-operative, intra-operative, and post-operative? How will you induce anesthesia? What are your concerns about the patient's intra-operative positioning? What will you do to mitigate the risks? Do you plan to extubate the patient at the end of the case?

## Clinical Issues

### Nonexpansible Space

1.  The posterior fossa contains the medulla, pons, cerebellum, motor and sensory pathways, respiratory and cardiovascular centers, and cranial nerve nuclei.
2.  Mass effect from tumors, bleeding, and edema can cause profound neurological damage, leading to obstructive hydrocephalus and brainstem compression.

    a.  Obstructive hydrocephalus leads to increased intracranial pressure (ICP), which results in mental status changes, visual changes, headaches, nausea, and vomiting.

    b.  Brainstem compression leads to changes in the level of consciousness, depressed respirations, cardiac dysrhythmias, and cranial nerve palsies.

3.  It is not uncommon that a patient will require intubation pre-operatively for mental status changes and airway protection.

### Patient Positioning

1.  Sitting
2.  Horizontal

    a.  Lateral

    b.  Park bench

    c.  Three-quarters lateral

    d.  Prone

### Sitting Position (Fig. 42.1–42.2; Table 42.1)

1.  Risks

    a.  Venous air embolism (VAE): one of the most concerning risks of the sitting position is the increased incidence (45%) of VAE and the associated paradoxical air embolism (PAE). Both VAE and PAE are addressed in Chapter 43.

    b.  Hypotension

    i.  There is decreased venous return, resulting in a decrease in cardiac output and cerebral perfusion pressure (CPP).

    ii.  Impaired regulatory mechanisms: general anesthesia can impair baroreceptor (carotid sinus and aortic arch) and renin-angiotensin–aldosterone compensatory mechanisms. This lack of compensation is exaggerated in the elderly.

    iii.  Anesthetic agents and positive-pressure ventilation can directly decrease systemic vascular resistance (SVR), which is more pronounced in the sitting position.

    iv.  Arterial blood pressure monitoring is necessary not only to monitor cardiovascular changes but also to gauge CPP.

    (1)  Accurate CPP monitoring can be obtained with the transducer at the level of the head (CPP = MAP – ICP).

    v.  The severity of hypotension can be blunted with adequate hydration and gradual positioning, such as in placing the patient in a semi-recumbent (modified sitting) position.

    c.  Hyperflexion of the neck

    i.  Jugular venous obstruction can result in brain and facial swelling.

    ii.  Resulting quadriplegia or paraplegia from compromised blood flow to the cervical cord or direct compression of the cord

    (1)  This is more likely in the elderly and those with pre-existing cervical spine disease. It is exacerbated by hypotension.

    (2)  Head and neck range of motion should be assessed pre-operatively.

    (3)  Consider radiographic studies (lateral X-ray, CT scan) to assess the width of the cervical canal.

    iii.  Flexion of the head can also cause the endotracheal tube to migrate deeper.

A

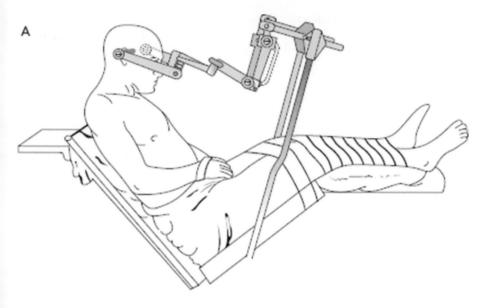

B

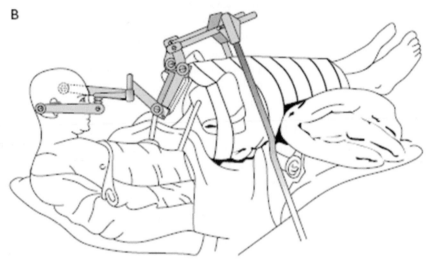

**Figure 42.1** Sitting positioning: (A) classic sitting position (B) modified sitting (semi-recumbent) position. Source: This figure has been reprinted with permission from *Youmans and Winn Neurological surgery, 7th Edition*, Richard H. Winn and Julian R. Youmans, Positioning for Cranial Surgery, Page e122–e126, Copyright Elsevier (2017).

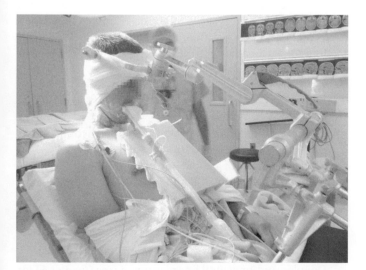

**Figure 42.2** Image of tumor removal from posterior fossa. Source: Allurimd (https://commons.wikimedia.org/wiki/File:Sitting_craniotomy.jpg).

(1) Equal breath sounds should be verified after positioning to ensure that the tube is not in the right mainstem.

iv. There should be at least a two-finger-breadth distance between the mandible and the sternum to ensure the neck is not over-flexed.

d. Peripheral nerve injuries: especially for the ulnar, peroneal, and sciatic nerves

e. Pneumocephalus: air enters the cranium through the craniotomy and can get trapped in the supratentorial space. Imagine an inverted soda pop bottle.

i. It has been advised to discontinue nitrous oxide (which will expand the air volume) before dural closure and to continue to avoid it for 2 weeks if more surgery is necessary.

ii. Can develop into tension pneumocephalus post-operatively

**Table 42.1** Pros and cons of sitting position

| Pros | Cons |
|---|---|
| Superior surgical exposure | VAE, PAE |
| Improved venous and CSF drainage | Possible CV instability |
| Reduced facial and conjunctival edema | Jugular venous obstruction |
| Improved ventilation | Quadriplegia, paraplegia |
| Better access to airway, chest, extremities | Peripheral nerve injuries |
| | Pneumocephalus |

Adapted from Barash PG, Cullen BF, Stoelting RK. *Clinical Anesthesia*, 8th ed. Philadelphia: Lippincott Williams & Wilkins, 2017, pp. 822–5; Miller RD *Miller's Anesthesia*, 9th ed. Philadelphia: Elsevier, Churchhill Livingstone, 2019, pp. 1868–910; Schubert A. *Clinical Neuroanesthesia*. Newton: Butterworth-Heinemann, 1997, pp. 31–42.

**Table 42.2** Pros and cons of lateral positioning

| Pros | Cons |
|---|---|
| Less VAE | Challenging surgical exposure |
| Improved CV stability | Cerebellar edema |
| | Hemorrhage |
| | Ischemic optic neuropathy |

Adapted from Barash PG, Cullen BF, Stoelting RK. *Clinical Anesthesia*, 8th ed. Philadelphia: Lippincott Williams & Wilkins, 2017, pp. 822–5; Miller RD *Miller's Anesthesia*, 9th ed. Philadelphia: Elsevier, Churchhill Livingstone, 2019, pp. 1868–910; Schubert A. *Clinical Neuroanesthesia*. Newton: Butterworth-Heinemann, 1997, pp. 31–42.

(1) When the patient is placed supine post-operatively, the beneficial effects of the sitting position are lost. There is no longer superior venous and cerebral spinal fluid (CSF) drainage. In addition, the effects of hypocapnia and osmotic diuresis may be lost post-operatively. The brain, blood, and CSF volume increase, which, combined with trapped air, can result in tension pneumocephalus.

(2) This should be considered with the patient who has delayed awakening or mental status changes.

2. Benefits

   a. The sitting position provides the best surgical access to the infratentorial fossa, requiring less aggressive surgical retraction, which has been reported to result in fewer cranial nerve deficits.

   b. Edema and hemorrhage: there is less potential for swelling of the brain and hemorrhage secondary to the superior venous and cerebrospinal fluid drainage of the head aided by gravity.

      i. Blood drains away easily from the operative site, which gives surgeons a superior surgical field.

      ii. There is less facial and conjunctiva swelling than is seen in patients who have been in the prone position.

   c. Ventilation is improved in the sitting position due to increased functional residual capacity (FRC) and better ventilation–perfusion matching.

## Horizontal Positions (Table 42.2)

1. Risks

   a. There is poor access to the airway, chest, and extremities.

   b. Cerebellar edema and hemorrhage are possible.

   c. Surgical access is less ideal and may require more aggressive surgical retraction, which can result in more post-operative neurologic dysfunction.

   d. The prone position especially has been associated with facial and tongue swelling and ischemic optic neuropathy.

   e. Peripheral nerve injuries are not uncommon.

2. Benefits

   a. There is a lowered risk of VAE.

   b. Cardiovascular stability is improved.

   c. Cervical cord injury risk is decreased.

## Summary of Patient Positioning

Both positions have advantages and disadvantages, and both can be used safely when proper precautions are taken. The decision on position should be made between the anesthesiologist and surgeon after careful evaluation of the patient's medical history, tumor size and location, and the risks and benefits associated with the position. The ideal choice will balance surgical comfort against the risks related to the patient. There is no clear best position; the decision should be individualized for each patient.

## Monitoring

1. EKG and arterial blood pressure monitoring is essential.

   a. Surgical manipulation can result in arrhythmias, compromising blood pressure.

   b. In addition, an arterial line can aid in the measurement of CPP and is necessary to monitor changes associated with VAE.

2. If the sitting position is chosen, a plan to monitor for VAE needs to be established pre-operatively and requires a transesophageal echocardiogram (TEE), precordial Doppler, and/or central line placement (see Chapter 43 for more on VAE).

3. Somatosensory evoked potentials (SSEPs) and brainstem auditory-evoked potentials (BAEPs) may be considered to monitor brainstem- or position-related ischemia.

## Post-operative Management

1. The decision for extubation must be made carefully since there may have been damage to respiratory centers, causing temporary or permanent central apnea.
2. In addition, due to possible manipulation of cranial nerves IX, X, and XII, the patient may be at risk for aspiration and have difficulty swallowing.
3. Frequent neurological assessments, arterial blood pressure monitoring, and EKG should be continued for at least 24 hours post-operatively due to the significant risk of neurologic, cardiac, and respiratory deterioration.
4. Any bleeding or edema that occurs in the post-operative period can result in hypertension, bradycardia, and loss of consciousness due to increased ICP, bleeding, and brainstem compression or infarction.

## KO Treatment Plan

### Pre-operative

1. Perform a complete history and physical on the child, with careful attention to neurologic function including any cranial nerve deficits, mental status, volume status, or signs of increased ICP (headache, vomiting, blurry vision, mental status change, hypertension).
2. The size of the tumor, vascularity, and surgical access are issues that need to be addressed with the surgeon.
3. The decision on position needs to be made based on weighing surgical access and the safety of the patient.
4. Typed and crossed blood, baseline hematocrit, and electrolytes to assess volume status are necessary.
5. An arterial line is essential and possibly a central line, especially if the sitting position is required as it may be necessary to aspirate air from the right atrium.
6. Consider precordial Doppler when the risk of VAE is increased.

### Intra-operative

1. Induction agent choices should be based on cardiovascular history, ICP status, and volume status, especially if the sitting position is chosen.

2. A rapid-sequence induction may be appropriate if there is a recent history of vomiting. The risk of transiently increased ICP with succinylcholine must be weighed against the risk of aspiration.
3. The endotracheal tube should be well secured, and any gastric tubes should be placed before positioning.
4. Patient positioning should be done gradually and after adequate hydration, especially when changing to the sitting position.
5. Extremities and pressure points need to be adequately padded.
6. The eyes must be free and clear.
7. Be prepared for hemodynamic instability as well as arrhythmias during dissection. These may be signs of VAE or brainstem compression.

### Post-operative

1. When considering extubation, remember the risk of aspiration from cranial nerve injury and central apnea from respiratory center damage.
   a. Injury to nerves IX, X, and XII can result in loss of control and patency of the upper airway.
   b. Swelling of the brainstem can result in impairment of both cranial nerve function and respiratory drive.
2. The candidate for extubation should have had an uncomplicated surgery, be hemodynamically stable, awake, spontaneously breathing adequate tidal volumes, and displaying adequate strength, as well as have intact airway reflexes.
3. The post-operative management should focus on frequent neurological exams and monitoring for cardiovascular and respiratory instability.
   a. Any alterations in these systems, especially mental status changes, hypertension, or bradycardia, could be an indication of bleeding, edema, or brainstem compression. Immediate re-exploration should be considered.
   b. For the nonawakening patient, consider bleeding, edema, and tension pneumocephalus, especially if the operation was completed in the sitting position.

## Bibliography

Barash PG, Cullen BF, Stoelting RK, et al. *Clinical Anesthesia*, 8th ed. Philadelphia: Lippincott Williams & Wilkins, 2017, pp. 822–5.

Gropper MA. *Miller's Anesthesia*, 9th ed. Philadelphia: Elsevier, 2020, pp. 1868–910.

Rozet I, Vavilala MS. Risks and benefits of patient positioning during neurosurgical care. *Anesthesiol Clin* 2007;**25**(3):631–53.

Schubert A. *Clinical Neuroanesthesia*. Newton: Butterworth-Heinemann, 1997, pp. 31–42.

# Venous Air Embolism

Brian M. Osman

## Sample Case

A 77-year-old, 120 kg female presents for a craniotomy and resection of her posterior fossa tumor. The surgeon prefers her to be placed in the sitting position for the operation. She has a medical history significant for diabetes (DM), hypertension (HTN), congestive heart failure (CHF), and gastroesophageal reflux disease (GERD). She is a nonsmoker with unknown exercise tolerance due to her decreased mobility secondary to osteoarthritis (OA) of her knees. What pre-operative labs and studies would you like? What monitors will you use? Should the procedure be done in the sitting position? Is venous air embolism (VAE) a concern? Will you use $N_2O$? How would you identify a VAE? Can you prevent a VAE? How would you treat a VAE?

## Clinical Issues

### Incidence and Risk of VAE

1. VAE can occur when the operative field is greater than or equal to 5 cm above the level of the right atrium or more specifically when there is more than a 5 cm $H_2O$ gradient between noncollapsible venous openings (e.g., diploic veins and dural sinuses) and the right atrium.

   a. With a VAE, the surgical site is elevated such that the pressure at that height is greater than the central venous back pressure, therefore setting the environment to entrain air.

2. Risk of occurrence is 25% and 45% during sitting cervical laminectomies and sitting posterior fossa procedures, respectively, using Doppler detection, and up to 76% during sitting posterior fossa procedures using transesophageal echocardiography (TEE) detection.

   a. It can also occur in the horizontal, lateral, supine, and prone positions. The reported incidence is 12%.

3. Hemodynamic consequences of air is approximated to occur at a cumulative volume of 1 mL/kg in animal studies.

   a. The lethal dose increases with slower entry of the air and decreases with a faster accumulation of air.

### Pathophysiology of a VAE

1. Air bubbles mechanically obstruct the pulmonary vasculature. This leads to hypoxemia and resultant vasoconstriction, V/Q mismatch, increased pulmonary artery pressure (PAP), and reduced cardiac output.

   a. The increase in pulmonary dead space will lower the end-tidal carbon dioxide ($ETCO_2$) and increase the arterial carbon dioxide ($PaCO_2$).

2. The air bubbles cause a release of vasoactive mediators, which lead to increased vascular permeability and interstitial pulmonary edema, further contributing to the increased pulmonary vascular resistance (PVR) and decrease in cardiac output.

3. Small volumes of air can be cleared by the pulmonary vasculature without hemodynamic signs.

4. Increased filling pressures, decreased cardiac output, hypotension, and the classic "mill wheel" murmur are late findings with a VAE.

5. Large volumes of trapped air in the right heart can cause an airlock.

   a. Increasing right ventricular (RV) afterload and decreasing left ventricular (LV) filling results in cardiovascular (CV) collapse.

### Paradoxical Air Embolism (PAE)

1. The reported risk is 5–10%.

2. Air from a VAE can cross into the arterial system via a probe patent foramen ovale (PPFO), right to left intracardiac shunt, or transpulmonary passage.

   a. The incidence of PPFO is 20–30% in adults and 50% in children less than 5 years old.

   b. Air on the left side of the heart can pass into the cerebral, coronary, or renal arterial systems, causing stroke, myocardial infarction (MI), or renal injury.

3. PAE is more likely when the right heart pressures exceed the left.

   a. When a VAE occurs, PVR increases due to increased right heart pressures.

      i. This can result in air passage to the left heart via a PPFO or an intracardiac shunt.

   b. In the sitting position, it has been estimated that 50% of patients have an increased right heart pressure over the left.

i. The normally decreased right atrial pressure (RAP) to pulmonary capillary wedge pressure (PCWP) gradient is said to reverse within 1 hour in the sitting patient, but can be partially attenuated by volume loading.

ii. The sitting position increases the risk of VAE and PAE.

iii. The sitting position should be avoided in patients with known intracardiac shunts.

c. Generous fluid administration can reduce the RAP to left atrial pressure (LAP) gradient.

d. Positive end expiratory pressure (PEEP) will increase the RAP to LAP gradient.

    i. In contrast, PEEP can also increase the central venous pressure (CVP), which can be helpful in preventing the initial and further entrainment of air. However, the benefit does not outweigh the risk of VAE from the associated increase in RAP.

    ii. Avoid PEEP in sitting procedures.

e. Valsalva can also increase the RAP to LAP gradient and should therefore be avoided.

f. PAE can also occur via transpulmonary passage.

    i. Large volumes of air can overcome the pulmonary vascular filter and result in air passage via the bronchial vessels and Thebesian veins.

4. Consider pre-operative TEE to rule out patent foramen ovale (PFO) or intracardiac shunt when planning a surgery in the sitting position.

## Detection of a VAE (Fig. 43.1)

1. Monitors: listed from the most sensitive to the least sensitive and therefore also listed from clinically significant to insignificant

a. Transesophageal echocardiography (TEE)

    i. Most sensitive, but invasive and bulky

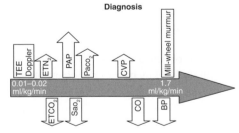

**Figure 43.1** Detection of a VAE. Changes in detection parameters for VAE with increasing volumes of air. BP, blood pressure; CO, cardiac output; CVP, central venous pressure; $ETCO_2$, end-tidal carbon dioxide; $ETN_2$, end-tidal nitrogen; $PaCO_2$, partial pressure of carbon dioxide; PAP, pulmonary artery pressure; $SaO_2$, arterial oxygen saturation; TEE, transesophageal echocardiography. The "mill wheel" murmur is the characteristic sound of turbulent flow heard on Doppler when the agitated saline (air) enters the right heart chambers. This figure was published in Faust's Anesthesiology Review (2015).

    ii. The only monitor that can show venous and arterial embolisms and therefore can diagnose VAE/PAE

b. Precordial Doppler

    i. Most sensitive noninvasive monitor

    ii. Can detect air volumes as small as 0.25 mL

    iii. High-pitched Doppler sounds indicate turbulent flow.

        (1) The transducer is placed at the right sternal border between the third and sixth intercostal spaces, where the audible signals from the right atrium (RA) are maximized.

        (2) Cannot differentiate clinically significant sounds versus clinically insignificant sounds with precordial Doppler alone

c. Pulmonary artery catheter (PAC)

    i. Will detect increases in PAP secondary to pulmonary vasoconstriction

        (1) The PAC will not be able to detect VAEs that are hemodynamically insignificant.

        (2) The increase in the PAP will correlate to the volume and severity of the VAE.

    ii. The PAC will be able to detect when the RAP is greater than the PCWP.

        (1) The patient can then receive a fluid bolus or be repositioned to attenuate this gradient.

d. Capnography

    i. $ETCO_2$ will decrease.

        (1) From V/Q mismatch caused by intravascular air

        (2) From reduced cardiac output caused by possible RV outflow obstruction/airlock

        (3) $ETCO_2$ can be used with precordial Doppler to help differentiate clinically significant sounds.

e. Cardiac output (decrease) and CVP (increase)

    i. A central venous catheter (CVC) can be used to aspirate air from the RA (see below).

f. Mass spectrophotometer

    i. End-tidal nitrogen ($ETN_2$) will be increased.

        (1) Air trapped in the vasculature will permeate the capillary/alveolar membrane, and the exhaled air will have an increased concentration of $N_2$.

        (2) Will probably not be helpful until near cardiovascular collapse

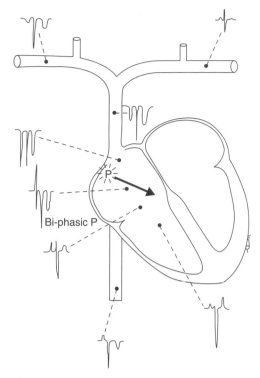

**Figure 43.2** CVC line placement. The P indicates the sinoatrial node. The heavy black line indicates the P wave vector. Source: Gropper MA. *Miller's Anesthesia*, 9th ed. Philadelphia: Elsevier, 2020, p. 1881. Reprinted with permission.

    g.    Decreased blood pressure and a "mill wheel" murmur: a loud, machine-like murmur caused by the air in the heart

## Central Venous Catheter (Fig. 43.2)

1.    A properly placed CVC can be used to aspirate embolized air from the RA.

    a.    For optimal recovery of air: a multi-orifice catheter should be positioned 2 cm below the superior vena cava (SVC)–RA junction and a single-orifice catheter 3 cm above the SVC–RA junction.

        i.    When there are large volumes of air in the RA, a catheter anywhere in the RA would suffice.

        ii.    A multi-orifice catheter is superior to the single-orifice catheter for aspirating air.

    b.    Confirmation of proper placement of the CVC can be made by:

        i.    Radiograph

        ii.    Monitoring the CVP: ensure the tip is in the RA by looking at the waveforms and pressures.

        iii.    Intravascular ECG: use electrical signals from the catheter to place the tip in the correct part of the RA.

           (1)    Use a commercially available kit with an ECG adapter or make your own by

attaching the left leg ECG lead to the catheter hub by clipping onto a metal stopcock.

           (2)    Fill the CVC with an electrolyte solution; bicarbonate is suggested.

           (3)    Monitor lead II and advance the catheter.

               (a)    The P wave will become increasingly negative as the catheter approaches the SVC–RA junction due to the proximity to the sinoatrial (SA) node.

               (b)    The P wave will become increasingly positive as the catheter goes past the SA node.

               (c)    The point where the P wave becomes biphasic (equal positive and negative deflections) is indicative of the mid-atrial position.

               (d)    The multi-orifice catheter is in the correct position when the P wave produces the most negative deflection, which indicates the SVC–RA junction. If using a single-orifice catheter, pull the catheter back from this position 2–3 cm.

               (e)    Avoid microshock: disconnect any unnecessary electrical equipment from the patient.

2.    The decision to use a CVC should be based on risks of VAE, procedure (likelihood of open venous channels), position (essentially all procedures in the sitting position should be accompanied by a CVC), the patient's medical history, and physiologic reserve.

3.    If the concern for VAE is large enough to use a precordial Doppler or TEE, consider a CVC to have a way to remove the air that may collect.

## Nitrous Oxide

1.    Can diffuse into trapped air and expand it, possibly making the effects of a VAE worse

2.    Can be used in procedures where VAE is a risk. However, it must be immediately discontinued should a VAE occur.

3.    Some would argue based on the above to avoid it all together and to eliminate $N_2O$ as part of the equation should a VAE occur.

## Prevention of a VAE

1.    Early detection

2.    Minimize elevation of the head

3.    Use of bone wax: minimize open venous channels

4.    Maintain euvolemia

5.    Avoid PEEP/Valsalva

## KO Treatment Plan

### Pre-operative

1. Complete history and physical
   a. Assess for any history of intracardiac shunts or PFO.
2. Discuss with the surgeon concerns of VAE and together weigh the risks and benefits of the sitting position.
3. Consider pre-operative TEE if the sitting position is absolutely necessary.
   a. TEE is used to rule out a PFO or intracardiac shunt.

### Intra-operative

1. Choose monitors.
   a. Arterial line
   b. CVC
   c. TEE vs. precordial doppler + PAC or $ETCO_2$
      i. The addition of PAC or $ETCO_2$ to precordial Doppler will help differentiate clinically significant air before a significant hemodynamic response occurs.
2. Prevention is key.
   a. Bone wax
   b. Avoid head-up positioning
   c. Proper hydration
3. If a VAE is suspected:
   a. Notify the surgeon and call for help.
   b. Flood the surgical field with saline, use bone wax, and pack the surgical field.
   c. Discontinue $N_2O$.
   d. Compress the neck veins.
      i. Increases venous pressure
      ii. May prevent further air entry
   e. Place the patient in a Trendelenburg and left lateral decubitus (LLD) position to help release air from the RV outflow tract if an airlock is suspected.
      i. The RV is the most anterior part of the heart.
   f. Aspirate air from a properly positioned CVC.
   g. Chest compression/percussion to release air lock or trapped air
   h. Avoid PEEP and Valsalva.
   i. Supportive therapy
      i. Maintain euvolemia.
      ii. May need pressors for blood pressure support

## Case Discussion

### Pre-operative

1. Order a complete blood count (CBC) and basic metabolic panel to investigate any end-organ damage from the patient's HTN and DM.
2. Consider how well controlled the patient's HTN and DM are when formulating an anesthetic plan.
3. Assess the patient's current volume status and rule out any active CHF.
4. Order a chest X-ray for current evaluation and for a baseline since the patient is at risk for intra-operative and post-operative CHF exacerbation.
5. Obtain a baseline EKG in this patient, who likely has some element of coronary artery disease based on her age and comorbidities.
6. If the patient has poor exercise tolerance, order a stress echocardiogram prior to surgery.
   a. The patient may benefit from revascularization; however, it may not be safe to delay the tumor resection for coronary artery stenting or cardiac bypass surgery.
   b. Consider using the stress test results to guide your anesthetic plan.
      i. Ejection fraction (EF): history of CHF
      ii. Presence of PFO
      iii. Patient's physiologic reserve
      iv. Remember that hydration is one way to keep the RA pressure greater than the PCWP.
      v. In this patient, hydration may not be a tool that can be utilized secondary to the history of CHF. Consider a PAC if the patient presents with low EF and chronic CHF.

### Intra-operative

1. I would induce with etomidate because of its stable hemodynamic profile.
2. A balanced maintenance technique using a volatile anesthetic, opioid, and a muscle relaxant can be used to maintain hemodynamic stability.
   a. Consider short-acting opioids and desflurane secondary to their rapid onset and offset, and therefore less long-term effect on hemodynamic stability.
3. Arterial blood pressure monitoring is indicated secondary to the patient's history of HTN, CHF, and DM.
   a. The patient will require tight blood pressure control to avoid a CHF exacerbation.
   b. This will be difficult with a blood pressure cuff alone, especially with her history of HTN.

c. In addition, the patient may need hourly glucose monitoring via an arterial blood draw and an insulin infusion.

4. If VAE is a concern, choose a way to detect it.

   a. The combination of precordial Doppler and $ETCO_2$ is appropriate.

**TKO:** Make it easy for yourself! Say, "assuming this patient has well-controlled DM and HTN and has a normal EF … " and "assuming this patient had a recent echocardiogram with no signs of PFO, I would consider the sitting position only after the surgeon and I weighed the risk of VAE versus the need for sitting position."

# Bibliography

Barash PG, Cullen BF, Stoelting RK, et al. *Clinical Anesthesia*, 8th ed. Philadelphia: Lippincott Williams & Wilkins, 2017, pp. 1016–18, 1271–2.

Black S, Ockert DB, Oliver WC, Cucchiara RF. Outcome following posterior fossa craniectomy in patients in the sitting or horizontal positions. *Anesthesiology* 1988;**69**:49–56.

Gropper MA. *Miller's Anesthesia*, 9th ed. Philadelphia: Elsevier, 2020, pp. 1868–910.

Murray M, Harrison B, Mueller JT. *Faust's Anesthesiology Review*, 4th ed. Philadelphia: Saunders, 2015 pp. 322–4.

Schubert, A. *Clinical Neuroanesthesia*. Newton: Butterworth-Heinemann, 1997, pp. 363–72.

# Cerebral Aneurysm Surgery

Cory Rene Brune and Jessica A. Lovich-Sapola

## Sample Case

A 60-year-old woman presents to the emergency department with a history of "the worst headache of her life." Paramedics report that although she is presently drowsy, she did briefly lose consciousness in the ambulance. Her blood pressure is 175/80 mm Hg with a heart rate of 60. Her other vital signs are all stable. A CT scan reveals a grade 3 subarachnoid hemorrhage (SAH). The neurosurgical team posts the case as an aneurysm clipping scheduled for the following morning. What are your concerns? How will you evaluate the patient? How will you induce and maintain general anesthesia in this patient?

## Clinical Issues

### Incidence of a Subarachnoid Hemorrhage

1. About 8–10 per 100,000
2. Predominantly occurring in the 55–60-year-old age group

### Pathophysiology

**Unruptured Aneurysms**

1. Present with prodromal symptoms as the aneurysm progressively enlarges
2. Headache is the most common symptom.
3. Third-nerve palsy is the most common physical sign.
4. Other symptoms:
   a. Visual field defects
   b. Trigeminal nerve dysfunction
   c. Cavernous sinus syndrome
   d. Seizures
   e. Hypothalamic–pituitary dysfunction
5. Treatment is a coiling or clipping of the aneurysm.

**Ruptured Aneurysms**

1. Usually present acutely
2. Sudden severe headache without focal deficits
3. Nausea and vomiting
4. Transient loss of consciousness secondary to the sudden rise in intracranial pressure (ICP) and drop in cerebral perfusion pressure (CPP) (Fig. 44.1)

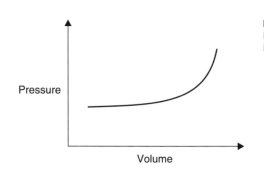

**Figure 44.1**
Pressure vs. volume in ICP.

a. The aneurysm rupture leads to an expanding mass effect of the hemorrhage and edema development that leads to an increase in ICP.
b. If the ICP does not drop rapidly, death will follow.
c. This increase in ICP leads to:
   i. Headache
   ii. Altered mental status, up to and including a loss of consciousness
   iii. Possible motor and sensory deficits

5. Rising ICP leads to a reactive increase in systemic mean arterial pressure (MAP) to maintain the cerebral perfusion; classically referred to as the Cushing reflex.
   a. CPP = MAP – ICP

6. Eventually the increase in ICP leads to a decrease in cerebral blood flow, limiting further leakage of blood from the aneurysm.

7. Delayed complications
   a. Delayed cerebral ischemia (DCI):
      i. Cerebral vasospasm is not the primary cause of DCI, as once believed.
      ii. Other causes include: cortical spread of depolarization and microthrombosis.
      iii. Treated with $Ca^+$ channel antagonist nimodipine
   b. Symptomatic vasospasm
      i. Nimodipine
      ii. If no response, begin the "Triple H" therapy
         (1) Hypervolemia (volume expansion)
         (2) Hemodilution
         (3) Hypertension

(4) "Triple H" therapy has recently been questioned and may be replaced with hypertension and euvolemia, in order to promote cerebral perfusion without excess strain on other organ systems.

    iii.  Catheter-delivered vasodilators

      iv.  Angioplasty

c. Re-rupture
d. Hydrocephalus

## Diagnosis

1. MRI
2. Angiography
3. Helical CT angiogram

## Rebleeding

1. Rebleeding is the most serious complication following SAH and is the primary cause of mortality.
2. Treatment involves early control of the vasculature and strict avoidance of hypertension.
3. Four percent incidence within the first day. After 48 hours, the incidence is 1.5% per day, with a cumulative rebleeding rate of 19% by the end of 2 weeks. Highest risk of rebleed is within the first 72 hours.

## Transcranial Doppler Monitoring (TCD)

1. Direct and noninvasive monitor of cerebral blood flow (CBF)
2. Indications
   a. Determine the severity of cerebral vasospasm after a subarachnoid hemorrhage.
   b. Measure the CBF during carotid artery clamping in a carotid endarterectomy.
   c. Detection of emboli after an arterial repair or during cardiopulmonary bypass
   d. Brain death diagnosis

## KO Treatment Plan

### Pre-operative

1. Hunt and Hess classification of patients with SAH: describes the clinical course of disease. Higher grades are associated with the presence of cerebral vasospasm, intracranial hypertension, and increased surgical mortality.
   a. Grade 0: unruptured aneurysm
   b. Grade I: asymptomatic or minimal headache and slight nuchal rigidity
   c. Grade II: moderate to severe headache, nuchal rigidity, no neurologic deficit other than cranial nerve palsy

d. Grade III: drowsiness, confusion, or mild focal deficit
e. Grade IV: stupor, moderate to severe hemiparesis, early decerebration, vegetative disturbance
f. Grade V: deep coma, decerebrate rigidity, moribund

2. Fischer grading of acute SAH: describes the appearance of the SAH on CT scan. This scale provides an index of vasospasm risk, but does not prognosticate clinical outcome.
   a. Grade 1: no blood detected
   b. Grade 2: diffuse thin layer of subarachnoid blood (≤1 mm thick)
   c. Grade 3: diffuse thick layer of subarachnoid blood (>1 mm thick) or localized clot
   d. Grade 4: intracerebral or intraventricular blood with diffuse or no subarachnoid blood

3. Neurogenic pulmonary edema (NPE)
   a. Nearly 17% of SAH patients develop severe pulmonary dysfunction (range 8–29%).
   b. NPE occurs with sympathetic activation secondary to the rise in ICP, leading to pulmonary and systemic vasoconstriction. This leads to an increase in pulmonary blood volume and a decrease in left ventricular compliance, with a concomitant rise in pulmonary capillary pressure and pulmonary capillary permeability.
   c. Treat with immediate surgical or pharmacologic relief of intracranial hypertension, supportive respiratory care, and careful fluid management.

4. Cardiac dysrhythmias and EKG abnormalities
   a. Due to excessive catecholamine release triggered by the SAH
   b. Severity of cardiac dysfunction correlates with degree of neurologic injury: more severe SAH leads to more severe changes on the EKG.
   c. Commonly presents with:
      i. Very deep, widely splayed T wave inversions
      ii. Long QT
      iii. Prominent U wave
      iv. ST segment depression
   d. May also cause:
      i. Systemic and pulmonary hypertension
      ii. Myocardial dysfunction and injury: 30% of acute SAH patients have elevated troponin levels.
      iii. Neurogenic stunned myocardium
   e. An increase in cardiac troponin during SAH is associated with myocardial injury and may herald a poor outcome.

5. Electrolyte abnormalities
   a. Hyponatremia

i. Occurs in 30–40% of patients with SAH
ii. Cerebral salt-wasting syndrome (CSWS) or syndrome of inappropriate antidiuretic hormone (SIADH)

   (1) CSWS is treated with isotonic or hypertonic saline to replace lost sodium and volume. Fludrocortisone is used to combat natriuresis and diuresis.
   (2) SIADH is treated with fluid restriction to suppress antidiuretic hormone (ADH) secretion.

   b. Other electrolyte abnormalities such as hypokalemia, hypocalcemia, and hypomagnesemia may occur secondary to diuretic therapy in an attempt to lower the ICP with loop or osmotic diuretics.

6. Calcium channel blockers (CCB)

   a. CCBs, most specifically nimodipine, have been utilized for the treatment and prevention of morbidity from cerebral vasospasm after subarachnoid hemorrhage.
   b. Incidence of angiographically detected vasospasm is not reduced.
   c. Mechanism of benefit in this setting is unknown, but all patients are recommended to start a CCB as soon as possible after SAH.

# Intra-operative

1. The goals of intra-operative management of these patients are to avoid aneurysm rupture, maintain CPP, maintain transmural aneurysm pressure, and provide a "slack brain." The anesthetic management provided below attempts to maintain these goals.

   a. The induction agents can vary depending on the patient's clinical status.
   b. The patient should be considered a "full stomach" and requires a rapid-sequence intubation.
   c. Blunt the sympathetic response to laryngoscopy with IV fentanyl (3 μg/kg) and/or IV lidocaine (1.5 mg/kg).
   d. Pretreatment with a small dose of rocuronium prior to giving succinylcholine helps to prevent the associated increase in ICP.
   e. Etomidate is the induction agent of choice secondary to its hemodynamic stability and decreasing effect on ICP; however, propofol can be used in judicious doses, aiming to prevent hypotension and resultant decreases in CPP, given the increased ICP.
   f. Maintenance of anesthesia is achieved with total IV anesthesia or inhalational agents, plus appropriate doses of opioid for analgesia.

2. IV access requires two large-bore IV catheters.

   a. The large IVs are important if the aneurysm ruptures and large volumes of replacement blood are required.

   b. Be careful to avoid giving the patient large amounts of crystalloid during a controlled case with minimal blood loss.

3. Type and cross for blood products.
4. Standard monitoring should be geared to the patient's needs.

   a. Standard ASA monitors and continuous arterial blood pressure monitoring are standard of care.
   b. A central venous pressure (CVP) catheter may be inserted for guidance of intravascular volumes in the face of severe cardiac instability, or when peripheral venous access is inadequate.
   c. Pulmonary artery catheter (PAC) monitoring is justified in the setting of myocardial dysfunction and post-operative "Triple H" therapy.

5. Treatment of increased ICPs

   a. Techniques to decrease ICP

      i. Hyperventilation
      ii. Osmotic diuresis with mannitol or hypertonic saline
      iii. Administration of increased levels of anesthetic gases and/or propofol
      iv. Lumbar cerebral spinal fluid (CSF) drainage. Use caution to avoid excessive drainage: decreasing the ICP too much too quickly increases the aneurysmal transmural pressure and increases the risk of bleeding.
      v. Position patients in reverse Trendelenburg (head-up) and ensure no jugular vein compression.

6. Neurophysiologic monitoring may be beneficial in areas potentially affected by the aneurysm clipping.
7. Induced hypotension

   a. This has been abandoned in routine practice due to the risk of cerebral hypoperfusion, but may still be used for brief periods of time to facilitate clip application to the aneurysm, or in cases of bleeding, preventing visualization by the surgeon.
   b. Use of a rapid-acting vasodilator such as sodium nitroprusside may accomplish brief periods of extreme hypotension to facilitate the surgery.
   c. Adenosine may be administered for temporary circulatory arrest.

8. Induced hypertension

   a. May be requested during periods of temporary vessel occlusion to increase collateral cerebral perfusion
   b. Phenylephrine is usually the medication of choice in this instance.

9. Temporary vessel occlusion and induced hypothermia

   a. Induced hypothermia does not improve neurologic outcomes in aneurysm clipping.

Cory Rene Brune and Jessica A. Lovich-Sapola

b. It is only useful in the setting of temporary vessel occlusion, or temporary clipping.

   i. A temporary clip may be placed proximal to the aneurysm on the feeding vessel, as well as distal to the aneurysm to isolate it.
   ii. This is more commonly used in large aneurysms.
   iii. Limited in time duration due to distal ischemia from clipping. Generally, periods less than 14 minutes are considered safe, whereas periods longer than 31 minutes are always associated with ischemia.

## Post-operative

1. The goals at emergence are to avoid coughing, straining, hypercarbia, and hypertension, as all of these will lead to an increase in ICP.

   a. Patients who were Hunt Hess grades I and II pre-operatively, with no intra-operative complications, may have the endotracheal tube removed upon conclusion of surgery.
   b. Patients who arrived in the operating room with decreased mentation should remain intubated until their neurologic status improves.

c. Other neurosurgical indications for maintaining post-operative intubation and ventilation are prolonged temporary vessel occlusion and severe intra-operative vasospasm.

2. Post-operative monitoring for severe hypertension, hypotension, and vasospasm must be initiated.

   a. Severe hypertension occurs from pre-existing hypertensive disorders, pain, $CO_2$ retention, or "Triple H" therapy.

      i. It may lead to cerebral edema or hematoma formation, leading to increased ICP and vasospasm.

   b. Hypotension must be avoided as the decreased blood pressure leads to decreased CPP, leading to neurologic compromise.

      i. The goal is to increase CBF, increase CPP, and improve CBF with decreased blood viscosity.
      ii. Systolic blood pressure is raised to 160–200 mm Hg in clipped aneurysms only.
      iii. Monitor patients with concomitant cardiac dysfunction, myocardial injury, or respiratory impairment carefully.

# Bibliography

Barash PG, Cullen BF, Stoelting RK, et al. *Clinical Anesthesia*, 8th ed. Philadelphia: Lippincott Williams & Wilkins, 2017, pp. 1018–19.

Butterworth JF, Mackey DC, Wasnick JD. *Morgan & Mikhail's Clinical Anesthesiology*, 6th ed. New York: McGraw-Hill Education, 2018, pp. 612–14.

Gropper MA. *Miller's Anesthesia*, 9th ed. Philadelphia: Elsevier, 2020, pp. 1886–90, 2683–5.

Muroi C, Keller M, Pangalu A, et al. Neurogenic pulmonary edema in patients with subarachnoid hemorrhage. *J Neurosurg Anesth* 2008;**20**(3):188–92.

Priebe HJ. Aneurysmal subarachnoid haemorrhage and the anaesthetist. *Br J Anaesth* 2007;**99**(1):102–18.

Sriganesh K, Venkataramaiah S. Concerns and challenges during anesthetic management of aneurysmal subarachnoid hemorrhage. *Saudi J Anesth* 2015:**9**(3):306–13.

200

# Syndrome of Inappropriate Antidiuretic Hormone Secretion, Cerebral Salt-Wasting Syndrome, and Diabetes Insipidus

**Chapter 45**

Jessica A. Lovich-Sapola

## Sample Case

A 50-year-old male is 24 hours status post transsphenoidal resection of a pituitary tumor. He is producing less than 50 mL/h of urine for several hours and is complaining of thirst. What is the likely etiology of this process and what laboratory values are expected? How should this patient be managed if he returns to the operating room emergently?

## Syndrome of Inappropriate Antidiuretic Hormone (SIADH)

## Clinical Issues

### Definition

1. Syndrome of excess release of antidiuretic hormone (ADH) from the posterior pituitary gland or another source
2. The release of ADH is then not inhibited by the resulting reduction in plasma osmolality.
3. State of hyponatremia in combination with elevated urine osmolality, excessive sodium secretion, and decreased serum osmolality
   a. Condition of excess water and not a sodium deficiency
   b. Patients are usually hypervolemic.
4. Cells secreting ADH are dysregulated and water absorption from the distal collecting tubules is enhanced.

### Incidence

1. Hyponatremia
   a. Defined as a plasma sodium concentration less than 135 mEq/L
      i. The most common electrolyte derangement in hospitalized patients
      ii. Incidence may be as high as 30%.
   b. A serum sodium concentration below 130 mEq/L is found in fewer than 3% of all hospitalized patients.
   c. ADH dysregulation is the most common etiology of hyponatremia.

### Etiology

1. Idiopathic: most common
2. Post-operative

3. Central nervous system disease
   a. Head trauma or intracranial bleeding
   b. Tumors and cerebrovascular accidents
   c. Delirium tremens
4. Neoplastic
   a. Lung: small cell
   b. Pancreas
   c. Ovary
   d. Lymphoma
   e. Thymoma
5. Endocrine
   a. Glucocorticoid insufficiency
   b. Hypothyroidism
6. Pulmonary disease
   a. Pneumonia
   b. Positive-pressure ventilation
   c. Chronic obstructive pulmonary disease (COPD)/asthma
   d. Tuberculosis
   e. Abscess
7. Medications
   a. Chlorpropamide
   b. Cyclophosphamide
   c. Tricyclic antidepressants (TCAs)
   d. Selective serotonin reuptake inhibitors (SSRIs)
   e. Nicotine
   f. MDMA drugs ("ecstasy" or "molly")
   g. Phenothiazine
   h. Opioids
   i. NSAIDS
   j. Vasopressin
8. Infectious
   a. Cytomegalovirus
   b. Mycobacteria associated with AIDS
   c. Brain or lung abscess

### Signs and Symptoms

1. Anorexia
2. Nausea and vomiting

3. Malaise
4. Headache
5. Confusion, stupor, and coma
6. Seizures

### Differential Diagnosis

1. Adrenal insufficiency
2. CSWS (cerebral salt-wasting syndrome)
3. Congestive heart failure
4. Diabetes mellitus
5. Hypopituitarism
6. Hypothyroidism
7. Nephrotic syndrome
8. Polydipsia
9. Simple hyponatremia

### Testing and Diagnosis of SIADH

1. Hyponatremia: serum sodium <130 mEq/L
   a. Often a diagnosis of exclusion for euvolemic hyponatremia, defined as serum sodium <135 mEq/L.
2. Plasma osmolality <270 mOsm/kg.
3. Urine sodium concentration >20 mEq/L
   a. Concentrated urine with a low flow rate and associated hypervolemia
   b. Urine osmolality is usually >100 mOsm/kg and sodium osmolarity is >40 mEq/L.
   c. Urine sodium excretion is generally equal to intake.
4. Low
   a. Blood urea nitrogen
   b. Creatinine
   c. Uric acid
      i. Hypouricemia and increased fractional excretion of uric acid may normalize after the correction of hyponatremia.
   d. Albumin
5. Exclude pseudohyponatremia by evaluating serum proteins, lipids, and glucose.
6. Normal serum bicarbonate and potassium levels

## Treatment

1. Treat the underlying cause if possible.
2. Primarily fluid (water) restriction
   a. 800–1000 mL per day
3. Intravenous (IV) saline
   a. Used for very symptomatic patients
   b. Hypertonic saline (5%) 200–300 mL IV over 3–4 hours
4. Medications

a. Diuretics
b. Demeclocycline
   i. Used for chronic cases when fluid restriction is difficult to maintain
5. The water imbalance should not be corrected too rapidly.

## Cerebral Salt Wasting

### Clinical Issues

#### Definition

1. State of hyponatremia with increased natriuresis
2. Hyponatremic dehydration owing to intracranial pathology
   a. Excessive renal sodium excretion secondary to a centrally mediated process
   b. The patients are usually dehydrated and hypovolemic (unlike SIADH, where the patient is usually hypervolemic).
3. There is some debate over whether this is a form of SIADH or a unique disease.

#### Incidence

1. The incidence of CSWS is unknown.
   a. Affects patients of all ages
   b. Up to 60% of patients with intracranial tumors or brain injuries develop hyponatremia, and CSWS may be responsible for an imbalance in sodium as frequently as SIADH.
   c. Some experts question the existence of this syndrome and consider it an extension of SIADH.

#### Etiology

1. Head injury
2. Intracranial tumor or surgery
3. Intracerebral bleed or stroke
4. Meningitis

#### Signs and Symptoms

1. Similar to SIADH

#### Differential Diagnosis

1. Idiopathic hyponatremia
2. SIADH

#### Testing

1. Serum chemistry shows hyponatremia.
2. Dilute urine with a high flow rate
3. Random urine sodium greater than 40 mEq/L
4. Urine sodium excretion greater than intake: negative sodium balance

5. Hypouricemia and increased fractional excretion of uric acid persist after correction of hyponatremia.

## Treatment

1. Fluids
2. Correction of the low sodium
   a. Normal or hypertonic saline
3. Medications
   a. Fludrocortisone: mineralocorticoid

# Diabetes Insipidus (DI)

## Clinical Issues

### Definition

1. State of hypernatremia with a normal total body concentration of sodium
2. Most common cause of hypernatremia in awake patients with a normal total body sodium content
3. An inability to concentrate urine due to either renal resistance to ADH, known as nephrogenic DI, or a decrease in ADH secretion known as central DI
4. Excretion of large amounts of extremely dilute urine, which does not decrease when the fluid intake is decreased
5. Polyuria without glycosuria

### Incidence

1. DI has an estimated prevalence of 1:25,000 in hospitalized patients.

### Etiology

1. Central DI
   a. Traumatic
      i. Surgical
      ii. Accidental
   b. Neoplasm
      i. Lymphoma
      ii. Craniopharyngioma
      iii. Metastasis
   c. Granulomatous disease
      i. Histiocytosis X
      ii. Sarcoidosis
   d. Idiopathic
   e. Infectious
      i. Meningitis
      ii. Encephalitis
   f. Vascular
      i. Cerebral aneurysms
      ii. Sheehan's syndrome
2. Nephrogenic DI
   a. Metabolic
      i. Hypokalemia
      ii. Hypercalcemia
   b. Infectious
      i. Pyelonephritis
   c. Post-renal obstruction release
   d. Vascular
      i. Sickle cell anemia
   e. Granulomatous disease
      i. Sarcoidosis
   f. Drug effects
      i. Lithium
      ii. Amphotericin B
      iii. Demeclocycline
      iv. Methoxyflurane
      v. Ifosfamide
      vi. Mannitol
   g. Genetic
      i. X-linked
      ii. Polycystic kidney disease

### Signs and Symptoms

1. Excessive urination: day and night
2. Extreme thirst
3. Some patients will develop signs of dehydration.
4. May present with fever, vomiting, and diarrhea

### Differential Diagnosis

1. Untreated diabetes mellitus type 1
2. Psychogenic polydipsia
3. Osmotic diuresis

### Testing

1. Diagnosis is often made clinically.
2. Check the patient's serum electrolytes.
   a. Sodium
   b. Glucose
   c. Bicarbonate
   d. Calcium
3. Urinalysis
   a. Dilute urine
   b. Low specific gravity: less than 1.005 and urine osmolality less than 200 mOsm/kg

4. Random plasma osmolality is often >287 mOsm/kg.

5. Water deprivation test can be used to determine if the DI is caused by the following:

    a. Excessive intake of fluid

    b. A defect in ADH production

    c. A defect in the kidney's response to ADH

        i. The test measures the patient's weight, urine output, and urine composition when fluids are withheld.

6. Desmopressin stimulation test

    a. Used to distinguish between nephrogenic and central DI

    b. Central DI: the patient has a reduction in urine output and increased urine osmolarity.

    c. Nephrogenic DI: no change in the urine output or urine osmolarity

## Treatment

1. Central DI

    a. Aqueous vasopressin: IM or SubQ

        i. Acute treatment of DI

    b. Desmopressin (DDAVP): IV, nasal spray, or tablet

    c. Adequate hydration

2. Nephrogenic

    a. Thiazide diuretic: hydrochlorothiazide (HCTZ)

    b. Indomethacin

    c. Adequate hydration

    d. Sodium and protein restriction

    e. Treat the underlying cause.

## KO Treatment Plan

The patient in the case stem question is likely experiencing SIADH associated with the transsphenoidal resection of his pituitary tumor. SIADH after resection is not uncommon and typically presents with hyponatremia, decreased serum osmolarity, and increased urine sodium along with complaints of thirst.

### Pre-operative

1. Patients with sodium level greater than 125 mEq/L are generally asymptomatic.

2. A serum sodium less than 105 mEq/kg is life-threatening.

3. Electrolytes should be checked pre-operatively and optimized if possible.

4. Pre-operative sedation should be administered judiciously in patients with associated mental status changes.

5. Fluid balance should also be optimized pre-operatively if possible.

### Intra-operative

1. Induction agents should be chosen with consideration to volume status.

2. A urinary bladder catheter should be placed to help monitor the patient's volume status.

3. Consider an arterial catheter if:

    a. Frequent laboratory values will be checked.

    b. There is a concern of hemodynamic lability.

    c. They aid in fluid resuscitation via pulse pressure variation.

4. Fluid replacement should commence judiciously due to the concern of central pontine myelinolysis.

    a. Central pontine myelinolysis is a noninflammatory demyelination of the pons, associated with a rapid correction of hyponatremia.

    b. Patients may have sudden quadriparesis, dysphagia, dysarthria, diplopia, and loss of consciousness.

    c. The patient may experience a "locked-in syndrome," where cognitive function is intact but all muscles are paralyzed except for eye blinking.

### Post-operative

1. The patient should be discharged to an appropriate level of care setting where resuscitation needs can be adequately met.

2. Hyponatremia associated with SIADH should be corrected with hypertonic saline in the symptomatic patient or a patient with serum sodium less than 110 mEq/L.

    a. The rate of correction should be less than 0.5 mEq/L/h.

        i. More severe circumstances allow for a more rapid correction.

        ii. Should not exceed 15 mEq correction over a 24-hour period

    b. Serum electrolytes must be closely monitored.

    c. Furosemide (Lasix) may be considered since water loss from Lasix is relatively greater than sodium loss.

## Bibliography

Barash PG, Cullen BF, Stoelting RK, et al. *Clinical Anesthesia*, 8th ed. Philadelphia: Lippincott Williams & Wilkins, 2017, pp. 398–404.

Butterworth JF, Mackey DC, Wasnick JD. *Morgan & Mikhail's Clinical Anesthesiology*, 6th ed. New York: McGraw-Hill Education, 2018, pp. 1140–8.

Fleisher, LA. *Anesthesia and Uncommon Diseases*, 5th ed. Philadelphia: Saunders Elsevier, 2006, pp. 430–2.

Yao, FSF. *Yao and Artusio's Anesthesiology*, 6th ed. Philadelphia: Lippincott, Williams, & Wilkins, 2008, pp. 601, 826–7.

# Spinal Cord Injury

## 46

Melvyn J. Y. Chin, Kamaljit K. Sidhu, and Jessica A. Lovich-Sapola

## Sample Case

A 32-year-old male with a spinal cord injury (SCI) at the level of T4 from a motor vehicle accident nine months ago presents for a pre-surgical anesthesia evaluation. He will be undergoing a lithotripsy for bladder stones. He has no sensation below the level of T4. Apart from the SCI, he has no other medical problems. What are your considerations for this patient? If this patient has autonomic dysreflexia, how would this change your anesthetic plan?

## Clinical Issues

### Acute SCI

1. Airway management/respiratory

   a. Cervical stabilization: your goal is to prevent further SCI.

      i. Manual in-line stabilization
      ii. GlideScope
      iii. Awake fiber-optic intubation

   b. Lesions above C5 usually require intubation and mechanical ventilation.

      i. The phrenic nerve arises from C3 to C5.

   c. Injuries below the cervical region may still require mechanical ventilation due to respiratory difficulties: weak accessory respiratory muscles.

   d. Supine positioning improves spontaneous respiration compared to an upright position in SCI patients.

      i. Paradoxical respiration (chest wall collapse with inspiration) may occur from the loss of chest wall and abdominal muscle tone.
      ii. In the upright position, the abdominal contents are not being pushed up against the diaphragm because of the loss of abdominal wall muscle tone. Since the diaphragm sits lower, the diaphragmatic excursion and vital capacity are reduced.

   e. SCI patients are more prone to hypoxemia and pneumonia.

      i. Atelectasis
      ii. Unopposed vagal tone

         (1) Increased airway secretions

      iii. Weak accessory respiratory muscles
      iv. Ineffective cough
      v. Pulmonary edema: catecholamine surge that occurs after an acute trauma to the spinal cord

   f. Post-operative respiratory care

      i. Aggressive bronchial hygiene: suctioning, positive pressure, and assisted cough mechanisms
      ii. Incentive spirometry
      iii. Percussion and vibration
      iv. Frequent position changes
      v. Intermittent positive-pressure breathing
      vi. β-agonist therapy (i.e., albuterol)

2. Spinal shock

   a. Definition:

      i. Loss or depression of all or most of the spinal reflex activity below the level of spinal injury
      ii. The loss of sympathetic tone results in unopposed parasympathetic stimulation.

   b. Timeline: duration can be 24 hours to 3 months after the initial injury, but on average it only lasts 3 weeks post-injury.

   c. Clinical manifestations: injuries above T6 are more likely to result in autonomic changes.

      i. Hypotension
      ii. Bradycardia: loss of activity in the T1–T4 cardioacceleratory fibers
      iii. Decreased preload
      iv. Decreased peripheral vascular resistance

   d. Management

      i. Fluids
      ii. Catecholamine infusion
      iii. May require temporary transcutaneous cardiac pacing
      iv. The ideal mean arterial pressure (MAP) that allows for maximal cord perfusion is uncertain; therefore, it is recommended that the patient be kept normotensive (MAP >80–90 mm Hg).

### Chronic SCI

1. Autonomic dysreflexia

a. Definition

    i. Noxious stimulus below the level of injury causes a massive reflex sympathetic discharge.

    ii. Occurs in patients with an SCI lesion at T6 or above

    iii. Sympathetic discharge is unopposed because of the interruption of descending sympathetic control, and the receptors below the level of injury are hypersensitive.

b. Timeline

    i. Develops after the resolution of spinal shock

    ii. It usually develops within the first 6 months to 1 year after the initial SCI.

c. Clinical manifestations

    i. Noxious stimulus below the level of the spinal cord lesion results in an uninhibited sympathetic response.

    ii. The autonomic dysreflexia will occur independently of the patient's sensation or lack of sensation.

    iii. Symptoms

      (1) Hypertension: secondary to sympathetically mediated vasoconstriction of the splanchnic, muscle, and skin vasculature

      (2) Reflex bradycardia: carotid response to the hypertension

      (3) Headache

      (4) Malaise

      (5) Piloerection

      (6) Sweating and flushing above the level of the SCI

d. Common noxious stimuli

    i. Bladder distension

    ii. Bowel distension

    iii. Infection

    iv. Labor

    v. Any abdominal emergency

    vi. Fracture: occult or obvious

    vii. Surgery at a site below the level of the lesion

e. Management: if untreated, it may lead to a cerebral vascular accident (CVA), subarachnoid hemorrhage (SAH), seizure, retinal hemorrhage, or death.

    i. Sit the patient up.

    ii. Identify and remove the noxious stimulus (see above).

    iii. Treat the hypertension:

      (1) Nitroglycerine (paste, SL, IV)

      (2) Hydralazine

      (3) Nifedipine

      (4) Clonidine

      (5) Nitroprusside

      (6) Spinal anesthesia

f. Prevention

    i. Preventing the development of autonomic dysreflexia is better than having to treat it.

    ii. Examples: general anesthesia/epidural/spinal for laboring patients or surgical procedures, even if the patient has no sensation of pain

    iii. An SCI patient with a lesion above T6 having surgical procedures below the level of the injury will require adequate anesthesia (neuraxial or general) to prevent autonomic dysreflexia.

g. Succinylcholine should be avoided after the first 48 hours post-cord injury.

    i. Risk of sudden, severe hyperkalemia leading to cardiac arrest

    ii. This has been reported in patients with thoracolumbar SCI and muscle denervation.

    iii. The massive efflux of potassium into the serum is presumed to be due to the proliferation of the extra-junctional acetylcholine receptors and its subsequent depolarization.

# KO Treatment Plan

## Pre-operative

1. Standard history and physical

    a. Level of injury

    b. Length of time of injury

    c. History of prior autonomic dysreflexia

    d. Baseline blood pressures

    e. Respiratory status

    f. Recent infections/pneumonias

    g. Prior anesthetic complications

## Intra-operative

1. Despite the fact that the patient lacks sensation below T4, anesthesia is still required to prevent the onset of autonomic dysreflexia.

    a. This can be accomplished by either neuraxial or general anesthesia.

2. One should have vasodilators readily available (i.e., nitroglycerin, nitroprusside).

## Post-operative

1. Routine monitoring in the post-anesthesia care unit with special attention to respiratory status and signs and symptoms of autonomic dysreflexia

## Bibliography

Barash PG, Cullen BF, Stoelting RK, et al. *Clinical Anesthesia*, 8th ed. Philadelphia: Lippincott Williams & Wilkins, 2017, pp. 1023–4.

Cuccurullo S. *Physical Medicine and Rehabilitation Board Review*, 4th ed. New York: Springer, 2019, pp. 556–7, 563–6, 655–7.

Hines M. *Stoelting's Anesthesia and Co-Existing Disease*, 7th ed. Philadelphia: Elsevier, 2018, pp. 305–14.

Lin, V. *Spinal Cord Medicine: Principles and Practice*. New York: Demos Medical Publishing, 2003, pp. 113–21, 189.

Chapter

# 47

# Acute Kidney Injury

Sennaraj Balasubramanian and Jessica A. Lovich-Sapola

## Sample Case

An 83-year-old male is post-operative on day one after a coronary artery bypass graft (CABG). His urine has decreased to 15 mL/h for the last 2 hours. Is this oliguria? What are the possible causes? How would you diagnose and treat this finding? How do you determine between pre-renal, renal, and post-renal causes of acute renal failure (ARF)?

## Clinical Issues

### Definition of Acute Kidney Injury

Acute kidney injury (AKI) is a syndrome of abrupt decline in renal excretory and homeostatic function. This results in bloodstream accumulation of products of nitrogenous metabolism and failure to regulate body fluid volume, electrolyte concentrations, and acid–base balance.

### Stages of AKI

The Improving Global Outcomes guidelines stage AKI according to severity:

1.  Stage 1: characterized by one of the following:

    a.  Serum creatinine level increase of 1.5–1.9 times the baseline (Tables 47.1 and 47.2)

    b.  Serum creatinine level increase of 0.3 mg/dL or more

    c.  Urine output less than 0.5 mL/kg/h for 6–12 hours

2.  Stage 2: characterized by one of the following:

    a.  Serum creatinine level increase of 2–2.9 times the baseline

    b.  Urine output less than 0.5 mL/kg/h for 12 hours or more

3.  Stage 3: characterized by one of the following:

    a.  Serum creatinine level increase of three times the baseline

    b.  Serum creatinine level increase of 4 mg/dL or more

    c.  Urine output of less than 0.3 mL/kg/h for 24 hours or more

    d.  Anuria for 12 hours or more

    e.  Any requirement for initiation of renal replacement therapy

    f.  In patients younger than 18 years, a decrease in estimated glomerular filtration rate (GFR) to less than 35 mL/min/1.73 m$^2$

**Table 47.1** Normal values

| GFR | Blood urea nitrogen (BUN) | 10–20 mg/dL |
| --- | --- | --- |
| | Creatinine (CR) | 0.5–1.5 mg/dL |
| | Creatinine clearance (CRCL) | 85–125 mL/min (women) 95–140 mL/min (men) |
| Tubular function | Specific gravity (SG) | 1.002–1.030 |
| | Osmolality (mOsm/kg) | 50–1400 |
| | Urine sodium (mEq/L/day) | 130–260 |

Adapted from Stoelting RK, Dierdorf SF. *Anesthesia and Co-Existing Disease*, 4th ed. Philadelphia: Churchill Livingstone, 2002; Miller RD, Fleisher LA, Johns RA, et al. *Anesthesia*, 6th ed. New York: Churchill Livingstone, 2005; Barash PG, Cullen BF, Stoelting RK. *Clinical Anesthesia*, 5th ed. Philadelphia: Lippincott Williams & Wilkins, 2006.

**Table 47.2** Pre-renal versus renal lab values

| | Pre-renal | Renal |
| --- | --- | --- |
| Urine output (cc/kg/h) | <0.5 | <0.5 |
| Urine sodium (mEq/L) | <25 | >35 |
| Fractional excretion of sodium (%) (FENa) | <1 | >1 |
| Urine osmolality (mOsm/kg) | >500 | <350 |
| Urine/plasma creatinine | >30:1 | <10:1 |
| Urine/plasma osmolality | >1.8:1 | <1.1:1 |
| Urine/plasma urea | >20:1 | <3:1 |
| BUN/CR | >20:1 | <10:1 |

Adapted from Stoelting RK, Dierdorf SF. *Anesthesia and Co-Existing Disease*, 4th ed. Philadelphia: Churchill Livingstone, 2002; Miller RD, Fleisher LA, Johns RA, et al. *Anesthesia*, 6th ed. New York: Churchill Livingstone, 2005; Barash PG, Cullen BF, Stoelting RK. *Clinical Anesthesia*, 5th ed. Philadelphia: Lippincott Williams & Wilkins, 2006.

4. Staging is carried out retrospectively when the episode is complete. Patients are classified according to the highest possible stage where the criterion is met, either by creatinine level rise or by urine output.

## Diagnosis

The diagnosis of AKI is usually made based on identification of one of the following:

1. An increase in serum creatinine concentration of more than 0.3 mg/dL within 48 hours
2. An increase of at least 1.5 times the baseline creatinine within a 7-day period
3. Abrupt decrease in urine output to less than 0.5 mL/kg/h for a 6–12 h period or 500 mL/day
4. A decrease in urine output does not necessarily accompany all cases of AKI.

## Incidence

1. AKI occurs in 5–25% of patients admitted to hospital.
2. Incidence in intensive care has been reported in more than 50% of patients.

## Mortality

1. AKI mortality ranges from 10% to 35% for mild AKI.
2. AKI in the ICU setting is associated with a 50–80% mortality rate.

## Risk Factors for AKI

1. Coexisting renal disease
2. Advanced age
3. Congestive heart failure (CHF)
4. Symptomatic cardiovascular disease
5. Major operative procedures
   a. CABG
   b. Abdominal aneurysm repair
   c. Emergency surgery
   d. Intraperitoneal surgery
   e. Liver transplant surgery
6. Sepsis
7. Multiple organ system dysfunction
8. Iatrogenic causes
   a. Inadequate fluid replacement
   b. Delayed treatment of sepsis
   c. Nephrotoxic drugs or dyes
9. Hypotension
10. Male sex
11. Limited cardiorespiratory reserve

## Etiology

1. Pre-renal: usually reversible with an improved circulatory status
   a. Absolute decrease in renal blood flow
      i. Dehydration
      ii. Acute hemorrhage
         (1) Hypovolemia
         (2) Hypotension
      iii. Gastrointestinal (GI) fluid loss
      iv. Trauma
      v. Surgery
         (1) Mechanical restriction of renal blood flow by aortic or renal artery clamping
      vi. Burns
      vii. Renal artery or vein thrombosis
      viii. Excessive diuretic use
   b. Relative decrease in renal blood volume
      i. Septic shock
      ii. Hepatic failure
      iii. Allergic reaction/transfusion reaction
      iv. Vasoconstriction
      v. CHF
      vi. Decreased cardiac output
      vii. Aortic/renal artery clamping
2. Renal: most serious form, which often requires hemodialysis to treat
   a. Acute glomerulonephritis
      i. Goodpasture's syndrome
      ii. Wegener's granulomatosis
      iii. Acute lupus nephritis with systemic lupus erythematosus
      iv. Post-infectious glomerulonephritis
      v. Berger's disease
      vi. Henoch-Schonlein purpura
      vii. Drugs
         (1) Allopurinol
         (2) Hydralazine
         (3) Rifampin
   b. Interstitial nephritis
      i. Pyelonephritis
      ii. Sarcoidosis
      iii. Allergic drug reaction (nonsteroidal anti-inflammatory agents [NSAIDs], aspirin)
   c. Acute tubular necrosis (most common in surgical patients)
      i. Ischemia (50% of cases)

(1) Episode of hypotension

(2) Shock (cardiogenic, septic, hemorrhagic)

  ii. Embolic event or aortic cross clamp

  iii. Mechanical damage

(1) Trauma

  iv. Nephrotoxic drugs (35% of cases)

(1) Radiographic contrast dyes

(2) Aminoglycoside antibiotics

(3) Anesthetic agents

(4) NSAIDs

(5) Chemotherapeutic agents

  v. Solvents

  vi. Myoglobinuria/rhabdomyolysis/hemolysis

  vii. Transfusion reaction

  viii. Hypoxia

  d. Vasculitis

  e. Chronic kidney disease

    i. Diabetes

    ii. Hypertension

  f. Multiple myeloma

3. Post-renal: found in <5% of the cases. It is usually reversible with the treatment of the obstruction. The obstruction is usually secondary to stones, strictures, infection, clots, tumors, surgical ligation, and edema. The obstruction can also be due to medications that interfere with normal bladder emptying.

  a. Upper urinary tract obstruction

    i. Renal pelvis

    ii. Ureter

  b. Lower urinary tract obstruction

    i. Bladder outlet

    ii. Foley catheter

    iii. Urethral

    iv. Prostatic hypertrophy or cancer

    v. Cervical cancer

## Complications of ARF

1. Neurologic

  a. Confusion

  b. Asterixis

  c. Somnolence

  d. Seizures

2. Cardiovascular

  a. Hypertension/hypotension

  b. CHF

  c. Pulmonary edema

  d. Cardiac dysrhythmias

3. Gastrointestinal

  a. Anorexia

  b. Nausea/vomiting

  c. Ileus

  d. GI bleeding

4. Infection

  a. Respiratory

  b. Urinary tract

5. Metabolic derangements

  a. Metabolic acidosis

  b. Hyperkalemia

## KO Treatment Plan

The sample patient can be considered to be oliguric if this low urine output continues. A urine output of 15 mL/h over 24 hours is only 360 mL/day (less than the designated 500 mL/day for the diagnosis of oliguria). It is important to diagnose and treat the cause of the ARF.

1. Check vital signs.

2. Determine whether the AKI is pre-renal, renal, or post-renal.

3. Determine and treat the underlying cause.

  a. Pre-renal

    i. Look for signs of decreased cardiac output, shock, or hypovolemia by assessing the intravascular volume status.

    ii. Central venous pressure (CVP)

    iii. Pulmonary artery catheter (PAC)

    iv. Transesophageal echocardiography

    v. Fluid challenge

  b. Renal

    i. Check urine for blood or myoglobin.

    ii. Check the electrolytes.

    iii. Check BUN/CR.

    iv. Check FENa.

    v. Send a blood and urine specimen for sodium, osmolality, creatine, and urea.

    vi. Discontinue nephrotoxic drugs.

  c. Post-renal

    i. Renal ultrasound is best to diagnose post-renal obstruction.

    ii. Check the Foley catheter.

    iii. Palpate the bladder.

4. Resuscitate the patient until he or she is normotensive with a normal cardiac output.

  a. Fluids

    i. Guided by a Foley catheter – urinary output and CVP monitoring

b. Inotropes

    i. Norepinephrine IV

    ii. Dobutamine IV

    iii. Vasopressin

5. Furosemide IV to maintain urine output in hypervolemic ARF, because a non-oliguric ARF is usually considered better than an oliguric ARF.

6. Hemodialysis every 2–4 days as needed

## Bibliography

Barash PG, Cullen BF, Stoelting RK. *Clinical Anesthesia*, 5th ed. Philadelphia: Lippincott Williams & Wilkins, 2006, pp.1017–18.

Gropper MA. *Miller's Anesthesia*, 9th ed. New York: Churchill Livingstone, 2020, pp. 1340–53.

Hines RL, Jones SB. *Stoelting's Anesthesia and Co-Existing Disease*, 8th ed. Philadelphia: Churchill Livingstone, 2022, pp. 415–38.

Jamie L, Gross M, Prowle JR. Perioperative kidney injury.

*Br J Anaesth Edu* 2015;**15**(4):213–18.

Ronco C, Bellomo R, Kellum JA. Acute kidney injury. *Lancet* 2019;**394**:1949–64.

# Chapter 48

# Chronic Renal Failure

Brian Wheatley and Jessica A. Lovich-Sapola

## Sample Case

A 43-year-old male presents to the operating room for a revision of his arteriovenous dialysis graft. He missed his dialysis yesterday because he did not have transportation. His last dialysis was 4 days ago. Does he need dialysis prior to surgery? What lab values would you like? What if his potassium is 6.4 mEq/L? What would you do? Do you want an EKG? Why? What if his hematocrit is 27%? What would you do? Does he need a blood transfusion? When you do the surgery, what is your choice of anesthetic?

## Clinical Issues

### Definitions

1. Uremic syndrome
   a. Most extreme form of chronic renal failure (CRF)
   b. Glomerular filtration rate (GFR) <10 mL/min
   c. Inability of the kidneys to regulate volume and composition of the extracellular fluid
   d. Inability of the kidneys to effectively excrete waste products
   e. Leads to multiple system organ dysfunction
   f. Requires frequent or continuous dialysis

2. End-stage renal disease (ESRD): a clinical syndrome characterized by multiple-organ dysfunction that would prove fatal without dialysis.
   a. GFR <10 mL/min

3. Renal insufficiency
   a. GFR of 25–40 mL/min
   b. Abnormal creatinine and blood urea nitrogen (BUN) values
   c. At this functional level, one almost always becomes symptomatic. Nocturia is fairly common.

4. Mild kidney insufficiency
   a. GFR of 40–60 mL/min
   b. May have symptoms

5. Decreased kidney reserve
   a. GFR of 60–100 mL/min
   b. Asymptomatic
   c. Normal blood levels of creatinine and urea

## Complications of Uremic Syndrome

1. Electrolyte abnormalities occur usually below GFR of 25 mL/min
   a. Hyponatremia
   b. Hyperkalemia
      i. Peaked T waves, prolongation of the QRS complex and PR interval, heart block, and ventricular fibrillation can be seen on the EKG.
      ii. If the serum potassium is greater than 6.5 mEq/L or if the EKG changes are present, the hyperkalemia should be treated.
      iii. Treat the hyperkalemia with IV calcium, glucose, insulin, bicarbonate, and/or emergency dialysis.
      iv. Most common in GFRs <5 mL/min
   c. Hypocalcemia: commonly in alkalosis
   d. Hyperphosphatemia
   e. Hypermagnesemia
   f. Metabolic acidosis
      i. Treat a pH <7.3 with IV bicarbonate, assuming the patient has appropriate ventilation.

2. Cardiovascular
   a. Heart failure secondary to hypervolemia
   b. Hypertension
      i. Treat with diuretics in pre-dialysis patients.
      ii. Treat with hemodialysis.
   c. Uremic pericarditis/cardiac tamponade
   d. Myocardial dysfunction
   e. Arrythmias
   f. Accelerated peripheral vascular disease/coronary artery disease

3. Respiratory
   a. Pulmonary edema
   b. Central hyperventilation secondary to metabolic acidosis

4. Hematologic
   a. Normochromic, normocytic anemia
      i. Treat with recombinant human erythropoietin (epoetin alpha/Epogen/Procrit).

ii. Parenteral iron

iii. Avoid blood transfusions if possible.

b. Platelet dysfunction

c. Coagulopathy

d. Uremic bleeding

i. Treat with cryoprecipitate to provide factor VIII and/or DDAVP (desmopressin).

5. Gastrointestinal (GI)

a. Delayed gastric emptying

b. Anorexia

c. Nausea/vomiting

d. Hemorrhage/peptic ulceration has 10–30% prevalence

e. Increased incidence of hepatitis B/C

6. Neuromuscular

a. Encephalopathy

b. Seizures

c. Tremors

d. Myoclonus

e. Polyneuropathy

f. Autonomic dysfunction

7. Endocrine/metabolism

a. Osteodystrophy

i. Treat with antacids to bind the phosphorus in the GI tract, oral calcium supplements, and vitamin D therapy.

b. Glucose intolerance

c. Increased atherosclerosis

d. Fatigue

e. Pruritus

## Associated Causes

1. Systemic hypertension

2. Glomerulopathies

a. Primary

b. Associated with a disease

i. Diabetes mellitus

ii. Amyloidosis

iii. Systemic lupus erythematosus

iv. Wegener's granulomatosis

3. Tubulointerstitial disease

a. Sarcoidosis

4. Hereditary disease

a. Polycystic kidney disease

5. Renal vascular disease

6. Obstructive uropathy

7. Human immunodeficiency virus (HIV)

## KO Treatment Plan

### Pre-operative

1. This surgery is not an emergency. He very likely has a temporary dialysis catheter in place.

2. This patient should have dialysis prior to this surgery. The hemodialysis should correct his elevated potassium.

3. While waiting for dialysis, the patient should have a 12-lead EKG to look for any changes secondary to the hyperkalemia. If he has EKG changes, his hyperkalemia should be treated immediately and not wait for his dialysis.

a. 10 mL of 10% calcium chloride IV infused over 10 minutes

b. Glucose (D10 W) IV and 5–10 units of regular insulin for every 25–50 g of glucose given

c. Sodium bicarbonate 50–100 mEq IV over 5–10 minutes

d. $\beta_2$ agonist (albuterol)

4. His hematocrit may be low secondary to hemodilution from fluid overload due to missing his dialysis. Review any old records. Repeat a hematocrit after his dialysis. These patients typically tolerate a lower hematocrit. I would not transfuse for a hematocrit of 27% if the patient is normally anemic.

### Intra-operative

1. This is a low-risk surgery. It should be able to be done under regional technique or local block with sedation.

2. If the patient requires general anesthesia, remember that he is considered "full stomach" secondary to his associated delayed gastric emptying. If he has had hemodialysis and has a normalized potassium level, a rapid-sequence induction with succinylcholine can be safely done. His potassium will increase only about 0.5 mEq/L, the same as in normal healthy patients. If the patient was an emergent surgery and was not able to have his dialysis, then succinylcholine should be avoided.

**TKO:** Pick one induction agent and defend it. Do not give a list of all the induction agents that can be used. Don't say "I could . . . " – say "I would use this drug and this is why."

3. Safe induction agents

a. You may choose etomidate because of the presumed associated cardiovascular issues with this patient and the fact that renal failure does not seem to affect its clinical effects.

b. You may choose propofol because of the uremia-associated nausea/vomiting, decreased gastric emptying, and the fact that it also has an unchanged clinical profile in renal failure patients.

c. Ketamine is also a good choice because poor renal function does not tend to alter its pharmacokinetic or clinical profile.

4. Intra-operative opioids

a. Fentanyl is an excellent choice and is recommended secondary to its primary liver metabolism and lack of active metabolites.

b. Remifentanil is also good secondary to its rapid metabolism by blood and tissue esterases.

c. A single small dose of morphine is acceptable, but chronic dosing is not acceptable, secondary to the accumulation of its metabolite, 6-glucuronide, which leads to prolonged respiratory depression and sedation.

d. Meperidine has a metabolite, normeperidine, which is neurotoxic and can lead to convulsions when used in a renal failure patient.

5. All volatile anesthetics can be used safely, but sevoflurane does have a theoretical risk secondary to the plasma inorganic fluoride concentrations approaching nephrotoxic levels (50 μmol/L) after prolonged inhalation. However, no evidence of gross changes in renal function has been found in humans.

6. Nitrous oxide can be employed, but to maximize arterial oxygenation it is beneficial to maintain $FiO_2$ above 50%.

7. Muscle relaxants

a. Succinylcholine is safe if the potassium value is known.

b. Cisatracurium and atracurium are degraded by plasma ester hydrolysis and Hoffman elimination, and are excellent choices for renal failure patients.

c. Vecuronium and rocuronium effects can be prolonged in patients with kidney disease, but are still safe in severe kidney disease.

8. Reversal agents

a. Neostigmine and edrophonium half-lives are at least as long as reversal agents thereby reducing the chance of "recurarization."

b. Sugammadex is eliminated in unmetabolized form by the kidney but may exist for days in the plasma and is not yet recommended for ESRD according to the package insert.

i. Despite this, sugammadex is still used in ESRD patients in some clinical settings.

# Bibliography

Barash PG, Cullen BF, Stoelting RK, et al. *Clinical Anesthesia*, 8th ed. Philadelphia: Lippincott Williams & Wilkins, 2017, pp. 1410–15.

Butterworth JF, Mackey DC, Wasnick JD. *Morgan & Mikhail's Clinical Anesthesiology*, 6th ed. New York: McGraw-Hill, 2018, pp. 675–91.

Gropper MA. *Miller's Anesthesia*, 9th ed. Philadelphia: Elsevier, 2020, pp. 1043–6.

Stoelting RK, Dierdorf SF. *Anesthesia and Co-Existing Disease*, 4th ed. Philadelphia: Churchill Livingstone, 2002, pp 344–9.

# Dialysis

Maureen Keshock, Lisa L. Bethea, and Jessica A. Lovich-Sapola

## Sample Case

A 49-year-old male with type II diabetes mellitus, hypertension, end-stage renal disease (ESRD), and chronic obstructive pulmonary disease presents for a laparoscopic hemicolectomy for colon polyps. The patient usually receives hemodialysis (HD) 3 days per week. What are the major concerns in the pre-, intra-, and post-operative periods? If surgery is scheduled on the day of dialysis, should the patient receive dialysis prior to the surgery? How will this affect your anesthetic management before, during, and after surgery?

## Clinical Issues

Definition: dialysis is used as a substitute for the kidney when the kidney cannot perform its usual functions, including fluid and electrolyte balance and toxin/drug removal.

## Modalities

1.  HD – intermittent and continuous
    a.  Removes both solutes and fluids from the body
    b.  This is done by diffusive and convective clearance for solutes and ultrafiltration for fluids.
    c.  Solute clearance is determined by the molecular size of the solutes, concentration gradient, membrane surface area, membrane permeability, and flow rate of blood and dialysate.
    d.  Ultrafiltration is determined by the transmembrane pressure.
    e.  Continuous HD or continuous renal replacement therapy (CRRT) is recommended for hemodynamically unstable patients.

2.  Peritoneal dialysis
    a.  Removal of fluids and solutes through use of the patient's own peritoneal membrane
    b.  Solute removal is via diffusion across a concentration gradient, whereas fluid removal is via osmotic ultrafiltration.

3.  Patient survival is equal between the two forms of dialysis, but in the United States HD is the most common ESRD modality.

## Indications for Dialysis

1.  Absolute indications
    a.  Metabolic acidosis

b.  Electrolyte abnormalities
    i.  Hyperkalemia
    ii.  Hypercalcemia
    iii.  Hyperphosphatemia
    iv.  Hypermagnesemia
    v.  Hypernatremia or hyponatremia

c.  Intoxication/drug overdose: this is not a complete list – just examples of some of the more commonly used drugs for anesthesia that are dialyzable. Propofol, fentanyl, and rocuronium are not dialyzable.
    i.  Acetaminophen
    ii.  Aspirin
    iii.  Antibiotics
        (1)  Amoxicillin
        (2)  Ampicillin
        (3)  Cefazolin
        (4)  Cefepime
        (5)  Cefotaxime
        (6)  Cefoxitin
        (7)  Penicillin
    iv.  Acyclovir
    v.  Allopurinol
    vi.  Most β-blockers
        (1)  Atenolol
        (2)  Esmolol
        (3)  Metoprolol
    vii.  Most angiotensin-converting enzyme inhibitors (ACEIs)
        (1)  Captopril
        (2)  Enalapril
        (3)  Lisinopril
    viii.  Vitamins
        (1)  Ascorbic acid
        (2)  Edetate calcium
        (3)  Folic acid
    ix.  Mannitol
    x.  Metformin
    xi.  Nitroprusside
    xii.  Phenobarbital

d. Fluid overload/pulmonary edema
e. Uremia
f. Encephalopathy
g. Pericarditis

2. Relative indications

  a. Blood urea nitrogen (BUN) and creatinine (Cr) values should be used only as a guide.

    i. BUN >100 mg/dL or Cr >10 mg/dL values are used when initiating chronic dialysis.

  b. Glomerular filtration rate (GFR) less than 15 mL/min/1.73 m$^2$

3. General

  a. Acute renal failure
  b. Chronic renal failure
  c. ESRD
  d. Uncontrolled hypertension

## Access

1. Hemodialysis

  a. Vascular access

    i. Native arteriovenous fistula (AVF)

      (1) Connection between the radial artery or brachial artery and the cephalic or basilic veins
      (2) This allows blood flow rates of 400 mL/min.
      (3) Matures in 6–8 weeks
      (4) Longest survival after maturation
      (5) Fewest complications

    ii. Artificial arteriovenous graft (AVG)

      (1) Synthetic graft used when AVF cannot be placed
      (2) Easier to place
      (3) Higher rate of complications, including infection, stenosis, and thrombosis

    iii. Percutaneous double-lumen catheter

      (1) Placed in the internal jugular or femoral vein and usually tunneled under the skin
      (2) Catheters have been placed in the subclavian vein in the past, but they were found to be associated with central venous stenosis.

2. Peritoneal dialysis

  a. Access via catheter in the abdominal cavity, placed between the anterior abdominal wall and the omentum/bowel loops.
  b. The catheter is either a silicone or polyurethane material.
  c. The catheter is cuffed.

## Complications

1. Hemodialysis

  a. Vascular access problems

    i. Infection
    ii. Bleeding from the puncture site
    iii. Thrombosis
    iv. Stenosis
    v. Aneurysm
    vi. Arteriovenous access steal

  b. Hypotension

    i. Decreased intravascular volume
    ii. Hemorrhage
    iii. Septicemia
    iv. Cardiogenic shock
    v. Dysrhythmia
    vi. Anaphylactoid reaction
    vii. Air embolism

  c. Hemorrhage with resultant cardiac symptoms

    i. Symptomatic angina
    ii. Congestive heart failure
    iii. Patients are typically treated with epoetin prior to dialysis to prevent severe anemia.

  d. Gastrointestinal bleed

    i. Angiodysplasia
    ii. Peptic ulcer disease

  e. Cardiovascular

    i. Acute pericardial tamponade
    ii. Chest pain

      (1) Most dialysis patients have coronary artery disease (CAD); therefore, ischemic origin of chest pain must be ruled out.

  f. Electrolyte abnormalities

    i. Hypo-/hyperkalemia
    ii. Hypo-/hypercalcemia
    iii. Hypermagnesemia
    iv. Hypo-/hyperglycemia

  g. Shortness of breath due to volume overload
  h. Neurologic dysfunction

    i. Disequilibrium syndrome: headache, malaise, nausea, vomiting, and muscle cramps. This may progress to seizures and coma.
    ii. Cerebrovascular accident
    iii. Subdural hematoma
    iv. Hypertensive encephalopathy

2. Peritoneal dialysis

a. Peritonitis is due to bacterial contamination, usually from a *Staphylococcus* species.

b. Catheter contamination

c. Catheter leakage

d. Abdominal wall or inguinal hernia due to the associated increased intra-abdominal pressure

e. Infection of catheter exit site

f. Pneumoperitoneum from air that enters during exchange therapy

g. Mechanical problems

    i. Inability to drain dialysate completely because of catheter kinking or obstruction

h. Volume overload may lead to worsening blood pressure control or acute pulmonary edema.

i. Volume depletion

    i. Poor oral intake

    ii. Increased gastrointestinal loss

j. Metabolic problems (e.g., hyperglycemia) from absorption of glucose from the dialysate fluid (hyperosmolar solution)

**TKO:** Dialysis patients have an increased risk of morbidity and mortality. This risk is further enhanced in the setting of surgery.

## Increased Risk of Morbidity and Mortality

1. Higher likelihood of CAD and cardiac abnormalities

2. Electrolyte and fluid imbalances, especially in the presence of worsening kidney function

    a. Patients with renal failure tend to have fluid overload/pulmonary edema as well as increases or decreases in potassium, magnesium, calcium, and/or glucose levels.

3. Problems with drug excretion and metabolism, which interferes with anesthetic dosing

    a. Drugs that are renally metabolized/excreted take longer to be removed from the body and therefore can build up and cause toxicity.

4. Bleeding complications

    a. Impaired platelet function

        i. Prolonged bleeding time

        ii. Platelet dysfunction is most often seen in the presence of uremia because toxins are not properly removed from the body.

5. Blood pressure fluctuations, depending on when dialysis was last received

    a. If too much fluid has been removed, then the blood pressure tends to be low from volume depletion.

b. If too little fluid has been removed or it has been days since the last treatment, then the blood pressure is elevated from volume overload.

6. Require more medical management: prolonged ICU/hospital time and mechanical ventilation.

## KO Treatment Plan

### Pre-operative

1. Start with a history.

    a. Complaint of chest pain or shortness of breath

    b. New or worsening headache, nausea/vomiting, malaise

    c. Medical problems and current medications

    d. Dialysis schedule and when last received

    e. Dry weight

2. Physical exam

    a. Check vital signs: blood pressure, heart rate, respiratory rate, temperature, and oxygen saturation.

    b. Listen to the patient's heart and lungs.

    c. Look for signs of fluid overload: extremity edema, jugular venous distension, and use of accessory muscles of respiration.

    d. Assess for signs of volume depletion: poor skin turgor, dry mucous membranes, hypotension, and tachycardia.

    e. Assess bruit in fistula, if indicated.

3. Labs

    a. Laboratory values must be monitored closely prior to any surgical intervention. The patient's baseline electrolyte, hemoglobin, coagulation panel, and platelet values are important.

        i. Check prior lab values to assess patient trends. If there are significant increases or decreases, further treatment may be necessary.

        ii. Potassium less than 6.0 mEq/L is usually acceptable unless there are cardiographic changes on the electrocardiogram.

          (1) Peaked T waves

          (2) Prolonged PR interval

          (3) Widened QRS complex

        iii. Anemia is present in ESRD patients (usually chronic) and procedures are usually well tolerated with hematocrit levels of 20–24%.

          (1) If the procedure is nonemergent, the patient can receive erythropoietin to help stimulate red blood cell production. For emergent procedures, IV desmopressin is recommended.

        iv. Glucose

(1) Must consider NPO status, decreased activity level, and comorbid conditions that might affect glucose metabolism.

   v. Bleeding problems must be corrected with blood transfusions, platelets, desmopressin, or cryoprecipitate.

      (1) Heparin should be avoided in the days leading up to surgery.

4. Cardiovascular evaluation will assess for CAD and myocardial dysfunction.

  a. No further evaluation is needed for low-risk patients; no history of CAD, myocardial ischemia, or chest pain.

  b. An EKG can help determine whether cardiovascular effects of hyperkalemia are present as well as assess for arrhythmias.

    i. A baseline EKG will help evaluate the patient for changes intra-operatively and post-operatively.

  c. An echocardiogram and/or stress test is used to evaluate myocardial function and determine whether ischemia develops in the presence of stress.

    i. This is a noninvasive way of determining whether the patient can handle the stress of surgery and helps determine whether further procedures (angiography, cardiac catheterization) are needed.

5. Nutrition status is the key to good healing.

  a. Check the patient's protein catabolic rate and/or albumin concentration.

  b. Eliminate drugs that hinder appetite.

  c. Give drugs that inhibit or treat gastroparesis.

6. Good blood pressure control leading up to the surgery is important. This will allow for less labile pressures, hopefully preventing instances of hypertension and hypotension during the surgery.

  a. Hypotension is usually due to too much fluid removed during dialysis or inappropriate dosages of antihypertensive medications.

    i. Adjust medication dosages as needed.

    ii. This may also be treated with judicious fluid boluses.

    iii. If this does not help, vasopressors (phenylephrine, ephedrine) may be needed.

  b. Hypertension should be treated with antihypertensive agents such as β-blockers, hydralazine, diltiazem, and nitroglycerin.

7. A more intensive dialysis regimen prior to surgery may be beneficial.

  a. Patients receiving intermittent hemodialysis may benefit from daily dialysis several days prior to surgery (more beneficial for cardiac surgery).

  b. Those receiving peritoneal dialysis may benefit from an additional exchange every day for the entire week leading up to surgery.

8. Dialysis should be provided the day prior to surgery.

  a. Dry weight

  b. Ensure normalization of electrolytes.

  c. Optimize fluid status.

  d. Having dialysis on the day of surgery could cause volume depletion if too much fluid is removed. This would cause significant hypotension during surgery, which is worsened in the presence of vasodilatation already produced by anesthesia.

9. Antibiotics, if necessary, should be adjusted for renal function.

10. IV access

  a. Avoid any sites that may be needed for dialysis access in the future.

  b. Subclavian access should be avoided because of the increased risk for stenosis.

  c. Awareness of the patient's vascular anatomy is important.

## Intra-operative

1. Drugs/anesthetic agents are not metabolized the same in patients with renal failure. Maintain caution to avoid overdosing and/or toxic levels.

  a. Pre-induction agents

    i. Benzodiazepines have increased protein binding, which may lead to increased free fraction in the presence of renal failure.

    ii. Smaller doses should be used.

  b. Induction agents

    i. Propofol is metabolized by the liver and is therefore not contraindicated in renal failure.

  c. Neuromuscular blockers

    i. Depolarizing agents

      (1) Succinylcholine can cause hyperkalemia, which can be a significant problem in patients with renal failure.

        (a) Succinylcholine raises serum potassium about 0.5 mEq/L.

        (b) This increase is not significant in normal patients but can be potentially dangerous in the presence of renal failure.

(c) Typically, if the serum potassium is less than 5 mEq/L, then succinylcholine is acceptable to use.

ii. Neuromuscular blocking agents

(1) Pancuronium is a long-acting nondepolarizer and is renally excreted. It should be avoided in these patients due to the risk of prolonged blockade.

(2) Atracurium is excreted via extra-renal mechanisms (Hoffman elimination) and is therefore a preferred neuromuscular blocking agent.

2. Monitors

a. Standard ASA monitors including heart rate, blood pressure, pulse oximetry, and temperature

b. Arterial line

i. Watch for excessive alterations in blood pressure.

ii. Glucose monitoring helps maintain a glucose level within normal limits.

3. Maintenance

a. Anesthesia can be maintained with isoflurane, $O_2$, and air.

b. $N_2O$ is contraindicated in laparoscopic procedures because it can diffuse into spaces and cause distension of the bowel. This would hinder visualization for the surgeon.

c. Isoflurane may decrease renal blood flow but not more or less than any other anesthetic agent. There are no contraindications in renal failure.

d. All volatile anesthetics can be used safely, but sevoflurane does have a theoretical risk secondary to the plasma inorganic fluoride concentrations approaching nephrotoxic levels (50 μmol/L) after prolonged inhalation. However, no evidence of gross changes in renal function has been found in humans.

e. Opiates can be used intra-operatively for pain control.

i. Fentanyl is preferred because of its short redistribution phase and lack of active metabolites.

4. IV fluids

a. Normal saline is preferred because it does not contain additional electrolytes such as potassium, calcium, and magnesium, which are found in Lactated Ringer's solution.

b. Providing fluids with additional electrolytes can cause electrolyte imbalances post-operatively.

c. Judicious amounts of fluids should be given to prevent fluid overload.

## Post-operative

1. Recovery depends on the nature of the surgery. Patients do not need to go to the ICU unless the procedure itself requires this.

2. Blood pressure monitoring must continue in the post-operative period.

a. Treat hypotension with vasopressors (phenylephrine, norepinephrine, and vasopressin) as necessary.

b. Avoid giving too much fluid.

c. If vasopressors are needed, an ICU setting is preferred.

d. Treat hypertension with antihypertensive agents such as hydralazine, β-blockers, or nitroglycerin.

i. If the hypertension cannot be controlled, dialysis may be required to remove excess fluid.

3. Labs should be checked immediately post-operatively and daily to assess electrolyte abnormalities. Follow glucose levels closely, especially if the patient has an NPO status.

4. Fluid status can be evaluated by following the patient's dry weight and/or monitoring urine output if the patient still produces urine.

5. Dialysis should be resumed post-operatively. The timing depends on patient fluid status, electrolyte balance, and hemodynamic stability. When dialysis is used in the post-operative period, heparin must be avoided for 24–48 hours.

6. Analgesics, such as opiates and acetaminophen, may be used for post-operative pain relief.

a. Acetaminophen has no renal effects and can be used without adjustments.

b. Because of its short redistribution phase and lack of active metabolites, fentanyl is a good choice.

c. Morphine's sedative effects are prolonged in the presence of renal failure because its metabolites are renally excreted. Morphine should therefore be used with caution.

d. Meperidine is broken down to its active metabolite, normeperidine, whose half-life is prolonged in renal failure. Build-up of this metabolite can lead to myoclonic jerks, seizures, and respiratory depression. Therefore, meperidine should not be used.

## Bibliography

Ferri FF. *Practical Guide to the Care of the Medical Patient*, 7th ed. Philadelphia: Elsevier Mosby, 2007, pp. 682–6.

Goldman L, Ausillo D. *Cecil's Medicine*, 23rd ed. Philadelphia: Saunders Elsevier, 2007, pp. 936–41.

Golper TA, Fissell R, Fissell WH, et al. Hemodialysis: core curriculum 2014. *Am J Kidney Dis* 2014;**63**(1):153–63.

Humes HD. *Kelley's Textbook of Internal Medicine*, 4th ed. Philadelphia: Lippincott Williams and Wilkins, 2000, pp. 1290–7.

Kaplan AA. Peritoneal dialysis or hemodialysis: present and future trends in the United States. *Contrib Nephrol* 2017;**189**:61–4.

Kidney Disease: Improving Global Outcomes (KDIGO) Acute Kidney Injury Work Group. KDIGO clinical practice guideline for acute kidney injury. *Kidney Int* 2012;**2012**(suppl.):1–138.

Kohli MS. *Perioperative Medicine: Medical Consultation and Co-Management.* Hoboken: Wiley-Blackwell, 2012, p. 197.

Lok CE, Huber TS, Lee T, et al. KDOQI clinical practice guideline for vascular access: 2019 update. *Am J Kidney Dis* 2020;**75**(4)(suppl. 2): S1–S164.

Marx JA, Hockberger RS, Walls RM, et al. *Rosen's Emergency Medicine: Concepts and Clinical Practice*, 6th ed. Philadelphia: Mosby Elsevier, 2006, pp. 1546–54.

Selby NM, Kazmi I. Peritoneal dialysis has optimal intradialytic hemodynamics and preserves residual renal function: why isn't it better than hemodialysis? *Semin Dial* 2019;**32**(1):3–8.

Soundararajan R, Golper TA. Medical management of the dialysis patient undergoing surgery. In Berns JS, O'Connor MF, eds., *UpToDate* (accessed January 6, 2023).

Tandukar S, Palevsky PM. Continuous renal replacement therapy: who, when, why, and how. *Chest* 2019;**155**(3):626–38.

Wijeysundera DN, Finlayson E. *Miller's Anesthesia*, 9th ed. Philadelphia: Elsevier, 2020, pp. 960–1.

**Chapter 50**

# Transurethral Resection of the Prostate and TURP Syndrome

Elvera L. Baron, Lisa L. Bethea, and Jessica A. Lovich-Sapola

## Sample Case

A 55-year-old male with hypertension, chronic obstructive pulmonary disease, and benign prostatic hypertrophy (BPH) presents for a transurethral resection of the prostate (TURP). Pre-operative vital signs include a blood pressure of 145/70 mm Hg, a pulse of 90 beats/min, respiration rate of 20, and a temperature of 36.4 °C. The procedure is performed under spinal anesthesia. After placement of the spinal and proper positioning of the patient, the procedure is begun without incident. About 1 hour into the procedure, the patient complains of a headache and difficulty breathing. The blood pressure is noted to be 90/50 mm Hg. Other vital signs include respirations of 25, heart rate of 65 beats/min, and an oxygen saturation of 97% on 3 L nasal cannula. What are your major concerns? Are there any laboratory tests to order? Should the procedure have been done under general anesthesia instead? How should the patient's headache and breathing difficulties be treated?

## Clinical Issues

### Definition

1. Transurethral resection of the prostate

   a. Surgical procedure in which enlarged prostate tissue is resected via the urethra using cystoscopy

   b. Used for the treatment of bladder outlet obstruction due to BPH

   c. Indications for a TURP:

      i. Obstructive uropathy

      ii. Bladder calculi

      iii. Recurrent episodes of urinary retention

      iv. Urinary tract infections

      v. Hematuria

      vi. Patients with prostate cancer who are not candidates for a radical prostatectomy may have a TURP to relieve urinary obstruction.

   d. The procedure involves distending the bladder with irrigation fluid and cauterizing the prostatic tissue with electrical current.

      i. The irrigation fluid washes out the debris and helps keep the bladder distended for improved visualization of the prostate.

      ii. Several irrigation fluids are available, including glycine, sorbitol, mannitol, glucose, and cytal.

      iii. The irrigating solution must be isotonic, sterile, nontoxic, and not conduct electricity.

2. TURP syndrome

   a. A group of signs/symptoms caused by the absorption of irrigating fluids into the prostatic veins during prostate resection.

      i. Circulatory overload

      ii. Water intoxication

      iii. Toxicity from the irrigating fluids

   b. This can result in hyponatremia, hypo-osmolality, hyperglycinemia, hyperammonemia, hypervolemia, and metabolic acidosis.

   c. Incidence of TURP syndrome is estimated at ~0.8–1.4% of patients undergoing TURP, and is significantly decreased by use of newer techniques such as laser prostatectomy.

   d. Mortality rate has been reported as high as 25% for severe TURP syndrome.

## Risk Factors for Development of TURP Syndrome due to Increased Risk of Irrigation Fluid Absorption

1. Prostate >45 g
2. Prolonged resection time greater than 90 minutes
3. High inflow irrigating fluid pressure
4. Noncontinuous irrigating fluid
5. Pre-operative hyponatremia
6. Smoking history

## Triggers for TURP Syndrome

1. Absorption of irrigating fluid is the primary cause, which can lead to iatrogenic water intoxication and resultant hyponatremia.
2. The resection time has a profound effect on the amount and rate of irrigation solution absorption (10–30 mL fluid absorbed/min of resection time).

## Clinical Features of TURP Syndrome

The symptoms usually present with prolonged procedures, increased irrigating fluid or bladder pressure, and/or a serum sodium concentration of <120 mEq/L.

1. Neurologic
   a. Early: headache, nausea, irritability, apprehension, confusion, restlessness
   b. Late: visual disturbances, somnolence, seizure, coma, death
2. Cardiovascular
   a. Early: hypertension, reflex bradycardia
   b. Intermediate: negative inotropy, hypotension, dysrhythmias
   c. Late: widened QRS, ST segment elevations, ventricular arrhythmias, congestive heart failure, cardiovascular collapse
3. Respiratory
   a. Early: tachypnea, oxygen desaturation
   b. Late: hypoxemia, pulmonary edema, Cheyne–Stokes breathing, respiratory arrest
4. Metabolic
   a. Early: hyponatremia, hyperglycinemia, hyperammonemia, hypo-osmolality
   b. Late: metabolic acidosis
5. Other
   a. Renal failure
   b. Hemolysis or disseminated intravascular coagulation (DIC)

TKO: TURP syndrome is characterized by acute shifts in intravascular fluid volume. This can lead to significant electrolyte abnormalities, which can contribute to the above symptoms. If the patient becomes symptomatic, stop the procedure, provide supportive care, and check serum sodium level as well as serum osmolality.

## Other Complications of a TURP

### Most Common

1. Clot retention
2. Failure to void
3. Uncontrolled acute hematuria
   a. Dependent on the prostate size, 20–50 mL/g of prostate
   b. Dependent on resection time, 2–5 mL/min of the resection time
4. Urinary tract infection
5. Chronic hematuria

### Less Common

1. TURP syndrome
2. Bladder perforation
   a. Caused by overdistension of the bladder or the resectoscope going through the bladder wall.
   b. Intraperitoneal versus extraperitoneal
   c. Signs and symptoms may include: abdominal pain, shoulder pain, pallor, sweating, nausea/vomiting, hypotension, and acute, vagally mediated bradycardia.
   d. Decreased return of irrigating fluid from the bladder is an early sign.
   e. Diagnosis with cystourethrography
   f. Treatment is a suprapubic cystostomy.
3. Hypothermia
   a. Occurs secondary to the use of irrigating fluids at room temperature
   b. Warming fluids can prevent this problem.
   c. Post-operative shivering can dislodge clots.
   d. Post-operative hypothermia can promote bleeding.
4. Transient bacteremia and sepsis
   a. Due to prostatic bacteria entering through the prostatic sinuses
   b. Treat with antibiotics and supportive care.
5. Coagulopathy
   a. Clinical (1% of cases) versus subclinical (6% of cases)
   b. Causes: fibrinolysis, dilution of coagulation factors/platelets, DIC
6. Toxicity of irrigating fluids
   a. Glycine toxicity: transient blindness, T wave depressions or inversions on EKG
   b. Ammonia toxicity: neurologic sequelae, nausea, vomiting, convulsions, coma

# KO Treatment Plan

## Pre-operative

1. Formulate an appropriate anesthetic plan. Regional anesthesia is preferred because it provides the ability to do the following:
   a. Monitor the patient's mental status
   b. Detect hyponatremia early
   c. Detect other complications of TURP syndrome early
   d. Decrease the rate of deep venous thrombosis (DVT)
   e. Decrease blood loss due to the sympathetic block and decreased central venous and peripheral venous pressures
   f. Improve post-operative pain control, with decreased narcotic requirements
2. Correct pre-operative electrolyte abnormalities.

TKO: Spinal anesthesia is considered the anesthetic technique of choice when traditional TURP is performed. If regional anesthesia is performed, you must ensure at least a T9–10 sensory level to have adequate coverage of the bladder (T11–12) and prostate (T11–12) as well as coverage of the pelvic floor and perineum (S2–S4). Blockage above T9 is not recommended because it will obscure any symptoms that may develop if a bladder perforation were to occur.

**TKO:** TURP syndrome is currently rare due to advances in technology, but it still makes for a really good test question.

1. Low-voltage bipolar TURP allows the use of isotonic saline irrigation fluid, which can therefore avoid TURP syndrome.
2. Laser resection has no requirement for nonconductive fluid, so 0.9% saline may be used to avoid the complications of TURP syndrome.

## Intra-operative

1. Monitor the patient closely for any signs of mental status changes.
2. Note any significant alterations in vital signs and provide supportive measures.
3. Have the surgeon stop or expedite the procedure as soon as possible if any complications develop.
4. Restrict IV fluids.
5. Use loop diuretics (furosemide) to get rid of excess free water.
6. Check the serum sodium level. If severe hyponatremia develops with neurologic symptoms, treat with 3% saline IV. Replace the sodium deficit slowly as to avoid central pontine myelinolysis.

a. Correction of the sodium deficit: dose = weight (kg) × (140 – current sodium concentration) × 0.6
b. Correct at a rate of 0.6–1.0 mmol/L/h until the serum sodium is 125 mEq/L.
c. Replace half of the deficit over the first 8 hours and the rest over the next 1–3 days.
d. Monitor the sodium level frequently.

7. Supplemental oxygen and/or tracheal intubation/mechanical ventilation, as needed
8. Demeclocycline 150 mg qid or 300 mg bid if fluid restriction alone is inadequate

## Post-operative

1. Follow all labs and vital signs closely, including serial serum electrolyte concentrations.
2. Monitor the patient's urine output.
3. Monitor the patient's mental status for changes.
4. Watch for signs of DIC, including thrombocytopenia, hemolysis, and abnormal bleeding.
5. Assess for metabolic acidosis with an arterial blood gas and treat as needed.
6. A TURP procedure is usually done on an inpatient basis. Following the procedure, the patient is admitted to a general floor for recovery. However, if the patient exhibits any signs/symptoms of TURP syndrome, the patient should be monitored overnight in the ICU to allow for closer monitoring.

## Bibliography

Barash PG, Cullen BF, Stoelting RK, et al. *Clinical Anesthesia*, 8th ed. Philadelphia: Lippincott Williams & Wilkins, 2017, pp. 1472–30.

Butterworth JF, Mackey DC, Wasnick JD. *Morgan & Mikhail's Clinical Anesthesiology*, 6th ed. New York: McGraw-Hill Education, 2018, pp. 698–701.

Gropper MA. *Miller's Anesthesia*, 9th ed. Philadelphia: Elsevier, 2020, pp. 1942–6.

Hines RL, Marschall KE. *Stoelting's Anesthesia and Co-Existing Disease*, 5th ed. Philadelphia: Saunders, 2008, pp. 425–48.

Leslie, SW. Transurethral resection of the prostate. eMedicine. 2006. https://emedicine.medscape.com/article/449781-overview (accessed January 6, 2023).

# Emesis on Induction and Aspiration

**51**

Jessica A. Lovich-Sapola and Michael Leeds

## Sample Case

A 35-year-old male is scheduled for a left knee arthroscopy. He denies anything to eat or drink since midnight. He is an otherwise healthy ASA 1. Your plan is for a general anesthetic with a laryngeal mask airway (LMA). After the placement of the LMA the patient coughs and starts vomiting. What do you do? How will you treat the patient immediately? Do you secure the airway? Do you cancel the case? What medications will you give the patient? Does the patient need antibiotics? Steroids? Will you do a bronchial lavage?

## Clinical Issues

### Minimum Fasting Guidelines for Healthy Patients Undergoing Elective Procedures Requiring General Anesthesia, Regional Anesthesia, or Procedural Sedation and Analgesia

1. Clear liquids: 2 hours
   a. Water
   b. Fruit juice without pulp
   c. Carbonated beverages
   d. Clear tea
   e. Black coffee
   f. No alcohol

2. Breast milk: 4 hours
3. Infant formula and nonhuman milk: 6 hours
4. Light meals: 6 hours
   a. Toast without butter

5. Regular meals: 8 hours
6. Fried and fatty foods or meat: >8 hours

## Definitions

1. Aspiration: inhalation of gastric contents into the tracheobronchial tree
2. Aspiration pneumonia: aspiration of a substance containing bacteria
3. Aspiration pneumonitis: chemical injury of the lungs from sterile gastric contents and particulate antacids. The severity depends on the acidity and volume of the aspirate.
   a. Occurs in 1 in 3,000 patients receiving general anesthesia
   b. Mortality is high

   c. 10–30% of all deaths related to anesthesia are due to aspiration.
   d. Stage 1: symptoms peak after a few hours secondary to direct caustic effects of the aspirate.
   e. Stage 2: after 6 hours, the symptoms are due to an inflammatory process.

4. Mendelson syndrome: acute chemical aspiration pneumonitis. It presents with immediate respiratory distress with bronchospasm, cyanosis, tachycardia, and dyspnea. It is followed by a partial recovery and then a gradual return of respiratory dysfunction. It is associated with a very high mortality.

5. Chemical pneumonitis is more likely if the aspirate has a pH <2.5 or the volume of the aspirate is >0.4 mL/kg (about 25 mL in an adult). This results in atelectasis, edema, bronchospasm, and hypoxia within 10 minutes. The patient's chest X-ray may remain normal for hours before developing possible bilateral, perihilar, or basal atelectasis.

## Predisposing Factors for Aspiration

1. Pregnancy
   a. Increased gastric acid secondary to placental gastrin
   b. Delayed gastric emptying and decrease in lower esophageal sphincter tone secondary to progesterone
   c. Stomach contents after 4 hours in a nonpregnant patient and a nonlaboring pregnant patient are the same.
   d. A laboring patient can have solids in her stomach for up to 24 hours after eating.

2. Morbid obesity
   a. Increased volume of gastric contents
   b. Increased acidity of gastric contents

3. Emergency surgery
4. Decreased level of consciousness
5. Hiatal hernia
6. Scleroderma
7. Presence of a nasogastric tube
8. Diabetic gastroparesis
9. Uremia
10. Alcohol abuse
11. Drug abuse
12. Head trauma
13. Seizures

14. Neurologic disorders
15. Administration of sedatives
16. Esophageal cancer/incompetent gastroesophageal junction
17. Bowel obstruction
18. Repeated vomiting
19. Induction and recovery from anesthesia
20. Impaired laryngeal reflexes
21. Muscle weakness and paralysis
22. Trauma

    a. Full stomach secondary to the ingestion of food or liquids prior to the trauma
    b. Full stomach secondary to swallowed blood from an oral or nasal injury
    c. Delayed gastric emptying secondary to the stress of the trauma
    d. Liquid contrast medium given for CT scanning
    e. Distracting concerns
    f. Potential difficult airway/cervical collar
    g. Pain
    h. An emergency has a four times greater risk of aspiration than an elective case.

23. Acute intoxication
24. ASA 4 and 5

    a. 1.1% risk with ASA 1 versus a 29% risk with an ASA 4 or 5.

25. Bedridden patients/prolonged hospitalization

## Signs/Symptoms of Aspiration

1. Arterial hypoxemia is the earliest and most consistent clinical manifestation.
2. Visualization of gastric contents
3. Increased peak inspiratory pressures
4. Copious tracheal secretions
5. Pulmonary hypertension
6. Hypercarbia and acidosis
7. Wheezing/rales/rhonchi
8. Dyspnea
9. Apnea
10. Tachypnea
11. Coughing
12. Cyanosis
13. Bronchospasm/laryngospasm
14. Pulmonary edema
15. Shock
16. Radiographs

    a. Most commonly show infiltrates and atelectasis in the dependent areas of the lung, especially the right lower lobe (Fig. 51.1)
    b. 15–20% have unremarkable chest X-rays.
    c. Often takes 6–12 hours to develop.

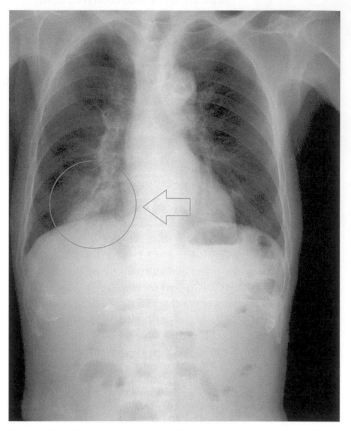

**Figure 51.1** Aspiration pneumonia right side lower lobe chest X-ray. Source: Melvil (https://commons.wikimedia.org/wiki/File:Aspiration_pneumoni a201711-3264.jpg).

## Differential Diagnosis of Aspiration

1. Hypoxia secondary to an obstructed endotracheal tube
2. Bronchospasm
3. Pulmonary edema
4. Pulmonary embolism
5. Pneumonia
6. Acute respiratory distress syndrome (ARDS)

## KO Treatment Plan

### Pre-operative

1. Pre-operative fasting
2. Avoid general anesthesia.
3. Delay nonemergent surgeries until NPO for 6–8 hours.
4. Pretreatment medications

    a. Nonparticulate antacid

        i. Sodium citrate or sodium bicarbonate
        ii. Reduces the level of acidity
        iii. Does not reduce the gastric volume
        iv. Decreases the severity of the aspiration
        v. Effectiveness is lost by 30–60 minutes after the ingestion.

b. Histamine-2 (H2) receptor antagonists (famotidine)

    i. Competitive inhibitor of histamine which prevents binding to parietal cells

    ii. Decreases gastric volume

    iii. Decreases gastric acidity

    iv. Works best if given the night before and again 2 hours before surgery.

    v. Some forms of H2 receptor antagonists have been discontinued recently due to breakdown into NDMA, a carcinogen.

c. Metoclopramide (10–20 mg IV)

    i. Onset 3–5 minutes

    ii. Gastrointestinal stimulant

    iii. Increases lower esophageal sphincter tone

    iv. Enhances gastric emptying

    v. Decreases volume of gastric fluid

    vi. No effect on acidity

d. Proton pump inhibitors (omeprazole)

    i. Bind to the proton pump of parietal cells in the gastric mucosa

    ii. Inhibit secretion of hydrogen ions

e. Transdermal scopolamine patch

    i. Best for motion sickness

    ii. Must be placed several hours prior to the surgery

    iii. Side effects include dry mouth, somnolence, mydriasis, and dizziness.

5. Optimize the airway.

6. Effective cricoid pressure

7. Intubate the trachea and inflate the cuff as quickly as possible.

8. Consider an awake tracheotomy with local anesthetics or an awake fiber-optic intubation.

## Intra-operative Treatment of Aspiration

1. Trendelenburg: head of the bed down 30 degrees with a right lateral tilt

2. Apply cricoid pressure once the patient is finished vomiting. Do not apply cricoid pressure until the patient has lost consciousness.

3. Suction the airway before intubation.

4. Secure the airway with a cuffed endotracheal tube (ETT).

5. Suction the ETT before giving positive-pressure ventilation.

6. Minimize exposure of the aspirate to the lungs.

7. Ensure adequate oxygenation and ventilation.

8. Supportive treatment for hypoxia and cardiovascular instability: give 100% oxygen, positive end expiratory pressure (PEEP), and inotropes as needed.

9. Bronchoscopy with irrigation only if particulate aspiration of the obstructive type occurs. Sample the aspirate for pH, gram stain, and culture.

10. Antibiotics if fecal material is aspirated and bacteria identified on a culture

11. Steroids are not recommended. They have no proven benefit and can impair long-term healing.

12. Cancel elective cases.

13. Bronchodilators

14. Send an arterial blood gas (ABG).

15. Nasogastric suction prior to extubation

16. Extubate only after the recovery of the protective laryngeal reflexes.

## Post-operative

1. A patient with suspected aspiration requires at least 24 hours of observation. The symptoms will likely worsen over the next few hours.

2. The treatment is purely symptomatic.

3. Follow serial chest X-rays.

4. Continuous pulse oximetry is recommended.

# Bibliography

Apfelbaum JL, Agarkar M, Connis RT, et al. Practice guidelines for preoperative fasting and the use of pharmacologic agents to reduce the risk of pulmonary aspiration: application to healthy patients undergoing elective procedures. *Anesthesiology* 2017;**126**(3):376–93.

Barash PG, Cullen BF, Stoelting RK, et al. *Clinical Anesthesia*, 8th ed. Philadelphia: Lippincott Williams & Wilkins, 2017, pp. 1550–1.

Butterworth JF, Mackey DC, Wasnick JD. *Morgan & Mikhail's Clinical Anesthesiology*, 6th ed. New York: McGraw-Hill Education, 2018, pp. 276–81, 782–4.

Gropper MA. *Miller's Anesthesia*, 9th ed. Philadelphia: Elsevier, 2020, p. 1381.

Stoelting RK, Dierdorf SF. *Anesthesia and Co-Existing Disease*, 4th ed. Philadelphia: Churchill Livingstone, 2002, pp. 580–1.

# Post-operative Jaundice

Jagan Devarajan and Jessica A. Lovich-Sapola

## Sample Case

Three days after a reportedly uneventful bilateral mastectomy, the patient's bilirubin is 7 mg/dL and she appears jaundiced. The patient is told that her jaundice is due to her anesthesia, and is referred to you to evaluate. How do you approach the patient? What do you say to the patient? What do you say to the surgeon? What tests or exams do you order? What are the management options available?

## Clinical Issues

### Definition of Jaundice

1. Jaundice is a clinical condition associated with elevated levels of serum bilirubin more than 3 mg/dL (51.3 μmol/L).
2. Bilirubin levels above 1.2 mg/dL is considered abnormal; however, it will not be clinically evident as jaundice until the level exceeds 3 mg/dL.
3. Jaundice is manifested by yellowish discoloration of skin, sclerae, and mucous membranes.
4. Jaundice occurs when there is excess production of bilirubin or when the liver is unable to properly metabolize or excrete bilirubin, a breakdown product of hemoglobin.

### Incidence of Post-operative Jaundice

1. 25–75% of patients undergoing surgery experience post-operative hepatic dysfunction. This can range from mild elevations of liver biochemical tests to hepatic failure.
2. Post-operative jaundice has also been reported to occur in over 25–35% of patients undergoing certain cardiac operations and conferred a higher mortality rate in those cases.
3. Jaundice has been reported in almost 50% of patients with underlying cirrhosis in the post-operative period.
4. Patients undergoing upper abdominal surgeries are at the highest risk of post-operative liver dysfunction.
5. In general, it is uncommon to observe clinically significant increase in bilirubin in patients without underlying hepatic disorders.

### Causes of Post-operative Jaundice

The etiology of post-operative jaundice is multifactorial and the manifestation is worsened by concomitant renal failure.

The causes are divided into three categories based on pathophysiology.

- Pre-hepatic: increased bilirubin production and abnormal metabolism
- Intrahepatic: hepatocellular dysfunction
- Post-hepatic: extrahepatic biliary obstruction

1. Pre-hepatic
   a. Anything that causes an increased rate of hemolysis
   b. Laboratory findings
      i. Normal to increased total bilirubin
      ii. Increased serum unconjugated/indirect bilirubin
      iii. Serum alkaline phosphatase and alanine transaminase (ALT) are often normal.
      iv. Elevated reticulocytes and schistocytes in peripheral blood smear
      v. Elevated lactate dehydrogenase (LDH) and rarely aspartate aminotransferase (AST)
   c. Examples (due to increased production or abnormal metabolism of bilirubin)
      i. Breakdown of transfused erythrocytes (hemolysis) from multiple transfusions
      ii. ABO incompatibility transfusion reaction
      iii. Resorption of hematomas
      iv. Hemolytic anemia: drug-induced
      v. Glucose-6-phosphate dehydrogenase (G6PD) deficiency
      vi. Hemolysis caused by cardiopulmonary bypass and aortic cross clamping
      vii. Malaria
      viii. Gilbert's syndrome (glucuronyltransferase deficiency)
      ix. Sickle cell anemia
      x. Spherocytosis
      xi. Kidney diseases leading to hemolytic uremic syndrome

2. Decreased hepatic clearance secondary to hepatic hypoperfusion
   a. Noncardiogenic shock/bacteremia/infection/sepsis
   b. Cardiogenic shock (heart failure)
   c. Endotoxemia

3. Hepatic
   a. Direct hepatocellular injury
   b. Laboratory findings
      i. Increased total bilirubin
      ii. Markedly elevated aminotransferases (up to 200%) along with LDH elevation
      iii. Predominant serum ALT elevation
      iv. Conjugated bilirubin present in the urine
      v. Normal alkaline phosphatase
      vi. Similar or somewhat less marked aminotransferase elevation is seen with toxic injury, congestive hepatopathy, and hepatocellular necrosis after liver transplantation.
   c. Examples
      i. Acute viral hepatitis and other unrecognized chronic liver diseases
      ii. Acute post-transfusion hepatitis
      iii. Alcoholic liver disease
      iv. Hypotension
      v. Hypovolemia
      vi. Peri-operative hypoxia
      vii. Sepsis-induced hyperbilirubinemia
      viii. Benign post-operative cholestasis
      ix. Ischemic hepatitis: shock liver
      x. Hepatic allograft rejection
      xi. Hepatic artery thrombosis
      xii. Primary biliary cirrhosis
      xiii. Gilbert's syndrome
      xiv. Crigler–Najjar syndrome
      xv. Metastatic carcinoma
      xvi. Hepatotoxicity
         (1) Hepatotoxic drugs:
            (a) Antibiotics
               (i) Tetracycline
               (ii) Cephalosporins
               (iii) Penicillin
               (iv) Rifampin
            (b) Inhalational anesthetics: halothane
            (c) Sodium thiopental
            (d) Ranitidine
            (e) Insulin
            (f) Antihypertensive medications
               (i) Hydralazine
               (ii) Labetalol
               (iii) Alpha-methyldopa
            (g) Procainamide
            (h) Phenothiazine
            (i) Heparin
            (j) Acetaminophen
            (k) Nonsteroidal anti-inflammatory drugs (NSAIDs)
               (i) Salicylates
               (ii) Ibuprofen
            (l) Steroids
            (m) Alcohol
            (n) Oral contraceptives
            (o) IV contrast media
            (p) Prolonged total parenteral nutrition (TPN)
            (q) Carbamazepine
            (r) Niacin

4. Post-hepatic
   a. Obstructive jaundice/cholestatic jaundice
   b. Caused by an interruption to the drainage of the bile in the biliary system
   c. Patients may present with pale stools, dark urine, and severe itching.
   d. Laboratory findings
      i. Increased total bilirubin
      ii. Increased direct/conjugated bilirubin
      iii. Markedly elevated serum alkaline phosphatase
      iv. Mild to moderate rise in aminotransferase
      v. Presence of bile salts in urine
   e. Examples
      i. Mechanical obstruction of the common bile duct
         (a) Gallstone
         (b) Stricture
         (c) Biliary atresia
         (d) Duct ligation
         (e) Surgical injury
         (f) Sphincter of Oddi dysfunction
         (g) Tumor: pancreatic cancer at the head of the pancreas, pancreatitis, pancreatic pseudocysts, ductal carcinoma
         (h) "Liver fluke" parasites (Trematoda)
      ii. Sepsis
      iii. Prolonged cardiopulmonary bypass
      iv. Acalculous cholecystitis
      v. Cholangitis
      vi. Biliary sludge
      vii. Prolonged TPN
      viii. Dubin–Johnson syndrome
      ix. Drugs causing post-hepatic obstruction
         (a) Amoxicillin-clavulanate
         (b) Erythromycin
         (c) Trimethoprim-sulfamethoxazole
         (d) Chlorpromazine
         (e) Warfarin

x. Acute exacerbation of infiltrative liver diseases such as sarcoidosis, lymphoma, amyloidosis can cause both intra- and extrahepatic cholestasis.

## Clinical and Laboratory Signs and Symptoms of Post-operative Jaundice

1. Jaundice most often manifests within 3 weeks after the surgery.
   a. Hyperbilirubinemia due to ischemic hepatitis manifests within 24 hours, whereas jaundice due to surgical obstruction, transfusion, and benign intrahepatic cholestasis occurs within 1–2 weeks.
   b. Drug-, toxin-, and viral-induced hyperbilirubinemia may present after 3 weeks.
2. Anemia
3. Yellowish discoloration of the skin, sclerae, and mucous membranes
4. An associated fever, rash, and eosinophilia are often present with drug-/toxin-induced hyperbilirubinemia or due to halothane anesthetic toxicity.
5. Hypotension is often present in patients with ischemic hepatitis.
6. Imaging
   a. Abdominal ultrasonography or CT scanning can be used to demonstrate ductal dilatation or any evidence of choledocholithiasis.
   b. It is often difficult to visualize bile stones in the duct by ultrasound, hence magnetic resonance cholangiopancreatography is helpful to delineate extrahepatic obstruction.

## Inhalational Anesthetic-Induced Jaundice

1. Halothane
   a. Rare syndrome of acute hepatotoxicity, usually after repeat exposures
      i. First exposure incidence: 0.3–1.5 per 10,000
      ii. Incidence after multiple exposures: 10–15 per 10,000
   b. Halothane is rarely used in the United States but is commonly seen in other countries.
   c. Presents with fever, eosinophilia, jaundice, myalgias, ascites, gastrointestinal hemorrhage, and hepatic necrosis a few days to weeks after the anesthesia.
   d. More frequent in females (2:1)
   e. Mortality rate is 10–80% in the pre-transplantation era. Much lower mortality with a liver transplant.
   f. Associated risk factors:
      i. Age 40 years or older
      ii. Female
      iii. Repeat exposures
      iv. Obesity
      v. Family predisposition

g. Spontaneous recovery of symptoms can occur.
2. Isoflurane, sevoflurane, and desflurane
   a. The quantity of metabolized volatile anesthetic contributes to hepatotoxicity.
   b. Hepatotoxicity is extremely rare because these volatile anesthetics exhibit a much lower degree of metabolism compared to halothane.

## Benign Post-operative Cholestasis

1. Benign post-operative cholestasis is a poorly understood condition in which there is progressive rise in conjugated bilirubin starting at day 2 and peaking in 10 days.
2. Bilirubin levels often reach as high as 10–40 mg/ dL.
3. Often associated with 2–4-fold elevation of alkaline phosphatase and normal aminotransferase.
4. The condition more commonly follows thoracic or major abdominal surgery complicated by hypovolemia, blood transfusion, or post-operative sepsis.
5. Diagnosis is often by exclusion of other conditions causing cholestasis.
6. Recovery depends on the patient's underlying condition.

## KO Treatment Plan

## Post-operative Evaluation

### Conversation with the Patient and Surgeon

It should be emphasized that the jaundice is less likely due to anesthesia. It is often related to the systemic inflammatory response related to surgery and the post-operative condition of the patient. Halothane can cause anesthetic-related jaundice but is rarely used today. The jaundice could very likely be secondary to an acute peri-operative event.

Tell the patient that you will carefully examine her and her peri-operative records to help to determine a possible cause of her jaundice. The patient will be reassured and provided all forms of management options.

A discussion should be held with the surgeon about the possible causes. If obstructive jaundice is suspected, she should be immediately notified so further surgical evaluation can be immediately instituted.

1. Perform a history and physical exam.
   a. Age
   b. Sex
   c. Latency/onset of the jaundice
   d. Does the patient have a fever?
   e. Does the patient have a rash?
   f. History of hepatomegaly?
   g. History of any pre-existing liver problems?
   h. Look for the following signs of chronic liver disease:
      i. Spider telangiectasias
      ii. Gynecomastia
      iii. Palmar erythema

iv. Caput medusa
v. Dupuytren's contractures
vi. Hepatomegaly (in patients without cirrhosis)
vii. Splenomegaly
ix. Ascites.

i. Does the patient have large bruises or hematomas as a source of unconjugated bilirubin elevation?
j. Coagulopathy?

2. Review the peri-operative record for events that can lead to jaundice.

a. Did the patient receive a transfusion?
b. Make a list of all of the medications given in the peri-operative period that may be hepatotoxic.
c. Note any hypoxic events.
d. Note any significant hypotensive events.

3. Order appropriate labs and tests.

a. Liver function tests
b. Check for serum eosinophilia.
c. Hemoglobin and hematocrit to check for hemolysis
d. Coagulation panel
e. Send a urine and stool sample. Check the urine for signs of hemolysis.
f. Abdominal ultrasound: liver, gallbladder

4. Management

a. Consult a gastroenterologist
b. Management should be focused on the suspected underlying cause of the hyperbilirubinemia.
c. Supportive treatment together with optimizing hepatic perfusion by avoiding hypovolemia and hypoxia.
d. Avoid hepatotoxic medications and fluid overload to prevent further injury and hepatic congestion, respectively.
e. If acetaminophen toxicity is suspected, serial acetaminophen levels should be checked and N-acetylcysteine administration should start immediately.
f. Refrain from giving any medications (particularly NSAIDs) which either cause or worsen hemolysis.
g. If liver function is severely impaired, lactulose 30 g PO several times a day, titrated to 3–4 bowel movements per 24 h should be given to prevent encephalopathy.
h. Consider an endoscopic retrograde cholangiopancreatography (ERCP), ballooning, and biliary stent to relieve biliary duct obstruction.
i. Start antiviral therapy if the jaundice is due to viral-induced hepatitis.

# Bibliography

Feldman M, Friedman LS, Brandt LJ. *Sleisenger & Fordtran's Gastrointestinal and Liver Disease*, 8th ed. Philadelphia: Saunders Elsevier, 2006, pp. 1853–5.

Goldman L, Aussiello D. *Cecil Medicine*, 23rd ed. Philadelphia: Saunders Elsevier, 2008, chapters 150, 151, 153, 159.

Gropper MA. *Miller's Anesthesia*, 9th ed. Philadelphia: Elsevier, 2020, pp. 427–36.

Hung OL, Kwon NS, Cole AE, et al. Evaluation of the physician's ability to recognize the presence or absence of anemia, fever, and jaundice. *Acad Emerg Med* 2000;**7**(2):146–56.

Mastoraki A, Karatzis E, Mastoraki S, et al. Postoperative jaundice after cardiac surgery. *Hepatobiliary Pancreat Dis Int* 2007;**6**(4):383–7.

Sandha GS, Bourke MJ, Haber GB, Kortan PP. Endoscopic therapy for bile leak based on a new classification: results in 207 patients. *Gastrointest Endosc* 2004;**60**(4):567–74.

Stoelting RK, Dierdorf SF. *Anesthesia and Co-Existing Disease*, 3rd ed. New York: Elsevier.

Sullivan JI, Rockey DC. Diagnosis and evaluation of hyperbilirubinemia. *Curr Opin Gastroenterol* 2017;**33**(3):164–70.

Wang MJ, Chao A, Huang CH, et al. Hyperbilirubinemia after cardiac operation: incidence, risk factors, and clinical significance. *J Thorac Cardiovasc Surg* 1994;**108**(3):429–36.

# Ascites

**Chapter 53**

Taylor Bowman

## Sample Case

A 50-year-old man with a history of liver cirrhosis secondary to alcohol abuse presents for an exploratory laparotomy for a suspected bowel obstruction. His blood pressure is 100/50 mm Hg and his heart rate is 92. His abdomen is severely distended with ascites. How does his liver cirrhosis and ascites affect your anesthetic plan? Would you like any pre-operative tests? Should his ascites be drained prior to the surgery?

## Clinical Issues

### Definition of Ascites

1. Accumulation of fluid in the peritoneal cavity
2. Common sequela of many forms of cirrhosis
3. Factors that contribute to its formation:
    a. Portal hypertension: increased pressures in portal vessels leads protein-containing fluids to leak from the liver/intestines, with accumulation in the abdomen.
    b. Hypoalbuminemia: reduced plasma oncotic pressure favors the extravasation of fluid from plasma to the peritoneal fluid.
    c. Sodium and water retention

### Theories of Pathogenesis of Ascites in Cirrhosis

1. Underfilling hypothesis
    a. Portal hypertension leads to sequestration of fluid in the splanchnic vascular bed, which decreases blood volume available to other organs, giving the sense that the blood volumes are "underfilled."
    b. This decreases the effective intravascular volume, activating the renin–angiotensin aldosterone system (RAAS), resulting in sodium and water retention by the kidney.
2. Overflow hypothesis
    a. In spite of the intravascular hypervolemia that occurs with cirrhosis, the activation of the RAAS leads to sodium and water retention.
    b. This combination "overflows" the vasculature, as the increased portal hydrostatic pressure leads to translocation of fluid from the splanchnic circulation into the peritoneal cavity.

3. Peripheral vasodilation hypothesis
    a. Sequestered blood flood in the splanchnic vascular bed due to portal hypertension leads to an accumulation of nitric oxide and activation of nitric oxide synthase. Nitric oxide leads to increased peripheral vasodilation, decreasing perfusion to all other organs, including the kidneys.
    b. Decreased kidney perfusion activates the RAAS, leading to renal sodium and water retention, with ascites as described above.

## New-Onset Ascites

1. Evaluation
    a. Hepatic
        i. Liver function tests
        ii. Coagulation tests
        iii. Abdominal ultrasound
        iv. Abdominal CT scan
        v. Liver biopsy
    b. Cardiac
    c. Renal function
        i. Serum creatinine and electrolytes
        ii. Urinary sodium and protein
    d. Analysis of ascitic fluid
        i. Cell count
        ii. Bacterial culture
        iii. Total protein
        iv. Other: albumin, glucose, lactate dehydrogenase, amylase, triglycerides

## Common Treatment Theme

1. Decrease sodium intake.
2. Diuretic therapy
    a. Spironolactone: aldosterone antagonist
        i. Maximum diuresis should not exceed 1 L/day or 1 kg/day.
    b. Loop diuretics may be administered if spironolactone and sodium restriction are ineffective.

232

3. LeVeen peritoneovenous shunt

    a. Routes ascitic fluid subcutaneously from the peritoneal cavity to the internal jugular vein

4. Large volume paracentesis

    a. Removal of large amounts of ascitic fluid in treatment of refractory ascites: 4–6 L/day

    b. Physiologic effects

        i. Initial improvement in hemodynamic status occurs with the release of pressure on the inferior vena cava and right atria, resulting in an increase in cardiac output.

        ii. Subsequent paracentesis-induced circulatory dysfunction (PICD)

            (1) The increased cardiac output triggers a reflex sympathectomy and nitric oxide release, with subsequent vasodilation and hypotension.

            (2) Ensuing hypotension may be prevented by the concurrent administration of a plasma expander.

                (a) Albumin: 6–8 g of albumin should be administered for every liter removed greater than 5 L.

                (b) Colloid

                (c) Dextran

                (d) Hetastarch

## KO Treatment Plan

## Pre-operative

1. Full history and physical examination in regard to the patient's liver dysfunction are critical, even in an emergency situation. Systemic effects to consider include:

    a. Cardiovascular abnormalities

        i. High cardiac output

        ii. Low peripheral vascular resistance

        iii. Low blood pressure

        iv. Increased stroke volume

        v. Elevated heart rate

    b. Hepatic circulatory dysfunction with portal hypertension

    c. History of variceal hemorrhage

    d. Pulmonary dysfunction

        i. Resultant hypoxemia

            (1) Intrapulmonary shunting

            (2) Fluid retention

            (3) Concurrent obstructive airway disease

            (4) Elevation of the diaphragm secondary to ascites causes decreased lung volumes, especially functional residual capacity (FRC).

    e. Renal dysfunction

    f. Disorders of coagulation

        i. Decreased amounts of vitamin K-dependent clotting factors (II, VII, IX, and X)

            (1) Parenteral vitamin K should be given if the patient has a prolonged prothrombin time.

        ii. Thrombocytopenia

    g. Hepatic encephalopathy

    h. Dehydration

        i. Secondary to the use of diuretics to control ascites formation

    i. Electrolyte abnormalities: order a serum electrolyte panel.

        i. Hypoglycemia

**TKO:** Maximize hepatic oxygen delivery and prevent and treat associated complications: encephalopathy, cerebral edema, coagulopathy, hemorrhage, and portal hypertension.

2. Consider pre-operative drainage of tense ascites.

    a. The ascites may impede the patient's respiratory function.

    b. The ascites may increase the patient's risk for aspiration.

        i. Patients with acute deterioration of pulmonary function or tense ascites may benefit from pre-operative drainage in a semi-urgent or elective situation.

        ii. In a true emergency, the laparotomy itself will lead to loss of ascitic fluid.

            (1) Be prepared for circulatory collapse after the drainage of the ascites.

                (a) Give concomitant intravenous plasma expander solutions during the ascites drainage.

                (b) Re-equilibration of the intravascular volume will occur 6–8 hours after the removal of a large volume of ascitic fluid.

## Intra-operative

1. Standard ASA monitors with consideration given to the placement of an arterial line and possible central line

    a. Arterial line

        i. Immediate measurement of the patient's hemodynamic status in the setting of large volume shifts

            (1) Similar hemodynamic changes to those seen during large volume paracentesis may be anticipated in the setting of emergent laparotomy in the face of tense ascites.

        ii. Frequent blood draws

b. Central line

   i. Provides an indication of cardiac filling pressures

   ii. Placement may be difficult in patients with coagulopathy and known pulmonary dysfunction.

   iii. Monitoring of intravascular fluid volume, especially in situations of

      1. Underlying cardiovascular instability

      2. Hepatorenal syndrome

      3. Dehydration

      4. Anticipated large intercompartmental fluid shifts

c. Foley catheter

2. A rapid-sequence intubation should be performed to minimize the possibility of aspiration.

a. In this sample case, the ascites increases intra-abdominal pressure, while the bowel obstruction also independently increases the probability of aspiration.

b. Must consider paralytic options in a rapid-sequence induction.

   i. Renal dysfunction or elevated potassium may preclude the use of succinylcholine.

   ii. The duration of action of succinylcholine is decreased in the setting of low pseudocholinesterase levels secondary to decreased liver function.

3. Maintenance drugs

a. Any maintenance regimen may be used as part of a balanced anesthetic technique.

b. Drugs requiring hepatic metabolism may require lower doses and have increased durations.

c. Muscle relaxants

   i. Because of the altered volume of distribution, coupled with the altered hepatic metabolism in patients with end-stage liver disease (ESLD), train-of-four stimuli need to be monitored.

   ii. Cisatracurium and rocuronium may be beneficial in order to avoid issues with hepatic metabolism. (Please refer to the liver transplant chapter for further information.)

d. Opioids

   i. Half-lives of opioids would be likely prolonged, leading to respiratory depression in the PACU or ICU.

## Post-operative

1. Post-operative care is guided by the patient status before and during the case.

2. Most likely, however, this patient will need ICU monitoring to prevent cardiac decompensation in the subsequent 6–12 hours post-surgery, as intercompartmental fluid shifts occur.

## Bibliography

Barash PG, Cullen BF, Stoelting RK, et al. *Clinical Anesthesia*, 8th ed. Philadelphia: Lippincott Williams & Wilkins, 2017, pp. 1313–14.

Butterworth JF, Mackey DC, Wasnick JD. *Morgan & Mikhail's Clinical Anesthesiology*, 5th ed. New York: McGraw Hill. 2013, pp. 707–18

Gropper MA. *Miller's Anesthesia*, 9th ed. Philadelphia: Elsevier, 2020, pp. 433–7.

Hines M. *Stoelting's Anesthesia and Co-existing Disease*, 5th ed. New York: Churchill Livingstone, 2008, chapter 11.

Lindsay AJ, Burton J, Ray CE. Paracentesis-induced circulatory dysfunction: a primer for the interventional radiologist. *Semin Intervent Radiol* 2014;**31**:276–278.

# Physiologic Changes of Pregnancy

## 54

Marcos Izquierdo and Jessica A. Lovich-Sapola

## Sample Case

A 24-year-old female presents for a repeat cesarean section. She is otherwise healthy. She is deathly afraid of needles and demands a general anesthetic. It is important that you give her an informed consent for her anesthetic. Please explain to her your anesthetic of choice, and why. Discuss with her the physiologic changes that occur in pregnancy, and how they affect your anesthetic plan.

## Clinical Issues

### Cardiovascular System

1. Increases

   a. Cardiac output (CO)

      i. Increases from the fifth week of pregnancy
      ii. Maximum level at 32 weeks of pregnancy
      iii. Increases by 30–50% during pregnancy
      iv. CO increases secondary to an increase in stroke volume and heart rate
      v. Results in increased perfusion to uterus, kidneys, and skin
      vi. The cardiac output continues to increase by 60–85% during labor and in the postpartum period secondary to autotransfusion and the removal of aortocaval compression by evacuating the uterus.
      vii. The cardiac output will return to nonpregnant values over the next 12 weeks postpartum.

   b. Stroke volume (SV)

      i. Increases by 20–50% at term from nonpregnant values

   c. Heart rate (HR)

      i. An increase in resting HR can be seen by 4 weeks' gestation and rises as much as 20% over the gestational period.

   d. Blood volume

      i. Increases by 45% over nonpregnant values

2. Decreases

   a. Systemic vascular resistance (SVR)
   b. Systemic blood pressure – nadir at 20 weeks' gestation
   c. Pulmonary vascular resistance

3. No change

   a. Central venous pressure (CVP)
   b. Pulmonary capillary wedge pressure
   c. Pulmonary artery pressure
   d. Left ventricular function
   e. Ejection fraction

4. Variable

   a. Contractility

5. EKG changes associated with pregnancy

   a. Sinus tachycardia
   b. Left axis deviation
   c. Ectopic beats
   d. Inverted or flattened T waves
   e. Q waves in lead III

6. Minor changes in the cardiovascular system are considered normal. Further investigation is warranted if the patient has:

   a. Chest pain
   b. Syncope
   c. Hemodynamically significant arrhythmias
   d. Severe shortness of breath or hypoxia
   e. Systolic murmur more than grade 3
   f. Diastolic murmur

### Hematologic System

1. Physiologic anemia

   a. Plasma volume increases by a higher percentage (50%) compared to cell volume (30%), which will decrease hematocrit.

      i. Oxygen transport is not compromised by this physiologic anemia due to the patient's:

         (1) Increase in CO
         (2) Increased partial pressure of arterial oxygen
         (3) Rightward shift of the oxyhemoglobin dissociation curve

   b. This physiologic anemia occurs to:

      i. Allow adequate perfusion to vital organs, including the fetus
      ii. Prepare for blood loss associated with delivery

2. Average hemoglobin of 11.6 g/dL
3. Average hematocrit of 35.5%
4. Platelet count is usually unchanged.
5. Leukocytosis up to 13,000/mm$^3$ is normal and unrelated to infection
6. Hypercoagulable state
   a. Increased levels of most coagulation factors, including I (fibrinogen), VII, VIII, IX, X, and XII
   b. Largest increase in factor VII and fibrinogen
   c. Thromboelastography (TEG)
      i. Decrease in R and K values
      ii. Increase in alpha angle and maximum amplitude
7. Plasma proteins
   a. Albumin levels decrease
   b. Decrease in the colloid oncotic pressure

# Respiratory System

1. Increases
   a. Minute ventilation: 50% increase due to increased respiratory center sensitivity and drive
      i. Increase in tidal volume with a minimally increased respiratory rate
      ii. The increased respiratory drive is believed to be due to the elevation in serum progesterone, a direct respiratory stimulant.
   b. Tidal volume increases by 40–45%.
      i. The patient has an increased oxygen demand and requirement for carbon dioxide elimination.
   c. Respiratory rate increases by 0–15%.
   d. Work of breathing
   e. Pulmonary blood flow with increased pulmonary capillary blood volume
      i. Pulmonary edema
   f. Oxygen-carrying capacity
   g. Oxygen consumption: increased metabolic demands
2. Decreases
   a. Functional residual capacity (FRC)
   b. Expiratory reserve volume
   c. Chest wall compliance: enlarging uterus
3. No change
   a. Closing capacity
   b. Vital capacity
   c. Forced expiration
      i. Forced expiratory volume in 1 second ($FEV_1$) is not affected by pregnancy.
4. Compensated respiratory alkalosis

a. Normal arterial blood gas (ABG) in pregnancy
   i. pH 7.44
   ii. $PaO_2$ 103 mm Hg
   iii. $PaCO_2$ 30 mm Hg
   iv. $HCO_3^-$ 20 mEq/L
   v. p50 30 mm Hg
5. Rapid hypoxia secondary to:
   a. Decreased FRC
   b. Decreased FRC/closing capacity (CC) ratio resulting in faster small airway closure when the lung volume is reduced
   c. Increased oxygen consumption
6. Capillary engorgement of the mucosa is due to increased blood volume and increased estrogen.
   a. Edema of the oropharynx, larynx, and trachea
   b. Increased risk of difficult intubation
      i. Use a smaller endotracheal tube than usual.
   c. Any airway manipulation may result in:
      i. Edema
      ii. Bleeding
      iii. Upper airway trauma
   d. The nasopharynx mucosa is particularly friable; therefore, all instrumentation of the nose should be avoided.
7. Normal chest X-ray in a pregnant patient
   a. Mild cardiomegaly
   b. Widened mediastinum
   c. Increased anterior–posterior diameter
   d. Prominence of the pulmonary vasculature

# Gastrointestinal System

1. Progesterone
   a. Relaxes smooth muscle
   b. Impairs esophageal and intestinal motility
   c. Reduces lower esophageal sphincter tone
   d. Increases the placental production of gastrin: increases gastric acidity
2. Gastric emptying is not delayed in a normal pregnancy.
3. Delayed gastric emptying is found in:
   a. Laboring patients/painful labor
      (i) Placentally derived gastrin
   b. Patients receiving parenteral opioids
   c. Patients receiving large doses of epidural opioids
4. Increased risk of aspiration when sedated after about 16 weeks' gestation
5. Lab values in pregnancy

a.  Increased: alkaline phosphatase levels

   i.  Due to placental production

b.  Decreased: pseudocholinesterase, transaminase, and bilirubin levels

## Renal System

1.  Affected by the increase in progesterone and the mechanical effects of compression by the enlarging uterus
2.  Increases

   a.  Urea clearance
   b.  Creatinine clearance
   c.  Uric acid clearance
   d.  Renal plasma flow (RPF): secondary to the increase in CO
   e.  Glomerular filtration rate (GFR): secondary to the increase in CO
   f.  Risk of urinary tract infection, nephrolithiasis, and pyelonephritis
   g.  Frequency, urgency, and incontinence

3.  Decreases

   a.  Plasma creatinine and urea

      i.  Secondary to:

         (1)  Dilutional effect of plasma volume expansion
         (2)  Increase in GFR

      ii.  "Normal" renal indices in pregnancy are lower than in the nonpregnant state.

## Central Nervous System

1.  Increased sensitivity to both regional and general anesthetics

   a.  Decreased minimum alveolar concentration (MAC) for volatile anesthetics
   b.  Mechanism is unclear

   i.  Possibly due to the increased progesterone levels
   ii.  Possibly due to the increased concentrations of endorphins and dynorphins which results in an altered pain threshold
   iii.  Mechanical effects of the enlarging uterus
   iv.  Decrease in spinal cerebral spinal fluid volume

      (1)  Increase in epidural fat volume
      (2)  Increase in epidural vein volume

## KO Treatment Plan

### Pre-operative

1.  Regional anesthesia is the preferred choice for a cesarean section in an otherwise healthy patient.

   a.  Rapid hypoxia
   b.  Capillary engorgement of the mucosa
   c.  Increased risk of aspiration

      i.  Edema of the oropharynx, larynx, and trachea
      ii.  Increased risk of difficult intubation
      iii.  Any airway manipulation may result in:

         (1)  Edema
         (2)  Bleeding
         (3)  Upper airway trauma

      vi.  Avoid instrumentation of the nose.

### Intra-operative

1.  Understand that a patient refusal is the number one contraindication to a regional anesthetic.

   a.  If after your long explanation of why you would choose a regional anesthetic she still chooses a general anesthetic, then put her to sleep.

      i.  Assuming she has a normal airway exam, perform a rapid-sequence induction/intubation.

## Bibliography

Chestnut DH, Wong CA, Tsen LC, et al. *Chestnut's Obstetric Anesthesia: Principles and Practice*, 6th ed. Philadelphia: Elsevier, 2020, pp. 13–37.

Gropper MA. *Miller's Anesthesia*, 9th ed. Philadelphia: Elsevier, 2020, pp. 2006–41.

Wise RA, Polito AJ, Krishnan V. Respiratory physiologic changes in pregnancy. *Immunol Allergy Clin North Am* 2006;**26**(1):1–12.

# Preeclampsia

Hoaky Lam

## Sample Case

A 26-year-old female, G1P0 at 34 3/7 weeks, presents with complaints of severe right upper quadrant pain. She has had no prior issues with this pregnancy. Her blood pressure (BP) is 160/90 mm Hg, heart rate (HR) 75, respiratory rate is 20, and temperature 36.6 °C. On exam, the patient has some tenderness in her right upper abdominal quadrant and moderate pedal edema. She has a Mallampati (MP) class 3 airway. Laboratory analysis reveals platelets 100, AST 156, ALT 174, and creatinine 1.0. She is scheduled for an urgent cesarean section. What are your concerns? Do you want any more laboratory tests? Would you use a regional or general anesthetic? If a general anesthetic was required, how would you induce anesthesia? What monitors would you use?

## Clinical Issues

### Definition

1.  Preeclampsia
    a.  Hypertension (BP >140/90 mm Hg, two elevated BPs taken four hours apart) with proteinuria **or** any of the other severe features:
        i.   Severe hypertension (SBP >160 mm Hg or DPB >110 mm Hg)
        ii.  Thrombocytopenia (platelet count $<100 \times 10^9$/L)
        iii. Impaired liver function: elevated blood concentrations of liver transaminases to twice the normal)
        iv.  Renal insufficiency (serum creatinine (CR) >1.1 mg/dL or doubling of baseline serum CR in the absence of other renal disease)
        v.   Pulmonary edema
        vi.  New-onset cerebral or visual disturbances
    b.  Proteinuria
        i.   Proteinuria >300 mg over 24 hours
        ii.  Protein/creatinine ratio of 0.3 mg/dL or more
        iii. Dipstick reading of 2+
    c.  Symptoms of preeclampsia
        i.   Placental ischemia
        ii.  Systemic vasoconstriction
        iii. Increased platelet aggregation

d.  Unique to human pregnancy
e.  Unknown etiology
    i.    This is a disease process in which the basic underlying etiology is unclear, but it is likely to involve both maternal and fetal/placental factors. It is thought to begin with abnormal implantation of myometrial spiral arteries that results in suboptimal uteroplacental blood flow and hypoxic trophoblast tissue. This results in a state of exaggerated oxidative stress for the placenta which then adversely affects the villous angiogenesis.
    ii.   As the pregnancy advances, the placenta increasingly secretes antiangiogenic factors such as soluble FMS-like tyrosine kinase-1 [sFlt-1] and endoglin into the maternal circulation, which bind vascular endothelial growth factor (VEGF) and placental growth factor (PlGF).
    iii.  This results in widespread maternal vascular inflammation, endothelial dysfunction, and vascular injury.
    iv.   Endothelial cells become dysfunctional with an excess production of thromboxane and a decrease in prostacyclin and nitrous oxide production by the placenta.
    v.    Thromboxane leads to vasoconstriction, platelet aggregation, increased uterine activity, and decreased uteroplacental blood flow.
    vi.   In a normal pregnancy, these effects are equally opposed by the actions of prostacyclin.
    vii.  In preeclampsia the widespread arteriolar vasoconstriction causes hypertension, tissue hypoxia, and endothelial damage.
    viii. Placental ischemia leads to a release of thromboplastin with subsequent deposition on the already constricted glomerular vessels, which in turn leads to proteinuria.
    ix.   Renal damage may continue with decreased renal blood flow and a decreased glomerular filtration rate.
    x.    Right upper quadrant pain may be secondary to a subcapsular hematoma of the liver (rare). Rupture of this liver hematoma carries an 80% mortality rate.
    xi.   Cerebral edema and small foci of degeneration may develop.

2. HELLP syndrome is a form of severe preeclampsia characterized by **h**emolysis, **e**levated **l**iver enzymes, and **l**ow **p**latelets.
3. Eclampsia

   a. The occurrence of convulsions and/or coma unrelated to preexisting neurologic disease
   b. Seizures may occur before, during, or after the delivery.
   c. 25% of all postpartum eclampsia-related seizures occur between 48 hours and 4 weeks postpartum.
   d. Once a seizure occurs, it is usually self-limited.

      i. Magnesium sulfate is preferred over benzodiazepines or phenytoin for prophylaxis and treatment of eclamptic seizures.
      ii. A bolus of IV magnesium sulfate, 4–6 g, should then be administered, followed by an initial infusion of 1–2 g/h.

   e. An airway must be established.

      i. Administer supplemental oxygen.
      ii. Bag and mask ventilate as needed.

   f. Pulse oximetry, EKG, and BP should be monitored.
   g. The only "cure" for preeclampsia/eclampsia is delivery of the fetus and placenta.

**TKO:** Typically, in preeclampsia and HELLP syndrome, the obstetrical management strategies should focus on the stabilization of the mother until the fetus is mature. With severe preeclampsia, if the patient is stable, she may be followed until the fetus is viable or at least until 48 hours of steroid benefit can be achieved. Progression to eclampsia or fetal deterioration mandates immediate delivery of the fetal/placental unit.

## Thrombocytopenia

1. Circulating platelets adhere to the damaged or activated endothelium.
2. The thrombocytopenia is usually moderate, and clinical bleeding is rare unless disseminated intravascular coagulation (DIC) develops.
3. The choice of anesthetic technique depends upon the mode of delivery, fetal gestational age, coagulation status, history of recent/current bleeding, and other medical issues.
4. The risk of an epidural hematoma is estimated to be about 1:150,000 after epidural analgesia.
5. A platelet count of 100,000 is considered safe for performing an epidural block, although there are no supporting data.
6. Hematologists suggest that a platelet count of over 50,000 is safe for surgery and neuraxial blockade, provided the function of the existing platelets is normal.
7. Many anesthesiologists would agree that a platelet count of 80,000 would be safe for a central neuraxial block, as the benefits of regional anesthesia far outweigh the risks of a general anesthetic. It is important to follow the trend of the patient's platelets.

8. Available platelet function tests include:

   a. Thromboelastogram (TEG)
   b. Aggregometry
   c. Flow cytometry
   d. Platelet function assay (PFA)-100

      i. The most rapid and simple assessment of platelet aggregation
      ii. Uses epinephrine and ADP

## Magnesium

1. This is the first-line therapeutic drug used for controlling preeclampsia and eclampsia.
2. Properties of magnesium

   a. Central nervous system depressant and anticonvulsant effects
   b. Vasodilation with increased uterine and renal blood flow
   c. Bronchodilator
   d. Decreased platelet aggregation
   e. Tocolysis
   f. Decreased fetal heart rate variability
   g. Generalized muscle weakness
   h. Decreased muscle tone and lower APGAR scores in neonates
   i. Increased maternal sensitivity to both depolarizing and nondepolarizing muscle relaxants

      i. Magnesium inhibits the release of acetylcholine at the neuromuscular junction.
      ii. Decreases the sensitivity of the motor endplate to acetylcholine
      iii. Decreases the muscle membrane excitability

3. Therapeutic levels of magnesium are 4–6 mEq/L.

   a. Deep tendon reflexes are lost at 10 mEq/L.
   b. Sinoatrial and atrioventricular block occurs concurrent with respiratory paralysis at 15 mEq/L.
   c. Cardiac arrest occurs around 20 mEq/L.

4. Calcium gluconate counteracts the cardiac effects of magnesium.
5. Treatment of magnesium toxicity

   a. Stop the magnesium infusion.
   b. Intravenous calcium gluconate 1 g or calcium chloride 300 mg
   c. Ventilate and intubate if respiratory failure occurs.

## KO Treatment Plan

Be prepared to defend your choices. The following is representative of how the authors might manage this patient. However, be prepared to be taken down a total/high spinal pathway or a difficult airway pathway as alternatives. Multiple anesthetic techniques are acceptable, but be prepared to defend your choice.

## Pre-operative

1. Prepare for surgery with consideration of a 500 mL fluid bolus of crystalloid to expand her intravascular volume, depending on a current assessment of her volume status.

   a. Remember that a patient who is currently on a magnesium drip has a tenuous fluid status and an increased risk of pulmonary edema.

2. Order a repeat platelet count to determine the trend and rate of change in the platelet count.

3. Given that this is an urgent cesarean section, spinal anesthesia would be appropriate.

4. In the face of a difficult airway, it is defensible to perform a neuraxial anesthetic technique down to a platelet count of about 80,000, assuming no recent rapid decrease in the platelet number.

5. Provide aspiration prophylaxis with an $H_2$-blocker and administer 30 mL of a nonparticulate antacid.

6. Consider an arterial line prior to the placement of the neuraxial technique if the severely preeclamptic patient has uncontrolled BP, in order to better monitor the BP changes.

## Intra-operative

1. Be prepared to treat large swings in BP that may occur due to the spinal anesthetic.

2. Treat hypotension with oxygen via face mask, left uterine displacement, hydration, and IV phenylephrine or ephedrine.

3. Remember that the pre-eclamptic patient is more sensitive to the effects of pressors.

4. Raise the lower extremities to facilitate venous return.

## The Airway

1. Difficulty with intubation occurs at a higher rate in pregnant than nonpregnant women, and patients with preeclampsia have additional considerations.

2. Often, upper airway narrowing occurs in these patients during sleep.

3. Reduced plasma proteins due to proteinuria and marked fluid retention make the tongue larger and less mobile.

4. Multiple direct laryngoscopy attempts may lead to laceration and bleeding of the pharyngeal structures.

5. Swelling can be severe enough to cause total airway obstruction.

**TKO:** Please review the difficult airway section to consider the various scenarios examiners may present in the obstetric patient.

## Epidural versus Spinal Anesthesia

1. There has been concern that the intravascular volume contraction that has been noted in preeclamptic patients could result in severe hypotension with the onset of a sympathectomy.

2. Historically, epidural anesthesia has been used in these patients in order to better control the sympathectomy with a more gradual onset. Recent studies, however, are showing no significant difference in the incidence of hypotension in severely preeclamptic women with spinal or epidural anesthesia.

3. Spinal anesthesia in stable, noncoagulopathic, severely preeclamptic women is a reasonable alternative to an epidural block, especially in emergency situations, and is preferred as an attempt to avoid general anesthesia.

## General Anesthetic

1. If there is a contraindication for a regional anesthetic, a general anesthetic must be performed.

2. Give aspiration prophylaxis.

   a. Oral nonparticulate antacid

   b. H2-blocker

   c. Metoclopramide

3. Preoxygenate and denitrogenate with 100% oxygen.

4. Labetalol or nitroglycerin can be given pre-induction to blunt the sympathetic response to direct laryngoscopy and intubation.

5. Perform a rapid-sequence induction with propofol and succinylcholine, assuming the patient does not have a "difficult airway."

   a. This patient's airway exam revealed a Mallampati 3 score; therefore, have a video laryngoscope available and be prepared to perform a fiber-optic intubation.

6. Have smaller endotracheal tubes available secondary to the associated airway edema.

7. Remember that the magnesium sulfate will potentiate the effects of both depolarizing and nondepolarizing muscle relaxants.

8. Consider a pre-induction arterial line in any patient with severe preeclampsia.

## Post-operative

1. Be aware of the post-operative development of eclampsia.

2. Continue magnesium therapy in the post-operative setting for 24–48 hours.

3. Monitoring must be continued for 24–48 hours after delivery due to the potential development of eclampsia as well as the risks associated with magnesium therapy. The location of management (labor and delivery, ICU, or floor) is at the discretion of the managing physician and should be guided by the patient's clinical status.

4. An additional 24 hours of BP monitoring in the postpartum unit once the magnesium drip is completed is also recommended.

# Bibliography

ACOG. Gestational hypertension and preeclampsia, *Obstet Gynecol* 2020;**135**(6): e237–e260

Barash PG, Cullen BF, Stoelting RK, et al. *Clinical Anesthesia*, 8th ed. Philadelphia: Lippincott Williams & Wilkins, 2017, pp. 1155–9.

Chestnut DH, Wong CA, Tsen LC, et al. *Chestnut's Obstetric Anesthesia: Principles and Practice*, 6th ed. Philadelphia: Elsevier, 2020, p. 840.

Hughes SC, Levinson G, Rosen MA, eds. *Shnider & Levinson's Anesthesia for Obstetrics*, 4th ed. Philadelphia: Lippincott Williams & Wilkins, 2001, pp. 297–315.

Ives CW, Sinkey R, Rajapreyar I, Tita ATN, Oparil S. Preeclampsia: pathophysiology and clinical presentations. *J Am Coll Cardiol* 2020;**76**(14):1690–702.

Kam PCA, Thompson SA, Liew ACS. Thrombocytopenia in the parturient. *Anaesthesia* 2004;**59**:255–64.

Mandal NG, Surapenemi S. Regional anaesthesia in pre-eclampsia: advantages and disadvantages. *Drugs* 2004;**64**(3):223–36.

Munner U, deBoisblanc B, Suresh MS. Airways problems in pregnancy. *Crit Care Med* 2005;**33**(10): S259–68.

Santos AC, Epstein JN, Chaudhuri K. *Obstetric Anesthesia*. New York: McGraw Hill, 2015, pp. 317–329.

Yao FSF, Fontes ML, Malhorta V. *Yao and Artusio's Anesthesiology: Problem-Oriented Patient Management*, 6th ed. Philadelphia: Lippincott Williams & Wilkins, 2008, pp. 917–18, 923.

**Chapter 56**

# Obstetrical Antepartum Hemorrhage

Marcos Izquierdo and Jessica A. Lovich-Sapola

## Placental Abruption

### Sample Case

A 22-year-old female presents to labor and delivery at 34 weeks' gestation. She reports bleeding for several hours. She has mild abdominal tenderness. A toxicology screen is positive for cocaine. Would you recommend regional or general anesthetic for her cesarean section?

### Clinical Issues

#### Definition

1. Partial or complete separation of the placenta from the uterus before delivery of the fetus
2. Occurs in 0.4–1% of all pregnancies
3. Usually occurs in the final 10 weeks of gestation

#### Pre-existing Conditions

1. Chronic hypertension
2. Gestational hypertension
3. Preeclampsia
4. Maternal cocaine use
5. Excessive alcohol intake
6. Smoking
7. Multiparity
8. Advanced age
9. Premature rupture of membranes
10. Trauma: especially blunt trauma to the abdomen

#### Presentation

1. Painful vaginal bleeding of dark, clotted blood
2. Uterine tenderness
3. Increased uterine activity/hypertonus
4. Blood loss can be concealed behind the placenta and therefore underestimated.
5. Blood loss of >2 L can result in maternal hypotension and tachycardia.
6. Fetal bradycardia and death

#### Associated Complications

1. Maternal
   a. Up to a 30% risk of developing disseminated intravascular coagulation (DIC)
   b. Acute renal failure
   c. Hemorrhage and shock
   d. Anterior pituitary necrosis: Sheehan's syndrome
   e. Couvelaire uterus: extravasated blood dissects between the myometrial fibers
   f. 2–11% maternal mortality
2. Fetal
   a. Fetal growth restriction
   b. Fetal demise secondary to hypoxia
   c. Up to 50% fetal mortality

#### Obstetrical Management

1. Large-bore IV access
2. Draw baseline blood samples: hematocrit, coagulation studies, blood typing, and cross-matching.
3. Continuous monitoring of the fetal heart rate
4. Supplemental oxygen
5. Placement of a Foley catheter
6. Left uterine displacement
7. Deliver the fetus and placenta.
8. Correct the patient's blood volume and coagulation with blood components.
   a. Fresh frozen plasma
   b. Cryoprecipitate
   c. Platelets
   d. Packed red blood cells
9. Mild cases, with no evidence of fetal distress and a favorable cervix, can be managed by the induction of labor with oxytocin and the artificial rupture of the amniotic membranes.
10. Emergency cesarean section required if:
    a. Nonreassuring fetal heart rate
    b. Maternal hemodynamic instability
    c. Coagulopathy
11. Mild cases with a pre-term fetus may warrant a delay of delivery and observation in the hospital to allow time for fetal lung maturation.

## KO Treatment Plan

### Labor and Vaginal Delivery

1. A continuous epidural anesthetic has been successfully used in patients with normal coagulation studies and no intravascular volume deficit.

### Intra-operative

1. General anesthesia is usually preferred in the setting of coagulopathies, uncontrolled hemorrhage, and hemodynamic instability.

   a. IV ketamine (1 mg/kg) or etomidate are the preferred choices for the induction of anesthesia. Propofol may precipitate hypotension in a patient with unrecognized hypovolemia.

2. Depending on the severity of the abruption, an arterial line and/or central venous pressure (CVP) monitor may be necessary to guide volume resuscitation.

3. Monitor closely for postpartum hemorrhage as these patients are at high risk of uterine atony and coagulopathy.

# Placenta Previa

## Sample Case

A 33-year-old patient presents to labor and delivery with painless vaginal bleeding. This is her fifth pregnancy, and two were delivered by cesarean section. She is awake and alert. Her lab values are all normal. She is hemodynamically stable. Since she is 37 weeks pregnant, her obstetrician decides to perform an elective cesarean section. Would you do regional or general anesthesia?

## Clinical Issues

### Definition

1. Low implantation of the placenta into the uterus
2. The placenta either is overlying or encroaching on the cervical os.
3. Present in about 0.1–1% of all pregnancies

### Diagnosis

1. Painless, bright red vaginal bleeding
2. The bleeding usually occurs after the seventh month of pregnancy.
3. Lack of pain or abnormal uterine tone favors placenta previa above placental abruption.

### Increased Risk

1. Multiparous women
2. Advanced maternal age
3. Previous cesarean section or other uterine surgery
4. Previous placenta previa
5. Smoking history

## Obstetrical Management

1. Diagnosed by ultrasound
2. Avoid a vaginal exam due to the possibility of inducing bleeding.
3. If the bleeding stops spontaneously, conservative treatment is recommended.

   a. Fetal demise is uncommon with the first episode of bleeding.

   b. Tocolysis: medications may be used to suppress premature labor.

   c. Regular monitoring of hemoglobin with blood transfusions as needed

   d. Serial ultrasounds

   e. Nonstress test and biophysical profile

   f. Corticosteroids to accelerate fetal lung maturity if between 24–34 weeks' gestation

4. Persistent bleeding, active labor, or a mature fetus require delivery of the fetus by cesarean section.

   a. Send a type and cross for packed red blood cells (PRBC).

   b. Send labs for hematocrit.

   c. Place at least one large-bore IV.

   d. Begin volume resuscitation with normal saline or lactated Ringer's solution.

5. Increased risk of postpartum hemorrhage

   a. Susceptible to uterine atony

   b. Associated with placenta accreta

   c. Hysterectomy may be required.

## KO Treatment Plan

1. A parturient presenting with hemorrhage may require emergent intervention.
2. A concise history and physical should be performed focused on the airway exam and intravascular volume status.

### Intra-operative

#### Double Setup

1. The vaginal examination is performed in the operating room if you are dealing with a marginal previa or a low-lying placenta, as these may sometimes be delivered vaginally. If the patient has a known complete or partial previa, this will automatically require a cesarean section.
2. Obstetrics, anesthesia, and the neonatologist are present in the operating room.
3. Make a full preparation for a cesarean section.

   a. Two large-gauge IVs

   b. Administration of a nonparticulate antacid

   c. Sterile prep and draping of the abdomen

   d. Two units of PRBCs in the operating room

4. A cesarean section is performed if the obstetrician confirms the placenta previa.

5. This double-setup technique is rarely performed anymore since the accuracy of ultrasound has significantly improved the diagnoses of placenta previa.

### Cesarean Section

1. Obtain large-bore IV access.
2. Type and cross-match the patient for two units of blood, and have them available in the operating room.
3. Regional anesthesia is recommended for the patient unless contraindicated (i.e., coagulopathy, patient refusal).
4. If the patient has significant blood loss and is hemodynamically unstable, general anesthesia should be considered.
    a. Use a rapid-sequence induction of anesthesia.
    b. Ketamine (0.5–1 mg/kg) or etomidate (0.2–0.3 mg/kg) are your best choices for induction agents. If you choose to use propofol, use a reduced dose.
    c. Anesthesia can be maintained with 50% nitrous oxide, 50% oxygen, and a low concentration of volatile anesthetic in patients with modest bleeding and no pre-existing fetal distress. In patients with fetal distress, consider omitting the nitrous oxide.
    d. Post-delivery, give IV oxytocin, reduce the volatile anesthetic, and resume 70% nitrous oxide plus a small dose of an opioid IV.
5. The patient may require a hysterectomy if the placenta does not separate from the uterus.
    a. Consider a central venous catheter for rapid fluid replacement.
    b. Consider an arterial line for frequent blood draws and the continuous beat-to-beat measurement of the blood pressure.

# Uterine Rupture

## Sample Case

A 32-year-old female is scheduled for a vaginal birth after a cesarean section. Her first pregnancy ended in a normal vaginal delivery. She had an emergent cesarean section for her second pregnancy for fetal decelerations. She has a good, working epidural. The obstetrical nurse notes that she has recently been having trouble monitoring contractions, and she also noticed a bulge in her abdomen. The obstetrician is called, and on examination he notes a loss of station of the fetal presenting parts. The patient is currently hemodynamically stable. Would you do regional or general anesthesia?

## Clinical Issues

### Definition

1. Complete nonsurgical disruption of all uterine layers in a gravid uterus
2. Resulting fetal distress and/or maternal hemorrhage

### Incidence

1. Increasing incidence, secondary to the increasing number of cesarean sections nationally
2. Incidence in vaginal birth after a cesarean (VBAC) with a known transverse lower uterine segment incision is <1%. Patients with a prior classical uterine incision have a 4–9% risk of uterine rupture and thus should have a repeat cesarean section and not be offered a VBAC.
3. Maternal and fetal morbidity and mortality is about 10–25%.

### Precipitating Factors

1. Trial of labor after a prior cesarean section
2. Prior uterine surgery
3. Multiparity
4. Advanced maternal age
5. Multiple gestations
6. Trauma – including excessive fundal pressure
7. Induction or augmentation of labor with oxytocin
8. Inter-delivery interval less than 12–16 months
9. Placenta percreta
10. Uterine tumors
11. Fetal malposition, anomaly, or macrosomia

### Diagnosis

1. Nonspecific symptoms
2. Fetal heart rate abnormalities are the first sign in >80% of patients.
3. Maternal hypotension
4. Loss of function of the uterine pressure monitors
5. Constant abdominal pain (possibly concealed by a labor epidural)
6. Change in the uterine shape
7. Cessation of contractions
8. Vaginal bleeding
9. Loss of station of fetal presenting parts
10. Suspected clinically, but confirmed surgically with a laparotomy

### Obstetrical Management

1. Repair of the uterus
2. Arterial ligation: O'Leary or hypogastric artery ligation
3. Hysterectomy

## KO Treatment Plan

### Intra-operative

1. Emergency laparotomy
2. Regional anesthesia can be used if a good working epidural is already in place and the patient is hemodynamically stable.
3. If the patient does not have an epidural catheter *in situ*, general anesthesia is indicated.

4. You must explain to the patient that it is likely that she may still require general anesthesia depending on the findings of the laparotomy. Uterine rupture can lead to significant damage to the surrounding organs, especially the bladder.
5. Aggressive volume replacement
6. Maintain urine output

# Vasa Previa

## Clinical Issues

### Definition

1. Velamentous insertion of the umbilical vessels so that they run through the amniotic membranes traversing between fetal presenting part and the cervical os.
2. These vessels are very fragile and susceptible to trauma during labor.
3. The associated bleeding is fetal in origin.
4. Uncommon (1 in 3000 deliveries)
5. High fetal mortality secondary to the fetus's small blood volume (50–75%)
6. No threat to the mother

### Diagnosis

1. Ultrasound can identify vasa previa prior to hemorrhage.
2. Vaginal bleeding immediately on rupture of the amniotic membranes
3. Fetal heart rate abnormalities

### Increased Risk

1. Multiple gestation, especially with triplets
2. Low-lying placenta, placenta previa

### Obstetrical Management

1. Early diagnosis and treatment
2. Immediate delivery
3. Can be managed conservatively with delivery at 34 weeks if identified early

## KO Treatment Plan

1. Emergency cesarean section in the case of ruptured vasa previa
2. Use the fastest technique possible for the induction of anesthesia. This is usually general anesthesia. If you believe that you can get a spinal in the lateral position faster (rapid-sequence spinal) than inducing general anesthesia, do that. If you already have a continuous spinal or epidural, use that. Use whatever is the fastest and safest technique.
3. Remember, the bleeding is fetal and not maternal. The mother should not be hypotensive from the blood loss. She also should not require significant volume replacement.
4. The neonate will require rapid volume replacement after delivery. The physician may transfuse some of the baby's own blood drawn from the umbilical–placental vessels into a heparinized syringe.

# Bibliography

Barash PG, Cullen BF, Stoelting RK, et al. *Clinical Anesthesia*, 8th ed. Philadelphia: Lippincott Williams & Wilkins, 2017, pp. 1159–61.

Chestnut DH, Wong CA, Tsen LC, et al. *Chestnut's Obstetric Anesthesia: Principles and Practice*, 6th ed. Philadelphia: Elsevier, 2020, pp. 901–36.

Gropper MA. *Miller's Anesthesia*, 9th ed. Philadelphia: Elsevier, 2020, pp. 2006–41.

Landon MB, Galan HL, Jauniaux ERM, et al. *Gabbe's Obstetrics: Normal and Problem Pregnancies*, 8th ed. Philadelphia: Saunders, 2020, chapters 18, 24.

# Obstetrical Postpartum Hemorrhage

Marcos Izquierdo and Jessica A. Lovich-Sapola

## Placenta Accreta

### Sample Case

A 33-year-old female presents in labor for her fifth pregnancy. She reports three prior cesarean sections. What are your anesthetic concerns?

### Clinical Issues

#### Definition

1. The placenta becomes abnormally adherent to the implantation site.
2. Can cause life-threatening hemorrhage as the placenta is delivered
3. Classified by the degree of placental penetration of the myometrium
   a. Placenta accreta: the placenta is adherent to the myometrium.
   b. Placenta increta: the placenta invades the myometrium.
   c. Placenta percreta: the placenta extends through the myometrium and may adhere to the surrounding structures.

#### Associated Risk Factors

1. Previous cesarean section
2. Current placenta previa

#### Diagnosis

1. Ultrasonography
2. Magnetic resonance imaging (MRI)
3. Often not recognized until the obstetrician has difficulty separating the placenta from the uterus

#### Obstetric Management

1. Intrauterine balloon tamponade
2. Cesarean hysterectomy – must keep placenta intact
3. Arterial embolization under radiographic guidance in the case of persistent bleeding

### KO Treatment Plan

#### Intra-operative

1. Large-bore IV access; consider central venous access
2. Arterial line

3. Type and cross at least four units of packed red blood cells (PBRC).
4. Consider intra-operative blood salvage in case of massive hemorrhage.
5. General anesthesia is usually required for patient comfort and adequate operating conditions.
6. Neuraxial anesthesia can be performed in carefully selected patients; avoid a single-shot spinal and consider placement of a combined spinal epidural or continuous epidural for the ability to extend the duration of the block while minimizing sympatholysis.
7. A continuous epidural can be used, but the timing of the epidural catheter removal is controversial secondary to the possibility of an associated massive hemorrhage and transfusion-precipitated disseminated intravascular coagulation (DIC).

## Uterine Atony

### Sample Case

A 25-year-old-female delivered her seventh baby. Twenty minutes after delivery, the nurse reports a lot of vaginal bleeding. Manual uterine massage does not seem to be helping. IV oxytocin is running as ordered. What are your concerns? What are your recommendations for treatment?

### Clinical Issues

#### Definition

1. Most common cause of early postpartum hemorrhage (80% of cases of hemorrhage)
2. Ineffective uterine muscle contraction
3. Occurs in 1 in 20 deliveries.

#### Risk Factors

1. Prolonged or rapid labor
2. Prolonged oxytocin use
3. Over-distended uterus: fetal macrosomia, multiple gestation, polyhydramnios
4. Infection: chorioamnionitis
5. Grand multiparity
6. Placenta previa
7. Administration of drugs that relax the uterus
   a. Halogenated anesthetics
   b. β-sympathetic agonists

c. Magnesium sulfate

d. Nitroglycerin

**Diagnosis**

1. Rapid uterine bleeding
2. Lack of myometrial tone

## KO Treatment Plan

1. Bimanual uterine massage
2. Uterotonic therapy
   a. Oxytocin (Pitocin)
      i. First-line therapy
      ii. Given intravenous (IV) or intramuscular (IM)
      iii. Side effects: hypotension, nausea, emesis, water intoxication
      iv. Usually given by continuous IV infusion
   b. Prostaglandins
      i. PGF$_2\alpha$ (hemabate/carboprost)
         (1) IM or intrauterine (IU)
         (2) Side effects: nausea, vomiting, flushing, chills, and bronchospasm
         (3) Contraindicated in patients with active cardiac, pulmonary, renal, or hepatic disease
      ii. PGE (misoprostol)
         (1) Rectal (PR) or oral (PO)
         (2) Side effects: tachycardia and fever
   c. Methylergonovine (methergine)
      i. IM or IU
      ii. Blood vessel constrictor and smooth muscle agonist
      iii. Side effects: profound hypertension, nausea, and vomiting
      iv. Contraindicated in patients with chronic hypertension, preeclampsia, peripheral vascular disease, and ischemic heart disease
3. When the uterine atony is due to a tocolytic therapy such as magnesium sulfate, treat with 1 g of calcium gluconate IV.
4. Uterine tamponade
5. Selective arterial embolization
6. Surgical intervention
   a. Arterial ligation
   b. Uterine suturing
   c. Hysterectomy

## Uterine Inversion

## Clinical Issues

**Definition**

1. Rare

2. Uterine fundus inverts through the cervix into the vagina.

**Risk Factors**

1. Uterine atony and over-distension
2. Fetal macrosomia
3. Prolonged labor
4. Uterine malformations
5. Short umbilical cord
6. Excessive umbilical cord traction
7. Ehlers–Danlos syndrome
8. Inappropriate fundal pressure

**Diagnosis**

1. Hypotension is usually seen before significant blood loss.
2. Sudden onset of vaginal bleeding
3. Diagnosed with a bimanual exam and ultrasound

## KO Treatment Plan

1. IV fluid therapy
2. Provide uterine relaxation.
   a. Stop all uterotonics.
   b. β-sympathomimetic agents
   c. Magnesium
   d. Nitroglycerin
   e. The agent of choice depends solely on the patient's hemodynamic status.
3. Restore the uterus to its normal position.
4. If these initial attempts fail, rapid-sequence induction with cricoid pressure, endotracheal intubation, and the administration of a halogenated anesthetic may be necessary to provide sufficient uterine relaxation.
5. Once the uterus is in place, oxytocin should be given to induce uterine contraction.

## Retained Placenta and Products of Conception

## Clinical Issues

**Definition**

1. Placental tissue and amniotic membranes remain in the uterus after delivery and can inhibit the uterus from contracting adequately, resulting in hemorrhage.
2. Occurs in about 0.5–1.0% of deliveries

**Associated Risk Factors**

1. Mid-trimester delivery
2. Chorioamnionitis
3. Accessory placental lobe

## KO Treatment Plan

1. This usually only requires manual exploration and ultrasound diagnostics. This can be done in the birthing room if the patient has an epidural in place.
2. Some patients will require a uterine curettage in the operating room.
3. Light sedation may be adequate to allow for exploration and extraction of the retained products.
4. Neuraxial anesthesia should be considered in patients who are hemodynamically stable.

5. The surgeon may require complete uterine relaxation. This can be accomplished with general anesthesia or nitroglycerin (IV or sublingual).
   a. Perform rapid-sequence induction of general anesthesia followed by high-dose volatile anesthetic to relax the uterus.
   b. Risk of failed intubation and aspiration

### Non-uterine Causes of Postpartum Hemorrhage

1. Genital tract lacerations
2. Vulvar and vaginal hematoma
3. Retroperitoneal hematoma
4. Maternal coagulopathy

## Bibliography

Chestnut DH, Wong CA, Tsen LC, et al. *Chestnut's Obstetric Anesthesia: Principles and Practice*, 6th ed. Philadelphia: Elsevier, 2020, pp. 901–36.

Gropper MA. *Miller's Anesthesia*, 9th ed. Philadelphia: Elsevier, 2020, pp. 2006–41.

Landon MB, Galan HL, Jauniaux ERM, et al. *Gabbe's Obstetrics: Normal and Problem Pregnancies*, 8th ed. Philadelphia: Saunders, 2020, chapters 18, 21.

# Other Obstetrical Complications

Monica Cheriyan and Jessica A. Lovich-Sapola

## Umbilical Cord Prolapse

### Sample Case

A 25-year-old female, G2P1, in labor has a cervix dilated to 6 cm. You have placed an epidural and are verifying the level when the obstetrical resident comes in to rupture the patient's membranes. Upon rupture, the fetal heart rate drops suddenly. The obstetrical resident notes that she can now feel the umbilical cord. What is the diagnosis? What is your anesthetic plan for this emergent cesarean section?

### Clinical Issues

#### Definition

1. The umbilical cord prolapses through the cervical os.
2. This leads to significant cord compression and sudden fetal bradycardia.

#### Incidence

1. Rare
2. 0.1–0.6% of cephalic term pregnancies
3. Increased risk with breech, transverse lie, multiple gestations, and long umbilical cord
4. Increased risk with polyhydramnios

#### Diagnosis

1. Suspect cord prolapse when there is a sudden drop in the fetal heart rate immediately after the membranes are ruptured.
2. Confirm by palpation of the umbilical cord on vaginal exam below the presenting fetal part.

### KO Treatment Plan

#### Pre-operative

1. Manual replacement of the cord
2. Fetal head elevation until operative delivery
3. Avoidance of cord compression by the presenting fetal parts
4. Emergent cesarean section

#### Intra-operative

1. Use a regional technique if an epidural catheter is *in situ*. In this patient, I would use my recently placed catheter

and dose with local anesthetic to achieve a T4–T6 level. It is important to ask the obstetrical resident to monitor the fetal heart rate by palpating the cord.

2. General anesthesia is usually the first choice if there is associated fetal compromise. If the obstetrical resident noted a loss of fetal heart tones prior to achieving a proper level with the epidural catheter, I would induce general anesthesia. Always remember that the mother is your first priority. If you believe that she will be a difficult intubation, wait for your epidural level, or if this is inadequate, an awake intubation prior to general anesthesia may be required.

## Fetal Heart Rate Decelerations

### Sample Case

A 22-year-old female, G1P0, is scheduled for an urgent cesarean section at 37 weeks' gestation. She has gestational hypertension. The fetal heart rate tracing shows late decelerations. Her blood pressure is 170/100 mm Hg and her hemoglobin is 9.5 g/dL. What is a late deceleration? Is it significant? Are there other tests that can be done to assess fetal well-being?

### Clinical Issues

1. Early decelerations (Fig. 58.1)
   a. Definition
      i. Shallow, symmetric, uniform decelerations with a gradual onset and return to baseline, resulting in a U-shaped deceleration
      ii. They begin early in the contraction; their nadir coincides with the peak of the contraction and returns to baseline by the time the contraction is over.

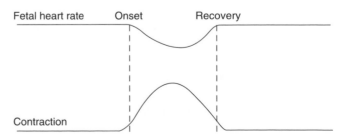

**Figure 58.1** Early deceleration. Figure credit: J. Lovich-Sapola, MD, MBA, FASA.

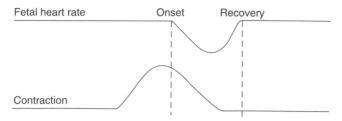

Fetal heart rate    Onset    Recovery

Contraction

**Figure 58.2** Late deceleration. Figure credit: J. Lovich-Sapola, MD, MBA, FASA.

   iii. Usually occurs when the patient's cervix is dilated between 4 and 6 cm.

   iv. They do not indicate fetal hypoxia and are benign.

   v. Occur in 5–10% of all labors

  b. Cause

   i. Fetal head compression by the uterine cervix as it overrides the anterior fontanel of the cranium

   ii. This results in altered fetal cerebral blood flow, precipitating a vagal reflex, with resultant slowing of the fetal heart rate.

2. Late decelerations (Fig. 58.2)

  a. Definition

   i. Gradual onset and return to baseline

   ii. U-shaped

   iii. Delayed in timing relative to the contraction

   iv. Begin about 30 seconds after the onset of the contraction or even at or after its peak

   v. The nadir is after the peak of the contraction.

   vi. Late decelerations *always* indicate fetal hypoxia.

  b. Causes

   i. Uteroplacental insufficiency causing relative fetal brain hypoxia during the contraction

   ii. Uteroplacental perfusion is temporarily interrupted during the peak of a strong contraction.

   iii. Any compromise in delivery, exchange, or uptake in fetal oxygen, other than umbilical cord compression, can result in a late deceleration if the insult is sufficient.

   iv. Excessive uterine contractions (seen with IV oxytocin)

   v. Spinal or epidural secondary to either systemic or local hypoperfusion/hypotension

   vi. Post-maturity

   vii. Maternal hypertension

   viii. Collagen vascular disease

   ix. Advanced diabetes mellitus

   x. Placental abruption

   xi. Severe maternal anemia or hypoxemia

   xii. Chronic fetal anemia

  c. Diagnosis

   i. Fetal scalp pH

    (1) Used to determine fetal acidosis

    (2) Technically difficult

    (3) Used infrequently

    (4) The patient must be at least 4–5 cm dilated, vertex, and −1 station.

    (5) A pH <7.20 is consistent with fetal acidosis and requires an emergent cesarean section.

    (6) A pH of 7.20–7.25 is considered borderline and should be repeated if the late deceleration pattern persists.

    (7) A pH greater than 7.25 is considered adequate for the fetus. Continue to closely monitor the mother and fetus, and repeat the pH as needed.

  d. Treatment

   i. Call for help.

   ii. Administer supplemental oxygen.

   iii. Change the maternal position: lateral or knee–chest.

   iv. Treat maternal hypotension with IV fluids or vasopressor administration.

   v. Consider tocolysis to treat uterine tetany or hyperstimulation.

   vi. Discontinue the oxytocin infusion.

   vii. Consider an amnioinfusion.

   viii. Determine whether an assisted vaginal delivery or cesarean section is required.

    (1) *In situ* epidural, spinal, or general anesthesia are all viable options for the induction of anesthesia, depending on the pattern and depth of decelerations.

3. Variable decelerations

  a. Definition

   i. Most common decelerations

   ii. Variable size, shape, depth, duration, and timing relative to the contraction

   iii. Caused by umbilical cord compression

   iv. Continued cord compression leads to a progressive increase in fetal $CO_2$ and a resulting respiratory acidosis. This can worsen over time into a combined respiratory and metabolic acidosis.

   v. Usually has a favorable outcome

  b. Causes

   i. Umbilical cord compression and stretch

   ii. Initially a reflex response to changes in pressure and not hypoxia

   iii. Can be seen in fetuses with no change in oxygen saturation

   iv. Oligohydramnios in early labor

v. Nuchal cord at 8–9 cm dilated

vi. Umbilical cord prolapse

# Molar Pregnancy

## Sample Case

A 32-year-old female presents with a 2-week history of lower abdominal pain, nausea, vomiting, and vaginal bleeding. She has a 16-week-sized uterus. She is scheduled for an evacuation of her molar pregnancy. What potential problems could be anticipated? Three hours after the evacuation, she complains of chest pain, cough, and tachypnea. What is the differential diagnosis? How would you diagnose and manage her care?

### Definition

1. Vesicular swelling of placental (choroid) villi
2. Absence of an intact fetus
3. Gestational trophoblastic disease that originates in the placenta

## Diagnosis

1. Ultrasound
2. Abnormally elevated human chorionic gonadotrophin (hCG) levels for gestational age

### Symptoms and Signs

1. Abnormal bleeding in early pregnancy
2. Can mimic an incomplete or threatened abortion
3. Large uterus for dates
4. Nausea and vomiting
5. Late first and early second trimester signs of toxemia (prior to 24 weeks)
6. Laboratory manifestations of hyperthyroidism
7. Lower abdominal pain
8. Absent fetal heart tones or fetal parts

### Associated Complications

1. Anemia
2. Pregnancy-induced hypertension
3. Pulmonary insufficiency
   a. Acute dyspnea
   b. Cyanosis
4. Congestive heart failure
5. Hyperthyroidism/thyrotoxicosis
   a. hCG is identical to a sub-unit of the thyroid-stimulating hormone (TSH) but has a weak thyroid-stimulating effect in normal pregnancies.
   b. Molar thyrotropin is responsible for the associated thyrotoxicosis with molar pregnancies.
6. Disseminated intravascular coagulation (DIC)
7. Pulmonary embolism (trophoblastic embolization)

### Obstetrical Management

1. The molar pregnancy must be evacuated from the uterus using suction curettage.

## KO Treatment Plan

### Pre-operative

1. Complete history and physical
2. Laboratory test
   a. CBC: high risk for anemia secondary to vaginal bleeding
   b. Electrolytes
   c. Arterial blood gas
   d. Thyroid function tests: high risk for thyrotoxicosis
   e. Chest X-ray
3. Treat any associated hyperthyroidism with intravenous iodine and β-adrenergic receptor blockers.
   a. It is not possible to get the patient into a euthyroid state prior to the surgical procedure.
   b. Focus on controlling the sympathetic activity.
4. Avoid excessive fluid resuscitation to prevent pulmonary edema.

### Intra-operative

1. General anesthesia is recommended.
   a. Secure the airway with a rapid-sequence intubation.
   b. Regional anesthesia is not recommended secondary to the associated DIC.
2. An arterial line is recommended for continuous monitoring of the patient's blood pressure and frequent blood draws.

### Post-operative

1. The patient should be monitored closely in the ICU for 12–24 hours.
2. Observe for pulmonary embolus, congestive heart failure, DIC, and thyrotoxicosis.

# Amniotic Fluid Embolism (AFE)

## Sample Case

A 33-year-old female, G9P4, presents for a scheduled cesarean section. After delivery, the obstetrician lifts the uterus for examination. One minute later you notice hypotension and the patient complains of difficulty breathing. What is the diagnosis?

## Clinical Issues

### Definition

1. AFE is a life-threatening emergency.
2. It can occur at any time throughout pregnancy.
   a. Typically during vaginal or cesarean delivery

3. If left untreated it will lead to hemodynamic collapse and death.

   a. Even with treatment, the mortality is reported at 40–80%.

### Incidence

1. Incidence between 1.7 and 7.7 per 100,000 deliveries

### Risk Factors

1. Multiparity
2. Advanced maternal age
3. Abruption
4. Placenta previa
5. Cervical laceration
6. Uterine rupture
7. Induction of labor
8. Cesarean section

## Symptoms and Signs

1. Restlessness and confusion
2. Dyspnea, cyanosis, and respiratory arrest
3. Cardiovascular

   a. Hypotension
   b. Arrythmia

      i. PEA, bradycardia, asystole, and ventricular fibrillation

4. Uterine atony
5. Consumptive coagulopathy (DIC)

   a. Low fibrinogen
   b. Low platelets
   c. High fibrin split products
   d. Abnormal prothrombin time (PT) and partial thromboplastin time (PTT)

6. Fetal distress and death

### Diagnosis

1. Previously diagnosed by fetal squamous cells in the maternal pulmonary circulation but this is also present at time of delivery in healthy patients
2. Diagnosis of exclusion

   a. Differentiate from venous or pulmonary embolism, cardiac dysfunction, massive hemorrhage, or pulmonary aspiration.

3. No diagnostic laboratory test exists.
4. The mechanism is unclear, but is thought to be anaphylactoid rather than embolic.

## KO Treatment Plan

1. Early recognition and communication with obstetrician
2. Aggressive resuscitation; establish large-bore IVs or central venous access.
3. Resuscitation priorities include oxygenation, hemodynamic support, and correction of coagulopathy.
4. A-OK management is based on the hypothesis that the emergent treatment of an amniotic fluid embolism should include therapy that targets the serotonin and thromboxane A2 pathways.

   • A: Atropine 1 mg: vagal response

      a. Decreases vasoconstriction in the pulmonary vasculature
      b. Treats bradycardia and heart block

   • O: Ondansetron 8 mg: serotonin
   • K: Ketorolac 30 mg: thromboxane A2

      a. Inhibits clot formation and the extension of the clot
      b. Decreases the cascade of inappropriate clotting

# Shoulder Dystocia

## Sample Case

A 29-year-old female, G3O2, with gestational diabetes and polyhydramnios, is in the second stage of labor. During delivery, the obstetric resident delivers the head but is unable to deliver the rest of the fetus and you hear an overhead call for help. What is the diagnosis?

## Clinical Issues

### Definition

1. Shoulder dystocia occurs when, after delivery of the head, the shoulders cannot be delivered past the pelvis.
2. Obstetric emergency associated with prolonged gestation, fetal macrosomia, and obesity
3. No causal relationship exists with epidural analgesia.
4. Associated with an increased risk of postpartum hemorrhage and fourth-degree lacerations

## KO Treatment Plan

1. Epidural analgesia allows for manipulation in the case of shoulder dystocia.
2. The obstetrician may try different maneuvers to extract the infant from the pelvis.
3. The anesthesiologist can provide small doses of nitroglycerin to relax the uterus and aid with delivery.
4. If unsuccessful, the fetus may be pushed back into the pelvis and emergent cesarean delivery may be required.

## Bibliography

Chestnut DH. *Obstetric Anesthesia: Principles and Practice*, 3rd ed. Philadelphia: Mosby, 2004, pp. 119, 662–76.

Copper PL, Otto MP, Leighton BL. Successful management of cardiac arrest from amniotic flid embolism with ondansetron, metoclopramide, atropine, and ketorolac: a case report. Paper presented at SOAP 2013.

Erol DD, Cevryoglu AS, Uslan I. Preoperative preparation and general anesthesia administration with sevoflurane in a patient who develops thyrotoxicosis and cardiogenic dysfunction due to a hydatidiform mole. *Internet J Anesthesiol* 2004;**8**(1).

Gabbe SG, Niebyl JR, Simpson JL. *Obstetrics: Normal and Problem Pregnancies*, 5th ed. Philadelphia:

Churchill Livingston & Elsevier, 2007, chapters 15, 18.

Gropper MA. *Miller's Anesthesia*, 9th ed. Philadelphia: Elsevier, 2020, pp. 2006–41.

Katz VL, Lentz GM, Lobo RA, et al. *Comprehensive Gynecology*, 5th ed. Philadelphia: Mosby Elsevier, 2007, chapter 35.

# Difficult Obstetrical Airway

Nicholas Bigler

## Sample Case

An obese, 25-year-old woman, G1P0, presents for an elective cesarean section secondary to breech presentation of the fetus. She has a medical history significant for asthma and morbid obesity, with a BMI of 42. She had a prior laparoscopic cholecystectomy, at which time she states that she awoke with an incredibly sore throat and a chipped front tooth. She states that she had been told there was some difficulty in putting her to sleep, but is unable to provide further details. What is your plan? Which would you recommend: regional anesthesia, or a general anesthetic approach? Assuming you have to induce general anesthesia, how will you secure the airway?

## Clinical Issues

### Difficult Intubation

1. Difficult intubation occurs in 3.3% of obstetric patients and is not anticipated in two-thirds of those cases.
2. A difficult airway cart must be available in any area where airway management in an obstetric patient may occur.
3. Studies in obstetric populations having both cesarean and noncesarean delivery show a rate of failed intubation at about 1:230, vs. 1:2000 in the general population. The working definition of a failed tracheal intubation is a failure to achieve successful tracheal intubation within three attempts, regardless of the techniques utilized (i.e., direct vs. video laryngoscopy).

## Characteristics of an Obstetrical Airway That Lead to an Increased Incidence of Difficult Intubations

1. Airway edema: There is capillary engorgement of the mucosa throughout the entire respiratory tract. This increases the risk and severity of bleeding in the airway.
2. The Mallampati score will often advance by one or two classes due to increased pharyngeal edema and fatty infiltration of the pharyngeal tissue.
3. Associated morbid obesity
4. Patients with preeclampsia and eclampsia retain fluids, often making the tongue size larger and the neck area more edematous and stiffer (see Chapter 55).
5. Increased breast size leads to difficult mask ventilation and increases the difficulty of insertion of a standard size laryngoscope handle.

6. Uterine enlargement with ensuing cephalad displacement of the diaphragm decreases functional residual capacity (FRC), decreasing the apneic time interval before desaturation occurs.

## Ways to Prepare to Help Prevent Difficult Intubations

1. Proper position of head and neck
   a. Elevation of shoulders
   b. Flexion of cervical spine
   c. Extension of atlanto-occipital joint
2. Have readily available a variety of laryngoscopes blades, short handle, multiple endotracheal tube sizes, laryngeal mask airway (LMA), video laryngoscope, fiber-optic bronchoscope, and the ability to do transtracheal jet ventilation.

## Aspiration

1. Obstetric patients are at high risk for pulmonary aspiration, with incidence increasing to 8%, compared with 1% in case-matched controls.
2. A delay in gastric emptying can be demonstrated by the end of the first trimester.
3. Lower esophageal sphincter tone is generally reduced due to increased circulating progesterone (as progesterone decreases smooth muscle tone, including uterine tone to prevent early labor).
4. The angle of the gastroesophageal junction is altered due to displacement of the stomach by the gravid uterus.
5. A rapid-sequence induction of anesthesia with proper cricoid pressure and use of a cuffed endotracheal tube is required for any general anesthetic after the 12th week of gestation.

## KO Treatment Plan

### Pre-operative

1. Anticipation of a difficult airway may help reduce the risk of a failed intubation. Airway history and exam are critical in the assessment of every pregnant woman. Exam should include:
   a. Mouth opening (Mallampati classification)

b. Thyromental distance
c. Atlanto-occipital extension
d. Upper lip bite test
e. Neck
f. Dentition
g. History of a difficult intubation

## Intra-operative

1. Because of the airway problems that are associated with general anesthesia, regional anesthesia should be used when possible.
2. It is recommended that early intervention with the placement of a functioning regional anesthetic (labor epidural) will minimize emergency induction of general anesthesia in parturients with difficult airways. Unexpected sequelae may still necessitate airway management (e.g., failure of block, high-level block, local anesthetic toxicity, cardiac arrest, hemorrhage).
3. In the event of an urgent or emergent cesarean section, establishment of a surgical block is often quicker than establishing adequate anesthesia via an awake intubation or, worse, securing an airway after a failed intubation.

## Labor and a Known Difficult Airway

1. A functioning epidural block minimizes the need for general anesthesia and resultant airway instrumentation.

## Cesarean Section with a Known Difficult Airway

1. Regional anesthesia is the best possible choice in most cases of an anticipated difficult airway.
   a. In a nonurgent situation, slow titration of an epidural block allows for the avoidance of any major hemodynamic and respiratory compromise.
   b. In a more time-sensitive situation, spinal anesthesia allows for rapid establishment of surgical anesthesia.

2. Aspiration prophylaxis in the form of H2-blockers and/or non-particulate antacid should be provided to all patients two hours prior to cesarean section.
3. Optimal positioning should be used in each patient.
4. An awake intubation allows for preservation of the natural airway and airway reflexes.
   a. A nasal fiber-optic intubation should be avoided due to the mucosal engorgement and the high risk of epistaxis, leading to a compromised airway.
   b. With adequate psychological and pharmacological preparation, patients can generally tolerate an awake intubation.
   c. Video laryngoscopy has become more standard of care, and may replace the need for an awake fiber-optic intubation in many situations.
5. Additional equipment should be immediately available to establish an airway in case a need arises. Equipment should include:
   a. Endotracheal tubes in smaller sizes, with stylets in place
   b. Short-handle laryngoscope
   c. LMAs of varying sizes
   d. Immediate availability of secondary airway equipment, based on practitioner familiarity, such as a fiber-optic scope, video laryngoscope, and/or a tracheotomy tray

## Cesarean Section and an Unknown Difficult Airway

1. In an urgent situation when perhaps there is not enough time to administer a regional anesthetic, a general anesthetic is performed. To reduce the risk of aspiration of gastric contents, a rapid-sequence induction with tracheal intubation is considered the gold standard of airway management.
2. Before induction of anesthesia, the anesthesiologist should discuss with the obstetric team whether to wake the woman or continue anesthesia in the event of failed tracheal intubation (Table 59.1).

**Table 59.1** Failed obstetric intubation recommendations

| Failed intubation | Inadequate ventilation | Adequate ventilation |
| --- | --- | --- |
| 1. Call for help.<br>2. Ventilate with 100% oxygen.<br>  a. Face mask and cricoid pressure<br>  b. LMA and cricoid pressure | 1. Nonsurgical airway<br>  a. LMA with cricoid<br>  b. Combitube<br>  c. Transtracheal jet ventilation<br>2. Surgical airway<br>  a. Cricothyrotomy<br>  b. Tracheotomy<br>3. Deliver the baby | 1. Assess the fetus<br>2. Fetal distress<br>  a. Spontaneous ventilation with sevoflurane and 100% oxygen<br>  b. LMA plus cricoid pressure<br>  c. Intubation through the LMA<br>3. No fetal distress<br>  a. Wake the patient<br>  b. Attempt an awake intubation or regional anesthesia |

Adapted from Difficult intubation in obstetric patients figure. In Butterworth JF, Mackey DC, Wasnick JD. *Morgan & Mikhail's Clinical Anesthesiology*, 6th ed. New York: McGraw-Hill Education, 2018, p. 877.

3. The overriding indications to proceed with general anesthesia are maternal compromise not responsive to resuscitation and acute fetal compromise secondary to an irreversible cause.

4. Oxygenation after failed intubation is critical. A second-generation supraglottic device should be available.

5. If the surgery needs to proceed despite failed intubation, mask ventilation with cricoid pressure should be attempted. In the presence of fetal distress, the surgery may proceed.

6. As this situation progresses, the Obstetric Anesthetists Association/Difficult Airway Society Master Algorithm should be followed.

7. None of these are popular techniques, but well-thought-out algorithms and equipment must be available to deal with airway emergencies during failed intubations of the obstetric patient.

# Bibliography

Alanoğlu Z, Erkoç SK, Güçlü ÇY, et al. Challenges of obstetric anesthesia: difficult laryngeal visualization. *Acta Clin Croat.* 2016;55(Suppl. 1):68–72.

Butterworth JF, Mackey DC, Wasnick JD. *Morgan & Mikhail's Clinical Anesthesiology*, 6th ed. New York: McGraw-Hill Education, 2018, pp. 875–8.

Kinsella SM, Winton AL, Mushami MC, et al. Failed tracheal intubation during obstetric general anaesthesia: a literature review. *Int J Obstet Anesth* 2015;24:356–374.

Law JA, Broemling N, Cooper RM, et al. The difficult airway with recommendations for management – Part 1: difficult tracheal intubation encountered in an unconscious/induced patient. *Can J Anaesth* 2013;60(11):1089–118.

Mandal NG, Surapeneni S. Regional anaesthesia in pre-eclampsia: advantages and disadvantages. *Drugs*, 2004;64(3):223–36.

Munner U, deBoisblanc B, Sursh MS. Airway problems in pregnancy. *Crit Care Med* 2005;33(10):S259–68.

Mushambi MC, Kinsella SM, Popat M, et al. Obstetric Anaesthetists' Association and Difficult Airway Society guidelines for the management of difficult and failed tracheal intubation in obstetrics. *Anaesthesia* 2015;70:1286–1306.

# Anesthesia for a Vaginal Delivery

Sarah Zach, Alma Hoxha, and Jessica A. Lovich-Sapola

## Sample Case

A 26-year-old female, G3P2, 39 weeks pregnant, comes to labor and delivery complaining of 6/10 pain with contractions and is asking for an epidural. Her medical history is only significant for the recent diagnosis of preeclampsia. Vital signs on admission include a blood pressure of 165/82 mm Hg, a heart rate of 98, a respiratory rate of 19, and a temperature of 36.3 °C. What kind of analgesia would you offer to this patient? Do you have any concerns?

## Clinical Issues

### Stages of Labor

1.  First stage of labor
    a.  Uterine contractions
    b.  Complete dilation of the cervix
    c.  Stretching of the lower uterine segment
    d.  Pain impulses are carried in visceral afferent C-fibers accompanying the sympathetic nerves.
        i.   Early stage: T11–T12
        ii.  Later stage: T10–L1

2.  Second stage of labor
    a.  Full cervical dilation to the delivery of the fetus
    b.  Additional pain impulses
        i.   Distention of the vaginal vault and perineum
        ii.  Impulses are carried via the pudendal nerves (S2–S4).

3.  Third stage
    a.  Delivery of the placenta

### Well-Conducted Obstetrical Analgesia

1.  Pain relief
2.  Reduced anxiety
3.  Many benefits for the mother
    a.  Blunts the increase in heart rate, cardiac output, and blood pressure
    b.  Blunts the release of catecholamines: epinephrine, norepinephrine
    c.  Pain relief may improve uterine blood flow.

d.  Blunts maternal hyperventilation–hypoventilation cycle
    i.   Indirectly benefits the fetus

## Mechanisms to Treat Labor Pain

1.  Psychologic techniques
    a.  Psychoprophylaxis
        i.   Lamaze: prepared childbirth
            (1)  Positive conditioning and education
        ii.  Works under the concept that a lack of knowledge, fear, and anxiety can increase a patient's perception of pain
    b.  Hypnosis
    c.  Acupuncture
    d.  Transcutaneous electrical nerve stimulation
    e.  Massage

2.  Systemic medications
    a.  Opioids
        i.   Meperidine: historically most commonly used, but in past decade use has decreased secondary to the side effects and lack of efficacy
            (1)  Given intravenously (IV): 25–50 mg
                (a)  Peak effect 5–10 minutes after administration
            (2)  Intramuscularly (IM): 50–100 mg
                (a)  Peak effect 40–50 minutes after administration
            (3)  Intrathecally 10–20 mg
                (a)  Effective labor analgesia in 2–12 minutes with a duration of 1–3 hours
            (4)  Good for the first and second stages of labor
            (5)  Side effects
                (a)  Nausea and vomiting
                (b)  Dose-related depression of ventilation
                (c)  Orthostatic hypotension
                (d)  Neonatal depression

(e) May decrease beat-to-beat variability of the fetus

(f) The placenta transfers the active metabolite normeperidine. It has a half-life of 13–23 hours in the parturient and up to three times longer in the neonate, which could lead to toxicity.

(g) Fetal exposure to the drug is highest at 2–3 hours after administration.

  ii. Fentanyl, remifentanil

    (1) Most commonly used

    (2) Potent medications

    (3) Provide complete analgesia without sympathectomy or motor blockade when used in a neuraxial block

    (4) Patient-controlled analgesia (PCA) is a better choice than bolus administration, but PCA has the potential for accumulation and increased risk of neonatal depression.

    (5) Remifentanil PCA may decrease side effects in the fetus, but may not provide enough pain relief to the parturient.

    (6) Must monitor oxygenation and respiration closely

  iii. Morphine

    (1) IV or IM administration

    (2) Produces more respiratory depression than meperidine in equianalgesic doses

    (3) Rarely used for labor pain

    (4) Used very early in labor, if used at all

    (5) Onset of 10–20 minutes

    (6) The active metabolite, morphine-6-glucuronide, has a longer half-life in neonates than parturient and can cause significant sedation and respiratory depression.

    (7) Histamine release that can cause rash and pruritis

  iv. Butorphanol and nalbuphine: given IV, IM, or SQ

    (1) Opioid agonist–antagonist

    (2) Decreased incidence of nausea and vomiting

    (3) Decreased dysphoria

    (4) Ceiling effect on the depression of ventilation

    (5) Side effects: high incidence of maternal sedation

    (6) Usually well tolerated

    (7) Avoid in patients on chronic opioids secondary to the risk of acute withdrawal.

b. Ketamine

  i. Potent analgesic

  ii. Side effects: unacceptable amnesia

  iii. If used at 0.2–0.4 mg/kg, it gives adequate analgesia with no neonatal depression.

c. Sedatives

  i. Recommended only in the very early phase of labor when delivery is not anticipated for more than 12–24 hours secondary to the associated significant fetal respiratory depression

    (1) Promethazine

      (a) Relieves anxiety

      (b) Decreases the opioid requirements

      (c) Controls emesis

    (2) Benzodiazepines

      (a) Rarely used

      (b) Sedation and anxiolysis

      (c) Should be given in very small doses

      (d) Usually recommended for use after the delivery of the fetus

d. Inhaled anesthetics

  i. Nitrous oxide: rarely used in the United States

  ii. 50% by volume

  iii. The mother intermittently self-administers the gas at the onset of the contraction.

  iv. Requires a waste gas scavenging system

3. Regional

a. Most effective techniques

b. Allows the mother to be awake and enjoy her labor

c. Studies have shown that neuraxial anesthesia early in labor does not increase the risk for a cesarean delivery

d. Complications

  i. Hypotension resulting from the sympathectomy (most common)

  ii. Cardiac arrest

  iii. Nerve damage

  iv. Total spinal anesthesia

  v. Postdural puncture headache

e. Contraindications

  i. Absolute

    (1) Patient refusal

    (2) Bacteremia/sepsis

    (3) Increased intracranial pressure (ICP)

    (4) Infection at the needle insertion site

    (5) Shock or severe hypovolemia

    (6) Coagulopathy or therapeutic anticoagulation

  ii. Relative

    (1) Pre-existing neurologic disease

    (2) Severe psychiatric disease or dementia

(3) Aortic stenosis

(4) Left ventricular outflow tract obstruction

(5) Various congenital heart conditions (see the related Chapter 63)

(6) Deformities or previous surgery of spinal column

f. Side effects of neuraxial analgesia

i. Hypotension

ii. Pruritus

iii. Nausea and vomiting

iv. Fever

v. Shivering

vi. Urinary retention

vii. Recrudescence of herpes simplex virus

viii. Delayed gastric emptying

g. Complications of neuraxial analgesia

i. Inadequate analgesia

ii. Unintentional dural puncture

iii. Intravascular injection of local anesthetic

iv. Respiratory depression

v. High block or total spinal anesthesia

vi. Extensive motor blockade

vii. Back pain

viii. Pelvic floor injury

h. Patient preparation

i. Start an IV line: 500 mL saline bolus.

ii. Have resuscitation equipment available.

iii. Medications

(1) Benzodiazepines/intralipid: seizures

(2) Ephedrine/phenylephrine: hypotension

(3) Naloxone: respiratory depression

iv. Complete history and physical examination

v. Understanding of the obstetric plan

vi. Understanding of the fetal status

vii. Appropriate monitors

viii. Informed consent

## Spinal Analgesia

1. Rarely used for a vaginal delivery

a. More commonly used for a cesarean section

2. Fast and reliable onset

3. Bolus or continuous

4. Opioid alone or in combination with bupivacaine

a. Most commonly lidocaine, bupivacaine, or tetracaine is used.

b. Lidocaine

i. Quickest onset and shortest duration of action

ii. Transient neurologic symptoms reported in 13–36% of patients receiving spinal lidocaine, especially for procedures performed in the lithotomy position.

c. Low-dose opioids can produce analgesia without a motor block or systemic opioid effects.

i. Morphine

ii. Sufentanil

iii. Fentanyl

iv. Meperidine

5. Risk of postdural puncture headache

6. The physiologic effects of a spinal anesthetic depend on the level of anesthesia, which itself depends on:

a. Volume of solution injected into the subarachnoid space

b. Concentration of the agent in the solution

c. Speed of injection of the solution

d. Site of injection

e. Specific gravity of the solution

f. Position of the patient

i. A saddle block (sacral nerve root block) occurs when the patient is allowed to sit up after the spinal anesthetic is placed so that the sacral nerve roots are blocked, resulting in anesthesia of the buttocks, perineum, and inner thighs. This can be used for an instrumental delivery.

g. Barbotage

i. Repeated injection and aspiration of a spinal anesthetic

h. Presence of increased intra-abdominal pressure

i. Height of the patient

7. The interruption of the spinal cord function begins caudally and proceeds in a cephalic direction.

a. It starts with the loss of the autonomic function, followed by sensory and then motor function.

8. Physiologic effects of spinal anesthesia

a. Cardiovascular

i. There is a 15–20% decrease in mean arterial pressure (MAP), central venous pressure, and total peripheral resistance in normal nonmedicated volunteers having spinal anesthesia.

ii. Minimal reduction in cardiac output, stroke volume, and heart rate

b. Respiratory

i. If the phrenic nerve is intact, resting ventilation is not impaired.

259

ii. If all spinal nerve roots are blocked, inspiratory capacity is decreased by 20%, and the expiratory reserve volume is decreased to zero.

c. Cerebral blood flow (CBF)

i. CBF is maintained due to autoregulation during spinal anesthesia as long as the MAP is kept above 60 mm Hg: the MAP should be higher in patients with hypertension and atherosclerotic disease.

d. Renal and genitourinary

i. Decrease in renal blood flow (RBF) secondary to arterial hypotension

ii. With a high spinal there is a 5–10% decrease in the glomerular filtration rate and RBF.

iii. The bladder is the last organ to recover from spinal anesthesia, making urinary retention very common.

## Dural Puncture Epidural

1. Emerging technique
2. Similar to combined spinal–epidural analgesia (CSE) access
3. No medication is directly administered through dural puncture.
4. Medication from epidural infusion is thought to migrate through a dural puncture.
5. Quicker onset of analgesia and decreased incident of asymmetric block

## Epidural Analgesia

1. Most common regional anesthetic used for a vaginal delivery
2. Blocks pain from the first stage (T10–L1) and second stage (S2–S4) of labor
3. Benefits

   a. Effective pain relief
   b. Blunts the hemodynamic effects of uterine contractions

      i. Reduction in maternal catecholamines: tachycardia, increased systemic vascular resistance, hypertension, and hyperventilation
      ii. Sudden increase in cardiac preload

   c. Continuous pain relief
   d. No dural puncture needed
   e. The technique can be used for surgical anesthesia if the patient suddenly requires a cesarean section.

4. Epidural test dose

   a. Used to verify the proper placement of the epidural; identify unintentional cannulation of a vein or subarachnoid space
   b. Injected after a negative aspiration test
   c. It consists of 45 mg of lidocaine and a 1:200,000 concentration of epinephrine.

i. Subarachnoid injection results in leg weakness and evidence of an anesthetic block.

   (1) A high spinal can occur even with this low concentration of lidocaine if the patient lies flat.
   (2) Be prepared to treat a high spinal.

ii. Intravascular injection presents with tachycardia, tinnitus (ringing in the ears), metallic taste in the mouth, and perioral numbness.

5. Epidural opioids

   a. Meperidine: 100 mg provides good analgesia that lasts for 2.5 hours.
   b. Fentanyl: 100–200 µg provides analgesia that lasts for 1–2 hours with few side effects.

6. A local anesthetic should be selected on the basis of

   a. Speed of onset
   b. Degree of motor blockade
   c. Duration of the surgical procedure

7. Bupivacaine, ropivacaine, lidocaine, and 2-chloroprocaine are the most commonly used local anesthetics.

   a. The dose should be 1–1.5 mL per segment blocked, with a reduced dose in parturient, elderly, and obese patients.
   b. Adding epinephrine can prolong the duration of a lidocaine nerve block by 50%.

      i. Less dramatic results occur with bupivacaine.

8. Local anesthetics

   a. Bupivacaine

      i. Most commonly used
      ii. Relatively long duration of action
      iii. Lack of tachyphylaxis
      iv. Low placental passage secondary to its being highly protein bound
      v. Effective at low concentrations, especially if combined with an opioid
      vi. Risk: cardiotoxicity

   b. Lidocaine

      i. Used more often for a cesarean section than for labor pain relief

   c. 2-chloroprocaine

      i. Rapid onset
      ii. Brief duration of action
      iii. Very little drug crosses the placenta.
      iv. Has significant antagonism with subsequently injected epidural opioids or bupivacaine

   d. Ropivacaine

      i. Amide local anesthetic similar to bupivacaine
      ii. Less cardiotoxic than bupivacaine

9. Complications
   a. Accidental dural puncture
   b. Intravascular injection
   c. Hypotension
   d. High spinal
   e. Epidural abscess and hematoma

## Combined Spinal–Epidural Analgesia

1. The CSE is the placement of a catheter into the epidural space along with a single shot administration of intrathecal anesthetics/analgesics.
2. Benefits
   a. Rapid onset
   b. Reliability
   c. Minimal drug toxicity
   d. Flexibility of dosing
   e. Duration
   f. Analgesic level of control
   g. Continuous analgesia
3. There is a 30% reduction of medication used with a CSE when compared to an epidural.
4. Caution should be taken when placing a CSE in an obese patient and patients with poor airways: high spinal risk.
5. Complications are the same as those with epidural and spinal anesthesia.

## Paracervical Block

1. Relieves pain during the first stage of labor
2. Associated with a high incidence of fetal asphyxia and poor neonatal outcomes
   a. Uterine artery constriction
   b. Increased uterine tone

## Paravertebral Lumbar Sympathetic Block

1. Can be used if there is a contraindication to a central neuraxial technique
2. Good for the first stages of labor
3. Decreased risk of fetal bradycardia when compared to the paracervical block
4. Increased risk of intravascular injection

## Pudendal Nerve Block

1. Pudendal nerves are derived from the lower sacral roots (S2–S4).
   a. Vaginal vault, perineum, rectum, and bladder
2. Good for a forceps delivery or an episiotomy repair

## KO Treatment Plan

### Pre-operative

1. Once the diagnosis of preeclampsia is made, it is important to get laboratory values.
   a. Platelet count
   b. Fibrinogen level
   c. Liver function tests
   d. Coagulation panel
2. Vaginal delivery may be performed if the fetus is not distressed.
3. Lumbar epidural analgesia provides pain relief and a method to help control the patient's blood pressure during labor.
   a. Rule out coagulopathy.
   b. Optimize the patient's fluid status.
      i. Bupivacaine, fentanyl, and dilute epinephrine are given as an initial bolus, and then as a continuous infusion.
4. With regional anesthesia there is
   a. Less increase in blood pressure
   b. Less need for opioid analgesics
   c. Improvement in placental and renal blood flow

### Intra-operative

(See Chapter 55 for more information.)

1. Cesarean section is indicated for delivery of a distressed fetus.
2. If an epidural catheter has been previously placed, it may be used to provide surgical anesthesia, assuming the patient's volume status has been optimized.
3. Although previously considered controversial, spinal anesthesia has been proven to be a safe technique for cesarean section for severely preeclamptic patients.
4. General anesthesia is an acceptable way to manage preeclamptic patients, but there are associated risks of pulmonary aspiration, airway compromise from edema, and acute blood pressure elevation during laryngoscopy.
   a. This can lead to a significant risk of cerebral hemorrhage and pulmonary edema.
   b. A rapid-sequence induction technique should be used.
      i. Intravenous hydralazine, lidocaine, sodium nitroprusside, nitroglycerine, and/or esmolol can be used to attenuate the hypertensive response to laryngoscopy.
      ii. Propofol plus succinylcholine (1.5 mg/kg) IV
      iii. Anesthesia can be maintained with a volatile agent, $N_2O/O_2$, and neuromuscular blockade as needed, guided by the peripheral nerve stimulator.

## Bibliography

Barash PG, Cullen BF, Stoelting RK, et al. *Clinical Anesthesia*, 8th ed. Philadelphia: Wolters Kluwer, 2017, pp. 1148–52.

Chestnut DH, Wong CA, et al. *Chestnut's Obstetric Anesthesia*, 6th ed. Philadelphia: Elsevier, 2020, pp. 476–94.

Faust RJ, Cucchiara RF. *Anesthesiology Review*, 3rd ed. Philadelphia: Churchill Livingstone, 2002, pp. 430–1, 438–40, 444–5.

Gropper MA, Miller RD, et al. *Miller's Anesthesia*, 9th ed. Philadelphia: Elsevier, 2020, pp. 2017–22.

# Chapter 61

# Anesthesia for a Cesarean Delivery

Elvera L. Baron and Jessica A. Lovich-Sapola

## Sample Case

A 30-year-old G1P0 patient with a history of asthma presents for an urgent cesarean section due to fetal breech positioning. She is in active labor, dilated to 6 cm. Would you administer general or neuraxial anesthetic? Provide risks and benefits for each choice.

## Clinical Issues

### Incidence of Cesarean Delivery

1. Most common hospital-based surgical procedure in the United States
2. As of 2018, 31% of all births in the United States

### Indications for a Cesarean Delivery

1. Fetal distress
2. Elective repeat cesarean sections
3. Failure to progress (i.e., arrest of active phase of labor)
4. Nonreassuring fetal status
5. Cephalopelvic disproportion
6. Malpresentation
7. Prematurity
8. Previous uterine surgery

## Neuraxial Anesthesia

### Advantages over General Anesthesia

1. Decreased risk of difficult and/or failed intubation or aspiration
2. Avoidance of depressant anesthetic agents
3. Ability of the mother to remain awake and witness the birth of her child
4. Earlier attempts at breastfeeding
5. Reduced operative blood loss
6. Decreased fetal exposure to drugs
7. Ability to continue pain control via neuraxial analgesia after surgery

### Complications

1. Hypotension
2. Decreased uteroplacental perfusion
3. Preventive measures
   a. Left uterine displacement
   b. IV fluid administration
   c. Liberal use of vasopressors

## Contraindications

### Absolute

1. Patient refusal
2. Sepsis
3. Severe aortic stenosis or mitral stenosis
4. Severe coagulopathy
5. Known increased intracranial pressures
6. Known allergy to local anesthetic (rare)

### Relative

1. Uncooperative patient
2. Infection near the site of needle insertion
3. Mild to moderate aortic stenosis or mitral stenosis
4. Risk of bleeding
5. Anticipated intra-operative major blood loss and fluid shifts
6. Prior surgery at the site of injection
7. Congenital abnormalities of spine or meninges
8. Pre-existing neurological deficits or demyelinating disorders
9. Hypovolemia
10. Insufficient time to induce neuraxial anesthesia for urgent delivery

## Spinal Anesthesia

1. Most common

### Advantages

1. Used for most straightforward cesarean sections
2. Rapid onset
3. Superior, dense block
4. Cost-effective
5. Little risk of anesthetic toxicity secondary to the low doses used
6. Minimal drug transfer to the fetus
7. Failure rate/patchy blocks are very rare
8. Decreased risk of gastric aspiration
9. Mother can be awake for the delivery of her baby

## Disadvantages

1. Duration is limited
2. High incidence of hypotension
3. Despite an adequate level
   a. Visceral discomfort
   b. Nausea and vomiting

## Technique

1. Hyperbaric bupivacaine (0.75%, 1.6–1.8 mL)
   a. Duration is approximately 1.5–2.5 hours.
   b. Usually use a set dose of 12–15 mg
   c. Patient's height, weight, and body mass index do not tend to correlate with the height of the block.
   d. Doses greater than 15 mg are not recommended secondary to the increased risk of complications, including a high block.
   e. The addition of 10–20 μg of fentanyl to the spinal can decrease intra-operative nausea and decrease the visceral pain associated with the exteriorization of the uterus and visceral traction.
   f. 0.1–0.25 mg of preservative-free morphine can also be added to the spinal for post-operative pain control.
2. Prehydration with up to 20 mL/kg of crystalloid solution
3. Position
   a. Sitting
      i. Optimal for obese patients
   b. Lateral
4. Goal is a bilateral T4 level

# Epidural Anesthesia

## Advantages

1. Offers flexibility
   a. Good for a prolonged cesarean section
   b. Ability to titrate the dose to the desired level
2. A previously placed epidural catheter can be used for labor pain.

## Disadvantage

1. Requires a larger dose of local anesthetic compared to a spinal, which can be potentially toxic
2. Catheter location can migrate into the intrathecal space or a blood vessel.
3. Slower onset of action

## Technique

1. Agents: 3% 2-chloroprocaine, 2% lidocaine with epinephrine, 0.5% bupivacaine, and 0.5% ropivacaine

2. Adjunct agents: added to improve the quality of the block.
   a. Bicarbonate: shortens the onset time (not effective for bupivacaine).
   b. Epinephrine (1:200,000 or 1:400,000): decreases the vascular absorption of the local anesthetic, improves the quality of the anesthesia, prolongs the duration of the block, and shortens the onset time (not effective for bupivacaine).
   c. Fentanyl 50–100 μg or sufentanil 10–20 μg: improves operative conditions by decreasing the patient's sensitivity to visceral stimulation.

# Combined Spinal–Epidural Technique (CSE)

## Advantages

1. Rapid onset of a dense surgical anesthetic while allowing the ability to prolong the block with an epidural catheter.
2. The block can be supplemented at any time.

## Disadvantages

1. Difficulty interpreting a "test dose" in the catheter
2. Possibility of a failed epidural catheter
3. Risk of enhanced spread of the previously injected spinal drug after the use of the catheter
4. Some consider it to be cumbersome and time-consuming.

# Continuous Spinal Anesthesia

## Advantages

1. Small doses can be given in an incremental fashion.
2. Good for patients with cardiac disease, respiratory disease, morbid obesity, and neuromuscular disease.

## Disadvantages

1. Postdural puncture headache

# General Anesthesia

## Indications

1. Acute maternal hemorrhage
2. Severe hypovolemia
3. Overt severe coagulopathy
4. Life-threatening fetal compromise that may occur without an emergent cesarean section in a patient without an existing labor epidural
5. Patient refusal of neuraxial anesthesia
6. Inadequate neuraxial block

## Advantages

1. Rapid speed of induction
2. Control of the airway

3. Good when intense uterine relaxation is necessary: breech and transverse presentation.

## Disadvantages

1. Increased mortality compared to a regional anesthetic for a cesarean section
2. Risk of failed intubation
3. Pulmonary aspiration of gastric contents
4. Neonatal depression
5. Maternal awareness
6. Increased peri-operative morbidity is documented in patients with asthma, upper respiratory infections, obesity, or history of difficult intubation.

## Induction of General Anesthesia

1. Verify good IV access
2. Nonparticulate antacid
3. Pre-oxygenate (3–5 minutes)
4. Position into left uterine displacement
5. Administer IV metoclopramide (10 mg) and ondansetron (4 mg).
6. Apply all standard ASA monitors.
7. Ensure that the surgical team performs sterile preparation and draping of the patient to minimize time from induction/intubation to surgical incision.
8. Assuming a favorable airway exam, perform a rapid-sequence induction with propofol (up to 2 mg/kg) or ketamine (up to 1 mg/kg) followed by succinylcholine (1–1.5 mg/kg).

9. Rocuronium (0.6 mg/kg) is a suitable alternative if succinylcholine is contraindicated.
10. Apply cricoid pressure and maintain it until the endotracheal tube is secured and its placement is verified.
11. Maintain anesthesia with 50% nitrous oxide and 50% oxygen plus 0.5 MAC of a volatile anesthetic or total IV anesthesia, as indicated. Volatile anesthetic can be increased to 2 MAC temporarily just prior to the delivery to assist in uterine relaxation.
12. After delivery, increase the percentage of nitrous oxide to 70% and decrease the volatile anesthetic (high doses of volatile anesthetics can lead to uterine relaxation and bleeding post-delivery). Add an IV opioid and a benzodiazepine as needed.

## KO Treatment Plan

1. For this patient with a history of asthma and a need for an urgent cesarean section for breech positioning, I would perform a spinal anesthetic. She is otherwise healthy, so we assume that she has no major coagulopathy. A spinal can be done quickly in the sitting or lying position.
2. Since she has asthma, she may be more sensitive to the decreased sensation of breathing with the T4 spinal level. Monitor her oxygen saturation. Treat with albuterol as needed.
3. General anesthesia could be done safely if one is unable to place a spinal/epidural, or if patient refuses neuraxial anesthesia. Albuterol pre-treatment may be warranted. Given her asthma, be prepared to treat potential bronchospasm during induction/intubation.

## Bibliography

Barash PG, Cullen BF, Stoelting RK. *Clinical Anesthesia*, 8th ed. Philadelphia: Lippincott Williams & Wilkins, 2017, pp. 1152–4.

Chestnut DH. *Obstetric Anesthesia: Principles and Practice*, 6th ed. Philadelphia: Mosby, 2020, pp. 568–626.

Manullang GTR, Christopher MV, Pace NL. Intrathecal fentanyl is superior to intravenous ondansetron for the prevention of perioperative nausea during cesarean delivery with spinal anesthesia. *Anesth Analg* 2000;**90**:1162–6.

Miller RD, Fleisher LA, Johns RA, et al. *Anesthesia*, 9th ed. New York: Churchill Livingstone, 2020, pp. 2006–41.

Urman RD, Kaye AD. *Obstetric Anesthesia Practice*. New York: Oxford University Press, 2021, pp. 203–13.

# Complications of Obstetric Regional Anesthesia

John George and Jessica A. Lovich-Sapola

## Hypotension

### Sample Case

You have just placed an epidural in a 19-year-old pregnant female with no prior medical history. After a negative test dose, the epidural is bolused with a bupivacaine and fentanyl mixture. After 10 minutes, the patient's blood pressure is 80/40 mm Hg. The fetal monitor is showing late decelerations. What do you do?

### Clinical Issues

#### Definition of Hypotension

1. Systolic blood pressure decrease to less than 100 mm Hg or to more than 20–25% less than baseline readings.
2. The incidence and severity depend on the height of the block and the position of the patient.

#### Causes

1. Increased venous capacitance and pooling of a major portion of the blood volume in the lower extremities and splanchnic bed
2. Decreased systemic vascular resistance

#### Prophylactic Actions

1. IV fluid bolus up to 20 mL/kg of Lactated Ringer's solution prior to the placement of the spinal or epidural
2. Left uterine displacement to avoid aortocaval compression
3. Vigilant monitoring of the blood pressure at frequent intervals after the placement of the regional anesthetic
4. Monitor the fetal heart rate.
5. Prophylactic IV vasopressors as needed: ephedrine or phenylephrine

### KO Treatment Plan

1. Rapid IV fluid bolus
2. Give 100% oxygen by mask.
3. Increased left uterine displacement
4. Trendelenburg positioning
5. IV bolus of phenylephrine (100–200 µg increments) or ephedrine (5–10 mg increments)
6. Evaluate the level of the block.
7. Call the obstetrical service for assessment of the mother and fetus.

## Accidental Dural Puncture

### Clinical Issues

#### Definition

1. Accidental puncture of the dura mater
2. "Wet tap"
3. Incidence is 3%.
4. Can lead to postdural puncture headaches (PDPH) in 50–70% of cases

### KO Treatment Plan

1. The traditional method was to reposition the epidural at a different interspace.
2. A recent recommendation is to pass the epidural catheter into the spinal space and use a continuous spinal technique.
   a. Rapid and effective pain relief
   b. Significant reduction in the PDPH and the need for an epidural blood patch
   c. Excellent labor analgesia
   d. Almost instant onset for anesthesia for a cesarean section

### Techniques to Decrease the Risk of PDPH after an Accidental Dural Puncture

1. Inject cerebrospinal fluid (CSF) from the epidural syringe back into the subarachnoid space through the epidural needle.
2. Insert the epidural catheter into the subarachnoid space.
3. Administer continuous intrathecal labor analgesia.
4. Leave the catheter in for a total of 12–24 hours.
5. Inject preservative-free normal saline through the catheter prior to its removal.

## Postdural Puncture Headache

### Clinical Issues

#### Incidence

1. Pregnant women are at a higher risk of developing PDPH secondary to their age and gender.
2. Incidence decreases with increasing age.

3. Incidence decreases with the use of a small-diameter spinal needle.
4. Women are at a greater risk than men.

### Postpartum Headache Differential Diagnosis

1. Headaches occur in 15% of pregnant patients who do not receive an epidural.
2. Headaches occur in 12% of pregnant patients who receive an epidural but show no sign of a dural puncture.
3. Nonspecific headache
4. Migraine
5. Hypertension
6. Pneumocephalus can occur if air is used for the loss of resistance (LOR) technique during the epidural placement.
7. Infection (sinusitis, meningitis)
8. Cortical vein thrombosis
9. Intracerebral pathology
10. Caffeine withdrawal
11. PDPH

### Definition of PDPH

1. Headache after a dural puncture
2. Headache is worsened by standing or sitting.
3. Headache is relieved by lying down.
4. The headache is characteristically fronto-occipital.
5. Can have associated cranial nerve symptoms (diplopia, tinnitus)
6. Some patients have nausea and vomiting.
7. The headache results from the loss of CSF through the meningeal needle hole resulting in decreased support for the brain. When upright, the brain sags and puts traction on the cranial nerves and pain-sensitive structures.

## KO Treatment Plan

Conservative treatment: indicated for mild to moderate discomfort. The symptoms usually resolve in a few days to a week if untreated.

1. Bed rest
2. Hydration
3. IV caffeine (500 mg) or oral caffeine (300–500 mg)
   a. Cerebral vasoconstrictor
   b. Transient relief
   c. Side effects: unable to sleep, anxious, seizures, and cardiac arrhythmias
4. Analgesics
5. Vasopressin
6. Theophylline
   a. Cerebral vasoconstrictor
7. Sumatriptan
   a. Serotonin agonist
   b. Cerebral vasoconstrictor

8. Adrenocorticotropic hormone (ACTH)

### Epidural Blood Patch

1. Used if the patient's symptoms are severe enough to limit her activity, if cranial nerve involvement is noted, or if conservative management has failed.
2. Most effective treatment for PDPH
3. Success rate of 75%
4. Immediate relief occurs in almost all patients, but only 61% have a permanent cure.
5. About 90% of patients who fail the first blood patch have good results with the second.
6. Possible mechanism
   a. Clotted blood obstructs the dural tear, thereby decreasing further CSF leakage.
   b. CSF pressure and cerebral vasoconstriction increase.

### Technique

1. Sterile epidural
2. Draw 20 mL of the patient's blood using a sterile technique.
3. Most practitioners inject 10–20 mL of blood and stop injecting if the patient has pain.
4. Place the blood patch as close as possible to the original dural puncture.
5. The patient should lie flat for at least an hour after the procedure.
6. Avoid heavy lifting for the next week.
7. The procedure may be repeated as necessary.

### Side Effects of an Epidural Blood Patch

1. Backache
2. Radicular pain
3. Transient bradycardia
4. Cranial nerve palsies

## Total Spinal Block
### Clinical Issues
#### Definition

1. Rare
2. Very serious complication
3. Excessive cephalad spread of the local anesthetic in the subarachnoid space
4. The local anesthetic spreads high enough to block the entire spinal cord and occasionally the brainstem.

#### Signs and Symptoms

1. Profound hypotension (complete sympathetic block)
2. Bradycardia (complete sympathetic block)
3. Respiratory arrest
4. Complete sensory and motor blockade
5. Hypotension

6. Unconsciousness
7. Loss of protective airway reflexes

**Causes**

1. Can result from a single-shot spinal or inadvertent intrathecal spread after an accidental dural puncture or catheter migration.
2. Subdural spread can also result in a high block.
   a. High sensory level
   b. Sacral sparing
   c. Incomplete or absent motor block
3. Single-shot spinal anesthetic after a failed spinal or patchy epidural; therefore, a spinal should not be performed after a failed spinal/epidural.

## KO Treatment Plan

1. Rapidly secure the airway with an endotracheal tube.
2. Positive-pressure ventilation with 100% oxygen
3. Treatment of the associated hypotension
   a. Left uterine displacement
   b. Trendelenburg positioning
   c. IV fluids
   d. Vasopressors (ephedrine or epinephrine)
   e. Atropine

## Accidental Intravascular Injection

### Sample Case

An 18-year-old healthy patient is receiving an epidural for labor pain relief. You identify the epidural space, place the epidural catheter, and give a test dose. Despite your negative test dose, the patient has a grand mal seizure after the initial bolus of bupivacaine and fentanyl. What is your differential diagnosis? How will you treat this problem? Would you recommend a cesarean section?

### Clinical Issues

**Consequences of an Accidental Intravascular Injection of Local Anesthetic**

1. Life-threatening convulsions
2. Cardiovascular collapse (increased risk with bupivacaine)

**Differential Diagnosis of Seizures in Pregnancy**

1. Eclampsia
2. History of previous seizures
3. Intravascular local anesthetic toxicity
4. Syncope
5. Hypoglycemia

### KO Treatment Plan

1. Primarily supportive

2. Stop any injection of local anesthetic.
3. Secure the airway and maintain oxygenation.
4. Treat the seizure with midazolam (2–5 mg), diazepam (5–10 mg), or propofol (1 mg/kg).
5. Succinylcholine can terminate the muscular activity to facilitate ventilation, but remember that it does not terminate the seizure.
6. Mild cardiovascular depression caused by lidocaine that leads to hypotension and bradycardia can be treated with IV ephedrine (10–30 mg) and IV atropine (0.4 mg).
7. If cardiovascular collapse occurs, likely secondary to bupivacaine, an emergent cesarean section may be necessary to relieve aortocaval compression and improve the efficacy of cardiac massage.
8. Resuscitation may require large doses of epinephrine, vasopressin, and amiodarone.
9. IV lipids have been recommended. Use a 20% lipid solution at a dose of 4 mL/kg followed by a 0.5 mL/kg/min infusion for 10 minutes.
10. Some patients have required cardiopulmonary bypass until the local anesthetic can be metabolized.

## Neurologic Complications

### Clinical Issues

**Incidence**

1. Rare
2. Neurologic complications are five times more common after childbirth itself than after regional blockade.
3. Most neurologic injuries that occur after delivery are obstetric in origin.
4. Postpartum back pain is equally common in patients who receive neuraxial anesthesia and in those who do not.

**Causes**

1. Related to anesthesia
   a. Epidural hematoma
   b. Epidural abscess
   c. Localized tenderness
   d. Nerve root irritation (may last weeks or months)
2. Unrelated to anesthesia
   a. Obstetrical instrumentation
   b. Nonanatomic positioning during labor
      i. Lithotomy
   c. Compression of sacral nerve roots by the fetal head during delivery

**Compression of the Lumbosacral Trunk (L4–L5)**

1. Presents with foot drop
2. Weakness with ankle dorsiflexion
3. L5 sensory deficits
4. Causes

a. Cephalopelvic disproportion
b. Prolonged labor
c. Difficult vaginal delivery

## Obturator Nerve Palsy

1. Presents with weakness of hip adduction and internal rotation
2. Sensory deficit over the inner thigh

## Femoral Nerve Palsy

1. Presents with inability to climb stairs
2. Causes

   a. Prolonged flexion
   b. Prolonged abduction
   c. Prolonged external rotation of the hips
   d. Excessive lithotomy position

## Meralgia Paresthetica

1. Neuropathy of the lateral femoral cutaneous nerve
2. It is a purely sensory nerve.
3. It presents with numbness, tingling, and/or burning over the anterolateral aspect of the thigh.
4. Causes

   a. Pregnancy (increased intra-abdominal pressure)
   b. Retractors during pelvic surgery

## Sciatic Nerve Palsy

1. Presents with a loss of sensation below the knee, with sparing of the medial side and an absence of movement below the knee
2. Causes

   a. Excessive sitting in one position

## Peroneal Nerve Palsy

1. Presents with foot drop, but the plantar flexion and inversion is preserved, unlike an L4–L5 lesion.
2. Causes

   a. Regional anesthesia
   b. Lithotomy position
   c. Improper or prolonged positioning in the stirrups
   d. Compression of the lateral knee against any hard object

## KO Treatment Plan

1. Go to see the patient.
2. Thorough history and physical
3. Neurological assessment
4. Rule out an epidural hematoma or abscess.
5. A neurology consult may be necessary.

# Lumbar Epidural Hematoma

## Sample Case

A 23-year-old female requested a lumbar epidural for labor pain relief. The patient's labor was progressing rapidly, so your colleague placed an epidural without any pre-procedure labs. The next morning you are called to see the patient. She is complaining of severe back pain and leg weakness and numbness that has not resolved since her epidural was removed. What should you do?

## Clinical Issues

1. Rare complication (1 in 150,000)
2. A hemostatic abnormality was present in 68% of the reported patients with an epidural hematoma.
3. Significantly increased risk with associated anticoagulant medications
4. Difficult or bloody placement of needles and catheters occurred in 25% of the reported cases of epidural hematoma.
5. Usually develops hours after the placement of the catheter
6. The incidence of a vessel puncture with the placement of the catheter is 1–10%.
7. Signs and symptoms

   a. Sciatic pain
   b. Persistent pain after the removal of the catheter
   c. Severe back pain, sometimes radiating to the legs
   d. Leg weakness
   e. Paraplegia
   f. Numbness
   g. Signals of the need for emergency imaging

      i. Significant delay in normal recovery
      ii. Deterioration of lower limb or bladder function

8. Increased risk

   a. Scoliotic patients
   b. Elderly with a narrow spinal canal
   c. Coagulation defect

## KO Treatment Plan

### Pre-operative Diagnosis

An epidural hematoma is a serious condition that requires immediate diagnosis and treatment to try to prevent long-term neurological complications. Any complaints of back pain after a spinal or epidural should be taken seriously. If an epidural hematoma is suspected, after a quick history and physical, neurosurgery should be consulted and MRI/CT should be arranged.

### Pre-operative Evaluation to Determine a Regional Anesthetic Candidate

1. An epidural/spinal is approved for patients taking nonsteroidal anti-inflammatory drugs (NSAIDs).

2. An epidural/spinal is also approved for patients on subcutaneous unfractionated heparin for deep vein thrombosis (DVT) prophylaxis.
3. It is contraindicated in patients taking thienopyridine derivatives (ticlopidine and clopidogrel) and GP IIb/IIIa antagonists.
   a. Ticlopidine should be discontinued for 2 weeks and clopidogrel for 1 week prior to the placement of an epidural/spinal.
   b. GP IIb/IIIa should be stopped for 24–48 hours before an epidural/spinal.
4. For the patient receiving low-molecular-weight heparin (LMWH), a neuraxial technique should be deferred for 10–12 hours in a patient who has received a low dose, and 24 hours for a patient that has received a higher dose of LMWH. An epidural catheter should not be removed until 10–12 hours after the last dose of LMWH, and the subsequent dose should not be given for at least 2 hours after the catheter removal.

### Intra-operative Treatment

1. Decompressive laminectomy within 8 hours of the symptoms

## Lumbar Epidural Abscess

### Sample Case

A 23-year-old female has an epidural placed for labor pain relief. On post-procedure day 2, the patient complains of a severe headache, fever, and back pain. What should you do?

### Clinical Issues

1. Rare complication
2. Usually presents 24–72 hours after the performance of an epidural block, but can take 4–10 days
3. Can develop spontaneously in up to 1 in 10,000 patients admitted to the hospital in the United States
4. 30% of patients have a history of back trauma.
5. Signs and symptoms
   a. Severe headache
   b. Local tenderness/severe back pain
   c. Paraspinal muscle spasm
   d. Fever

   e. Leukocytosis
   f. Meningismus
   g. Elevated erythrocyte sedimentation rate
   h. Localized infection
   i. Neck stiffness
   j. Headache
   k. Sensory and motor deficits in the legs
   l. Bladder complications
6. Sensory findings
   a. Absent or paresthesias only
7. Motor findings
   a. Flaccid skeletal muscle paralysis

### KO Treatment Plan

#### Pre-operative Prevention

1. Hand washing
2. Sterile "prep and drape"
3. Limit the number of people present in the room for the procedure.
4. Face mask and hair net for everyone present for the procedure
5. Some physicians are recommending sterile gowns.
6. Be especially careful to maintain the sterility of the epidural kit and the catheter.

#### Diagnosis

An epidural abscess is a serious condition that requires immediate treatment to try to prevent long-term complications. Any complaints of back pain after a spinal or epidural should be taken seriously. If an epidural abscess is suspected, after a quick history and physical, neurosurgery should be consulted and MRI/CT should be arranged.

1. MRI is the most sensitive modality.
2. CT is useful for determining the presence of extradural compression of the spinal cord.

#### Intra-operative Treatment

1. A decompressive laminectomy should be performed promptly to minimize the likelihood of permanent neurological deficits.
2. Continued antibiotic treatment

## Bibliography

Barash PG, Cullen BF, Stoelting RK, et al. *Clinical Anesthesia*, 8th ed. Philadelphia: Lippincott Williams & Wilkins, 2017, pp. 1154–5.

Chestnut DH, Wong CA, Tsen LC, et al. *Chestnut's Obstetric Anesthesia: Principles and Practice*, 6th ed. Philadelphia: Elsevier, 2020, pp. 498–507, 598–603.

Gilbert A, Owens BD, Mulroy MF. Epidural hematoma after outpatient epidural anesthesia. *Anesth Analg*, 2002;**94**:77–8.

Gropper MA. *Miller's Anesthesia*, 9th ed. Philadelphia: Elsevier, 2020, pp. 2026–9.

Sollmann WP, Gaab MR, Panning B. Lumbar epidural hematoma and spinal abscess following peridural anesthesia. *Reg Anaesth*, 1987;**10**(4):121–4.

Stoelting RK, Dierdorf SF. *Anesthesia and Co-Existing Disease*, 4th ed. Philadelphia: Churchill Livingstone, 2002, pp. 577–8.

# 63 Cardiovascular Disease in Pregnancy

Elvera L. Baron and Jessica A. Lovich-Sapola

## Cardiovascular Disease

### Clinical Issues

1. The prevalence of cardiovascular (CV) disease in pregnancy is about 0.4–4.1%.
2. Maternal outcome correlates with the New York Heart Association (NYHA) criteria.
   a. Class I or II have a <1% mortality.
   b. Class III or IV have a 5–15% maternal mortality rate and a 20–30% perinatal mortality rate.
3. Patients with CV disease should be followed closely by a cardiologist prior to pregnancy to determine a safe plan. This plan may include lifestyle or medication modifications, need for cardiac surgery prior or concomitant with delivery, or a plan to avoid pregnancy altogether. Medical decision-making for a woman with CV disease of childbearing age involves a multidisciplinary team, including an obstetrician, maternal–fetal medicine specialist, cardiologist, cardiothoracic and/or obstetric anesthesiologist, and/or cardiac surgeon, together with the patient.

#### NYHA Classification of CV Disease

1. Class I: the patient is not limited by her CV disease in her physical activity. Ordinary physical activity does not precipitate the occurrence of symptoms such as fatigue, palpitations, dyspnea, or angina.
2. Class II: the patient's CV disease causes a slight limitation in physical activity. The patient is comfortable at rest.
3. Class III: the patient's CV disease results in a marked limitation of physical activity. She is comfortable at rest. Less than ordinary activity precipitates symptoms.
4. Class IV: CV disease results in the inability to carry out physical activity without discomfort. Symptoms may be present at rest. Discomfort is increased with physical activity.

## Left-To-Right Shunts

### Clinical Issues

1. Left-to-right shunts are usually well tolerated in pregnancy.
2. Unrepaired arterial shunting results in right atrial and ventricular enlargement, potential right ventricular (RV) dysfunction, arrhythmias, and, in rare cases, paradoxical emboli or pulmonary hypertension.
3. Unrepaired arterial septal lesions have been implicated in increased risk of preeclampsia, small for gestational age neonates, and increased neonatal mortality.
4. Hemodynamically significant ventricular septal lesions cause left-sided volume overload, with potential ventricular dysfunction, arrhythmia, and, rarely, pulmonary hypertension.
5. Large patent ductus arteriosus may lead to pulmonary artery enlargement, left-sided volume overload, and pulmonary hypertension. Ductal flow decreases during pregnancy due to overall decrease in systemic vascular resistance (SVR).

### Causes

1. Small atrial septal defect (ASD) – most common congenital lesions in women of childbearing age.
2. Ventricular septal defect (VSD)
3. Patent ductus arteriosus (PDA)

## KO Treatment Plan

1. Avoid intravenous (IV) infusion of air bubbles.
2. Use loss-of-resistance (LOR) with saline (rather than air) technique for the placement of an epidural.
3. An early placement of an epidural is desirable. Pain can cause increased maternal catecholamines and lead to increased SVR, which may increase the severity of the left-to-right shunt, resulting in pulmonary hypertension and RV failure.
4. Slow onset of the epidural anesthesia is recommended because a rapid decrease in SVR could result in shunt flow reversal and maternal hypoxemia.
5. Supplemental oxygen should be given. Even mild hypoxemia can reverse the shunt flow.
6. Avoid hypercarbia and acidosis.

## Coarctation of the Aorta

### Clinical Issues

1. Congenital lesion
2. It is a fixed obstruction to the forward ejection of the left ventricular stroke volume. The most common complication is systemic hypertension.

271

3. An increase in cardiac output can be achieved by increasing the heart rate.
4. If the condition has been successfully surgically treated and she has normal arm and leg pressures, she does not need any special treatment or monitoring during pregnancy.
5. Patients with uncorrected coarctation are at a high risk for left ventricular failure, aortic rupture, aortic dissection, and/or endocarditis.
6. Fetal mortality in uncorrected patients may approach 20%.

## KO Treatment Plan

1. Maintain a normal to slightly elevated SVR, heart rate (HR), and intravascular volume status.
2. In uncorrected patients, vaginal delivery with epidural anesthesia is preferred. Systemic medications and inhalation anesthesia can be used, as well as a pudendal block.
3. Epidural or general anesthesia with blood pressure control can be used for a cesarean section.
4. Invasive hemodynamic monitoring (arterial line, central venous [CVP]) can help guide the administration of IV fluids.
5. The pressors of choice are dopamine and ephedrine to maintain SVR and HR.

# Tetralogy of Fallot (TOF)

## Clinical Issues

1. By definition, the lesion has four components:
   a. VSD
   b. RV hypertrophy
   c. Pulmonic stenosis with RV outflow tract obstruction
   d. Overriding aorta

2. Right-to-left shunt
3. Patients usually present with cyanosis.
4. Patients usually have had corrective surgery by the time they reach childbearing age. The hemodynamic lesions of concern in repaired TOF during pregnancy are pulmonary regurgitation, RV dilation, and RV dysfunction.
5. Even if the patient has been asymptomatic, an echocardiogram should be done before or during early pregnancy.
6. The increased blood volume, increased cardiac output (CO), and decreased SVR of pregnancy may unmask any previously asymptomatic complications from the earlier repair.
7. Most common cardiac maternal events include heart failure and atrial arrhythmias.

## KO Treatment Plan

1. 12-lead EKG
2. Avoid a decrease in SVR, which would increase right-to-left shunt.

3. Maintain adequate intravascular volume and venous return.
4. Perform a neuraxial block early in labor. Epidural is more favored over spinal, given slower medication titration via epidural and ability to maintain SVR appropriately.
5. Cesarean delivery should be done with a slowly titrated neuraxial anesthetic. A single-dose spinal is not recommended secondary to the abrupt decrease in SVR, which can lead to shunt reversal and hypoxemia.
6. General anesthesia is also an option for a cesarean delivery. Placement of an awake arterial line is recommended to determine baseline $PaO_2$ and provides the ability to address early signs of arterial hypoxemia throughout the case. Arterial hypoxemia worsens with increased right-to-left shunting. Pulse oximetry can also be used to reflect the changes in arterial oxygenation. Addition of minimal PEEP to ventilation parameters should be carefully monitored so as not to compromise CO.

# Eisenmenger Syndrome

## Clinical Issues

1. A chronic and uncorrected left-to-right shunt can produce RV hypertrophy, elevated pulmonary artery pressures, RV dysfunction, and ultimately Eisenmenger syndrome.
2. A reversal of the shunt flow occurs when the pulmonary artery pressure exceeds the level of the systemic pressure.
3. The primary left-to-right shunt becomes a right-to-left shunt.
4. The pulmonary vasculature does not respond to vasodilator therapy.
5. This combination of problems is not amenable to surgical correction.
6. These patients do not tolerate pregnancy well.

### Clinical Manifestations When Not Pregnant

1. Arterial hypoxemia
2. RV failure
3. Dyspnea at rest
4. Clubbing of the nails
5. Polycythemia
6. Engorged neck veins
7. Peripheral edema

### During Pregnancy

1. Decreased SVR associated with pregnancy exacerbates the right-to-left shunt.
2. These women are unable to respond to the increased demand for oxygen during pregnancy.
3. Maternal hypoxemia leads to decreased oxygen to the fetus and a high incidence of fetal demise.
4. Maternal mortality with pregnancy is 30–50%.
5. Maternal deaths can occur as late as 4–6 weeks postpartum due to massive fluid shifts and reabsorption, which are poorly tolerated by the failing RV and pulmonary hypertension.

## KO Treatment Plan

1. The patient should initially be counseled to avoid or terminate the pregnancy. If pregnancy is continued, elective cesarean delivery should be planned; active labor should be avoided, if possible.
2. Maintain SVR; phenylephrine is a pressor of choice.
3. Maintain intravascular volume and venous return.
4. Avoid aortocaval compression.
5. Prevent pain, hypoxemia, hypercarbia, and acidosis, which can lead to an increase in pulmonary vascular resistance (PVR) and exacerbate RV failure and arterial hypoxemia.
6. Avoid myocardial depression during general anesthesia.
7. Avoid the infusion of air through the tubing secondary to the increased possibility of paradoxical air embolus.

### Labor

1. Provide supplemental oxygen at all times.
2. Continuous pulse oximeter to look for changes in shunt flow
3. Arterial line to monitor $PaO_2$
4. Both CVP and a pulmonary artery catheter (PAC) monitoring are recommended. Post-delivery ICU admission should be planned. Potential risks of CVP ± PAC placement:
   a. Air emboli
   b. Infection
   c. Hematoma
   d. Pneumothorax
5. Also, the PAC rarely yields useful clinical information secondary to the presence of severe, fixed (i.e., unresponsive or minimally responsive to pulmonary vasodilating medications) pulmonary hypertension.
6. Pain control
   a. First stage: intrathecal opioids
   b. Second stage
      i. An epidural or intrathecal dose of a local anesthetic and an opioid. Titrate slowly to avoid decreases in SVR. Avoid epinephrine in the epidural solution.
      ii. If the patient has coagulation defects, then an IV infusion of remifentanil may be the next best option.

### Cesarean Section

1. Epidural anesthesia is the technique of choice.
2. Arterial line placement is recommended prior to epidural catheter placement.
3. The important thing is to employ incremental dosing while carefully correcting any hemodynamic changes.
4. Avoid aortocaval compression.
5. Maintain SVR, preload, and oxygen saturation.

6. General anesthesia may be required. Mode of delivery as well as specifics of operating room requirement (obstetric OR vs. cardiac OR vs. hybrid OR) and trained personnel (cardiac surgeon, cardiothoracic, and/or obstetric anesthesiologist) should be discussed in a multidisciplinary setting prior to delivery.
   a. Positive-pressure ventilation results in decreased venous return and compromised CO. Even minimal PEEP may not be hemodynamically tolerated.
   b. Volatile anesthetics can cause myocardial depression and further decrease SVR.
   c. Propofol boluses during a rapid sequence intubation (RSI) can cause a decrease in contractility and SVR, and, therefore, an exacerbation of the right-to-left shunt. RSI is usually avoided.
   d. Ketamine is often listed as the induction drug of choice.
   e. Conversely, a slow induction predisposes the patient to aspiration.
   f. Replace any large blood loss with crystalloid or appropriate blood products. Careful infusion is recommended as not to overwhelm a failing RV.
   g. Intra-operative transesophageal echocardiography (TEE) may be required if severe hemodynamic instability is encountered to help guide fluid and inotropic therapies.

## Primary Pulmonary Hypertension (PPH)

### Clinical Issues

1. Markedly elevated pulmonary artery pressure in the absence of an intracardiac or aortopulmonary shunt
2. Reactive pulmonary vasculature that initially responds to vasodilator therapy
3. Maternal mortality rate may be as high as 30–56%. Most deaths are due to congestive heart failure, which most often occurs in the early postpartum period.
4. High incidence of fetal loss (10–28%) and preterm delivery
5. Pregnancy is often contraindicated and preconception counseling should be provided.

### KO Treatment Plan

1. Prevent pain, hypoxia, acidosis, and hypercarbia because these conditions can cause an increase in PVR.
2. Maintain intravascular volume and venous return.
3. Maintain adequate SVR.
4. Avoid myocardial depression during general anesthesia.
5. Routine supplemental oxygen is recommended.
6. Arterial line placement prior to neuraxial or general anesthesia is recommended.
7. CVP monitoring can be helpful.
8. PAC placement may be beneficial if patient's pulmonary vasculature is responsive to vasodilators.

9. TEE may be necessary to help guide fluid and inotropic therapy during a cesarean section under general anesthesia.
10. Medical treatments may include:
    a. Inhaled nitric oxide
    b. Nitroglycerine
    c. Calcium channel blocking agents
    d. Prostaglandins
    e. Endothelin receptor antagonists

### Labor

1. An early placement of a continuous epidural is recommended:
   a. A slow induction of anesthesia with the epidural is important.
   b. Treat any resultant hypotension with IV fluids.
   c. Vasopressors, such as ephedrine, should be used with caution because they can further increase pulmonary artery pressure.
2. Avoid single-dose spinal administration due to potentially precipitous decrease of SVR.

### Cesarean Section

1. Avoid single-dose spinals.
2. An epidural or a spinal catheter placement and titrated medication administration has been used successfully to achieve surgical analgesia.
3. General anesthesia is often recommended, but it has associated risks:
   a. Increased pulmonary artery pressure during direct laryngoscopy and intubation.
   b. Positive-pressure ventilation has adverse effects on the venous return.
   c. Volatile anesthetics have a negative ionotropic effect.
4. Use a narcotic-based induction and maintenance anesthetic.
5. The patient requires at least one week of continued monitoring post-delivery secondary to the high incidence of sudden death during this period.

## Hypertrophic Obstructive Cardiomyopathy

## Clinical Issues

1. Severe left ventricular hypertrophy, in the absence of abnormal loading conditions, such as severe hypertension or valvular disease
2. Decreased left ventricular chamber size
3. Left ventricular dysfunction
4. Morbidity is predominantly related to left ventricle (LV) outflow tract obstruction and arrhythmias.
5. Sudden death is the major cause of mortality, secondary to ventricular arrhythmias.

6. Some patients tolerate pregnancy well, secondary to the increased blood volume of pregnancy.
7. Pregnancy-induced increase in HR, myocardial contractility, and decreased SVR may worsen the outflow obstruction.

## KO Treatment Plan

1. Women who are symptomatic or have a history of syncope should have a pacemaker or automatic implantable cardioverter defibrillator (AICD) placed before conception.
2. Slow the HR with a β-blocker throughout the pregnancy and delivery.
3. Modest expansion of intravascular volume is helpful to ensure adequate ventricular filling. Maintain hydration at all times.
4. Avoid increases in myocardial contractility.
5. Avoid decreases in SVR (arterial and venous vasodilators) since it tends to worsen the degree of outflow obstruction.
6. Maintain normal sinus rhythm. Atrial fibrillation is poorly tolerated and should be managed with cardioversion; digoxin is contraindicated due to its positive inotropic effects.
7. Avoid aortocaval compression.

### Labor

1. Most tolerate labor well.
2. Give oxytocin slowly. Avoid boluses.
3. Methylergovine may be a better alternative to oxytocin.
4. A combined spinal–epidural using intrathecal opioids is a good choice for pain relief.
5. Treat hypotension with phenylephrine.

### Elective Cesarean Section

1. Epidural anesthesia
2. A single-dose spinal is contraindicated since the rapid onset of a sympathectomy is hazardous.
3. These patients generally tolerate general anesthesia well, if needed.
   a. Volatile anesthetics decrease myocardial contractility, which is advantageous.

## Valvular Heart Disease

## Clinical Issues

1. Given the physiologic increase in HR and CO during pregnancy, stenotic lesions (aortic stenosis and mitral stenosis) are often poorly tolerated.
2. As a result of impaired forward flow with stenotic lesions, there is increased risk of intrauterine growth restriction, preterm delivery, and low birthweight.
3. In contrast, chronic regurgitant lesions are better tolerated due to physiologic reduction in SVR and afterload during pregnancy.

4. Women with regurgitant lesions are at higher risk for postpartum heart failure in the context of increased volume load and acute increase in SVR with delivery.

## Aortic Stenosis (AS)

### Clinical Issues

1. The lesion does not become symptomatic until the valve diameter is one-third of its normal size. The most common etiology is congenital bicuspid valve.
2. Normal aortic valve area is 2.5–3.5 $cm^2$.
3. The onset of angina, dyspnea, or syncope is ominous and signals a life expectancy of less than 5 years.
4. Associated with a coarse systolic murmur that radiates to the neck
5. The diagnosis should be made with echocardiography and it should be used to monitor the lesion throughout the pregnancy.
6. Those with bicuspid valve defects may have associated dilation of the ascending aorta and coarctation of aorta, resulting in an increased risk of dissection during pregnancy.
7. All patients with AS are at increased risk of heart failure and arrhythmias. Women with mild AS usually tolerate pregnancy well due to the associated increase in blood volume.
8. Patients with severe symptomatic AS, rapid progression of stenosis, or concomitant impaired LV function, should have corrective valvular surgery before conception.

### KO Treatment Plan

1. Maintain a normal HR and a sinus rhythm.
2. Maintain an adequate SVR.
3. Maintain the intravascular volume and venous return.
4. Avoid aortocaval compression.
5. Avoid myocardial depression during general anesthesia.

#### Labor

1. Labor and assisted vaginal delivery is preferred.
2. Place an arterial line early in labor.
3. Many anesthesiologists like to place a PAC, but others are concerned with the increased risk of ventricular arrhythmias and CV collapse. It is usually adequate to monitor the CVP only. Maintain the CVP and/or pulmonary capillary wedge pressure at high-normal levels.
4. A continuous spinal or epidural can be safely done. Titrate the anesthetic level slowly. Remove epinephrine from the epidural/spinal solution to avoid the risk of an inadvertent intravascular injection and tachycardia.

#### Cesarean Section

1. Reserved for obstetric indications
2. Moderate to severe AS is a relative contraindication to a single-dose spinal.

3. A continuous spinal or epidural can be safely done.
4. General anesthesia can be safely established using etomidate and an opioid for induction. Propofol can be used in titrated doses to avoid sudden myocardial depression, and ketamine is avoided because of its associated tachycardia.

## Mitral Stenosis (MS)

### Sample Case

You are called to evaluate a 22-year-old female for the placement of a labor epidural. She has a recent diagnosis of MS. Should a labor epidural be used in a patient with MS? What are the risks? What are the benefits? How do you minimize cardiac decompensation if a cesarean section is required? Would you use general or regional anesthesia for a cesarean section in this patient?

### Clinical Issues

1. Develops when the mitral valve surface area is <2 $cm^2$
2. Normal valve area is 4–6 $cm^2$.
3. Less than 1 $cm^2$ is considered severe and requires surgical intervention.
4. MS prevents the filling of the left ventricle, which results in a decreased stroke volume and CO.

#### Diagnosis

1. 25% of women are first diagnosed during pregnancy. Most common etiology is rheumatic disease.
2. Symptoms include dyspnea, hemoptysis, chest pain, right heart failure, and thromboembolism.
3. Diastolic murmur is heard with auscultation.
4. An EKG may show left atrial enlargement, paroxysmal atrial tachycardia, or atrial fibrillation.
5. Diagnosed by echocardiography
6. Increased incidence of pulmonary edema

#### Pregnancy

1. Pre-pregnancy consideration should be made for intervention for moderate to severe MS. Women with severe MS do not tolerate pregnancy well.
2. These patients are at an increased risk for pulmonary embolism or other thromboembolic events, particularly in the setting of concomitant atrial fibrillation.
3. The risk of maternal death is greatest during labor and in the postpartum period.

### KO Treatment Plan

1. β-blockers to prevent tachycardia
2. Aggressive treatment of atrial fibrillation with digoxin and/or β-blockers or cardioversion.
3. Heart failure should be treated with $β_1$-selective blockers and diuretic therapy when needed for volume overload.
4. Severe MS should be treated surgically prior to pregnancy. This can be done with a percutaneous mitral

commissurotomy (in NYHA III/IV or PAP >50 mm Hg on medical therapy) or a bioprosthetic valve replacement.

5. If symptoms become severe during the pregnancy, mitral commissurotomy should be performed in the second trimester. A percutaneous balloon valvuloplasty can also be done during pregnancy if the patient's valve is pliable enough.

6. Therapeutic anticoagulation may be needed in women with atrial fibrillation.

### Labor and Cesarean Section

1. Patients with symptomatic MS require hemodynamic monitoring.
2. Plan for a low forceps delivery or cesarean section if the patient has obstetrical conditions that require it.
3. Give supplemental oxygen for labor and delivery.
4. Left uterine displacement
5. Place a PAC before the induction of labor or in early labor.
6. Restrict fluids and maintain a pulmonary artery wedge pressure of approximately 14 mm Hg.
7. Prevent tachycardia. Maintain sinus rhythm and treat atrial fibrillation aggressively.
8. Maintain SVR.
9. Prevent pain by placing an epidural and maintain it until the immediate postpartum period to reduce preload and prevent postpartum pulmonary edema. A combined spinal–epidural can also be placed with an intrathecal dose of opioid given initially and a continuous infusion of a dilute solution of local anesthetic as a slow infusion for the later stages of labor.
10. Prevent hypoxia, hypercarbia, and acidosis.
11. Phenylephrine is the preferred vasopressor.
12. An epidural is recommended for a cesarean section
    a. IV fluid administration
    b. Slow induction of anesthesia
    c. Small boluses of phenylephrine or background phenylephrine infusion
    d. Avoid tachycardia by avoiding atropine, ketamine, and meperidine.
    e. A β-blocker and a dose of an opioid should be given pre-operatively.

## Transplanted Heart

### Clinical Issues

1. The transplanted heart has no afferent or efferent autonomic or somatic innervation.
2. Lack of vagal innervation causes the baseline HR to be 100–120 beats/min.
3. Reflex slowing of the HR does not occur. Atropine and neostigmine have no cardiac effect.
4. Isoproterenol can be used to produce chronotropic or ionotropic effects.

### KO Treatment Plan

1. Pre-anesthetic evaluation:
   a. Exercise tolerance
   b. Cardiac catheterization reports
   c. Echocardiograms
2. Stress dose of steroids
3. Strict aseptic technique
4. Avoid aortocaval compression.
5. Maintain adequate intravascular volume and venous return.
6. Slow induction with an epidural anesthetic can be done using a dilute solution of local anesthetic and opioid.
7. Treat the associated hypotension with phenylephrine or isoproterenol.
8. A CVP is rarely placed secondary to the risk of catheter-related sepsis.
9. An epidural is the preferred technique for a cesarean section.
   a. Give additional crystalloid to maintain adequate volume.
   b. Both a spinal and general anesthesia have been used successfully, however.
   c. Use ketamine instead of propofol for induction of general anesthesia.

## Peripartum Cardiomyopathy (PPCM)

### Clinical Issues

1. PPCM is a rare form of pregnancy-related systolic heart failure (LVEF <45% or fractional shortening <30%), distinct from dilated cardiomyopathy. It progresses rapidly and is associated with high morbidity and mortality.
2. Onset is either during the last month of pregnancy or in the first 5 months postpartum. Diagnosis requires exclusion of reversible causes of cardiomyopathy (e.g., myocarditis, hypertension, underlying valvular disease, toxin-induced, ischemia).
3. Presents with symptoms of a mild upper respiratory infection, chest congestion, and fatigue
4. Progresses to cardiac failure and low CO
5. 20% chance of relapse with a subsequent pregnancy

### Predisposing Factors

1. Multiple gestations
2. Multiparity
3. Comorbidities, such as preeclampsia, hypertension, obesity, diabetes
4. Family history, race/ethnicity
5. Advanced maternal age
6. Smoking, cocaine use, long-term (>4 weeks) use of β-adrenergic tocolytic therapy

## KO Treatment Plan

1. Provide supportive treatment with diuretics and digitalis.
2. Sodium and fluid restriction during pregnancy
3. Maintain rhythm control (β-blockers, digoxin).
4. Afterload reduction (hydralazine or nitrates)
5. Consideration of anticoagulation for LV thrombus
6. Prompt vaginal delivery or cesarean section
7. Continuous labor epidural is recommended for labor and vaginal delivery.
8. Perform general anesthesia with remifentanil and propofol for maintenance, or a slow induction of epidural anesthesia guided by pulmonary artery measurements.

# Cardiopulmonary Resuscitation (CPR) during Pregnancy

## Clinical Issues

### Epidemiology

1 in 20,000 pregnancies

### Differential Diagnosis of Cardiac Arrest in Pregnant Patient

1. Amniotic fluid embolus
2. Pulmonary embolus
3. Arrhythmia
4. Aortic dissection or hemorrhage
5. Myocardial infarction: pregnant women are at increased risk despite young age.
6. Congestive heart failure
7. Intracranial hemorrhage
8. Local anesthetic toxicity
9. High spinal anesthesia
10. Hypermagnesemia
11. Hypoxemia

## KO Treatment Plan

The general approach for most of the CPR and ACLS guidelines is the same as for nonpregnant patients.

1. Begin cardiopulmonary resuscitation (CPR).
2. Intubate the patient.
3. Prior to 24 weeks' gestation, the only concern should be saving the mother.
4. After 24 weeks' gestation, the team must consider both lives.
5. Maintain left uterine displacement.
6. Place the patient on a hard surface for more efficient cardiac compression.
7. Use all standard resuscitative measures, medications, and procedures without modification, including defibrillate unstable or pulseless.
8. If the initial resuscitative efforts are unsuccessful in a pregnant woman greater than 24 weeks, deliver the fetus. This should be done within the first 4–5 minutes of the resuscitation. This may save the fetus and facilitate resuscitation of the mother. Evacuation of the uterus allows for relief of aortocaval compression and restoration of venous return to the heart.
9. A cesarean section may be necessary even if the fetus is not viable.
10. If delivery of the fetus does not facilitate successful resuscitation, consider thoracotomy, open-chest cardiac massage, and cardiopulmonary bypass (CPB).
11. CPB is especially helpful in patients who have bupivacaine-induced toxicity, pulmonary embolus, or require rewarming.
12. Post-ROSC hypothermia

### Specific Differences in the Pregnant Cardiac Arrest Patient

1. Compression hand position: 1–2 interspaces higher than in the nonpregnant patient
2. Elevate the head of the bed to allow for better diaphragmatic excursion.
3. Left uterine displacement during CPR
4. Avoid amiodarone, if possible. It is a Class D medication.
5. Early airway management to mitigate increased aspiration risk and decrease duration of rapid desaturation.

# Bibliography

Chestnut DH, Wong CA, Tsen LC, et al. *Chestnut's Obstetric Anesthesia: Principles and Practice,* 6th ed. Philadelphia: Elsevier, 2020, pp. 987–1023.

Stoelting RK, Dierdorf SF. *Anesthesia and Co-existing Disease,* 4th ed. Philadelphia: Churchill Livingstone, 2002, pp. 664–8.

# Lactation and Anesthesia

Kara M. Barnett

## Sample Case

A 30-year-old female is scheduled for a melanoma excision of her left foot. She is currently breastfeeding a 6-month-old and asks if she can still breastfeed after surgery. What is your anesthesia plan? How will you counsel the patient?

## Clinical Issues

### Considerations

1. Child's age (actual and post-conceptual)

   a. Younger children require more breast milk than older children who are taking solids.

   b. Younger children have more immature guts.

2. Child's health

   a. Mothers of children with health concerns like apnea, hypotension, or hypotonia may benefit from a period of pumping and discarding post-operatively.

3. Patients should contact the child's pediatrician.

## KO Treatment Plan

### Pre-operative

1. Should be the earliest case possible to minimize fasting times

2. Counsel the patient on the safety of lactation and anesthesia.

   a. Typical anesthetic agents are compatible with lactation based on short peri-operative use once the patient is awake and alert in a full-term healthy neonate.

3. Consult evidence-based resources if unsure of medication compatibility with lactation.

   a. LactMed

   b. Medsmilk.com

   c. Infant Risk Center

4. The patient should breastfeed or express milk prior to surgery.

### Intra-operative

1. Prefer regional anesthesia whenever possible

   a. Local anesthetics are compatible with lactation.

   b. Minimize narcotics.

   c. Multimodal pain medications

2. Avoid betadine preparation of the skin if possible.

3. Increase IV fluids because of increased fluid requirement of lactation.

### Post-operative

1. Pain should be treated because pain will interfere with lactation.

   a. Judicious use of opioids

2. Patient should try to continue her typical lactation schedule in the post-operative period to avoid issues like engorgement, plugged duct, and decrease in supply.

3. Medications to avoid

   a. Codeine – risk of overdose if the mother is a fast metabolizer

   b. Meperidine – active metabolite

   c. Tramadol – active metabolite

4. Medications to limit

   a. Oxycodone – up to 30 mg/day

   b. Hydrocodone – up to 30 mg/day

5. Nonsteroidal anti-inflammatory drugs (NSAIDS), acetaminophen, and typical antiemetics are compatible with lactation.

6. While the patient is taking narcotics, another responsible adult should monitor the child for respiratory depression.

## Bibliography

American Society of Anesthesiology. Statement on resuming breastfeeding. Approved October 23, 2019. www .asahq.org/standards-and-guidelines/state ment-on-resuming-breastfeeding-after-anesthesia (accessed January 9 2023).

Reece-Stremtan S, Campos M, Kokajko L. ABM clinical protocol #15: analgesia and anesthesia for the breastfeeding mother, revised 2017. *Breastfeed Med* 2017;**12**(9):500–6.

Rieth EF, Barnett KM, Simon JA. Implementation and organization of a perioperative lactation program: a descriptive study. *Breastfeed Med* 2018;**13**(2):97–105.

**Chapter**

# 65

# The Basics of Pediatrics

Vijay R. Mohan

## Clinical Issues

### Airway

1. Anatomic differences

   a. Larger occiput with shorter necks. Neck flexion is not required to attain the "sniffing" position.

   b. Hypertrophied tonsil and adenoid tissue

   c. A more cephalad larynx

      i. C2–C3 in the premature infant

      ii. C3–C4 in the term infant

      iii. C4–C5 in the adult

   d. Narrower and relatively longer epiglottis. It is more anterior and superiorly located than in adults. The epiglottis is angled into the lumen of the airway, making it more difficult to displace anteriorly with direct laryngoscopy.

      i. Omega-shaped

      ii. Floppy

   e. The tongue is relatively larger in proportion to the oral cavity.

   f. The cricoid cartilage (subglottic) is the narrowest part of the upper airway (compared to the vocal cords in adults). This increases risk of post-extubation stridor.

   g. Infants are obligate nasal breathers through 6 months of age.

**TKO:** Despite these characteristics, unless syndromic facial anomalies exist, it is **extremely rare** that tracheal intubation cannot be accomplished in the prepubertal child.

2. Endotracheal tubes (ETTs)

   a. A variety of formulas exist for estimating the proper size ETT.

      i. Appropriate ETT size, **uncuffed** = 4 + [Age in years/4]

      ii. Appropriate ETT size, **cuffed** = 3.5 + [Age in years/4]

   b. Historically, uncuffed tubes have been used in children under the age of 8.

      i. Controversy still exists regarding the use of cuffed tubes in children, although trends are changing in favor of the use of cuffed tubes in younger children.

**Table 65.1** Pediatric pulmonary system

| Parameter | Infant | Adult |
|---|---|---|
| Tidal volume (mL/kg) | 7 | 7 |
| Dead space (mL/kg) | 2–2.5 | 2.2 |
| Alveolar ventilation (mL/kg/min) | 100–150 | 60 |
| FRC (mL/kg) | 27–30 | 30 |
| Oxygen consumption (L/min) | 7–9 | 3 |

Table adapted from Barash PG, Cullen BF, Stoelting RK. *Clinical Anesthesia*, 5th ed. Philadelphia: Lippincott Williams & Wilkins, 2006, pp. 1181–202.

      ii. Be prepared to defend a choice of cuffed versus uncuffed tubes if you intend to address this topic during your examination. These arguments are outside the scope of this review book.

### Physiology

1. Pulmonary system (Table 65.1)

   a. Infants are prone to peri-operative hypoxemia, secondary to increased oxygen consumption.

**TKO:** Desaturation occurs quickly in infants secondary to their increased oxygen consumption coupled with a relatively decreased functional residual capacity (FRC), leading to hypoxia and bradycardia.

   b. Smaller airway diameter, leading to increased work of breathing

   c. High closing volumes

      i. Lung volumes at which the alveoli close

   d. High MV/FRC ratio

      i. This leads to a rapid uptake of volatile anesthetics.

         (1) Faster inhalational induction

            (a) Increased MV/FRC ratio

            (b) Higher percentage of the neonate's body weight consists of vessel-rich tissues.

            (c) Greater cardiac output per kilogram of body mass

   e. Lower blood gas partition coefficient for volatile anesthetics

f. Pliable rib cage

  i. The diaphragm is the primary contributor to ventilation.

  ii. If the child has an increased oxygen demand, he or she responds by increasing the respiratory rate.

  iii. Increasing respiratory excursion by diaphragmatic contraction

  iv. This leads to negative intrathoracic pressure and retractions.

  v. This is an inefficient form of ventilation with a very high energy cost, especially if the patient develops an airway obstruction.

2. Cardiovascular system

a. Immature

b. Decreased ability to increase myocardial contractility

  i. The stroke volume (SV) is relatively fixed secondary to the pediatric noncompliant left ventricle.

**TKO:** The infant's cardiac output (CO) is heart rate (HR)-dependent: CO = HR × SV

c. Causes of decreased heart rate in infants

  i. Hypoxemia

  ii. Vagal stimulation

d. Poor ability to compensate for hypotension after volatile and intravenous anesthetics due to immature baroreceptor reflex

e. Temperature regulation

  i. Temperature regulation is maintained via brown fat metabolism (nonshivering thermogenesis), crying, and movement.

  ii. Infants do not shiver.

  iii. Poor ability to maintain normothermia secondary to a disproportionately large body surface area, increased metabolic rate, and a thinner layer of subcutaneous insulating body fat.

  iv. Operating room temperature must be kept higher, and warming blankets and fluid warmers must be used whenever possible.

3. Renal system

a. Decreased glomerular filtration rate (GFR) and renal blood flow (RBF)

  i. These values increase rapidly by 3 months of age.

  ii. This may clinically affect the clearance of certain medications.

    (1) Aminoglycosides

    (2) Muscle relaxants

b. Renal tubular function is also immature at birth.

  i. Limited ability to concentrate urine

4. Fluids and electrolytes

a. Maintenance fluid requirements

  i. 4 mL/kg/h for first 10 kg, plus

  ii. 2 mL/kg/h for second 10 kg, plus

  iii. 1 mL/kg/h for each remaining kilograms

b. Fluid deficits

  i. Estimated fluid deficit = estimated hourly maintenance (EHM) × the number of hours NPO

  ii. Estimated blood volume (mL/kg)

    (1) Premature: 100

    (2) Full term: 90

    (3) Infant to 1 year: 80

    (4) Child >1 year: 75

    (5) Adult: 70 (male) and 65 (female)

  iii. Glucose

    (1) Infants have increased metabolic demands and decreased glycogen stores; therefore, they are prone to hypoglycemia.

    (2) Intravenous dextrose (as D5 0.25%NS or D10 W) should be administered in all patients under 6 months of age, and in infants between 6 and 12 months if the surgery is anticipated to last longer than 1 hour.

    (3) Maintain serum glucose levels >40 mg/dL.

    (4) Other indications for IV dextrose administration include:

**Table 65.2** Age related vital signs

| | Newborn | 3 mos–2 yrs | 2–10 yrs | >10 yrs |
| --- | --- | --- | --- | --- |
| Respirations (breaths/min) | 45–60 | 30 | 25 | 20 |
| Heart rate (beats/min) | 100–180 | 80–150 | 70–110 | 50–90 |
| Minimum acceptable blood pressure | Mean BP ≥ PCA | SBP ≥70 + 2 × age | SBP ≥70 + 2 × age | SBP ≥~90 |

PCA, Post-conception age (weeks); SBP: systolic blood pressure
Table adapted from information at www.cchmc.org and Motoyama EK, Davis PJ, *Smith's Anesthesia for Infants and Children*, 7th ed. Philadelphia: Mosby Elsevier, 2006, pp. 798–9.

(a) History of liver disease
(b) Total parenteral nutrition (TPN) administration
(c) Severe systemic illness
(d) Newborn infants of diabetic mothers

iv. NPO guidelines

(1) Clear liquids: 2 hours
(2) Breastmilk: 4 hours
(3) Formula: 6 hours

(4) Nonhuman milk: 6 hours
(5) Meal with fat: 8 hours

v. Hemoglobin

(1) The oxyhemoglobin dissociation curve is shifted to the left.
(2) As the fetal hemoglobin decreases, there is a physiologic fall in the infant's hematocrit starting at 6–8 weeks and ending at about 12 weeks due to erythrocyte turnover.

# Bibliography

Barash PG, Cullen BF, Stoelting RK, et al. *Clinical Anesthesia*, 8th ed. Philadelphia: Lippincott Williams & Wilkins, 2017, pp. 1219–27.

Butterworth JF, Mackey DC, Wasnick JD. *Morgan & Mikhail's Clinical Anesthesiology*, 6th ed. New York: McGraw-Hill Education, 2018, pp 897–927.

Cincinnati Children's Hospital. Homepage. www.cchmc.org.

Gropper MA. *Miller's Anesthesia*, 9th ed. Philadelphia: Elsevier, 2020, pp. 2420–6.

Litman RS. *Pediatric Anesthesia: The Requisites in Anesthesiology*, 1st ed. Philadelphia: Mosby, 2004.

McNiece WL, Dierdor SF. The pediatric airway. *Semin Pediatr Surg* 2004:**13** (3):152–65.

Motoyama EK, Davis PJ. *Smith's Anesthesia for Infants and Children*, 7th ed. Philadelphia: Mosby Elsevier, 2006, pp 798–9.

# Neonatal Resuscitation

Cassandra Hoffmann and Jessica A. Lovich-Sapola

## Sample Case

You are taking care of a 24-year-old female, G1P0, for a cesarean section. Her epidural has been dosed with 20 mL of 2% lidocaine plus 1:200,000 of epinephrine. She had adequate prenatal care and had been laboring without progression for the previous 20 hours. When the baby is delivered, the child makes no sound and no attempts at breathing. The nurses turn to you for help. What will you do? Can you leave the mother to attend to the baby? Who do you have the ultimate responsibility to care for? Assuming you get a colleague to help care for the mother, how would you evaluate and resuscitate the baby?

## Clinical Issues

### Ethical Issues

1. The ASA standards for basic anesthetic monitoring state that "qualified personnel, other than the anesthesiologist attending the mother, should be immediately available to assume responsibility for resuscitation of the newborn."
2. While the primary responsibility of the anesthesiologist is to provide care for the mother, the guidelines for anesthesia care in obstetrics go on to state: "If the anesthesiologist is also requested to provide brief assistance in the care of the newborn, the benefit to the child must be compared to the risk of the mother."

### Transitional Physiology

1. Intrauterine fetal circulation
   a. General information
      i. Fetal shunts in utero
         (1) Ductus venosus
         (2) Foramen ovale
         (3) Ductus arteriosus
      ii. Pulmonary vascular resistance (PVR) is high.
      iii. Systemic vascular resistance is low.
   b. Pathway of fetal circulation
      i. Blood from the placenta travels to the baby through the umbilical vein.
      ii. The umbilical vein goes to the liver and splits.
         (1) About half of the blood bypasses the liver through the ductus venosus and goes directly to the vena cava, then to the heart.
         (2) The other half of the blood goes directly to the liver.
      iii. Once in the heart, the blood enters the right atrium.
         (1) The nonexpanded lungs of the fetus cause increased resistance and pressure in the pulmonary circuit so that the blood is shunted toward the systemic circuit due to pressure gradients.
         (2) Most blood then flows through the foramen ovale to the left atrium.
            (a) Blood then passes to the left ventricle and then to the aorta.
            (b) Blood from the aorta travels to the head and upper extremities.
         (3) The blood that does not enter the foramen ovale stays in the right heart and travels to the pulmonary artery.
            (a) Since the placenta does the work of oxygen exchange, the lungs are not used for this purpose in the fetus.
            (b) Most of the blood on its way to the lungs from the pulmonary artery is bypassed away from the lungs to the aorta through the ductus arteriosus.
      iv. The blood then travels from the aorta to the umbilical arteries, and back to the placenta.
2. Birth
   a. Arrest of the umbilical circulation removes the low resistance placental bed from circulation.
   b. Expansion of the lungs occurs as breathing is initiated within the first 30 seconds of life.
      i. By 90 seconds, sustained respirations are present.
      ii. The inflation of the lungs reduces the resistance to blood flow through the lungs, resulting in increased blood flow from the pulmonary arteries. Decreased PVR reverses the pressure gradients to stop and close the shunts.
         (1) PVR may remain elevated, resulting in a persistent fetal circulation.

(2) Causes of elevated PVR

    (a) Hypoxemia

    (b) Hypercarbia

    (c) Hypothermia

    (d) Hypovolemia

    (e) Acidosis

## Risk Factors for Fetal Distress and the Associated Need for Fetal Resuscitation

1. Maternal risk factors

    a. Diabetes

    b. Pregnancy-induced hypertension

    c. Previous stillbirth

    d. Infection

    e. Substance abuse

    f. Cesarean section delivery

    g. General anesthesia for delivery

    h. Narcotic or other substance use

    i. Chronic hypertension

    j. Previous Rh sensitization

    k. Bleeding in the second or third trimester

    l. Maternal infection

2. Fetal risk factors

    a. Post-term or pre-term gestation

    b. Multiple gestation

    c. Poly- or oligohydramnios

    d. Known fetal anomalies

    e. Abnormal fetal lie

    f. Nonreassuring fetal heart rate patterns

    g. Meconium-stained amniotic fluid

## Assessment of the Fetus during Labor

1. The fetal heart rate is the most reliable predictor of fetal well-being.

    a. It is ≥90% accurate in predicting a 5-minute APGAR score greater than 7.

    b. False positive rate of 35–50% in predicting fetal compromise

2. Fetal scalp pH can be used to confirm or exclude fetal acidosis.

    a. A pH of ≤7.20 is considered abnormal and indicates the need for immediate delivery.

## Assessment of the Fetus after Delivery

1. APGAR score (Virginia Apgar [1909–74], obstetric anesthesiologist)

    a. APGAR scoring is a useful method to evaluate the clinical status of the patient at 1 and 5 minutes after delivery.

    b. The scoring system is presented in Table 66.1.

    c. Do not wait for the 1-minute APGAR score to begin resuscitation if it is necessary.

    d. If the 5-minute APGAR score is less than 7, additional scores should be obtained every 5 minutes until 20 minutes have passed or 2 successive scores are more than 7.

    e. The current guidelines state that if more than 10 minutes of continuous and adequate resuscitative efforts produce no signs of life, then resuscitation should be discontinued.

## KO Treatment Plan

### Preparation for Resuscitation

1. Equipment

    a. Suction

        i. Bulb syringe

        ii. Mechanical suction

        iii. Suction catheters

        iv. Meconium aspirator

**Table 66.1** APGAR scoring

| Sign | 0 points | 1 point | 2 points |
| --- | --- | --- | --- |
| Appearance (skin color) | Pale, blue | Extremities blue | Completely pink |
| Pulse (heart rate) | Absent | <100 beats/min | >100 beats/min |
| Grimace (reflex irritability) | No response to stimulation | Grimace, weak cry with stimulation | Cough, sneeze, cry with stimulation |
| Activity (muscle tone) | Limp, floppy | Extremity flexion | Active motion, well flexed, and resisting extension |
| Respiratory effort | Absent, apneic | Slow, irregular breathing | Good, crying |

Adapted from Barash PG, Cullen BF, Stoelting RK. *Clinical Anesthesia*, 5th ed. Philadelphia: Lippincott Williams & Wilkins, 2006, pp. 1164–7, 1174–5; Gropper MA. *Miller's Anesthesia*, 9th ed. Philadelphia: Elsevier, 2020, p. 2423.

b. Intubation equipment

    i. Laryngoscope and blades (Miller #0 and #1)
    ii. Endotracheal tubes (2.5–4.0 mm)
    iii. Stylet

c. Bag and mask equipment

    i. Neonatal resuscitation bag with a pressure valve
    ii. Face masks in the appropriate sizes
    iii. Oral airways
    iv. Oxygen with a flowmeter

d. Extras

    i. Radiant warmer
    ii. Stethoscope

## Initial Treatment of All Infants

1. Warm and dry the infant.

    a. Goal axillary temperature of 36.5 °C (euthermia)

2. Position airway and aspirate the mouth, pharynx, and nose with a catheter to clear secretions.
3. Stimulate the infant by slapping the soles of the feet or rubbing the back.
4. Continue ongoing evaluation by verifying vital signs as per the above algorithm.

    a. Heart rate, respirations, and color

## Treatment of a Depressed Infant

1. If oropharyngeal suction reveals meconium or thick meconium-stained mucus, suction via an endotracheal tube before lungs are inflated, within 1–2 minutes of delivery.
2. If after stimulation and clearance of secretions the infant remains apneic or has a heart rate less than 100 beats/min, initiate positive-pressure ventilation (PPV) at a rate of 30–40 breaths/min, place an $SpO_2$ monitor, and consider an ECG monitor. Verify chest movement and ventilation corrective steps, and consider placement of an endotracheal tube or laryngeal mask airway (LMA) if needed.

    a. Recommendation is for PPV with room air, unless chest compressions or medications are needed; in this case use 100% oxygen.

3. If after 30 seconds of PPV the heart rate remains below 60 beats/min, intubate if not already performed, initiate chest compressions, and coordinate with PPV (3 compressions to 1 inflation, with 30 inflations per minute and 90 compressions per minute) using the two-thumb encircling-hands technique for compressions, place on 100% $O_2$, place an ECG monitor, and consider emergency umbilical venous access.
4. If heart rate continues to be less than 60 beats/min despite 60 seconds of chest compressions and adequate PPV, administer IV epinephrine, consider hypovolemia (in the setting of blood loss), and consider pneumothorax. When IV access is not feasible, an intraosseous route may be considered.

## Neonatal Resuscitation Medications

1. Sodium bicarbonate: 4.2% (0.5 mEq/mL)

    a. Sodium bicarbonate use is not recommended during brief cardiopulmonary resuscitation.
    b. If resuscitation is prolonged, in the face of a documented acidosis, with adequate ventilation and perfusion, 4.2% sodium bicarbonate may be infused to a total dose of 2 mEq/kg, via an umbilical catheter.

2. Naloxone: (0.4 mg/mL)

    a. A dose of 0.01 mg/kg may be injected intravenously (IV), intramuscularly (IM), subcutaneously (SQ), or via the endotracheal tube (ETT) once adequate ventilation is achieved in the setting of respiratory depression secondary to maternal opioid administration.
    b. Do not administer to infants of opioid-addicted mothers for fear of precipitating withdrawal.

3. Epinephrine: (1:10,000 concentration)

    a. Primary medication of neonatal resuscitation
    b. Give if the infant is in asystole or has a heart rate less than 60 beats/min 45–60 seconds after the initiation of PPV and chest compressions.
    c. Doses of 0.01–0.03 mg/kg may be injected IV or 0.1 mg/kg via the ETT. This dose can be repeated every 3–5 minutes as needed.

4. Atropine

    a. A dose of 0.02 mg/kg may be given IV or 0.03 mg/kg via the ETT to treat bradycardia.

5. Calcium gluconate

    a. A dose of 100 mg/kg may be infused over 5–10 minutes to treat low cardiac output.
    b. The neonate should be on continuous EKG monitoring.

6. Fluids: volume expanders, normal saline, dextrose 10%, and O-negative blood

    a. Acute volume expansion may be achieved with:

        i. O-negative blood or maternally cross-matched blood (10 mL/kg)
        ii. Normal saline or Lactated Ringer's (10 mL/kg)

    b. Albumin may be used, but the evidence of effectiveness is limited.

7. Severe acidosis (<7.0 pH) may decrease the effectiveness of the aforementioned medications.
8. Medications should be given with the smallest volume of fluid possible to decrease the risk of hypervolemia.

# Bibliography

Arkoosh, VA. Neonatal resuscitation. Annual Meeting Refresher Course Lectures, ASA Annual Meeting, 2006.

ASA. Standards for basic anesthetic monitoring (approved by ASA House of Delegates October 21, 1986 and last affirmed December 13, 2020 and last amended Ocotber 20, 2010). www.asahq.org.

Aziz K, Lee HC, Escobedo MB, et al. Part 5: Neonatal Resuscitation 2020 American Heart Association guidelines for cardiopulmonary resuscitation and emergency cardiovascular care. *Pediatrics*. 2020. doi:10.1542/peds.2020-038505E

Barash PG, Cullen BF, Stoelting RK. *Clinical Anesthesia*, 5th ed. Philadelphia: Lippincott Williams & Wilkins, 2006, pp. 1164–7, 1174–5.

Gropper MA. *Miller's Anesthesia*, 9th ed. Philadelphia: Elsevier, 2020, pp. 2524–37.

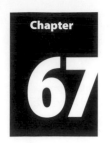
# Tracheoesophageal Fistula (TEF)

Sierra Ziska

## Sample Case

A 27-year-old female presents with an uncomplicated delivery of a male neonate at an estimated gestational age of 37 weeks. In the delivery room, the nurses observe that the baby is drooling excessively and appears to be coughing and choking. Upon initiating breastfeeding, the infant becomes cyanotic. Feeding is discontinued. A nasogastric catheter is passed, and a chest X-ray reveals a distal tracheoesophageal fistula. What are your concerns? How will you induce anesthesia? How would you intubate this patient? When would you extubate?

## Clinical Issues

### Epidemiology

1. Incidence is approximately 1 in 3000 live births.
2. Associated congenital anomalies are seen in approximately 50% of the cases.

   a. Other gastrointestinal malformation

   b. VACTERL association

      i. Vertebral/vascular

      ii. Anorectal

      iii. Cardiac: ventricular septal defect (VSD), atrial septal defect (ASD), and atrioventricular canal defects

      iv. Tracheoesophageal

      v. Radial/renal

      vi. Limb deformities

   c. Generalized chromosomal syndrome

3. Prematurity: 30% incidence

## Diagnosis

1. Prenatal: polyhydramnios, prominent esophageal pouch, small or absent stomach "bubble" with fluid-filled loops of bowel
2. The 3 Cs associated with TEF: choking (with initial feeds), coughing, and cyanosis (due to respiratory distress).
3. Neonatology will often diagnose TEF in a patient with excessive salivation in whom a catheter will not advance into the stomach.
4. Diagnostic imaging:

   a. Chest X-ray reveals the tip of the catheter in the superior mediastinum. Gas in the stomach and intestine indicate the presence of a distal fistula.

   b. Fluoroscopy with barium swallow or with water-soluble contrast will illustrate a proximal pouch.

## KO Treatment Plan

**TKO:** Please note that the majority of these cases are performed at regional pediatric surgical centers. The outline below illustrates basic management points with which every anesthesiologist should be familiar. These topics are more likely to be addressed in the short questions rather than a long stem due to the advanced nature of the procedure. Early or delayed surgical intervention is indicated, depending on the condition of the infant and the need to prevent further aspiration of gastric secretions or contents.

### Pre-operative

1. A complete pre-operative evaluation and treatment of the patient should include the following:

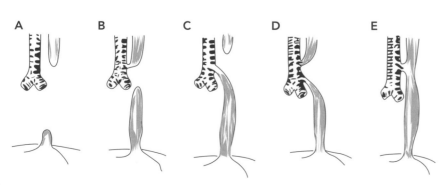

**Figure 67.1** Examples of tracheoesophageal fistula. Type A: Esophageal atresia (EA) without tracheoesophageal fistula (TEF); Type B: EA with proximal TEF; Type C: EA with distal TEF (85% of cases); Type D: EA with TEF between both esophageal segments and trachea; Type E: TEF without EA or H-type fistula. Source: Reprinted from Otolaryngologic Clinics of North America, Volume 40, Issue 1, Olga Achildi and Harsh Grewal, Congenital Anomalies of the Esophagus, Pages 219–44, 2007, with permission from Elsevier.

a. Evaluate respiratory complications secondary to infection or intrinsic lung disease associated with prematurity.

b. Verify the patient's hydration status.

2. Approximately 50% of the patients who have EA or TEF also present with additional birth defects; therefore, a complete evaluation should include the following:

a. Radiographs of the chest, abdomen, pelvis, and spine

b. Ultrasound of the spine and kidney

c. Echocardiography of the heart and aorta

3. Vascular access should be obtained.

4. Verify that a blood type and crossmatch are available.

5. Pre-operative management goals:

a. Reduce aspiration risk:

  i. Maintain NPO status.

  ii. Elevate the head of the bed.

  iii. Remove secretions via suction catheter in the proximal pouch.

b. Supplemental oxygen should be administered as needed to maintain oxygen saturation 88–93% in the neonatal patient.

## Intra-operative

1. Induction: awake intubation vs. rapid-sequence induction with tracheal intubation

a. Awake intubation with spontaneous ventilation is largely theoretical. It was previously thought that preservation of airway protective reflexes would decrease the risk of aspiration, with resultant avoidance of arterial desaturation after induction. However, it has been found to actually confer no benefits in preserving arterial oxygenation and has been generally abandoned.

b. In a modified rapid-sequence IV induction, positive-pressure ventilation is avoided in an attempt to prevent gastric distension secondary to the gases passing through the fistula into the stomach. Gastric inflation can lead to difficulty ventilating and arterial desaturation.

2. The endotracheal tube is intentionally placed into the mainstem bronchus in order to bypass the fistula. It is slowly withdrawn until positive-pressure breath sounds are bilateral.

3. Ventilation strategies:

a. Pressure control ventilation is more effective than volume control ventilation with regard to arterial oxygenation during one-lung ventilation. Intrapulmonary shunting is reduced.

b. Peak airway pressures should be maintained at 15–25 cm $H_2O$ to reduce the risk of barotrauma. Higher airway pressures may simply reflect the pressure needed to ventilate through a small-diameter tube.

c. Respiratory rate should be maintained around 35–40 breaths/min, with an I:E ratio of 1:2.5.

d. Intermittent airway suctioning may be necessary to clear secretions.

4. Surgical thoracoscopic approaches may lead to creation of an artificial pneumothorax with the continuous infusion of $CO_2$. Pressures of the artificial pneumothorax should be kept under 10 mm Hg to maintain hemodynamic stability.

5. 10% of surgeries convert to open thoracotomy, and considerations for post-operative analgesia should be evaluated. Most common reasons for conversion include: issues with ventilation, surgical knotting difficulties, and insufficient surgical exposure.

6. Other issues that may arise leading to desaturation or difficult ventilation:

a. Kinking or obstruction of the small endotracheal tube

b. Migration of the oral endotracheal tube into the fistula

c. Low lung compliance and high compliance of the fistula

## Post-operative

1. Usually the esophageal anastomosis is under tension and the infant is electively paralyzed and mechanically ventilated for up to 5 post-operative days.

2. Ventilation with a bag/mask should be avoided for several post-operative days, secondary to the fragility of the anastomosis.

3. Long-term complications include

a. Dysphagia

b. Gastroesophageal reflux disease (GERD)

c. Respiratory infections

d. Choking

e. Esophageal strictures

f. Symptomatic tracheomalacia

g. Recurrent TEF

h. Wheezing or bronchial hyperreactivity

i. Chest wall deformities

## Bibliography

Achildi O, Grewal H. Congenital anomalies of the esophagus. *Otolaryngol Clin N Am* 2007;**40**:219–44.

Cook-Sather SD, Tulloch H, Cnaan A, et al. A comparison of awake versus paralyzed tracheal intubation for infants with pyloric stenosis. *Anesth Analg* 1998;**86**:945–51.

Iaconoa R, Saxena V, Amulya K. Thoracoscopic repair of esophageal atresia with distal tracheoesophageal fistula (Type C): systematic review. *Surg Laparosc Endosc Percutan Tech* 2020;**30** (4):388–93.

Liu H, Le C, Chen J, et al. Anesthesia management of neonatal thoracoscopic surgery. *Transl Pediatr* 2021;**10**(8):2035–43.

Motoyama EK, Davis PJ. *Smith's Anesthesia for Infants and Children*, 7th ed. Philadelphia: Mosby Elsevier, 2006, pp. 550–2.

Spitz L. Oesophageal atresia. *Ophanet J Rare Dis* 2007;**2**:24–37.

# Pyloric Stenosis

Chapter 68

Luis A. Vargas-Patron

## Sample Case

A 3-week-old male infant, born 2 weeks premature and now weighing 4 kg, is scheduled for a pyloromyotomy. He has a history of nonbilious emesis for the past 5 days. He is limp and lethargic. His current vital signs are heart rate (HR) 168, respiratory rate (RR) 54, and blood pressure (BP) 72/35 mm Hg. His recent laboratory findings include an unremarkable complete blood count, $Na^+$ 130, $K^+$ 2.5, and $Cl^-$ 85. What are your concerns? Is this an emergency surgery? Should his electrolytes be corrected prior to surgery? What should they be corrected to? How would you induce anesthesia for this patient?

## Clinical Issues

### Acid–Base Balance and Electrolyte Abnormalities

Chronic emesis leads to the loss of hydrochloric acid (HCl) from the stomach. This eventually leads to a hypochloremic, hypokalemic metabolic alkalosis. With severe dehydration, a paradoxical aciduria may occur.

1. Hydrogen and chloride ions are lost from the stomach, which results in hypochloremic metabolic alkalosis.
2. The kidneys secrete potassium in exchange for hydrogen ions in an effort to maintain a normal arterial pH, causing hypokalemia.
3. As the kidneys exchange potassium for hydrogen ions, the infant becomes sodium-depleted from vomiting.
4. The kidney thus attempts to conserve sodium to maintain volume and exchanges sodium ions for potassium and hydrogen ions, causing a paradoxical aciduria.
5. The net result from the kidneys compensating for the emesis is a loss of hydrogen and potassium, which results in a hypokalemic metabolic alkalosis.
6. Because medullary chemoreceptors in the brainstem respond to changes in the hydrogen ion ($H^+$) concentration from diffusion of $CO_2$ in the cerebrospinal fluid, the decrease in $CO_2$ and less $CO_2$ diffusion across the cell membrane decreases the $H^+$ ion concentration inside the receptors and causes a compensatory respiratory depression and possible apnea in children. The respiratory depression is designed to compensate and correct the pH, but the risk of apnea is increased if the child is alkalotic and being ventilated during a surgery because the ventilator

delays the brain's effort to return to homeostasis. The apnea will be more likely to occur post-operatively due to this prevention of respiratory compensation during metabolic alkalosis.
7. To minimize the risk of post-operative apnea, this alkalosis must be corrected before surgery.

## Full-Stomach Precautions

1. The stomach is often filled with acidic gastric secretions, food contents, or barium.
   a. Ultrasound assessment of gastric contents can be made easily and quickly before the induction of anesthesia (Fig. 68.1).
2. The infant's *in situ* nasogastric (NG) tube should be suctioned prior to the induction of anesthesia.
   a. If an NG is not in place, most practitioners favor the placement of an orogastric (OG) or NG tube prior to the induction of anesthesia in a patient with pyloric stenosis in order to fully decompress the stomach contents.
3. Multiple laryngoscope handles and blades should be available.
4. Several sizes of endotracheal tubes with lubricated stylets in place should be ready.

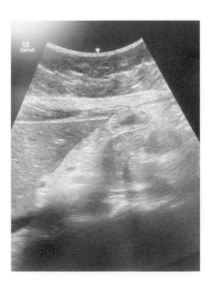

**Figure 68.1** Point of care gastric ultrasound to determine gastric volume before the induction of anesthesia. Image credit Luis Vargas Patron, MD.

Dark wedge (left) is the liver. White circle (right) is the gastric antrum.

## Airway Management

1. The best airway management for these full-stomach infants has been a matter of great debate.
2. Inhalational induction techniques following evacuation of the stomach contents via suctioning have generally been replaced by intravenous inductions in order to decrease the incidence of aspiration.
3. Induction of patients with pyloric stenosis has been historically hotly contested.
   a. Some anesthesiologists have recommended an awake tracheal intubation to maintain the protective airway reflexes due to concerns about undiagnosed airway abnormalities, risk of aspiration, and fear of desaturation following induction of anesthesia. However, awake endotracheal intubation is no longer recommended. Awake intubations have not been proven to prevent bradycardia, decrease arterial hemoglobin oxygen saturation, or even aspiration.
   b. Consensus advocates for a controlled, paralyzed tracheal intubation. This entails effective induction of sufficiently deep anesthesia, confirmation of complete muscle paralysis prior to tracheal intubation, and the use of gentle, pressure-limited mask ventilation (no more than 10–12 cm $H_2O$) with 100% oxygen.
   c. A controlled induction and intubation is favored over a rapid-sequence induction and intubation.
      i. Regurgitation and vomiting with potential aspiration are processes elicited by direct laryngoscopy under light anesthesia and incomplete muscle paralysis, which is more likely with a rapid sequence induction.
      ii. Neonates, infants, and small children have a reduced apnea tolerance in comparison with adults. This is due to the inability to sufficiently pre-oxygenate, a reduced functional residual capacity, and an increased oxygen demand.
      iii. Ensuring complete muscle paralysis and gentle ventilation prior to intubation results in significantly fewer episodes of hypoxemia and bradycardia, and has a higher rate of success with the first intubation attempt.

## Post-operative Apnea

1. There are many reports of apnea events following a pyloromyotomy.
   a. Patients are often less than 60 weeks post-conceptual age.
   b. It is thought that although the alkalemia is corrected, the cerebrospinal fluid alkalosis may take longer to correct and may play a role in post-operative ventilatory depression.
   c. For this reason, it is also wise to avoid administration of narcotics during the operative and post-operative periods.

   i. Pain control can often be adequately achieved with IV acetaminophen and the use of local anesthetic at the surgical site.

## KO Treatment Plan

### Pre-operative

1. Adequately volume-resuscitate the patient and replete electrolytes as needed. Usually a crystalloid solution containing sodium, chloride, potassium, and glucose is employed for slow correction of deficits.
2. Before proceeding with surgery, the patient's electrolytes **must** be normal!
   a. Normal electrolytes include a serum potassium level in the normal range (3.5–5.5 mEq/L) and a serum chloride level greater than 90 mEq/L or a urine chloride level greater than 20 mEq/L.
   b. Because the kidney will retain chloride as a result of volume contraction, a urine chloride greater than 20 mEq/L suggests that volume resuscitation has been adequate.
   c. Alkalosis should be corrected before surgery to a pH of 7.3–7.45.
3. This is a **medical**, not a surgical, emergency.
4. Assuming the patient is normovolemic with normal electrolytes, then proceed to the operating room.

### Intra-operative

1. Suction the stomach with a wide-bore catheter in the supine, right, and left lateral positions to remove as much of the stomach contents as possible.
2. Assuming the infant has a normal-appearing airway, some anesthesiologists will pre-treat with 20 µg/kg of atropine prior to induction of anesthesia. Intravenous anesthesia can be induced with propofol or another agent of choice, with either succinylcholine or an alternative nondepolarizing neuromuscular blocking drug.
3. Anesthesia is maintained with sevoflurane in a mixture of oxygen and air. Nitrous oxide is usually avoided because it can cause expansion of bowel gas. Isoflurane is associated with more episodes of post-operative apnea and longer recovery times than other agents, while desflurane is often unavailable and has negative environmental effects.
4. Additional doses of muscle relaxant are generally not indicated for the maintenance of anesthesia as this is a relatively short surgical procedure in which complete skeletal muscle relaxation is generally unnecessary.

### Post-operative

1. Extubate the patient when fully awake and displaying regular and adequate breathing patterns.
2. For pain control, acetaminophen can be administered intravenously or orally once the stomach can be used for oral intake.

3. Post-operative monitoring is vital.

   a. Persistence of electrolyte and fluid imbalances is possible.

   b. Often patients are less than 60 weeks post-conceptual age and are therefore more likely to exhibit post-operative ventilatory depression.

## Bibliography

Cook-Sather SD, Tulloch V, Cnaan A, et al. A comparison of awake versus paralyzed tracheal intubation for infants with pyloric stenosis. *Anesth Analg* 1998;**86**:945–51.

Craig R, Deeley A. Anaesthesia for pyloromyotomy. *BJA Edu.* 2018;**18**(6):173–7.

Engelhardt T. Rapid sequence induction has no use in pediatric anesthesia. *Pediatr Anesth* 2015;**25**:5–8.

Gagey AC, de Queiroz Siqueira M, Desgranges FP, et al. Ultrasound assessment of the gastric contents for the guidance of the anaesthetic strategy in infants with hypertrophic pyloric stenosis: a prospective cohort study. *BJA* 2016;**116**(5):649–54.

Jobson M, Hall NJ. Contemporary management of pyloric stenosis. *Semin Pediatr Surg* 2016;**25**:219–24.

Kamata M, Cartabuke RS, Tobias J. Perioperative care of infants with pyloric stenosis. *Pediatr Anesth* 2016;**25**:1193–206.

Litman RS. *Pediatric Anesthesia: The Requisites in Anesthesiology*, 1st ed. Philadelphia: Mosby, 2004, p. 233.

Schwartz D, Connelly NR, Manikantan P, Nichols JH. Hyperkalemia and pyloric stenosis. *Anesth Analg* 2003;**97**:355–7.

Stoelting RK, Dierdorf SF. *Anesthesia and Co-existing Disease*, 4th ed. Philadelphia: Churchill Livingstone, 2002, p. 700.

# Foreign Body Aspiration

Meaghan Fuhrmann

## Sample Case

A 2-year-old boy presents to the emergency department with new-onset irritability and coughing, and the parents report a sudden onset of difficulty breathing. The patient's parents deny history of asthma, recent fevers, or recent upper respiratory tract infection. The patient's parents report that he was in his usual state of health until an hour ago after he was found playing in his playroom alone. His temperature is 37.4 °C, heart rate 110 beats/min, respiratory rate 40 breaths/min, $SpO_2$ 85% on room air, and wheezing is noted on physical exam. What are your concerns? How will you induce anesthesia? Which inhaled anesthetic would you use and why? How would you maintain anesthesia for the procedure?

## Clinical Issues

1. Foreign body aspiration is a common event in children, and although it can occur at any age, it mostly presents in children from the ages of 6 months to 3 years.
2. Liquid aspiration is more commonly seen in infants, while solid food aspiration is more common in older children.
3. Even in the most stable patient, foreign body aspiration should be considered an emergency with the potential to progress to a life-threatening situation, and removal should not be delayed.
4. Rigid bronchoscopy remains the gold standard treatment for foreign body removal, and it is necessary for pre-operative intercommunication and planning between anesthesia and otolaryngology teams prior to the start of the procedure to allow for the best outcome for the patient.

## KO Treatment Plan

### Pre-operative

1. Asymptomatic and clinically stable patients with a suspected foreign body aspiration choking event should be sent for imaging.
   a. In the sample case, the patient stopped crying, his saturation improved, and he was stable enough to obtain an X-ray (Fig. 69.1).
   b. The X-ray showed that the child had ingested a screw and washer that was in the esophagus, but it could easily be coughed or vomited back into the airway.
   c. This case scenario requires an urgent procedure.

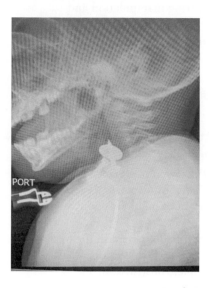

**Figure 69.1** X-ray of pediatric patient with a screw and washer located in the esophagus immediately distal to the laryngopharynx. Photo credit: MetroHealth Medical Center, Cleveland, Ohio.

2. Recommendations for removal in stable patients
   a. Bronchoscopy should be performed during daytime hours with experienced anesthesiologists and surgeons present under optimal conditions.
   b. Removal should not be delayed in unstable patients or to obtain images.

3. Be certain that all necessary bronchoscopes, endotracheal tubes, and emergency tracheotomy equipment are available.
   a. It is important to select the appropriately sized bronchoscope to avoid bronchospasm in this highly susceptible patient population.

4. A skilled otolaryngologist must be present and should always accompany an unstable patient once the diagnosis is suspected.
   a. Communication and planning of the procedure between both the otolaryngology and anesthesiology teams are necessary for best outcomes for the patient.

5. Concerns regarding a full stomach are theoretically reasonable as the children are not fasted. If the patient is stable, it is recommended to fast for 2 hours for liquids and 6 hours for solid food to decrease the risk of aspiration. If urgent or emergent removal is required, a gastric tube may be used to suction the stomach prior to induction of anesthesia to reduce the risk of aspiration.

## Intra-operative

1. Even if the child presents with intravascular access, it is easiest to maintain spontaneous ventilation with an inhalational induction.

   a. Be careful with preinduction sedatives (benzodiazepines) which may suppress the respiratory drive.

2. Steroids (dexamethasone 0.4–1 mg/kg) may be used to prevent airway edema during manipulation and bronchoscopy.

3. Administer nitrous oxide, oxygen, and sevoflurane for inhaled induction of anesthesia.

   a. Sevoflurane is preferred because it causes less irritation to the airways when compared to isoflurane and desflurane.

4. The child is permitted to deepen his/her level of anesthesia with spontaneous ventilation.

   a. A combination of IV (propofol, dexmedetomidine, ketamine) and inhaled anesthetics may be used; however, it is important to maintain spontaneous ventilation.

   b. Positive-pressure ventilation may push the foreign body further into the airway, converting a partial obstruction to a complete obstruction.

5. If the child did not present with IV access, access is now obtained, and standard ASA monitors placed.

6. With the patient deep and spontaneously ventilating, the otolaryngologist will perform a direct laryngoscopy and rigid bronchoscopy for examination of the airway and removal of the foreign object.

   a. It is appropriate to topicalize the epiglottis, vocal cords, and larynx with lidocaine prior to airway instrumentation to decrease the risk of laryngospasm and to maintain hemodynamic stability during the procedure.

7. Intubation may be necessary if airway control is needed emergently.

## Post-operative

1. The child should be observed closely immediately post-operatively, and after a short stay may be discharged home if no complications arise.

2. Admission and longer observation in a monitored unit may be necessary if the child suffered complications due to the initial foreign body aspiration or during the procedure.

   a. Examples of serious complications include laryngospasm, bronchospasm, complete airway obstruction with hypoxic episode, gastric content aspiration, pneumothorax, injury of the airway during removal of the object, and development of pneumonia.

## Bibliography

Bould MD. Essential notes: the anaesthetic management of an inhaled foreign body in a child. *BJA Edu* 2019;**19**(3):66–67.

Gropper MA. *Miller's Anesthesia*, 9th ed. Philadelphia: Elsevier, 2020, pp. 2552–3.

Kendigelen P. The anaesthetic consideration of tracheobronchial foreign body aspiration in children. *Journal of Thorac Dis* 2016;**8** (12):3803–7.

# Pheochromocytoma

**70**

Samuel DeJoy and Jessica A. Lovich-Sapola

## Sample Case

A 35-year-old male is admitted for resection of a pheochromocytoma, and you are consulted pre-operatively for management. His pre-operative hemodynamics are well controlled on metoprolol and phenoxybenzamine. What are your induction and maintenance plans? While the surgeon is resecting the tumor, the patient's mean arterial pressure (MAP) increases from 90 mm Hg to 160 mm Hg. How will you treat this? What can you use to prevent future episodes like this?

## Clinical Issues

### Definition

A pheochromocytoma is a catecholamine-producing, storing, and secreting tumor of ectodermal neural crest cell origin. Most tumors secrete norepinephrine and epinephrine, usually with norepinephrine as the major product. Pheochromocytomas are typically found in the adrenal medulla, but may develop in any area with chromaffin tissue. This can be anywhere from the skull base to the anus.

### Incidence

1. Pheochromocytomas are found in 0.005–0.1% of the population, with a peak occurrence in the third to fifth decade.
2. Traditional "Rule of 10s"
   a. 10% of pheochromocytomas are extramedullary (may be up to 24%).
   b. 10% of tumors are malignant (may be as high as 29%).
   c. 10% of tumors are bilateral adults and 25% are children.
   d. 10% are found in normotensive patients.
   e. 10–20% of patients have a familial history (may be up to 32%).
      i. 5% are inherited as a familial autosomal dominant trait.
3. 90% of the tumors are solitary, located in a single adrenal gland (usually right).
4. 95% are located in the abdomen with a small percentage in the thorax, bladder, or neck.
5. Pheochromocytomas account for 0.1% of all cases of diagnosed hypertension.

## Differential Diagnosis

1. Essential hypertension
2. Sympathetic stimulation: hypoxia, hypercarbia, pain, light anesthesia
3. Endocrine: thyroid storm, pheochromocytoma
4. Neurogenic: seizures, carotid sinus denervation, increased intracranial pressure
5. Renal disease: renal artery stenosis, nephritis
6. Miscellaneous: malignant hyperthermia, carcinoid syndrome, (pre)eclampsia

## Associated Syndromes

1. Von Hippel-Lindau disease: hemangioblastomas in retina, cerebellum, or other parts of the central nervous system and pheochromocytoma
2. Von Recklinghausen's neurofibromatosis: neurofibromas, café-au-lait spots, axillary freckling, optic nerve glioma, and pheochromocytoma
3. Multiple endocrine neoplasia (MEN) IIa: thyroid medullary carcinoma, pheochromocytoma, and parathyroid hyperplasia/adenoma
4. MEN IIb: thyroid medullary carcinoma, pheochromocytoma, mucosal neuromas, and marfanoid appearance

## Clinical Features

1. Classic triad of paroxysmal profuse sweating, palpitations/hypertension, and headache is more sensitive and specific than any laboratory test evaluating for pheochromocytoma.
2. Lethargy
3. Nausea
4. Weight loss
5. Pallor or flushing
6. Tremor
7. Anxiety
8. ST–T changes are often noted on EKG.
9. Catecholamine-induced cardiomyopathy occasionally manifests.
   a. Left ventricular (LV) hypertrophy can occur and progress to LV failure if the symptoms of the pheochromocytoma are not corrected.

b. Various forms of cardiomyopathy have been described, with hypertrophic cardiomyopathy as a result of chronic hypertension being the most frequent. There are also many case reports of inverted (atypical) Takotsubo cardiomyopathy.

10. Hyperglycemia reflects the β-effects of catecholamines and typically does not require insulin therapy.

11. Patients are often volume-depleted.

12. Hypomagnesemia and the associated dysrhythmias are often present.

13. Hypercalcemia is seen with MEN IIA patients with parathyroid adenoma.

## Triggers

1. Most pheochromocytomas are not under neurogenic control.

2. Physiologic factors affecting the pheochromocytoma

   a. Pain (this patient subset has been noted to have low pain tolerance)
   b. Light anesthesia
   c. Hypotension
   d. Hypoxia
   e. Hypercarbia
   f. Hypoglycemia
   g. Anger, fear, anxiety

3. Pharmacologic factors affecting the pheochromocytoma

   a. Direct and indirect sympathomimetics
   b. Histamine-releasing agents

## Diagnosis and Testing

1. 24-hour urine analysis for norepinephrine, epinephrine, dopamine, vanillylmandelic acid (VMA), and total metanephrines

   a. VMA is the metabolite of norepinephrine.
   b. Metanephrines are the products of epinephrine.

2. Total metanephrines have the highest true positive results at 98–99%.

3. If urine tests are negative or equivocal and a strong clinical suspicion exists, provocative testing can be performed with glucagon or suppression testing with clonidine.

   a. A three-fold increase in norepinephrine levels within 2 minutes after the glucagon is administered indicates a pheochromocytoma with high specificity.
   b. The clonidine suppression test is particularly useful in patients with increased plasma norepinephrine, in whom it is unclear whether the increase is due to sympathetic activation or catecholamine release from a tumor. Clonidine is administered, and a lack of a decrease in norepinephrine is highly suggestive of a pheochromocytoma.

4. Many patients are found to have died from complications of unknown pheochromocytoma at autopsy.

## Imaging

1. CT or MRI of the abdomen
2. Functional imaging (scintigraphy) is useful for extra-adrenal paragangliomas and pheochromocytomas.

## KO Treatment Plan

### Pre-operative (Table 70.1)

1. Identify tumor location(s) with imaging.

   a. Caution: dye used in arteriography can result in histamine release.

2. Pre-operative blood pressure control

   a. α-blockade

      i. Phenoxybenzamine

         (1) Nonselective, noncompetitive, long-acting α-blocker
         (2) May reduce the effects of catecholamine surges
         (3) May cause post-operative refractory (catecholamine-resistant) hypotension; therefore, it should be stopped 24–48 hours before surgery secondary to its long half-life
         (4) Side effects: reflex tachycardia, somnolence, headache, and nasal congestion

      ii. Doxazosin

         (1) Competitive, selective $\alpha_1$-blocker
         (2) Does not cause tachycardia or sedation
         (3) Reduced incidence of post-operative hypotension

   b. Calcium channel blockers (nicardipine)

      i. Inhibits norepinephrine-induced calcium influx
      ii. Used as an additional drug class to further improve control in those that are already α-blocked

   c. $\beta_1$-blockade (atenolol or metoprolol) may be considered but should not precede α-blockade.

      i. By blocking the β-receptors before the α-receptors, the unopposed α-effects may theoretically precipitate congestive heart failure.

**Table 70.1** Pre-operative preparation goals

Arterial blood pressure control
Reversal of chronic circulating volume depletion
Heart rate and arrhythmia control
Optimization of myocardial function
Reversal of glucose and electrolyte disturbances

d. Most patients receive 10–14 days of pretreatment and may be deemed ready for resection when there is:

i. No documented blood pressure above 160/90 mm Hg for 24 hours

ii. No demonstrated orthostatic hypotension

iii. No ST–T abnormalities on the EKG for 2 weeks

iv. There is no consensus on these criteria. Contemporary arterial pressure targets are tighter (seated arterial pressure of <130/80 mm Hg) and orthostatic hypotension is not a necessity. ST or T wave changes may reflect inverted Takotsubo cardiomyopathy rather than ischemia.

3. Consider pre-operative volume loading, as many patients with pheochromocytoma may be volume-depleted. Pre-operative optimization is of utmost importance. As α- and β-blockade are instituted, the patient is strongly encouraged to hydrate with oral electrolyte sport drinks.

a. The initiation of the α-blockade may reveal the volume depletion, if the volume depletion has not been properly treated.

4. Comorbid conditions related to pheochromocytoma, such as catecholamine-related cardiomyopathy, should be considered and appropriate pre-operative testing should be ordered.

5. Reversal of hyperglycemia

6. Reversal of hypercalcemia

## Intra-operative

1. Pre-operative sedation is essential.

2. General, regional, and combined techniques have all been described for intra-operative management.

3. Medications to avoid:

a. Desflurane
b. Ketamine
c. Morphine
d. Pethidine
e. Atracurium
f. Pancuronium
g. Ephedrine
h. Droperidol
i. Metoclopramide
j. Cocaine
k. Succinylcholine

4. In addition to standard ASA monitors, a pre-induction arterial line is highly recommended.

5. A pulmonary venous catheter and/or intra-operative transesophageal echocardiography can be placed as comorbid conditions dictate.

6. Short-acting hypotensive agents such as esmolol, sodium nitroprusside, nitroglycerin, and nicardipine infusions must be readily available.

7. Phentolamine is a reversible nonselective α-receptor antagonist, which primarily results in vasodilatation and can lead to reflex tachycardia. It is particularly useful to control surges in arterial pressure while establishing desired infusion rates of other drugs.

8. Intravenous lidocaine may blunt the response to laryngoscopy and decrease the incidence of arrhythmias.

9. Magnesium should be considered as a vasodilator and to control dysrhythmias.

a. It may also have analgesic properties.
b. Patients with pheochromocytoma are often magnesium-depleted.

10. Remifentanil is popular since it can be used to facilitate rapid titration and effect.

a. Good for blunting the hemodynamic response to pain, intubation, or abdominal insufflation

11. Induction should be a slow and careful process, regardless of the techniques or medications employed.

a. Adequate sedation and analgesia are required prior to intubation to minimize the sympathetic nervous system response to the airway manipulation.

12. Manipulation of the tumor may cause dramatic spikes in blood pressure and should be anticipated. If blood pressure spikes are extreme, ask the surgeon to pause tumor manipulation for a brief period to control the blood pressure spike.

a. A pneumoperitoneum, in the setting of a laparoscopic resection, may also cause increased catecholamine release.
b. Treat acute hypertensive crises with IV nitroprusside or phentolamine.
c. Tachydysrhythmia can be treated with infusion of the ultra-short-acting selective $\beta_1$-blocker esmolol.

i. Long-acting β-blockers should be avoided because the bradycardia and hypotension may persist after the tumor is removed.

13. Blood pressure may fall precipitously when the blood supply to the tumor is ligated during the surgical resection. Good surgical communication must occur at this critical period.

a. This can be controlled with adequate α-blockade and volume repletion prior to the ligation. Consider albumin and colloid expanders.
b. If hypotension still occurs, it should be treated with volume and IV phenylephrine, norepinephrine, or vasopressin.
c. Rule out surgical bleeding as the cause of the hypotension.
d. Monitor serum glucose frequently as hypoglycemia is a frequent result of lost β-stimulation.

14. Consider peri-operative glucocorticoid replacement, especially if both adrenals are removed.

## Post-operative

1. All patients should have invasive blood pressure monitoring for at least 24 hours after the procedure.

    a. Hypotension is often seen post-operatively. Hypovolemia and a decreased vasopressor response may be the cause, but bleeding should be considered.

    b. Persistent hypertension

        i. May signify incomplete tumor removal or metastatic disease

        ii. Pain

        iii. Co-existing essential hypertension

        iv. Urinary retention

        v. Fluid overload

        vi. Accidental ligation of the renal artery

2. Post-operative somnolence and decreased opioid requirements are frequently observed.

3. Hypoglycemia sometimes occurs after tumor removal when β-suppression is removed.

    a. Peri-operative glucose testing is mandatory.

    b. Glucose-containing IV fluids should be administered when indicated, and considered as a maintenance fluid.

4. Careful consideration should be given to the post-operative level of care; strongly consider a step-down unit minimally for observation overnight.

5. Intensive care unit monitoring is usually recommended.

6. Approximately 75% of patients become normotensive within 10 days of the surgery.

7. An uncommon post-operative complication is pulmonary edema from extreme blood pressure spikes and afterload increases that cause backflow through the mitral valve.

## Bibliography

Barash PG, Cullen BF, Stoelting RK, et al. *Clinical Anesthesia*, 8th ed. Philadelphia: Lippincott Williams & Wilkins, 2017, pp. 1340–3.

Conner D, Boumphrey S. Perioperative care of phaeochromocytoma. *BJA Edu* 2016;**16** (5):153–8.

Fleisher LA. *Anesthesia and Uncommon Diseases*, 5th ed. Philadelphia: Saunders Elsevier, 2006, pp. 440–3.

Yao Fsf. *Yao and Artusio's Anesthesiology*, 6th ed. Philadelphia: Lippincott Williams and Wilkins, 2008, pp. 767–81.

# Hyperthyroidism

Jessica A. Lovich-Sapola

## Sample Case

A 20-year-old female presents with untreated thyrotoxicosis for an emergency surgery. Her blood pressure is 180/100 mm Hg, pulse 125, and temperature 38 °C. What are her anesthetic risks? Would you do anything pre-operatively? Would a regional or general anesthetic be safer? How would you proceed if she refuses a regional anesthetic?

## Clinical Issues

### Definition

1. Hyperthyroidism is a spectrum of disorders that involve increased circulating blood levels of thyroid hormone. The spectrum ranges from an asymptomatic elevation in laboratory values to life-threatening multisystem organ dysfunction.
2. Thyroid storm
   a. Life-threatening exacerbation of hyperthyroidism
   b. Usually develops in the undiagnosed or untreated hyperthyroid patient because of the stress of surgery or a nonthyroid illness
   c. Symptoms
      i. Hyperpyrexia
      ii. Tachycardia
      iii. Dysrhythmias
      iv. Myocardial ischemia
      v. Congestive heart failure
      vi. Agitation and confusion
      vii. Hypotension
   d. Treatment
      i. Large doses of propylthiouracil (PTU)
      ii. Supportive measures to control the fever
         (1) Cooling blankets
         (2) Acetaminophen
      iii. IV fluids to restore intravascular volume
      iv. Sodium iodide
      v. Hydrocortisone
      vi. Meperidine to reduce shivering
      vii. Give digoxin for heart failure if the patient develops atrial fibrillation with a rapid ventricular response.
      viii. Propranolol or esmolol

## Incidence

1. Hyperthyroidism affects 0.2% of males and 2% of females.
2. Hyperthyroidism occurs in 0.2% of all pregnancies.

## Etiology

1. Graves' disease
   a. Most common etiology
   b. Autoimmune pathogenesis with diffuse goiter and ophthalmopathy
   c. IgG antibodies have effects similar to long-acting thyrotropin (thyroid stimulating hormone, TSH).
   d. Placental transfer is possible.
   e. Remits during pregnancy and is exacerbated after delivery.
2. Thyroid adenoma
3. Toxic multinodular goiter
4. Thyroiditis
5. Pregnancy
6. Pituitary tumors secreting TSH
7. Exogenous iodide exposure
8. Factitious illness
9. Thyroid cancer
10. Choriocarcinoma
11. Overdose of thyroid medication

## Signs and Symptoms

1. Anxiety or emotional instability
2. Exophthalmos
3. Diarrhea
4. Weight loss despite high caloric consumption
5. Increased bone resorption and hypercalciuria
6. Muscle weakness and fatigue
7. Heat intolerance
8. Mitral valve prolapse
9. Worsening angina or congestive heart failure
10. Atrial fibrillation or tachycardia
11. Hypertension
12. Increased cardiac output
13. Increased serum cortisol levels
14. Hyperactive reflexes

## Differential Diagnosis

1. Thyroid storm
2. Pheochromocytoma
3. Carcinoid syndrome
4. Malignant hyperthermia
5. Neuroleptic malignant syndrome
6. Anxiety
7. Infection
8. Cocaine intoxication
9. Strychnine poisoning
10. Anticholinergic exposure

## Testing

1. Decreased levels of TSH: presence of a normal level almost always excludes a diagnosis of hyperthyroidism.
2. Increased plasma levels of tetraiodothyronine (thyroxine, $T_4$)
3. If the TSH level is low and the $T_4$ is normal, evaluate the triiodothyronine ($T_3$) level for $T_3$ thyrotoxicosis.
4. Diagnosis during pregnancy is difficult because $T_4$-binding globulins are increased and thereby increase circulating $T_4$ concentrations.

## Hyperthyroidism Treatment

1. The most important goal is to make the patient euthyroid before any surgical procedure.
2. Nonemergent
   a. Antithyroid medications which inhibit thyroid hormone synthesis: can take 6–8 weeks
      i. Propylthiouracil (PTU)
         (1) Black box warning: risk of acute liver failure and death
         (2) Preferred in pregnancy
      ii. Methimazole
   b. Prevent hormone release
      i. Potassium
      ii. Sodium iodide
   c. Mask the signs of adrenergic overactivity with β-adrenergic antagonists
      i. Propranolol
   d. Radioactive iodine ($^{131}I$) destroys the thyroid cell function.
      i. Not safe during pregnancy
      ii. May result in hypothyroidism
   e. Surgery to remove the thyroid
   f. Glucocorticoids
      i. Used in the management of severe thyrotoxicosis

      ii. Reduce thyroid hormone secretion
      iii. Reduce the peripheral conversion of $T_4$ to $T_3$
3. Emergent
   a. β-blockers including propranolol
      i. Used to treat symptoms including rapid heart rate, sweating, and anxiety
      ii. β-blockers do not prevent thyroid storm.

# KO Treatment Plan

## Pre-operative

1. Elective surgery should be delayed in patients with poorly controlled hyperthyroidism. The patient should be clinically and chemically euthyroid.
   a. Normal $T_3$ and $T_4$ concentrations
   b. No resting tachycardia
2. Assess for airway compromise from an obstructing thyroid gland.
   a. Pre-operative CT or MRI can show mediastinal extension of the thyroid gland.
3. Consider judicious pre-medication with benzodiazepines, if indicated, to reduce the hemodynamic effects of anxiety.
4. Continue antithyroid medications through the morning of surgery.
5. Avoid the pre-operative use of atropine, scopolamine, and ketamine secondary to the associated tachycardia.
   a. Anticholinergics may cause tachycardia and further derangements in temperature regulation.

## Intra-operative

1. Consider pre-operative placement of an arterial line.
2. Blood gas and electrolyte levels should be monitored aggressively.
3. Large-bore peripheral IVs should be placed in patients with symptomatic thyrotoxicosis or thyroid storm.
4. Avoid ketamine.
5. MAC of volatile agents is not affected by hyperthyroidism but may appear so owing to the associated increase in cardiac output.
6. Exophthalmos warrants extra attention to eye protection.
7. Thyroid storm must be treated as soon as it is suspected and before lab values return.
8. Cooling may be necessary with cold lavage of body cavities, ice, and cooling blankets.
9. Consider a pre-induction central line and/or pulmonary artery catheter if the patient has a history of congestive heart failure, myocardial ischemia, pulmonary hypertension, renal failure, or significant hemodynamic instability.
10. Patients presenting for an emergent surgery may likely require a rapid-sequence endotracheal intubation.

A multi-tiered approach to airway management should be in place with all equipment present before induction. A reinforced endotracheal tube should be considered.

    a.   Avoid pancuronium because of the associated tachycardia.

11. The patient's hemodynamics should be appropriately treated before induction, so as to avoid the perils of extreme hyper- or hypotension during and immediately after laryngoscopy.

    a.   High-output heart failure may improve with β-blockers.

    b.   Short-acting agents such as nitroglycerine, nitroprusside, nicardipine, and esmolol should be used in treating the peri-operative blood pressure.

12. Sympathomimetic drugs used to treat hypotension may have an exaggerated effect and there is a theoretic concern that indirect sympathomimetics, such as ephedrine, may have lessened effect secondary to catecholamine depletion.

13. Regional anesthesia has the benefit of blocking the sympathetic nervous system. In patients without high-output heart failure, a regional anesthetic is a viable option. An epidural without epinephrine may be preferable to a spinal anesthetic because of its slower onset and less severe hemodynamic perturbations.

14. Choosing a regional anesthetic in an emergent procedure is situation-dependent, and the choice must take into consideration an unsecured airway, fluid shifts, and the location of the procedure.

## Post-operative

1. The decision to extubate should be based on the global clinical picture and the difficulty encountered during the initial intubation.

2. If there is concern for airway collapse, extubating over a fiber-optic bronchoscope and directly observing airway patency may be considered.

3. Thyroid storm typically does not occur in the operating room, but rather 6–24 hours after surgery. Patient disposition should be carefully considered.

4. Aspirin should be avoided because it raises free thyroid hormone levels by displacing some of the protein-bound fraction.

## Bibliography

Barash PG, Cullen BF, Stoelting RK, et al. *Clinical Anesthesia*, 8th ed. Philadelphia: Lippincott Williams & Wilkins, 2017, pp. 1327–31.

Butterworth JF, Mackey DC, Wasnick JD. *Morgan & Mikhail's Clinical Anesthesiology*, 6th ed. New York: McGraw-Hill Education, 2018, pp. 759–60.

Fleisher LA. *Anesthesia and Uncommon Diseases*, 5th ed. Philadelphia: Saunders Elsevier, 2006, pp. 440–3.

Stoelting, RK. *Anesthesia and Co-existing Disease*, 4th ed. Philadelphia: Churchill Livingstone, 2002, pp. 411–17.

Yao, FSF. *Yao and Artusio's Anesthesiology*, 6th ed. Philadelphia: Lippincott Williams and Wilkins, 2008, pp. 753–66.

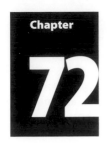

# Chapter 72

# Hypothyroidism

Jessica A. Lovich-Sapola

## Sample Case

A patient is scheduled for an emergency drainage of an abscess. Hypothyroidism was diagnosed 12 hours ago during her emergency room admission. Her total thyroxine ($T_4$) is less than 2 µg/dL (normal values are 4.5–10 µg/dL) and her thyroid-stimulating hormone (TSH) level is elevated. What are your anesthetic concerns? What anesthetic would you choose? What specific post-operative complications would you expect?

## Clinical Issues

### Definition

1. Hypothyroidism is a common endocrine disorder resulting from inadequate circulating levels of triiodothyronine ($T_3$), $T_4$, or both.
2. It is typically a primary process in which the thyroid gland produces insufficient amounts of thyroid hormone despite adequate TSH production.
3. It can also be secondary or tertiary.
   a. Secondary hypothyroidism occurs when the anterior pituitary gland does not produce enough TSH.
   b. Tertiary hypothyroidism occurs when the hypothalamus fails to produce enough thyrotropin-releasing hormone (TRH).
4. Patient presentation ranges from asymptomatic to comatose with multisystem organ failure.

### Incidence

1. 4.6% of the population is hypothyroid as defined by TSH levels (0.32% overt and 4.3% subclinical).
2. 1:4000 newborns are affected by congenital hypothyroidism (cretinism).
3. Hashimoto's thyroiditis is the most common presentation in the United States.
   a. Initial inflammation of the thyroid causes the release of excess thyroid hormone (hyperthyroidism).
   b. Over time, the inflammation prevents the thyroid from producing enough hormones (hypothyroidism).

### Etiology

1. Chronic thyroiditis (Hashimoto's disease)
   a. Chronic autoimmune disease that results in a progressive destruction of the thyroid
   b. The thyroid becomes enlarged and potentially distorts or obstructs the airway.
   c. Most common form of primary hypothyroidism in the United States
2. Iatrogenic
   a. Neck or brain irradiation
   b. Subtotal/total thyroidectomy
   c. Radioiodine therapy or severe iodine depletion
   d. Medications: amiodarone, methimazole, iodines, propylthiouracil, dopamine, and lithium
3. Genetic defects in hormone synthesis
4. Congenital defects in thyroid development
5. Anterior pituitary damage or destruction: Sheehan's syndrome
6. Hypothalamic dysfunction

### Differential Diagnosis

1. Addison's disease
2. Sleep apnea
3. Chronic fatigue syndrome
4. Depression
5. Fibromyalgia
6. Infectious mononucleosis
7. Iodine deficiency
8. Lymphoma
9. Syndrome of inappropriate antidiuretic hormone (SIADH)

### Signs and Symptoms

1. Fatigue and memory impairment
2. Hypothermia and cold intolerance
3. Depression and emotional lability
4. Weight gain and decreased appetite
5. Slowed speech and movements
6. Dry skin, coarse hair, or hair loss
7. Macroglossia
8. Goiter and hoarseness
9. May see systemic hypertension with a narrowed pulse pressure
10. Bradycardia

11. Pericardial effusion
12. Nonpitting edema (myxedema)
13. Hyporeflexia with delayed relaxation
14. Blurred vision
15. Nerve entrapment
16. Infertility
17. Constipation

## Testing

1. The measured TSH concentration is high when compared to the relatively low blood levels of $T_3$ or $T_4$ with primary hypothyroidism.
2. Reverse triiodothyronine uptake ($RT_3 U$) can be used to calculate the thyroid binding ratio. When multiplied by total $T_4$, the free $T_4$ estimate is obtained. This correlates closely with the metabolic status of the patient.
3. Serum thyroxine by radioimmunoassay ($T_4$-RIA) can yield the serum level of $T_4$.

   a. Normal values are 4.5–10 µg/dL.
   b. Since most $T_4$ is bound to thyroid binding-globulin (TBG), processes that affect TBG levels can affect total $T_4$ levels.

      i. Androgens, hypoproteinemia, and nephrosis can lower the TBG and thus $T_4$ since free $T_4$ is less stable.

4. Free serum triiodothyronine by radioimmunoassay ($T_3$-RIA) can detect serum levels of $T_3$, normally 75–200 ng/dL.

   a. The upper limit of normal declines with age.

## Clinical Features

1. Because lethargy and fatigue are common in hypothyroid patients, hypothyroidism is often not diagnosed until pre-operative testing since there may be a lack of motivation to see a primary care physician.
2. Cardiovascular changes are often the earliest clinical manifestation.

   a. Systolic and diastolic myocardial functions are impaired, and patients can occasionally experience congestive heart failure.
   b. The EKG may show prolonged PR, QRS, and QT intervals due to pericardial effusions.
   c. Torsades de pointes is possible.

3. Cortisol deficiency is possible secondary to the associated adrenal cortex atrophy.
4. The patient may be unable to excrete free water, leading to SIADH.

   a. Fluids should be replaced judiciously, as these patients are prone to hyponatremia.

5. Myxedema coma: medical emergency with a high mortality of up to 25–50%

   a. Rare
   b. Symptoms

      i. Loss of deep tendon reflexes
      ii. Hypothermia
      iii. Hypoventilation
      iv. Hyponatremia
      v. Hemodynamic instability
      vi. Congestive heart failure
      vii. Coma
      viii. Death

6. Hypothyroid patients with coronary artery disease are difficult to manage because establishing a euthyroid state may exacerbate angina.

   a. Coronary revascularization may be considered emergent in some circumstances.
   b. Thyroid replacement therapy must be cautiously undertaken.

## Myxedema Coma Treatment

1. Admit the patient to the ICU.
2. Correct hypovolemia and electrolyte abnormalities.
3. Intravenous (IV) levothyroxine ($T_4$) and liothyronine ($T_3$)
4. Rule out an infectious cause of the myxedema coma and treat with the appropriate antibiotics.
5. Give hydrocortisone 100 mg IV then repeat 25 mg IV every 6 hours.
6. Tracheal intubation and controlled ventilation as needed
7. Conserve body heat.
8. ECG monitoring

## Hypothyroidism Treatment

1. Nonemergent

   a. Levothyroxine (Synthroid) tablet
   b. IV or intramuscular (IM) dosing can be given if the oral route is precluded for long periods of time.
   c. Symptomatic treatment

# KO Treatment Plan

## Pre-operative

1. Elective surgery should probably be delayed for severe, symptomatic hypothyroidism to avoid the numerous associated peri-operative problems.

   a. Intra-operative hypotension
   b. Heart failure during cardiac surgery
   c. Gastrointestinal complications
   d. Neuropsychiatric complications

2. There is little reason to postpone an elective procedure in a patient with mild to moderate hypothyroidism.

   a. There has been no associated increase in blood loss, arrhythmias, hypothermia, hyponatremia, delayed recovery, poor wound healing, pulmonary complications, and/or hospital duration when studies have compared hypothyroid and euthyroid perioperative complications.

3. For elective procedures, patients should take their thyroid supplementation despite the long half-life of thyroxine.

4. Pre-operative cortisol supplementation should be considered because of the co-existing adrenal insufficiency.

5. Cautious pre-medication with opioids and benzodiazepines is advised due to a theoretical concern of increased sedation and respiratory depression.

6. A patient with severe uncorrected hypothyroidism requiring an emergent surgery should be treated with IV $T_3$ just prior to the induction of anesthesia.

## Intra-operative

1. The induction of anesthesia should be accomplished with a drug that has minimal hemodynamic affects.

   a. Ketamine has been considered the ideal induction drug in these patients because it increases myocardial contractility, heart rate, and systemic vascular resistance, which may be detrimentally lowered in the hypothyroid patient.

   b. Etomidate is also recommended as an option for induction.

   c. However, any induction drug can be used if given in a cautious and judicious manner.

2. Despite an elevated level of serum catecholamines, there is no evidence of a decreased response to exogenous catecholamines.

3. Volatile anesthetics should be titrated carefully due to the risk of cardiac depression.

4. The MAC is unaffected by hypothyroidism. It may appear decreased owing to a decrease in cardiac output (which may speed the rate of induction with an inhaled anesthetic) or due to the associated hypothermia.

5. Decreased production of $CO_2$ can make these patients prone to hypoventilation.

6. Use of an arterial line should be guided by the patient's clinical status and the procedure being performed.

7. Other intra-operative complications may include:

   a. Difficult intubation secondary to an enlarged tongue
   b. Hypoglycemia
   c. Anemia
   d. Hyponatremia
   e. Hypothermia

## Post-operative

1. Recovery from sedation may be prolonged and an extended post-anesthesia care unit stay may be required.

2. The inability to wean from mechanical ventilation may be due to over-sedation and hypothermia.

3. Despite the many concerns intra- and post-operatively, there is no evidence to suggest that patients with mild to moderate hypothyroidism experience more profound hypothermia or hypotension, require more cardiovascular support with vasopressors or inotropes, or need more post-operative ventilator support than a euthyroid patient.

## Bibliography

Barash PG, Cullen BF, Stoelting RK, et al. *Clinical Anesthesia*, 8th ed. Philadelphia: Lippincott Williams & Wilkins, 2017, pp. 1331–2.

Butterworth JF, Mackey DC, Wasnick JD. *Morgan & Mikhail's Clinical Anesthesiology*, 6th ed. New York: McGraw-Hill Education, 2018, pp. 760–1.

Fleisher LA. *Anesthesia and Uncommon Diseases*, 5th ed. Philadelphia: Saunders Elsevier, 2006, pp. 440–3.

Seeley RR, Stephens TD, Tate P. *Anatomy and Physiology*, 8th ed. New York: McGraw-Hill, 2008, p. 621.

# Peri-operative Diabetes Management

Zaid H. Jumaily and Jessica A. Lovich-Sapola

## Sample Case

A 19-year-old female is scheduled for a septoplasty. She is a type I diabetic. She says that her blood glucose is controlled by an insulin pump. Her endocrinologist is from an outside hospital. What are the pre-operative concerns? What labs would you request? What is your anesthetic plan?

## Clinical Issues

### Incidence of Diabetes Mellitus

1. Affects about 7–10% of the population of the United States
2. About 15–25% of hospitalized patients are diabetic, according to the American Diabetes Association.
3. Diabetics undergo surgery at a higher rate than nondiabetics.
4. Peri-operative morbidity and mortality are higher in diabetics.
   a. Tighter inpatient glycemic control tends to decrease the incidence of:
      i. Morbidity and mortality
      ii. Bloodstream infections
      iii. Acute renal failure
      iv. Transfusion requirements
      v. Critical illness polyneuropathy
5. More than 90% of diabetics are considered to be type II diabetics.
   a. Elderly
   b. Overweight
   c. Minority ethnicity
   d. Lower socioeconomic background
6. About 3–5% of pregnant women develop gestational diabetes.

### Etiology

1. Genetic susceptibility
2. Environmental triggers
3. Autoimmune

## Diagnostic Criteria According to the American Diabetes Association

1. Symptoms of diabetes plus a random glucose level >200 mg/dL
2. Fasting plasma glucose level >126 mg/dL
3. Two-hour plasma glucose level >200 mg/dL during an oral glucose tolerance test
4. Hemoglobin (Hb) A1c >6.5%

## Classification

1. Primary
   a. Diabetes mellitus type I
      i. Absolute deficiency in insulin production
         (1) Pancreatic β-cell failure
      ii. These patients will die without insulin secondary to the development of ketoacidosis.
      iii. Onset usually before age 30
      iv. Autoimmune destruction of the islet cells in the pancreas
   b. Diabetes mellitus type II
      i. Combination of:
         (1) Relative deficiency in insulin
         (2) Insulin resistance
         (3) Increased glucose production
      ii. Milder form
      iii. Affects all ages
      iv. Usually can be treated with diet, exercise, and oral hypoglycemic agents.
      v. These individuals are not as high risk for ketoacidosis.
2. Secondary
   a. Pancreatic disease
   b. Hormonal abnormalities
   c. Drug or chemically induced
   d. Insulin receptor abnormalities
   e. Genetic syndrome

3. Gestational diabetes

   a. Glucose intolerance first recognized in pregnancy

   b. Complicates about 4% of all pregnancies in the United States

4. Syndrome X (metabolic syndrome)

   a. Insulin resistance with hyperinsulinemia

   b. Rarely have hyperglycemia

## Complications

1. End-organ pathology secondary to chronic hyperglycemia

   a. Diabetic nephropathy leading to end-stage renal disease

   b. Cardiac

      i. Coronary artery disease

         (1) Myocardial infarction

         (2) Diabetes is an independent risk factor in post-operative myocardial ischemia among patients undergoing cardiac and noncardiac surgery.

      ii. Hypertension

      iii. Cardiac autonomic neuropathy

      iv. Microangiopathic cardiomyopathy

   c. Stroke

   d. Polyneuropathy

   e. Stiff joints

   f. Retinopathy

   g. Increased risk of infections

   h. Hypo-/hyperglycemia

   i. Diabetic ketoacidosis (DKA)

   j. Nonketotic hyperosmolar coma

   k. Compromised wound healing

## Treatment

1. Diabetes mellitus type I

   a. Exogenous insulin

      i. Rapid-acting

         (1) Insulin lispro injection (Humalog): not recommended to be given intravenously (IV)

            (a) Onset: 15–30 minutes (subcutaneous [SC])

            (b) Peak: 30–90 minutes (SC)

            (c) Duration 3–5 hours (SC)

         (2) Regular (Humulin, Novolin)

            (a) Onset: 15 minutes (IV) and 30–60 minutes (SC)

            (b) Peak: 15–30 minutes (IV) and 2–5 hours (SC)

            (c) Duration: 30–60 minutes (IV) and 8–12 hours (SC)

      ii. Intermediate-acting

         (1) Isophane (NPH)

            (a) Onset: 1–4 hours (SC)

            (b) Peak: 4–14 hours (SC)

            (c) Duration: 10–24 hours (SC)

      iii. Insulin analog

         (1) Glargine (Lantus)

            (a) Onset: 1–2 hours (SC)

            (b) Peak: none (constant concentration over 24 hours)

            (c) Duration: 24 hours (SC)

         (2) Aspart (Novolog)

            (a) Onset: 5–15 minutes (SC)

            (b) Peak: 1 hour (SC)

            (c) Duration: 2–4 hours (SC)

2. Diabetes mellitus type II

   a. Lifestyle modification

      i. Dietary modification

      ii. Exercise

      iii. Weight loss

   b. Oral hypoglycemic drugs

      i. Insulin secretagogues: stimulate insulin secretion.

         (1) Sulfonylureas (short-acting: glyburide, glipizide)

      ii. Biguanides: reduce hepatic glucose production and improve glucose utilization.

         (1) Metformin (often first-line therapy unless contraindicated)

            (a) Contraindication: renal failure secondary to the increased risk of lactic acidosis

      iii. α-glucosidase inhibitors: reduce postprandial hyperglycemia by delaying glucose absorption.

         (1) Miglitol/acarbose

      iv. Thiazolidinediones: reduce insulin resistance by binding to receptors in the nucleus of adipocytes.

         (1) Pioglitazone/rosiglitazone

      v. Glucagon-like peptide 1 (GLP-1) receptor agonists: daily/weekly injections, reduces weight and major adverse cardiovascular events.

         (1) Liraglutide/semaglutide/dulaglutide

      vi. Dipeptidyl peptidase 4 (DPP-4) inhibitor

         (1) Sitagliptin, saxagliptin, linagliptin, alogliptin

vii. Meglitinide (repaglinide): increases secretion of endogenous insulin by binding ATP-dependent $K^+$ channels of pancreatic beta cells.

viii. Pramlintide: amylin analog injected alongside insulin

c. Exogenous insulin

3. New therapies

   a. Transplantation of pancreatic tissue
   b. Islet cell transplant
   c. Immunosuppression
   d. Inhaled insulin

## Factors That Increase Endogenous Insulin Requirements

1. High-carbohydrate diet

   a. Total parenteral nutrition
   b. Tube feeds
   c. Dextrose-containing IV fluids

2. Infection
3. Sepsis
4. Stress
5. Medications

   a. Corticosteroids
   b. Thyroid preparations
   c. Oral contraceptives
   d. Thiazide diuretics
   e. Atypical antipsychotics
   f. Lithium
   g. Protease inhibitors
   h. Rifampin
   i. Phenytoin
   j. Medications mixed with dextrose-containing solutions

## Factors That Decrease Endogenous Insulin Requirements

1. Exercise
2. Coumadin
3. Decreased carbohydrate intake

   a. Fasting
   b. Nausea and vomiting

## Diagnosis and Treatment of Diabetic Ketoacidosis (DKA)

1. Acute medical emergency
2. Symptoms

   a. Acute abdominal pain
   b. Nausea and vomiting
   c. Lethargy
   d. Signs of hypovolemia

3. Absolute or relative deficiency of insulin that results in ketone acids in the blood

   a. Hyperglycemia
   b. Glucosuria
   c. Intracellular dehydration
   d. Acidosis
   e. Electrolyte imbalance

4. Diagnosis

   a. Serum ketone acids >7 mmol/L
   b. Decrease in serum bicarbonate to <10 mEq/L
   c. Decrease in pH level to <7.25

5. Labs that should be ordered

   a. Urinalysis
   b. Glucose level
   c. Serum electrolytes to determine the anion gap
   d. Serum ketone estimation
   e. Urea nitrogen level
   f. Complete blood cell count
   g. Arterial blood gas: acid–base balance

6. Treatment

   a. Fluids

      i. Restore intravascular volume

         (1) Start with 1 L of normal saline and continue an IV infusion of normal saline.

            (a) 0.45% normal saline should be used if the patient's osmolality is elevated.

         (2) 5% dextrose IV should be started once the serum glucose falls below 250–300 mg/dL to prevent secondary hypoglycemia.

      ii. Fluid therapy should be guided by urine output and central venous pressure monitoring if available.

   b. Insulin

      i. Regular insulin 10–20 units (or 0.2 units/kg) IV should be given initially.
      ii. Infusion of 1–2 units of regular insulin per hour (or 0.1 unit/kg/h) should be started, depending on the serum glucose level.
      iii. Goal rate of glucose level reduction should not exceed 50 mg/dL/h.

         (1) A rapid rate of reduction can lead to cerebral edema.

   c. Sodium bicarbonate

      i. Used to correct severe metabolic acidosis (pH <7.20)

   d. Potassium

      i. Potassium stores are often depleted.

ii. Serum potassium levels will decrease as a result of:

    (1) Hemodilution

    (2) The correction of acidosis results in the movement of potassium from the extracellular space to the intracellular space.

iii. Potassium should be added to the IV fluids 3–4 hours after the initiation of therapy.

e. Treat the underlying condition.

    i. Antibiotics for sepsis

## Diagnosis and Treatment of Nonketotic Hyperosmolar Coma

1. Syndrome of profound dehydration
2. Usually seen in patients with type II diabetes when they are unable to drink enough fluids to keep up with urinary losses secondary to glycosuria.
3. No ketoacidosis
4. Presents with:
   a. Extreme hyperglycemia: upwards of 1000 mg/dL
   b. Hyperosmolality
   c. Volume depletion
   d. Mental status changes
5. Mortality rate is around 50%.
6. Treatment
   a. Rapid administration of large amounts of IV fluid
   b. Insulin
   c. Dextrose
   d. Potassium

## Hypoglycemia

1. Blood glucose <50 mg/dL
2. Complications of hypoglycemia
   a. Arrhythmias: bradycardia
   b. Hypotension
   c. Seizures
   d. Irritability
   e. Cognitive defects
   f. Respiratory failure
   g. Death
3. Risk factors for hypoglycemia
   a. Decreased oral intake
   b. Renal insufficiency
   c. Liver disease
   d. Infection
   e. Pregnancy
   f. Cancer
   g. Burns
   h. Adrenal insufficiency

4. Risk factors for hypoglycemic unawareness
   a. β-blockade
   b. Sedation
   c. Advanced age
   d. Long history of diabetes
   e. Diabetic neuropathy
5. Treatment
   a. 15 g of fast-acting carbohydrate
      i. 4 oz of fruit juice or soda
      ii. 25 mL (one ampule) of 50% dextrose IV push
   b. Recheck the blood glucose after 15 minutes.
   c. Repeat the glucose administration if the glucose level is <80 mg/dL.
   d. Repeat the blood glucose check 60 minutes after the last glucose administration.

## Acute Hyperglycemia

1. Consequences
   a. Impaired wound healing
   b. Dehydration
      i. Osmotic diuretic effect of high-serum glucose levels
   c. Impaired immune system response
      i. Increased risk of post-operative infection
   d. Proteolysis

**TKO:** Anesthetic considerations:
1. Diabetes affects oxygen transport and can present with decreased oxygen saturation, especially in pregnant patients.
2. Commonly present with autonomic dysfunction
   a. Intra-operative hypothermia
   b. Inability to regulate blood pressure: orthostatic hypotension
3. Increased risk of coronary artery disease
   a. Patients more likely to have "silent cardiac ischemia."
   b. Consider peri-operative β-blocker therapy.
4. Delayed gastric emptying
   a. Diabetics should be considered to have a "full stomach."
5. More likely to have cerebrovascular accidents and peripheral vascular disease
6. The altered consciousness of anesthesia may mask the symptoms of hypoglycemia.

## Importance of Strict Glucose Control

1. Prevents DKA
2. Prevents hyper-/hypoglycemia

3. Prevents dehydration
4. Improves wound healing

## Serum Glucose Goals

1. Serum blood glucose <110 mg/dL in the ICU setting
2. Serum blood glucose <180 mg/dL in the non-ICU setting

   a. Pre-prandial blood glucose should be <110 mg/dL.

## KO Treatment Plan

### Pre-operative

1. Diabetes can affect every organ system.
2. Perform a complete history and physical examination.

   a. Evaluate the patient for symptoms of polyuria/polydipsia, and blurred vision.

   b. Cardiac history: asymptomatic cardiac ischemia is common.

      i. EKG
      ii. Stress test (as needed)
      iii. Echocardiography (as needed)

   c. Autonomic neuropathy

      i. Orthostatic hypotension
      ii. Lack of sweating
      iii. Early satiety
      iv. Gastroparesis

         (1) Gastric reflux
         (2) Nausea/vomiting
         (3) Regurgitation
         (4) Aspiration

      v. Lack of change in pulse with deep inspiration
      vi. Resting tachycardia
      vii. Painless myocardial ischemia

   d. Peripheral neuropathy
   e. Syncope
   f. Erectile or bladder dysfunction
   g. Cerebrovascular disease
   h. Renal dysfunction
   i. Airway exam

      i. Stiff joint syndrome

         (1) Limited atlanto-occipital joint mobility
         (2) Limited temporomandibular joint mobility
         (3) Limited cervical spine mobility
         (4) Positive prayer sign

      ii. Associated obesity

3. Check a HbA1c to determine the patient's chronic level of control.

   a. Used to assess the glucose level over the past 2–3 months
   b. A value >9% is an indicator of very poor control.

4. Check basic electrolytes and renal function tests.
5. Urinalysis for detecting glucose and ketones
6. Complete blood count
7. Arterial blood gas to determine acid–base status
8. Last intake of a meal?
9. Last dose of insulin?
10. Type I diabetics should be the first case of the day in order to disrupt their treatment regimen as little as possible.
11. Check the serum glucose and repeat again immediately pre-operatively.
12. If time allows, talk with the patient's endocrinologist about the preferred peri-operative diabetes management for the patient.

### Pre-operative Preparation

1. Diet-controlled diabetic

   a. Pre-operative fasting blood glucose on the morning of surgery
   b. Repeat check every 3 hours until oral intake is resumed.
   c. If the surgery is major or the patient has very poorly controlled blood glucose (>200 mg/dL), an IV infusion of insulin and dextrose should be considered.

      i. Hourly glucose monitoring

2. Diabetics requiring medical treatment

   a. Type II diabetic not taking insulin

      i. Discontinue or decrease the dose of the oral hypoglycemic agents 1–2 days pre-operatively (this should be determined by the prescribing practitioner).
      ii. Omit the morning dose of the oral hypoglycemic drugs.
      iii. Discontinue metformin at least 24 hours before surgery.

         (1) Metformin possesses a risk for the development of lactic acidosis.
         (2) It should be stopped 24 hours before and for at least 48 hours after any procedure using IV contrast dye.
         (3) Avoid completely in patients with renal dysfunction, congestive heart failure, recent myocardial infarction, any hypoxic state, current alcohol abuse, or impaired hepatic function.

      iv. Serum glucose should be checked immediately before and after the surgery.

         (1) For minor surgery, a blood glucose >200 mg/dL can be treated with 4–10 units of regular insulin subcutaneously.
         (2) For major surgery (lasting greater than 1 hour), IV insulin infusions should be

used with more frequent blood sugar checks.

v. Most oral agents should be restarted once the patient resumes eating.

(1) Metformin should be held for 48–72 hours following surgery for the infusion of any iodinated radiocontrast dye.

(a) Renal function should be evaluated and determined to be normal prior to the reinstitution of metformin.

b. Diabetic compliant with insulin therapy

i. There are many protocols, but no established consensus.

(1) Long-acting insulin, such as insulin glargine (Lantus), can be stopped 2 days prior to surgery.

(a) The patient should then begin a regimen of intermediate- and short-acting insulin.

(b) Recently, it has been determined that if the patient has been under good control, the long-acting Lantus can be continued throughout the day of surgery with a reduction of dose (25–50%).

(i) It maintains a stable glucose level for 24 hours.

(ii) It acts as a basal infusion.

(2) Often, patients are told to reduce their bedtime insulin dose once they are NPO and take a half-dose of their usual long- or intermediate-acting insulin on the morning of surgery.

(a) These patients require frequent glucose checks (hourly checks are preferred).

(b) They are to use short-acting insulin as needed.

(c) They may require a 5% dextrose IV infusion on the morning of surgery (2 mg/kg/min).

(i) This infusion is usually started at the time the patient would have had the next meal.

(3) Continuation of SC insulin infusion pump

(a) The pump may be stopped just prior to surgery or continued intra-operatively.

(i) Management is based on frequent blood glucose measurements.

(b) Glucose management often requires a continuous IV insulin infusion if the pump is stopped.

(4) SC regular insulin sliding scale with frequent blood sugar checks

(5) IV infusion plus frequent blood sugar checks

(a) The infusion rate can be determined by calculating insulin (units/h) = serum glucose (mg/dL)/150.

ii. A blood glucose level should be measured the morning of surgery.

(1) The blood glucose level should be <250 mg/dL before proceeding to surgery.

(2) The glucose level should be treated accordingly with regular insulin boluses or infusion.

iii. IV insulin infusions should be stopped and the usual insulin treatment resumed once oral intake is established.

3. Potassium infusion

a. The infusion of insulin and glucose induces an intracellular translocation of potassium, resulting in a potential hypokalemia.

4. Hydration

a. Avoid Lactated Ringer's.

b. Normal saline is the recommended fluid.

5. Antibiotics
6. Pre-medication

a. Metoclopramide: improves gastric emptying.

# Emergency Surgery

1. Rule out DKA and diabetic autonomic neuropathy of the gastrointestinal tract.

a. These can often present with abdominal pain.

b. Surgery can be prevented completely if this is the cause of the abdominal pain.

2. Obtain good IV access.
3. Send labs.

a. Glucose
b. Electrolytes
c. Acid–base assessment

4. Correct lab abnormalities as quickly as possible.
5. Life-saving surgery should not be delayed.

a. In a patient with DKA, the surgery should be delayed as long as safely possible in an attempt to correct the associated electrolyte abnormalities.

# Intra-operative

1. Standard ASA monitors

2. Surgery results in a stress response with a resultant increase in blood glucose levels.

   a. Plasma insulin levels remain constant.

   b. There is a phase of relative insulin resistance after surgery.

3. This patient should have a rapid-sequence induction and intubation secondary to her high risk of gastroparesis and aspiration.

4. Etomidate is recommended in patients with autonomic dysfunction.

   a. Less risk of induction-induced hypotension than with propofol

5. Consider the placement of an arterial line for frequent blood glucose and electrolyte measurements.

   a. Intra-operative hyperglycemia should be treated with IV regular insulin.

      i. Small doses up to 10 units of regular insulin can be bolused at a time.

      ii. Each unit of regular insulin lowers the serum glucose level by about 30 mg/dL.

      iii. A continuous infusion of regular insulin starting at 1–2 units per hour can be started and titrated to goal.

      iv. The goal glucose level should be <180 mg/dL

6. Maintenance

   a. Sevoflurane and isoflurane impair glucose tolerance to the same degree.

7. Check the serum glucose every 1–2 hours.
8. Maintain normothermia.

## Post-operative

1. Type I diabetics

   a. Continue an infusion of 5–10% dextrose–insulin–potassium, as determined by the blood glucose and potassium levels and the projected length of the NPO status or a "sliding scale" of subcutaneous regular insulin.

   b. Check electrolytes and serum glucose every 1–2 hours.

   c. Resume the patient's usual protocol once she resumes a regular diet.

   d. Once this sample patient is awake and alert, you can resume her SC insulin pump if stopped.

2. Type II diabetics

   a. Serum glucose level checks every 4 hours are usually sufficient.

## Bibliography

American Diabetes Association. Classification and diagnosis of diabetes: standards of medical care in diabetes – 2021. *Diabetes Care* 2021;**44**:S15

Dagogo-Jack S, George K. Management of diabetes mellitus in surgical patients. *Diabetes Spectrum* 2002;**15**:44–8.

Gropper MA. *Miller's Anesthesia*, 9th ed. Philadelphia: Elsevier, 2020, 955–6, 999–1007.

Goldman L, Ausiello D. *Cecil*, 23rd ed. Philadelphia: Saunders Elsevier, 2008, chapter 457.

Hirsch IB, Emmett M. Diabetic ketoacidosis and hyperosmolar hyperglycemic state in adults: treatment. In Nathan DM, ed., *UpToDate*. www.uptodate.com/contents/diabetic-ketoacidosis-and-hyperosmolar-hyperglycemic-state-in-adults-treatment (accessed October 30, 2021).

Inzucchi SE, Lupsa B. Clinical presentation, diagnosis, and initial evaluation of diabetes mellitus in adults. In Nathan DM, Wolfsdorf JI, eds., *UpToDate*. www.uptodate.com/contents/clinical-presentation-diagnosis-and-initial-evaluation-of-diabetes-mellitus-in-adults (accessed October 30, 2021).

Lor-Trivedi M. Perioperative management of the diabetic patient. eMedicine. 2008.

Marks JB. Perioperative management of diabetes. *Am Fam Physician* 2003;**67**:93–100.

Piccini JP, Nilsson KR. *The Osler Medical Handbook*, 2nd ed. Philadelphia: Saunders Elsevier, 2006, chapter 25.

Yao FSF, Fontes ML, Malhotra V. *Yao & Artusio's Anesthesiology: Problem-Oriented Patient Management*, 6th ed. Philadelphia: Lippincott Williams & Wilkins, 2008, pp. 782–95.

Chapter

# 74

# Rapid-Sequence Intubation

Ryan J. Gunselman and Jessica A. Lovich-Sapola

## Sample Case

Following a motor vehicle collision, a 24-year-old male is brought to the operating room for an emergent exploratory laparotomy due to a rigid abdomen and positive focused abdominal sonography for trauma (FAST) exam in the emergency department. The patient is awake and alert. However, he is in pain and is somewhat uncooperative. His blood alcohol content is 0.24%. The patient denies any significant medical history. He admits to binge drinking and smoking. The patient said he last ate around 2 hours ago while at a bar. His airway exam reveals a Mallampati 2 with a thyromental distance of 6 cm. How do you plan to secure this patient's airway? Does he need a rapid-sequence intubation (RSI)? If so, how would you do it? What are the situations in which a person would require an RSI? What are the contraindications to an RSI?

## Clinical Issues

### Definition of RSI

1. Technique used for rapid endotracheal tube placement (Fig. 74.1)
2. Performed in those patients who are at an increased risk for aspiration of gastric contents
3. The goal is for amnesia and intubating conditions within 30–60 seconds.
4. It is the most common method for securing an airway in trauma and emergency settings.

### Patient Identification

Identifying which patients are at risk for aspiration is the first and most important step in RSI.

1. Full stomach: <8 hours fasting
2. Last oral intake is unknown.
3. Morbid obesity
   a. These patients typically have gastroparesis in addition to increased intra-abdominal pressures, both of which increase the risk for aspiration.
4. Severe gastroesophageal reflux disease (GERD)
5. Decreased gastrointestinal motility
6. Intra-abdominal processes: abscess, obstruction, bleeding, etc.
7. Trauma

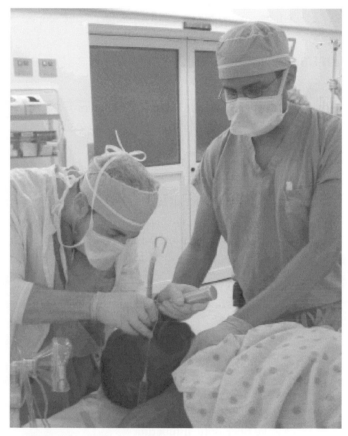

**Figure 74.1** Rapid-sequence intubation procedure. Photo credit: J. Lovich-Sapola, MD.

   a. NPO status is often unknown.
   b. The patient may be unable to protect his airway due to depressed mental status following head trauma.
   c. The patient has delayed gastric emptying immediately once the accident occurs.

8. Pregnancy
   a. Delayed gastric emptying
   b. More acidic gastric contents
   c. Increased intra-abdominal pressures

9. Decreased gag reflex or depressed mental status: unable to protect own airway

## Preparation for an RSI

1. History and physical exam, including complete airway exam and review of any drug-related allergies
2. Make sure that all emergency airway equipment is available.

   a. Laryngoscope blades
   b. Suction
   c. Oxygen
   d. Mask
   e. Oral and nasal airways
   f. Gum elastic bougie
   g. GlideScope/video laryngoscope/fiber-optic scope

## Contraindications to a RSI

1. Difficult airway

   a. History per the patient or medical record
   b. Short neck, limited range of motion, small chin
   c. Cervical collar in place
   d. Facial injuries
   e. Facial burn

2. Contraindication to succinylcholine

   a. Elevated potassium levels
   b. History of malignant hyperthermia
   c. Pseudocholinesterase deficiency

3. Cervical spine injury

   a. Cricoid pressure could cause increased damage to the cervical spine.
   b. An awake fiber-optic intubation is probably the best choice in this patient to avoid any additional cervical damage during the intubation.

**TKO:** If an RSI is contraindicated, then the risk of a failed intubation takes priority over the aspiration risk.

   c. Awake fiber-optic intubation
   d. Awake direct laryngoscopy
   e. Blind nasal intubation

## KO Treatment Plan

### Pre-operative

1. Proper emergency airway equipment available

   a. Laryngoscope blades
   b. Suction
   c. Oxygen
   d. Mask
   e. Oral and nasal airways
   f. Bougie
   g. GlideScope/video laryngoscope/fiber-optic scope
   h. Pillows/blankets to optimize sniffing position
   i. Intubating laryngeal mask airway

   j. Cricothyroidotomy kit
   k. Jet ventilation tubing

2. Adequate intravenous (IV) access
3. Medications

   a. Induction agent (propofol, etomidate, or ketamine), narcotic, succinylcholine (1.0–1.5 mg/kg), nondepolarizing muscle relaxant (rocuronium 0.9–1.2 mg/kg)
   b. If rocuronium is used, have sugammadex (16 mg/kg) available for emergent reversal if needed.

4. Placement of a nasogastric/orogastric (NG/OG) tube to suction the contents of the patient's stomach is not recommended.

   a. Will only be able to suction out some fluids, and not solid food
   b. It is believed that the NG/OG passing through the lower esophageal sphincter makes it incompetent and can actually "wick up" the gastric contents.
   c. If an NG/OG is currently in place, it should be suctioned prior to the RSI and should not be removed for the intubation.

### Intra-operative

1. Apply the standard ASA monitors.
2. Preoxygenate with 100% oxygen via a face mask for 3–5 minutes, refraining from any positive pressure that may introduce intragastric distension.

   a. This may be difficult in patients that are not cooperative or have limited functional residual capacity.

3. Cricoid pressure: Sellick's maneuver

   a. In most situations this is begun at the time of the induction agent administration, or immediately after due to the fact that it can be uncomfortable for an awake, conscious patient.
   b. Palpation of the cricoid cartilage is performed and approximately 8–10 pounds of posterior–cephalad pressure is applied by an assistant. The idea is that the application of pressure to the cricoid ring could obstruct the esophagus.
   c. Occlusion of the esophagus should help prevent aspiration of gastric contents.
   d. There has been recent debate over the effectiveness of this maneuver; however, most practitioners still utilize Sellick's maneuver for RSI.
   e. Cricoid pressure should be modified or removed if its use impedes intubation, bag mask ventilation, or insertion of the airway device, since securing the airway and ventilating is more important than the potential risk of aspiration.

4. Medication administration

   a. Induction with propofol, etomidate, or ketamine

i. Each agent can be used, but you must choose one and defend it.

ii. Assuming our sample case patient is hemodynamically stable, I would perform this RSI with propofol. He is an otherwise healthy, young male without any cardiac history.

iii. If the sample patient was hemodynamically unstable, I would choose ketamine or etomidate.

iv. Just pick one induction agent. The examiners want to know how you will induce, not all the different ways it can be done.

b. Paralytic is given immediately after the induction agent.

i. Succinylcholine is most commonly used for RSI.

ii. A fast-acting nondepolarizing muscle relaxant can also be used effectively (i.e., 1.2 mg/kg of rocuronium). This is becoming increasingly popular since the introduction of sugammadex for reversal.

iii. Depending on the agent used, one can monitor for fasciculations to cease or check the train-of-four to assess adequacy of paralysis to facilitate endotracheal intubation.

5. Do not ventilate the patient during the induction.

a. This increases the risk of aspiration by potentially filling the stomach with air.

b. If the patient absolutely requires ventilation, keep the peak airway pressures <20 cm $H_2O$.

6. Direct laryngoscopy

a. Once the patient is adequately paralyzed, visualization of the larynx is performed using a standard laryngoscope blade.

i. Direct laryngoscopy with other devices has been documented to have success (i.e., GlideScope or another video laryngoscope).

b. Once the vocal cords are visualized, an endotracheal tube is passed through and the balloon is inflated.

c. Cricoid pressure is maintained until end-tidal $CO_2$ is confirmed and breath sounds are auscultated bilaterally in the chest.

d. The endotracheal tube is then secured in the normal fashion.

## Post-operative

1. Extubation criteria should be met as in any other case.

2. Patients meeting the criteria should be completely awake and able to protect their airway prior to endotracheal tube removal as they are still at higher risk for aspiration.

3. Many practitioners will choose to suction the stomach contents with an NG/OG tube prior to extubation or waking the patient.

# Bibliography

Barash PG, Cullen BF, Stoelting RK. *Clinical Anesthesia*, 8th ed. Philadelphia: Lippincott Williams & Wilkins, 2017, pp. 786–8.

Gropper MA. *Miller's Anesthesia*, 9th ed. Philadelphia: Elsevier, 2020, pp. 1373–412.

Morgan GE, Mikhail MS, Murray MJ. *Clinical Anesthesiology*, 4th ed. New York: McGraw-Hill, 2006, pp 287–8.

Varon AJ, Smith CE. *Essentials of Trauma Anesthesia*, 2nd ed. Cambridge: Cambridge University Press, 2018, pp. 32–4.

# Cervical Spine Precautions

Jessica A. Lovich-Sapola and Michael Leeds

## Sample Case

A 27-year-old male presents to the operating room after falling off scaffolding at a concert 3 hours ago. He is having his left tibia repaired. He denies any other injury. His toxicology screen is positive for alcohol and cocaine. What would be an acceptable evaluation of his cervical spine?

## Clinical Issues

### Incidence

1. Roughly 2% of patients with a closed-head injury who survive to reach the hospital will have a fracture of the cervical spine.
2. The incidence of cervical spine injury is about 2–6% for all blunt trauma victims.
3. Ligamentous injuries are more common at C5 and C6, whereas fractures are often seen at C1 and C2.

### Cervical Spine Immobilization

1. Many trauma patients arrive with full spinal immobilization.
   a. Rigid cervical collar
      i. Not perfect to prevent spinal cord injury
      ii. Recommend to only use for a short period of time
      iii. Aspen- and Philadelphia-style collars with a transport vacuum mat are now being recommended.
   b. Plastic backboard
   c. Sandbags and tape

### Movement with Intubation

1. The goal is to secure the airway with as little movement of the cervical spine as possible.
2. The primary force applied by direct laryngoscopy is extension of the occiput on C1 combined with flexion at the lower vertebrae.
3. The more difficult the glottic exposure, the greater the force applied.
4. Thus, it is possible to aggravate or cause a serious spinal cord injury with the "hypnotic-relaxant-direct laryngoscopy" approach.

## How Is the Cervical Spine Cleared?

1. Alert, nonintoxicated patients without neck pain, depressed level of consciousness, intoxication, distracting injury, or neurologic abnormality or symptoms can be clinically cleared.
2. A patient's cervical spine cannot be cleared, even with appropriate radiographs, if he has a distracting injury. As in this sample case, cervical injury must be assumed and cervical spine precautions must be taken.
3. A normal cervical spine X-ray does not rule out cervical injury. A ligamentous injury will not always be identifiable on an X-ray.
4. A CT/MRI scan may be required to rule out ligamentous injury. There is rarely time for this testing in an emergency/trauma case.

## Inability to Clear Cervical Spine

1. Combative
2. Intoxicated
3. Obtunded
4. Distracting injuries

## Indications for Cervical Spine Precautions

1. All acute trauma patients with depressed level of consciousness
2. Patients reporting neck pain
3. Posterior midline cervical spine tenderness
4. Upper extremity paresthesia
5. Focal motor deficits
6. Whenever the pain of other injuries is likely to mask the neck pain
7. Falls, diving accidents, and high-speed motor vehicle accidents

## KO Treatment Plan

### Intra-operative

1. When there is any uncertainty regarding the airway or the cervical spine, direct laryngoscopy with atlanto-occipital extension should be avoided.
2. In patients with neurologic symptoms or a known spinal cord injury, awake flexible fiber-optic intubation is recommended in a cooperative patient. Complete

a neurologic exam after the intubation and prior to the induction of anesthesia.

3. If a rapid-sequence intubation is used, the standard approach should include in-line cervical stabilization. Be careful when applying cricoid pressure. Overly aggressive pressure might lead to cervical damage.

## In-line Stabilization

1. Hold the patient's occiput firmly on the backboard or operating table. This limits the amount of "sniff."

2. Immobilization of the cervical spine in a neutral position can be accomplished by using an assistant to provide manual in-line stabilization. A semi-rigid collar, sandbags placed on both sides of the head and neck, and the backboard can also help in maintaining the proper neck position. Note that well-fitted hard collars make it almost impossible to do direct laryngoscopy.

3. Hold the patient's head in-line with the cervical spine to prevent any cervical twisting.

4. Preoxygenate the patient, ideally for 2–3 minutes, but this time may have to be limited depending on the patient's condition.

5. Direct laryngoscopy will be more difficult with correct in-line stabilization.

6. Some physicians recommend leaving the posterior half of the cervical collar in place during laryngoscopy to act as a strut between the shoulders and the occiput and therefore serve to further limit the atlanto-occipital extension.

7. The gold standard for rapid-sequence intubation in the early stages of spinal cord injury is succinylcholine.

   a. Succinylcholine should be avoided on day 3 to 9 months after a spinal cord injury secondary to the risk of succinylcholine-induced hyperkalemia caused by denervation hypersensitivity.

   b. Rocuronium is an alternative choice.

8. While the cervical neck is immobilized, you can use different techniques to improve your success of intubation including: McCoy blade, Wu/Bullard scope, GlideScope, McGRATH, flexible fiber-optic, light wand, and retrograde intubation.

   a. In comparative studies of direct laryngoscopy, blind nasal intubation, and cricothyrotomy in patients with a known cervical cord or spine injury, or both, there was no difference in neurologic deterioration with the technique used and no evidence that direct laryngoscopy worsened the outcome.

   b. Therefore, use the technique that you are best at and will have the highest likelihood of rapid success.

9. If the cervical collar was removed during the intubation, it should be reapplied immediately after the intubation is confirmed.

## Bibliography

Barash PG, Cullen BF, Stoclting RK, et al. *Clinical Anesthesia*, 8th ed. Philadelphia: Lippincott Williams & Wilkins, 2017, pp. 1490–3.

Gropper MA. *Miller's Anesthesia*, 9th ed. Philadelphia: Elsevier, 2020, pp. 2161, 2221, 2123.

Smith CE. *Trauma Anesthesia*, 2nd ed. Cambridge: Cambridge University Press, 2015, p. 400.

Varon AJ, Smith CE. *Essentials of Trauma Anesthesia* 2nd ed. Cambridge: Cambridge University Press, 2018, pp. 34, 90.

# Head Trauma

Jeffrey Neurock and Jessica A. Lovich-Sapola

## Sample Case

A 40-year-old man presents to the trauma bay after a prolonged extrication, following an ATV accident. He is intoxicated, incoherent, and combative. The trauma team would like to sedate the patient for a CT scan to evaluate his head, abdomen, and pelvis. The patient's blood pressure is 170/90 mm Hg, heart rate is 48 beats/min, and temperature is 35.5 °C. What are your concerns in a traumatic brain injury (TBI) patient? How will you evaluate the patient? How will you induce and maintain general anesthesia in this patient?

## Clinical Issues

## Trauma Assessment and Emergency Therapy: ABCD

1.  Airway and breathing: secure the airway in any patient with a Glasgow Coma Scale <8 (Table 76.1).

    a.  The most expeditious approach to secure the airway, assuming that the patient does not have a difficult airway, is preoxygenation of the patient followed by a rapid-sequence induction (RSI) and intubation with cricoid pressure and maintenance of in-line cervical stabilization.

        i.  Cricoid pressure may inhibit the laryngeal view, and should be released if the initial attempt is unsuccessful.

    b.  Assume "full-stomach" in all head-injury patients.

        i.  In the setting of urgent airway securement, the benefits of the rapid onset and elimination of succinylcholine outweigh the risk of a transient increase in intracranial pressure (ICP).

        ii.  Rocuronium 1.2 mg/kg is an alternative to succinylcholine, with sugammadex readily available to reverse if needed to return to spontaneous ventilation.

    c.  There is a 1–3% incidence of cervical spine injury in the setting of known head injury.

        i.  In-line cervical stabilization requires an assistant to hold the occiput down on a backboard, with fingers on the mastoid process.

        ii.  The goal of in-line cervical stabilization is to prevent any further cervical injury during the

**Table 76.1** Glasgow Coma Scale

| Eyes open | Spontaneous | 4 |
| --- | --- | --- |
| | To speech | 3 |
| | To pain | 2 |
| | None | 1 |
| Best verbal response | Oriented | 5 |
| | Confused | 4 |
| | Inappropriate words | 3 |
| | Incomprehensible sounds | 2 |
| | None | 1 |
| Best motor response | Follows commands | 6 |
| | Localizes pain | 5 |
| | Withdrawal to pain | 4 |
| | Flexion to pain | 3 |
| | Extension to pain | 2 |
| | None | 1 |
| Maximum score/minimum score | | 15/3 |

Adapted from Miller RD. *Miller's Anesthesia*, 6th ed. Philadelphia: Churchill Livingstone, 2005.

intubation of the patient. Video laryngoscope offers improved laryngeal view with less cervical motion, although there is no evidence to support that direct laryngoscopy worsens outcomes.

    d.  Avoid nasal intubations in the face of basal skull fracture, severe facial fractures, or suspected bleeding diathesis.

2.  Circulation

    a.  Hypotonic solutions (0.45% NaCl) are more likely to increase brain water content with a large-volume fluid resuscitation secondary to a profound reduction in colloid oncotic pressure. This oncotic gradient leads to cellular swelling and brain edema.

b. Isotonic solutions (0.9% NaCl) prevent immediate increases in ICP and maintain plasma volume. Normal saline is typically the resuscitation fluid of choice in head trauma patients.

c. Hypertonic saline increases blood pressure and decreases overall fluid requirements. The use of 3% hypertonic saline is becoming more prevalent compared to mannitol because the saline gives more perfusion pressure support while still reducing ICP.

3. Disability

a. Evaluate for other injuries such as pneumothorax and intra-abdominal injury.

## Optimize Cerebral Perfusion

1. CPP = MAP – ICP (CPP, cerebral perfusion pressure; MAP, mean arterial pressure) (Fig. 76.1)

2. Maintain the CPP above 60–70 mm Hg (per Brain Trauma Foundation) to maintain cerebral blood flow and avoid cerebral desaturation.

3. A low CPP correlates with poor neurologic outcomes, as cerebral ischemia may occur at levels less than 50 mm Hg.

4. Aggressive use of pressors or volume expanders to maintain CPP above 70 mm Hg leads to systemic complications and does not improve general outcomes and therefore should be avoided.

5. An ICP monitor may be needed. ICP >22 mm Hg has increased mortality.

6. Temporary hyperventilation may be necessary to prevent herniation or to facilitate surgical access; however, this can lead to vasoconstriction and ischemia.

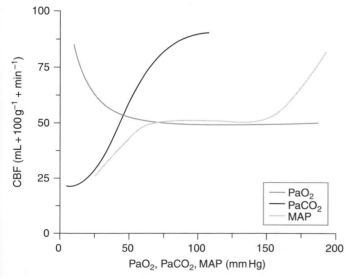

**Figure 76.1** Cerebral perfusion pressure. Source: This figure was published in RD Miller, LA Fleisher, RA Johns, et al. *Anesthesia*, 6th ed. Copyright Elsevier (2005). Reprinted with permission.

## Avoid Secondary Damage

1. Avoid hypoxia.

a. Hypoxia is significantly associated with increased morbidity and mortality.

2. Avoid hypercarbia.

a. Increased $CO_2$ leads to increased cerebral blood volume and flow via cerebral vasodilation.

b. In the setting of decreased intracranial compliance, ICP rises and CPP decreases.

3. Avoid hypotension.

a. A systolic blood pressure of 90 mm Hg is generally accepted as the lowest threshold.

b. A single episode of pre-hospital or in-hospital hypotension significantly increases mortality and morbidity.

c. Do not actively try to decrease the patient's elevated blood pressure.

d. Hypertension may be precipitated by the increase in ICP: Cushing's reflex.

e. A reduction in systolic blood pressure can aggravate cerebral ischemia by reducing CPP.

i. Again: CPP = MAP – ICP

4. Avoid anemia.

a. Hematocrit of 30–33% is recommended to maximize oxygen transport. The minimal acceptable hemoglobin level is 7 g/ dL.

5. Avoid hyperglycemia.

a. Hyperglycemia (blood glucose >200 mg/ dL) is correlated with the severity of injury and is associated with a poor outcome in regard to early mortality and functional recovery.

## Nonoperative Treatment of Diffuse Cerebral Swelling

1. Hyperventilation

a. Reduces ICP by causing vasoconstriction with a subsequent decrease in cerebral blood flow

b. Hyperventilation is no longer recommended to less than 35 mm Hg in the first 24 hours, as the vasoconstriction that is induced may lead to increased ischemia.

2. Mannitol

a. Osmotic diuretic

b. Onset is delayed 15–30 minutes after administration, with effects persisting for 90 minutes to 6 hours or more.

c. The immediate increase in plasma volume with administration leads to a decrease in hematocrit, reducing blood viscosity, increasing cerebral blood flow (CBF), and increasing oxygen delivery.

d. There is insufficient evidence to conclude whether continuous infusion or intermittent boluses are optimal in reducing ICP.

3. Hypertonic saline: there is some evidence of efficacy and relative benefit over mannitol for decreasing ICP while maintaining CPP.

   a. Effects of decreased ICP are due to osmotic movement of water across an intact blood–brain barrier.

   b. Leads to plasma volume expansion with improved blood flow

4. Barbiturate administration

   a. Because of the coupling of CBF to cerebral metabolic rate of oxygen consumption ($CMRO_2$), decreasing $CMRO_2$ leads to a decrease in ICP and decreased global cerebral perfusion.

   b. However, barbiturate therapy often results in a fall in blood pressure, offsetting any ICP-lowering effect on CPP. There is no evidence that this therapy improves outcomes.

5. Steroids do not improve outcome or lower ICP in severe TBI.

6. Hypothermia

   a. Hypothermia decreases $CMRO_2$. Theoretically, decreasing the temperature will decrease CBF, thus decreasing ICP. However, hypothermia is associated with significant other problems.

      i. Coagulopathy
      ii. Increased infection rate
      iii. Delayed emergence from anesthesia
      iv. Cardiac dysrhythmias

   b. Routine use of active cooling to less than 35°C is therefore **not** advocated.

7. Start basal caloric enteral feeding by day 7 post-TBI and consider early tracheostomy to prevent nosocomial pneumonia.

# KO Treatment Plan

## Pre-operative

1. Primary and secondary surveys must be completed in the trauma bay. The patient must be fully evaluated prior to proceeding to another setting.

2. Assuming that the patient has a normal airway, due to his combative nature, intoxication, and probable head injury, proceed with an RSI with manual in-line cervical stabilization to secure the airway with an endotracheal tube, prior to proceeding to the CT scanner.

   a. Obtaining lateral X-rays will only delay definitive airway control, and they are unreliable to rule out ligamentous injury.

   b. Again, succinylcholine leads to a transient increase in ICP, but the benefits of rapid airway securement outweigh this transient change.

3. Do not treat the hypertension. It is likely elevated in response to the increase in ICP (Cushing reflex).

4. Initiate nonoperative treatments to decrease the ICP. This decrease in ICP may result in a decrease in the patient's blood pressure, while maintaining the CPP.

## Intra-operative

**TKO:** Sometimes more script is revealed during the exam. Roll with the following punches . . . After the CT scan, it is discovered that the patient has a subdural hemorrhage and requires emergency surgery to decompress his brain.

1. In addition to standard ASA monitors, other monitors include:

   a. Foley catheter: if diuretics are to be given for ICP monitoring, a Foley is mandatory.

   b. Arterial line: close blood pressure monitoring is critical for reasons described above.

## Post-operative

1. Extubation should be carried out only when the patient is appropriately responsive. If the patient exhibited depressed mentation prior to the surgery, endotracheal intubation should be maintained through the initial post-operative time frame, until the patient's neurologic status improves.

2. Monitor the patient in an appropriate setting for possible systemic sequelae, including

   a. Cardiopulmonary issues

      i. Sympathetic hyperactivity is typical in the post-TBI setting, causing:

         (1) Left ventricular dysfunction which can lead to hypotension

         (2) Hypertension with resultant:

            (a) Trauma-associated acute lung injury (Fig. 76.2)
            (b) Neurogenic pulmonary edema
            (c) Subarachnoid hemorrhage

   b. Immune system depression leads to infectious complications.

      i. Pneumonia

   c. Pulmonary

      i. Trauma-associated acute lung injury

   d. Seizures

      i. Relatively common after TBI
      ii. Seizures increase the metabolic rate and increase ICP.

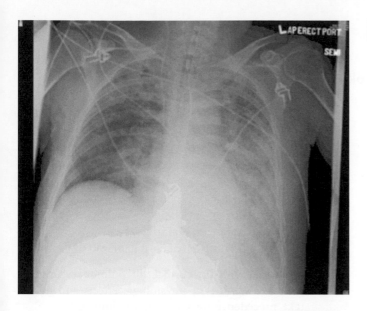

**Figure 76.2** Trauma-associated acute lung injury. Photo credit: MetroHealth Medical Center, Cleveland, OH.

iii. Antiepileptics are typically started in the immediate post-operative period.

e. Hematologic complications

i. Severe TBI patients are likely to develop a coagulopathy.

(1) Disseminated intravascular coagulation (DIC) can occur secondary to brain thromboplastin that is released into the systemic circulation after brain injury.

(2) Therapy is supportive, with treatment and resolution of the underlying problem, in order to control the consumptive coagulopathy that may develop.

# Bibliography

Barash PG, Cullen BF, Stoelting RK, et al. *Clinical Anesthesia*, 8th ed. Philadelphia: Lippincott Williams & Wilkins, 2017, pp. 1499–502.

Brain Trauma Foundation. Guidelines for the management of severe traumatic brain injury, 3rd ed. *J Neurotrauma* 2007;**24S**:1–95.

Gropper MA. *Miller's Anesthesia*, 9th ed. Philadelphia: Elsevier, 2020, pp. 1868–910, 2115–42, 2680–2.

Han C, Yang F, Guo S, et. al. Hypertonic saline compared to mannitol for the management of elevated intracranial pressure in traumatic brain injury: a meta-analysis. *Front Surg* 2022;**8**:765784

Lim HB, Smith M. Systemic complications after head injury: a clinical review. *Anaesthesia* 2007;**62**:474–82.

Moppett IK. Traumatic brain injury: assessment, resuscitation and early management. *Br J Anaesth* 2007;**99** (1):18–31.

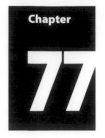

## Chapter 77

# Eye Trauma

Marcos A. Izquierdo and Michael Prokopius

## Sample Case

A 34-year-old man presents to the operating room follow-ing an open globe injury scheduled for operative repair. He was assaulted in a bar fight 2 hours prior to arrival and remains in a cervical collar. The ophthalmologist declared the case a surgical emergency. He is edentulous with a Mallampati class 3 score on exam. Vital signs are heart rate 112, respiratory rate 16, and blood pressure 105/56 mm Hg. What are your anesthetic concerns? How will you manage the airway?

## Clinical Issues

### Incidence

1. Approximately 2.5 million eye-related injuries occur on an annual basis in the United States, with construction injuries and sports injuries being the most common mechanisms.
2. Most common:
   a. Foreign body
   b. Open wound
   c. Contusion
   d. Burn

### Mechanisms of Ocular Injury

1. Direct injury to the eye globe
   a. Laceration
   b. Rupture
   c. Contusion
   d. Injury to the optic nerve
   e. Hypoperfusion of eye structures
   f. Loss of eyelid integrity
2. Open globe injury
   a. Full-thickness wound through eye wall, cornea, and sclera
3. Closed globe injury: ocular wall preserved

### Considerations for Eye Trauma Surgery

1. Associated injuries
   a. Consider the mechanism of trauma and the resulting associated injuries.

   i. Orbit
   ii. Face
   iii. Head: traumatic brain injury
   iv. Neck: cervical spinal cord damage
   b. Serious neurologic, cardiac, or pulmonary injuries can have significant physiologic effects and may take precedence over any ophthalmologic intervention.
   c. Maxillofacial injuries can result in difficult airway management.

2. NPO status/aspiration risk
   a. Trauma patients usually are not fasted, and delayed gastric emptying can contribute to increased aspiration risk.
   b. Emergent cases will require either awake intubation or rapid-sequence induction.

3. Management of intraocular pressure (IOP)
   a. Normal IOP is 8–21 mm Hg.
   b. Prolonged elevations greater than the normal range can lead to permanent blindness.
   c. Acute rises in IOP in the setting of an open globe injury can lead to extrusion of globe contents.
   d. Factors leading to increased IOP

      i. Coughing/bucking
      ii. Vomiting
      iii. Crying
      iv. Supine position
      v. External compression, bag mask ventilation
      vi. Succinylcholine
      vii. Hypertension
      viii. Light anesthesia
   e. Prevention of increased IOP

      i. Ensure a deep plane of anesthesia prior to laryngoscopy.
      ii. Reverse Trendelenburg position
      iii. Antiemetics
      iv. Gentle application of the facemask during preoxygenation
      v. Intravenous lidocaine
      vi. Opioids

## Airway Management

1. The goal is to rapidly secure the airway, prevent regurgitation and aspiration, and avoid deleterious rises in IOP.
2. Succinylcholine will provide ideal intubating conditions in the shortest amount of time, but will increase IOP by ~6–10 mm Hg for up to 10 minutes.
   a. Defasciculating with nondepolarizing relaxants is not effective in blunting the increase in IOP.
   b. Pretreating with IV lidocaine or opioids is advocated for blunting the increase in IOP.
3. High-dose rocuronium can be used for a modified rapid-sequence induction; however, coughing or bucking can increase IOP up to 40 mm Hg.
4. Balance the risk of a mild transient increase in IOP seen with succinylcholine with potentially inadequate neuromuscular blockade seen with rocuronium.
5. An awake fiber-optic intubation can significantly increase IOP if the patient coughs, bucks, or performs a Valsalva maneuver.
6. If a difficult airway is anticipated, the viability of the eye should be addressed with the surgeon.
   a. Viable – rapid-sequence intubation taking measures to prevent an increase in IOP
   b. Not viable – consider delaying the case. Plan for an awake fiber-optic intubation, assuming the patient is cooperative.

# KO Treatment Plan

## Pre-operative

1. Assess coexisting injuries and prioritize the management of those injuries.
   a. Perform a history and physical to assess comorbid conditions, mental status, or possible level of intoxication.
   b. Consult with the trauma surgery team regarding any concerns.
   c. Review the available imaging for spine injuries, rib fractures, intracranial injury, vascular injury, or anything that may preclude surgery or change management.
2. Perform a thorough airway assessment.
   a. Prolonged direct laryngoscopy can contribute to a significant sympathetic response and hemodynamic changes which can increase IOP.
   b. Consider using video laryngoscopy to decrease laryngeal stimulation.
3. Determine the urgency of the surgical procedure.
4. NPO status and the timing of the case will help determine airway management.
   a. There are few ophthalmologic surgical emergencies.
   b. The case may be able to wait until the patient has fasted for 8 hours.
5. Antiemetics and antacids
   a. Vomiting can severely increase IOP.
   b. Trauma patients are at increased risk of aspiration.
   c. Ondansetron – reduces the risk of emesis
   d. Metoclopramide – increases gastric emptying if given preemptively
   e. Sodium citrate – quickly reduces the pH of gastric contents
   f. H2-histamine antagonist such as famotidine

## Intra-operative

1. Induction medications
   a. Propofol can facilitate a decrease in IOP, but may also cause hypotension in the trauma patient.
   b. Etomidate would be a good choice in an unstable patient, but myoclonus on induction can also contribute to elevation of IOP.
   c. Ketamine does not increase IOP. It will maintain cardiac output by indirect sympathetic stimulation, but is a direct myocardial depressant in patients with exhausted sympathetic reserves.
   d. Rapid-sequence intubation can be performed with either succinylcholine or high-dose rocuronium. Succinylcholine will increase the IOP by about 6–10 mm Hg, but can provide better intubating conditions.
2. Intubation
   a. Options include rapid-sequence intubation with direct laryngoscopy, video laryngoscopy, or fiber-optic intubation.
   b. No matter which technique you choose, have backup airway equipment available; that is, laryngeal mask airway (LMA), intubating stylet, additional laryngoscope blades, anesthesia staff with airway experience.
3. Maintenance
   a. Inhalational agents will proportionally decrease IOP.
   b. Maintain normocapnia, normoxia, and mechanical ventilation.
   c. Consider a propofol infusion to further decrease IOP and decrease the risk of post-operative nausea and vomiting.
   d. Avoid nitrous oxide.
      i. Intravitreal gas may be used for retinal detachment and $N_2O$ can result in expansion of the bubble.
      ii. A preexisting pneumothorax can expand with positive-pressure ventilation and nitrous oxide use.

4. Emergence
    a. Balance the risk of aspiration and prevention of increased IOP.
        i. Awake extubation once airway reflexes return
        ii. Smooth emergence
    b. Lidocaine – endotracheal or IV

    c. Small boluses of esmolol to blunt the hemodynamic response
    d. Incremental dosing of opioids
    e. Continuous infusion of dexmedetomidine
    f. Prophylactic antiemetics
    g. Sugammadex does not increase IOP, where neostigmine and atropine can increase IOP.

## Bibliography

Gropper MA. *Miller's Anesthesia*, 9th ed. Philadelphia: Elsevier, 2020, pp. 2194–209.

Varon AJ, Smith CE. *Essentials of Trauma Anesthesia*, 2nd ed. Cambridge: Cambridge University Press, 2018, pp. 200–4.

# The Pregnant Trauma Patient

Jessica A. Lovich-Sapola

## Sample Case

A 25-year-old woman is brought to the trauma bay after injury in a motor vehicle accident. She was the restrained passenger in a head-on collision. She tells her caregivers she is 7 months pregnant and repeatedly asks, "Is my baby OK?" She is tachycardic to 120 and moderately hypotensive at 92/56 mm Hg, with complaints of abdominal tenderness. What concerns do you have in the trauma bay? How do you want to proceed?

## Clinical Issues

### Incidence

1. Approximately 5–10% of all pregnant women experience some type of trauma, with 8% occurring in the first trimester, 40% in the second trimester, and the remaining 52% in the third trimester.
2. Trauma is the leading cause of death for all women of childbearing age.
3. Most common cause of injury-related maternal death includes (in order):
   a. Motor vehicle collision
   b. Domestic violence: increases during pregnancy
   c. Falls: the physics of the growing abdomen results in imbalance.
   d. Penetrating injury
4. The primary cause of fetal death is maternal death.
5. Ensuring adequate maternal care is the best method of ensuring adequate care of the fetus.

### Mechanism of Injury

1. Blunt trauma
   a. Most common
   b. Maternal mortality 2%
   c. Fetal mortality 10%
   d. Injuries: preterm labor, maternal–fetal hemorrhage, direct fetal injury
   e. Pelvic fracture: most common maternal injury that results in fetal death
2. Penetrating trauma
   a. Gunshot and stab wounds
   b. Maternal mortality 7%

c. Fetal mortality is 75% secondary to direct trauma, uteroplacental disruption, or maternal shock.
3. Burns
   a. For second or third trimester patients, delivery may be indicated if the total body surface area (TBSA) burn is >50%, due to the high associated maternal mortality rate.
   b. Fetal compromise is common, with associated sepsis.
   c. Carbon monoxide poisoning
      i. Carbon monoxide crosses the placenta rapidly and fetal hemoglobin has more affinity for carbon monoxide than maternal hemoglobin.
      ii. Treat with oxygen/hyperbaric oxygen.

## Complications Associated with Pregnancy

1. Placental abruption
2. Uterine rupture
3. Preterm rupture of membranes
4. Preterm labor
5. Direct fetal injury

## Issues Specific to the Care of a Pregnant Trauma Patient

1. Presence of the obstetrical (OB) team immediately in trauma bay
2. Call a pediatrician or neonatologist immediately upon the patient's arrival.
3. Need for fetal monitoring
   a. Viable fetuses (estimated gestational age ≥23 weeks) are placed on continuous electronic fetal heart rate (FHR) monitoring in order to assess FHR variability.
      i. This requires continuous monitoring by the OB team.
   b. Fetal well-being is a reflection of adequate maternal blood flow and oxygenation.
      i. Proportional to maternal mean arterial pressure
      ii. Inversely proportional to uterine vascular resistance
   c. Even if the estimated fetal age is nonviable, FHR tracings may provide information regarding adequate

fetal perfusion and may indicate the need for more intensive maternal management.

    d. Prolonged decreased FHR or late decelerations may indicate the need for an immediate cesarean section.

4. Radiologic studies

    a. X-rays should be ordered on the basis of clinical need for information pertinent to diagnosis.

    b. Radiation effects are most deleterious during organogenesis in weeks 2–7.

    c. Avoid computerized tomography (CT) scans of the abdomen. If they are truly necessary, then it is advised to limit the area studied or the number of cuts.

5. Major obstetrical hemorrhage may be induced by trauma.

    a. Includes:

      i. Placental abruption

      ii. Uterine rupture

    b. Also consider nontrauma-related hemorrhage such as

      i. Placenta previa

      ii. Placenta accreta/increta/percreta

      iii. Vasa previa

      iv. Postpartum bleeding

        (1) Retained placenta

        (2) Uterine atony

        (3) Cervical/vaginal lacerations

## Causes of Maternal Cardiac Arrest

1. Pulmonary embolism
2. Severe preeclampsia/eclampsia
3. Hemorrhage
4. Trauma
5. Sepsis
6. Myocardial infarction
7. Congestive heart failure
8. Amniotic fluid embolism
9. Iatrogenic causes

    a. Hypermagnesemia

    b. Failed airway

    c. High spinal/local anesthetic toxicity

## ACLS for the Pregnant Patient

1. Left uterine displacement after 20 weeks' gestation
2. The remainder of her body is supine for effective chest compressions.
3. If the fetus has scalp electrodes, the lead should be disconnected from the fetal monitor prior to defibrillation.

## Emergency Cesarean Delivery during Cardiac Arrest

1. If ACLS is not successful after 4 minutes, emergency cesarean section is recommended for patients at 20 weeks' gestation or later.
2. Fetal anoxia begins at 5 minutes after maternal cardiac arrest, so plan for skin incision at 4 minutes for immediate delivery.

    a. Fetus survival rates after perimortem cesarean delivery

      i. 70% when delivered in <5 minutes

      ii. 13% when delivered within 6–10 minutes

      iii. 12% when delivered within 11–15 minutes

3. Chest compression and tracheal intubation may be easier after delivery of the fetus.

# KO Treatment Plan

## Pre-operative

1. A complete understanding of the hematologic, cardiovascular, pulmonary, and gastrointestinal system alterations secondary to pregnancy is necessary.
2. Primary survey: consistent with the review of all trauma patients, assessment begins with the ABCs – airway, breathing, and circulation – followed by a secondary survey. Special considerations in pregnant patients include:

    a. Increased risk for aspiration due to lower esophageal sphincter relaxation and cephalad displacement of the stomach. It may be necessary to intubate the trachea quickly to avoid aspiration.

    b. Increased risk of difficult airway secondary to:

      i. Weight gain

      ii. Increased breast tissue

      iii. Airway edema

      iv. Possible cervical neck and spine injuries from the trauma

    c. Need for lateral decubitus positioning to relieve aortocaval compression by the gravid uterus

      i. Aortocaval compression decreases maternal systolic blood pressure by up to 30 mm Hg and decreases stroke volume by 30%.

      ii. If cardiopulmonary resuscitation is needed:

        (1) Supine positioning is necessary.

        (2) Manual displacement of the gravid uterus to the left decreases uterine compression on the abdominal aorta and inferior vena cava.

        (3) Delivery of the fetus may need to be emergently performed in order to apply effective CPR and save the life of the mother.

    d. Confirmation of fetal heart tones

3. No difference between pregnant and nonpregnant patients exists in the decision to proceed with a trauma-related emergency surgery.
4. Imaging should not be withheld or deferred secondary to concerns for fetal radiation exposure.

   a. Ultrasound
   b. CT
   c. MRI

## Intra-operative

1. Consider regional and neuraxial techniques when feasible.
2. Goals are to maintain uteroplacental circulation and fetal oxygenation, with prevention of fetal distress.
3. Premedication with nonparticulate antacid and/or H2-receptor blockers to reduce the gastric pH in order to reduce or decrease the severity of the pneumonitis if aspiration occurs.
4. Elevate the patient's upper back, shoulders, and head to help with laryngoscopy; sniffing position.
5. Supplemental oxygen
6. Large-bore IV access placed above the diaphragm
7. Arterial line if indicated (goal SBP >100 mm Hg to maintain uteroplacental blood flow)

   a. Ephedrine and phenylephrine are safe in pregnancy.

8. Rapid-sequence induction with cricoid pressure
9. Review intra-operative management of pregnant patients for review of the best drugs to use or avoid in pregnant surgical patients. Of note:

   a. Hemodynamically unstable patients may be unable to tolerate volatile anesthetic agents during surgery.
   b. Ketamine increases uterine tone and decreases uteroplacental perfusion, thus making it a suboptimal drug, even in the situation of hemodynamic instability.
   c. Avoid nitrous oxide if risk for pneumothorax or first trimester pregnancy.

10. Fluid resuscitation

    a. Crystalloids
    b. Blood products

       i. Prefer cross-matched blood (type O Rh-negative if no time for cross-match)
       ii. Goal-directed therapy
       iii. Increased risk of developing disseminated intravascular coagulation (DIC)
       iv. Order the massive transfusion protocol if needed (Fig. 78.1).

11. Laboratory evaluation

    a. Complete blood count (CBC)
    b. Type and screen/cross
    c. Blood urea nitrogen (BUN), creatinine (CR)

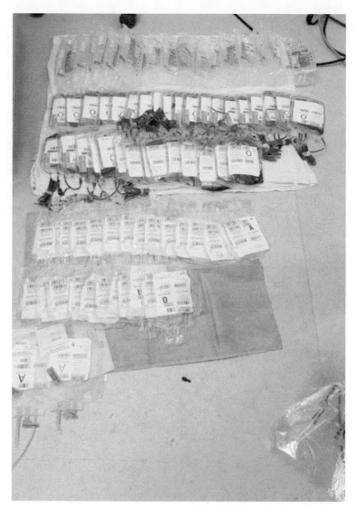

**Figure 78.1** Blood products and fluid used for a massive transfusion in a trauma patient. Photo Credit: Jessica Lovich-Sapola, MD, MBA, FASA.

    d. Glucose
    e. Liver function tests
    f. Lactate
    g. Toxicology
    h. Arterial blood gas
    i. Platelet levels
    j. Prothrombin
    k. Partial thromboplastin
    l. Fibrinogen
    m. Thromboelastography (TEG)
    n. Rotational thromboelastography (ROTEM)

12. Need for fetal resuscitation

    a. FHR monitoring should be continued throughout the surgery if the location of the surgical site allows.

## Post-operative

1. Fetal–maternal hemorrhage must be considered in cases of abdominal trauma.

a. Women who are Rh-negative must be treated with Rh(D)-immunoglobulin (Rhogam) within 72 hours to prevent maternal isoimmunization.

2. Continue FHR monitoring in the post-operative period.
3. Continue obstetrical team involvement.

a. Increased risk of preterm labor
b. Tocolytic administration may be necessary to prevent contractions leading to preterm delivery.

## Bibliography

Gropper MA. *Miller's Anesthesia*, 9th ed. Philadelphia: Elsevier, 2020, pp. 2149–50.

Hull SB, Bennett S. The pregnant trauma patient: assessment and anesthetic management. *Int Anesthesiol Clin* 2007;45 (3):1–18.

Jain V, Chari R, Maslovitz S. Guideline for the management of a pregnant trauma patient. *J Obstet Gynaecol Can* 2015;37 (6):553–71.

Krywko DM, Troy FK, Kahan ME, et al. Pregnancy trauma. In: *StatPearls* [Internet]. Treasure Island: StatPearls Publishing, 2022.

Mercier FJ, Van de Velde M. Major obstetric hemorrhage. *Anestheisol Clin* 2008;26:53–66.

Neufeld JD, Moore EE, Marx JA, et al. Trauma in pregnancy. *Emerg Med Clin North Am* 1987;5:623.

Prentice-Bjerkeseth R. Perioperative anesthetic management of trauma in pregnancy. *Anesth Clin North Am* 1999;17 (1):278–95.

Smith CE. *Trauma Anesthesia*, 2nd ed. Cambridge: Cambridge University Press, 2015, pp. 623–36.

Varon AJ, Smith CE. *Essentials of Trauma Anesthesia*, 2nd ed. Cambridge: Cambridge University Press, 2018, pp. 304–16.

**Chapter 79**

# Burn Anesthesia

Casey L. Kohler and Jessica A. Lovich-Sapola

## Sample Case

A 47-year-old male was upset with his girlfriend and poured gasoline on her house and set it on fire. While admiring his work he sat back and lit a cigarette. At this point he went up in flames. He presents to the emergency room with a 75% total body surface area (TBSA) burn. He is awake and talking. He has facial burns, singed nasal hair, and increased secretions. He is telling you that he will be fine, and doesn't need a breathing tube. Pulse ox reads 99%. What are your specific concerns? What is your plan for airway management? What is your plan for fluid therapy?

## Clinical Issues

### Airway

1. Upper airway inhalation injury is usually due to a heat injury, which leads to edema and upper airway obstruction. The most common site of laryngeal injury is the epiglottis and vocal folds. Lower airway inhalation injury is due to inhalation of chemicals and toxins.
2. Patients with significant burns to the face and neck are at increased risk of airway injury.
3. Predictive indicators of an inhalation injury include:
   a. History of a closed-space fire
   b. Impaired mental status
   c. Loss of consciousness
   d. Associated drug or alcohol use
   e. Facial burns
   f. Airway soot
   g. Singed nasal hair
   h. Abnormal finding on the nasopharyngoscopy and bronchoscopy
   i. Airway edema
   j. Carbonaceous material in the airway
   k. Abnormal flow-volume loops showing extrathoracic obstruction and an elevated carbon monoxide level >15%
4. Indications for early intubation in possible inhalation injuries:
   a. Hemodynamic instability
   b. Respiratory failure
   c. Central nervous system depression

d. Massive burns over 60% TBSA or extensive burns to face and neck
   e. Inability to protect airway
   f. Significant toxicity from carbon monoxide or cyanide
   g. Signs and symptoms of impending obstruction:
      i. Increasing respiratory rate
      ii. Increased secretions
      iii. Stridor
      iv. Dyspnea
      v. Use of accessory muscles
      vi. Dysphagia
      vii. Progressive hoarseness

5. Patients with minimal airway distress should be questioned as to the events associated with the burn, SAMPLE history, and other pertinent information prior to airway manipulation.
   a. Signs and symptoms
   b. Allergies
   c. Medications
   d. Pertinent history
   e. Last intake
   f. Events of the injury

6. With an upper airway injury with impending signs of obstruction, the patient will require rapid tracheal intubation as a stable airway can quickly become catastrophic.
7. It is best to intubate early, as the likelihood of airway edema increases significantly with massive fluid resuscitation.
8. Evaluate the patient's airway for a potential difficult intubation. Burn injuries can severely compromise mobility of the neck/mandible and cause edema of the airway, making visualization difficult and laryngeal injury possible. There may be potential signs of a difficult airway independent of the burn injury.

### Tracheal Intubation with a Normal-Appearing Airway

1. Usually accomplished with rapid-sequence intubation using an IV induction drug and a rapid-acting muscle relaxant

327

2. Succinylcholine is safe in the first 24 hours after a burn, but after that it can cause an exaggerated hyperkalemic response.
3. Rocuronium can be given safely at any time to a burn patient.
4. Always preoxygenate the patient with 100% oxygen prior to airway manipulation to ensure a good oxygen reserve during the patient's period of apnea.
5. If a cervical collar is in place, the patient will require manual in-line stabilization during airway manipulation.
6. Securing the endotracheal tube is difficult secondary to topical wound agents, continued swelling and edema of the face and neck, and fluid extruding through the facial burn. This is usually done with ties or wiring the tube to the teeth, as tape will not stick to the face.

## Tracheal Intubation with an Abnormal-Appearing Airway

1. Most often secured with the patient awake
2. The most important things to remember during an awake intubation are topical anesthesia, proper patient positioning, and supplemental oxygen.
3. Excessive opioid sedation may worsen the airway obstruction.
4. The safest technique depends on the operator's expertise.
5. If the patient will not cooperate with an awake intubation, then consider taking the patient to the operating room for an inhalational induction with continued spontaneous ventilation, or a surgical airway including retrograde techniques, transtracheal jet ventilation, cricothyroidotomy, or tracheostomy.
6. Inhalational induction with oxygen and sevoflurane is often necessary for children.

## Respiratory Physiology

1. Inhalation injury and resultant pneumonias increase mortality from 20% with inhalation injury alone to 60% when combined with pneumonia.
2. The first phase of inhalation injury (first 48 hours) may include asphyxia and acute toxicity. Granulocyte and mast cell infiltration, interstitial edema, loss of type-1 epithelial pneumocytes, damage to the tracheobronchial epithelium, hemorrhage, and submucosal edema also occur.
   a. Asphyxia occurs secondary to the lack of oxygen during combustion.
   b. Acute toxicity occurs with the inhalation of carbon monoxide and cyanide.
3. Carbon monoxide (CO) toxicity
   a. CO is a byproduct of combustion.
   b. It is responsible for 80% of deaths associated with smoke inhalation and accounts for the majority of deaths that occur at the scene of the fire.
   c. CO has an affinity for hemoglobin that is 250 times greater than oxygen, preventing oxygen from loading onto the molecule. Even very low partial pressures of CO result in a far-leftward shift on the oxygen dissociation curve, impairing oxygen delivery and resulting in tissue hypoxia and metabolic acidosis.
   d. CO poisoning is diagnosed with an arterial measurement of carboxyhemoglobin levels with co-oximeter blood analysis. The arterial oxygen pressure, pulse oximetry saturation, and arterial oxygen saturation may be normal and misleading because the carboxyhemoglobin is interpreted as oxyhemoglobin, therefore giving falsely elevated levels.
   e. Mixed venous oxygen saturation monitoring does not detect the presence of carboxyhemoglobin and progressively overestimates fractional oxyhemoglobin and carboxyhemoglobin increases.
   f. Patients with carbon monoxide poisoning may manifest no signs of peripheral cyanosis secondary to their characteristic "cherry red" appearance.
   g. CO saturation levels and resulting symptoms:
      i. CO level <15%: rarely has any signs or symptoms
      ii. CO level at 15–20%: the patient will likely have a headache, tinnitus, and confusion.
      iii. CO level at 20–40%: the patient will have nausea, fatigue, and disorientation.
      iv. CO level at 40–60%: the patient will have hallucinations, display combativeness, and show cardiovascular instability.
      v. CO level >60%: death
   h. Treatment consists of the administration of 100% oxygen using a face mask or endotracheal tube since it will accelerate the dissociation of carboxyhemoglobin by 50% every 30 minutes.
   i. Although rarely clinically practical, hyperbaric oxygen therapy can accelerate the dissociation more quickly and is most useful in patients who are comatose with carboxyhemoglobin levels greater than 30%. Hyperbaric oxygen treatment is not recommended if it will delay fluid resuscitation.
4. Cyanide toxicity
   a. Cyanide is produced by combustion of plastics, and impairs the mitochondria's utilization of oxygen in metabolism, causing tissue asphyxia.
   b. Signs and symptoms include: headache, dizziness, tachycardia, tachypnea, lethargy, seizures, and respiratory failure.
   c. Suspect cyanide poisoning in patients with persistent anion gap metabolic acidosis or high lactate levels despite oxygen administration.
   d. Treatment consists of high inspired oxygen concentration and a cyanokit (hydroxocobalamin).

5. The second phase of inhalation injury (24–96 hours) is the result of pulmonary parenchymal damage caused by chemical irritation.

   a. Airway edema, tracheobronchitis, pulmonary edema, atelectasis, increased airway resistance, and decreased static lung compliance are likely to occur.

   b. The patient often has dyspnea, rales, rhonchi, wheezing, and copious tracheal secretions and exudates.

   c. The secretions are often very viscous and may contain carbonaceous particles, pieces of mucous membranes, and casts.

   d. Impaired ciliary action decreases airway debris clearance and exacerbates airway obstruction.

   e. The clinical picture is almost identical to adult respiratory distress syndrome (ARDS) and ventilation with reduced tidal volumes is recommended.

   f. The initial inhalation injury and resultant pneumonias increase mortality from 20% with inhalation injury alone to 60% when combined with pneumonia.

# KO Treatment Plan

## Pre-operative

1. IV access

   a. Establishing vascular access is extremely important prior to burn excision and grafting procedures and can be difficult due to the extent of the burn.

   b. A minimum of two large-bore peripheral IV lines or one peripheral and one central line are necessary. Central trauma lines are excellent for rapid fluid administration and possible placement of pulmonary artery catheters.

   c. Pulmonary artery catheters are not routinely placed because of the risk of infection, but can be used in patients with ischemia or valvular heart disease to guide fluid administration.

   d. Site of central line placement is through unburned skin if possible. The use of an ultrasound probe for internal jugular and femoral venous catheters greatly decreases the risk of complications including pneumothorax, arterial puncture, hemothorax, hematoma, and nerve injury. The subclavian approach is still dependent on anatomic landmarks.

   e. Complications are the most significant in patients with coagulopathies, mechanical ventilation, poor pulmonary function, chronic IV use, and soft tissue edema, all of which are usually present in a burn patient.

   f. If a central venous line is not possible, then a small-bore peripheral vein can be dilated to a larger gauge using specially designed kits.

   g. Consider an intraosseous infusion to deliver drugs, fluids, and blood with a low incidence of complications until an IV line can be placed.

   h. IV lines can be safely placed through a burn site if the usual sterile technique is used.

   i. IV lines should be connected to high-efficiency rapid-infusion fluid warmers in the operating room to help prevent significant heat loss.

2. Pre-operative fasting guidelines

   a. Achieving adequate caloric intake in burn patients is difficult, so in patients with a protected airway it is recommended to continue enteral feedings.

   b. Patients without a secure airway should have enteral feedings held four hours prior to surgery.

3. Intubation

   a. Our sample patient requires immediate intubation for signs of inhalation injury and a greater than 60% TBSA burn. He may be awake and talking now, but he will become a near-impossible intubation once his edema progresses when his fluid resuscitation begins. Also, despite his pulse ox reading of 99%, he has a high likelihood of CO poisoning and therefore a significantly worse oxygenation status than the current picture presents. Get a rapid history and secure his airway. Send labs, including an arterial blood gas (ABG). Also, obtain a chest X-ray. Establish good IV access and start the fluid resuscitation.

## Intra-operative

1. Monitors and Foley catheter

   a. Vital signs and urine output are considered the minimum standard of care in the resuscitation of the burn patient. Invasive monitoring is reserved for high-risk patients and those failing resuscitation.

   b. EKG monitoring

      i. Use needle electrodes or surgical staples with an alligator clamp attached to monitor electrocardiogram in burned surfaces.

      ii. Most patients will have a satisfactory signal if you place the electrocardiogram pads under dependent parts of the body.

   c. Pulse oximetry:

      i. When peripheral perfusion is poor (as in states of hypovolemia, hypothermia, vasoconstriction, low cardiac output, and low mean arterial pressure), pulse oximetry readings become extremely unreliable or cease.

      ii. In burn patients, standard sites such as fingers and toes may be affected by the burn or unusable due to tourniquet placement.

      iii. Alternative sites (ear, nose, tongue) can be used with a standard pulse oximeter probe.

iv. Esophageal reflectance pulse oximetry may offer advantages if the skin sites for monitoring are limited.

v. Ultimately, the physician may have to rely on intermittent arterial blood samples and blood gas analysis.

d. Arterial blood pressure: should be monitored invasively during any large surgical debridement. Indications for an arterial line include:

i. Frequent arterial blood sampling

ii. Continuous real-time monitoring of blood pressures

iii. Failure to take indirect blood pressure measurements

iv. Intentional pharmacologic cardiovascular manipulation

v. Assessment of supplementary diagnostic clues

e. Pulmonary artery catheterization: may be indicated in patients who do not respond to fluid resuscitation or who have pre-existing cardiac disease.

f. Central venous pressure and pulmonary capillary wedge pressure: have been used as preload indicators to guide volume therapy. It is often required that the central venous catheter be placed through burned tissue and should be removed as soon as possible to minimize the risk of local and systemic infection.

g. The indication for extended hemodynamic monitoring is frequently present with a TBSA burn >50%.

h. Precordial and transesophageal echocardiography can be used to evaluate ventricular function and reliably estimate pulmonary artery capacitance.

i. A Foley catheter should be placed to evaluate hourly urine output even if a severe genitalia burn is present.

i. The use of silver-impregnated Foley catheters can significantly decrease the rate of urinary tract infection in the burn patient.

2. Thermal regulation

a. Temperature monitoring is essential because hypothermia is common and often difficult to prevent.

b. In the burn unit and the operating room, the patient's temperature should remain thermo-neutral to avoid further increases in the metabolic rate as burn patients already develop a hypermetabolic state in proportion to the severity of the burn.

c. Hypothermia can exacerbate coagulopathy and is particularly common in the burn patient due to the evaporative heat loss through the wounds.

d. Temperature regulation can be achieved by having the ambient temperature of the operating room greater than 28 °C, and having all topical and IV fluids warmed to 38 °C.

e. Nonoperative sites should be covered, and a forced-air warming device used. If available, over-the-bed warming lamps and hot water pads should be used.

3. Induction and maintenance of anesthesia

a. General anesthesia with the combination of an opioid, volatile anesthetics, and muscle relaxants is the most widely used technique for burn excision and grafting.

b. The induction agents are chosen based on the hemodynamic stability of the patient.

i. Ketamine offers the advantage of stable hemodynamics and analgesia. It is beneficial for dressing changes and bedside procedures. Its drawbacks include dysphoric reactions, which can be decreased with co-administration of benzodiazepines, and developing tolerance.

ii. In a hemodynamically unstable patient, etomidate is a reasonable alternative to ketamine. Etomidate should not be used for frequent dressing changes due to the possible adrenocortical suppressive effects of the drug.

iii. In patients who are adequately resuscitated and not septic, propofol may be used.

c. Opioids: supplemental opioids are important in burn patients secondary to the intense pain they experience. Burn patients usually require large doses of opioids to remain comfortable even in the absence of movement or surgical procedures, and therefore quickly become tolerant to these drugs.

d. Depolarizing muscle relaxants, including succinylcholine, have led to considerable debate concerning the timing and use in burn patients due to the potential for hyperkalemia and cardiac arrest.

i. Burn injury results in denervation of the tissue, which causes the entire skeletal muscle membrane, as opposed to the motor endplate only, to develop acetylcholine receptors.

ii. Upon administration of succinylcholine, an exaggerated number of acetylcholine receptors are depolarized, resulting in a massive efflux of potassium from the cell into the extracellular fluid.

iii. The hyperkalemia cannot be prevented by giving a defasciculating dose of nondepolarizer prior to the administration of the succinylcholine.

iv. The larger the TBSA of the burn, the higher is the likelihood of a hyperkalemic response.

v. The potassium concentration increases within the first minute after succinylcholine administration, peaks within 5 minutes, and starts to decline by 10–15 minutes.

vi. The hypersensitivity to the succinylcholine begins 48 hours after the burn, and peaks at 1–3 weeks and may persist for up to 2 years.

vii. Therefore, succinylcholine is safe for the first 48 hours, and is best avoided after that.

e. Nondepolarizing muscle relaxants (NDMRs) are often used during excision and grafting of burn patients.

   i. Patients with thermal injury are usually hyposensitive or resistant to the action of NDMRs and a marked resistance is seen in TBSA >30–40%.

   ii. This effect may take up to a week to develop and may be observed for as long as 18 months after the burn has healed.

   iii. Burn patients will require larger than normal doses of NDMR to achieve a desired effect and the duration of action will be shorter than normal.

   iv. Dose requirements can be increased by up to 250–500%. If muscle relaxants are being used, then neuromuscular function should be regularly monitored in the patient.

f. Volatile anesthetics

   i. Sevoflurane is an ideal agent for inhaled induction of anesthesia in burn patients with abnormal airways and is less irritating to the already damaged airways.

   ii. Isoflurane decreases cardiac output and oxygen consumption; however, the reductions parallel one another so the oxygen supply to the tissue remains sufficient to meet metabolic demands.

4. Estimated blood loss and fluid resuscitation during excision and grafting

a. Excisional treatment of burn wounds is usually associated with a large operative blood loss, approximately 100–400 mL for every 1% TBSA excised.

b. Aggressive fluid resuscitation is imperative to improving mortality, especially in the initial phase of treatment and during operative excision and grafting.

c. Blood loss is usually replaced with crystalloids, colloids, packed red blood cells, and fresh frozen plasma. Start the blood transfusion before the surgery begins in anticipation of the blood loss; it is very easy to fall behind. Communicate with the surgeon about the percentage of TBSA to be excised.

d. Hemodynamic changes after a burn are significant and must be managed carefully to optimize intravascular volume, maintain end-organ perfusion, and maximize the oxygen delivery to the tissues.

e. The initial goal of the cardiovascular resuscitation during excision and grafting is to correct or prevent hypovolemia.

f. IV fluid is usually given in proportion to the percentage of the TBSA burned and is guided by the clinical assessment, vital signs, and urine output. In a patient with normal renal function, the urine output should be at least 0.5 mL/kg/h in adults and 1 mL/kg/h in children.

g. Lactated Ringer's solution is the fluid of choice, except in patients younger than 2 years old, who should receive 5% dextrose Ringer's lactate.

h. Changes in the IV fluid should be made on a regular basis, at least hourly, based on the patient's hemodynamic response.

i. Failure to achieve this goal leads to burn shock with progressive oxygen debt, anaerobic metabolism, and lactic acidosis.

j. During the active fluid resuscitation in the operating room, frequent arterial blood samples should be sent to follow the changing levels of base excess and lactate levels.

## Post-operative

1. It is important to remember that the burn patient does not only have initial airway concerns but may have a compromised airway for life.

2. These patients often require frequent reconstructive surgeries long after the initial insult. Patients with healed burns of the neck, face, and chest may develop scar contractures that make direct laryngoscopy difficult. They also have a high incidence of laryngeal and tracheal strictures, and bronchial stenosis due to inhalation injury and prolonged intubation.

## Bibliography

Herndon D. *Total Burn Care*, 5th ed. New York: Elsevier, 2018, pp. 131–57.

Smith C. *Trauma Anesthesia*. New York: Cambridge University Press, 2015, pp. 666–88.

Chapter

# 80

# Malignant Hyperthermia and Masseter Muscle Rigidity

Luis A. Vargas-Patron and Jessica A. Lovich-Sapola

## Malignant Hyperthermia

### Sample Case

A 7-year-old male is scheduled for a herniorrhaphy. The child has no prior medical history. Per his parents, he had a previous tonsillectomy with no complications at age 2. He is adopted, so no family history is available. He has a mask induction with sevoflurane. After induction, an intravenous (IV) line is placed. Twenty minutes into the case the resident notes some mild tachycardia and a slowly increasing end-tidal $CO_2$ ($ETCO_2$). What are you concerned about? What tests would you order? Assuming this is malignant hyperthermia (MH), how would you treat it?

### Clinical Issues

#### Definition

1.  MH is a hypermetabolic disorder of skeletal muscle with varied presentations.
2.  MH is a pharmaco-genetic disease.
3.  Patients have a genetic predisposition for the development of the disease once exposed to the triggering agents (a halogenated inhalational anesthetic such as halothane, isoflurane, sevoflurane, or desflurane, or the paralytic agent succinylcholine) or stressful environmental factors.
4.  There are multiple associated modes of inheritance, but all have a presumed genetic defect in calcium release channels.
5.  Intracellular hypercalcemia in the skeletal muscle activates metabolic pathways that result in adenosine triphosphate (ATP) depletion, acidosis, membrane destruction, and cell death.

#### Incidence

1.  MH has been estimated to occur in 1:100,000 administered anesthetics in the general population. All ethnic groups in all parts of the world are affected. Reactions occur more frequently in males than females (2:1).
2.  Children under 19 years account for 45–52% of reported events. This is because the incidence of MH varies from 1:40,000 to 1:250,000 in adults but may be as high as 1:15,000 in children.

#### Risk Factors (Use MH Precautions and Nontriggering Agents)

1.  Muscle biopsy diagnosis of MH
2.  Family history of MH
3.  Central core disease
4.  King–Denborough syndrome
5.  Duchenne and Becker muscular dystrophy and related muscular dystrophies and myopathies

#### Possible Associations (Use MH Precautions and Nontriggering Agents)

1.  Sudden infant death syndrome (SIDS)
2.  Smith–Lemli–Opitz syndrome
3.  Charcot–Marie–Tooth syndrome
4.  Heatstroke
5.  Mitochondrial cytopathies
6.  Burkitt's lymphoma
7.  Osteogenesis imperfecta
8.  Myotonia congenita
9.  Neuroleptic malignant syndrome
10. Myelomeningocele
11. History of heat-, stress-, or exercise-induced rhabdomyolysis

#### Testing

1.  The most sensitive test for MH is the contracture test (skeletal muscle biopsies with *in vitro* contracture testing using halothane and caffeine separately). Negative results generally rule out the diagnosis. However, the contracture test is associated with a high incidence of false positive results (20%).
2.  Patients with a positive contracture test should undergo genetic testing to identify an MH mutation. If one is found, family members should be tested as well. However, not all mutations have been identified. Genetic testing has a very high false negative rate and low sensitivity.
3.  About 70% of susceptible patients have an increased resting plasma creatinine kinase (CK) concentration. Other patients may have a normal CK value; therefore, the test is not definitive and should not be used for screening purposes.

#### Triggers

1.  Succinylcholine and potent inhalational agents
2.  Local anesthetics used for spinals, epidurals, and nerve blocks are considered safe.

3. IV propofol, barbiturates, benzodiazepines, and etomidate are safe.
4. Nitrous oxide is safe.

## Clinical Features

1. Symptoms may develop within 10 minutes to hours after the beginning of the anesthetic.
2. Some cases of MH can even develop post-operatively.

## Early

1. The most reliable initial clinical sign is an unexplained increase in ETCO$_2$.
   a. Tachypnea (in spontaneously breathing patients)
   b. Breathing over the ventilator despite minute ventilation that would usually maintain normocarbia
   c. This is usually one of the earliest, most sensitive, specific, and consistent signs.
2. Sinus tachycardia
3. Irregular heart rate (cardiac dysrhythmias) including ventricular bigeminy, multifocal ventricular premature beats, and ventricular tachycardia
4. Masseter spasm or generalized muscle rigidity which may persist despite paralysis with a nondepolarizing muscle relaxant
5. Rapid exhaustion of the soda lime
6. Warm soda lime canister
7. PaCO$_2$ increases to 100–200 mm Hg
8. Metabolic and respiratory acidosis (pH 7.14 to 6.80)
9. Hyperkalemia and peaked T waves on the EKG
10. Unstable blood pressure

## Intermediate

1. Core body temperature increases at a rate of 1–2 degrees Celsius every 5 minutes.
2. Sweating and flushing
3. Cyanosis and a decrease in arterial and central venous oxygen saturation
4. Skin mottling
5. Dark blood is found in the surgical site secondary to increased plasma myoglobin.

## Late

1. Prolonged bleeding
2. Oliguria
3. Myoglobinuria (dark urine)
4. CK concentrations are elevated >1000 IU. The laboratory value often exceeds 20,000 in the first 12–24 hours.
5. Hypercalcemia
6. Hyperphosphatemia
7. Disseminated intravascular coagulation (DIC)
8. Pulmonary edema
9. Acute renal failure

10. Central nervous system damage, including blindness, seizures, coma, or paralysis
11. The blood gas analysis will show hypercarbia with a respiratory and metabolic acidosis without marked oxygen desaturation.
12. Lactacidemia

**TKO:** MH is characterized by signs and symptoms of hypermetabolism. If the patient develops any of the above symptoms, send an arterial blood gas, potassium level, and CK level.

## Preparation for an MH-Susceptible Patient

1. Ask about personal and family history of MH and any adverse anesthetic reactions, including unexplained fever or death.
   a. It is important to note, however, that up to 50% of patients who experience an MH episode have had an uneventful anesthetic in the past.
2. Pretreatment with dantrolene is not recommended secondary to the side effects and its inability to completely prevent MH.
3. Provide a nontriggering anesthetic to any patient with a history of MH susceptibility, including a family history.
4. A fully stocked MH cart should always be immediately available when using any potent volatile anesthetics or succinylcholine. This should include 36 vials of dantrolene, sterile water (without a bacteriostatic agent) to reconstitute the dantrolene, sodium bicarbonate, furosemide, dextrose, calcium chloride, regular insulin (refrigerated), and an antiarrhythmic.
5. Prepare the anesthesia machine.
   a. Ensure that the vaporizers are disabled by removing or taping them in the off position.
   b. Change the CO$_2$ absorbent.
   c. Apply a Vapor-Clean MH filter.
      i. If the Vapor-Clean MH filter is not available, set the O$_2$ flow to 10 L/minute for 20 minutes.
      ii. Attach a clean disposable breathing bag to the Y-piece of the circle system with the ventilator set to inflate the bag periodically.
      iii. Use a new disposable breathing circuit, and wait until the expired gas analyzer indicates the absence of any volatile agent within the circuit.
6. The patient should be sedated during the pre-induction period to reduce the chance of stress-induced MH.

## Post-operative Plan for an Uneventful Anesthetic in an MH-Susceptible Patient

Assuming an uneventful anesthetic, the patient may be discharged from the post-anesthesia care unit (PACU) if he or she presents with no signs of MH after a minimum of 1 hour of every-15-minute vital sign monitoring and 1.5 hours of phase 2 PACU monitoring.

## KO Treatment Plan

### Intra-operative

1. Call for help. Call for the MH cart and dantrolene. Also, have someone call the MH hotline at #1-800-MH-HYPER (#1-800-644-9737) for added assistance. Notify the surgeon.
2. Discontinue all triggering agents.
3. Change to a clean circuit not exposed to volatile anesthetic agents, using a new clean anesthesia machine or an oxygen tank with an Ambu bag. Alternatively, insert activated charcoal filters (Vapor-Clean) into the inspiratory and expiratory limbs of the anesthesia breathing circuit.
4. Hyperventilate with 100% oxygen.
   a. Maximize fresh gas flow. Increase minute ventilation (threefold normal minute ventilation).
   b. If the patient is not intubated, intubate using a nondepolarizing muscle relaxant if necessary and institute mechanical ventilation.
   c. Have the surgeon stop the surgery as soon as possible. Either expedite or abort the surgery. If anesthesia must be continued, use nontriggering IV agents (propofol, opioids, midazolam).
5. Start an IV dantrolene loading dose of 2.5 mg/kg IV (actual body weight) through a large-bore peripheral IV. Do not delay. Administer subsequent doses of 1 mg/kg IV every five minutes until the signs of acute MH begin to abate.
6. Place an arterial line for frequent lab testing.
7. Place two large-bore IVs or a central venous catheter.
8. Monitor and treat acidosis. Give IV sodium bicarbonate 1–2 mEq/kg guided by the pH and base deficit.
9. Cool the patient aggressively with cooling blankets, cold intravenous normal saline at a rate of 15 mL/kg, cold body cavity lavage (including the surgical wound, bladder, and down the nasogastric tube), and apply ice bags to the body.
   a. The goal of the cooling is to get the patient's temperature down to 38–39 °C.
10. Closely monitor urine output with a Foley catheter. Maintain a goal urine output of >1–2 mL/kg/h using fluids, furosemide (1 mg/kg IV), and mannitol (0.25 g/kg IV). Also watch for signs of myoglobinuria.
11. Send off frequent labs, including an arterial/venous blood gas, electrolytes, hepatic function, coagulation panel, CBC, CK, serum glucose, and urine myoglobin. These labs should be closely followed for 24–48 hours.

12. Treat hyperkalemia with a combination of 0.1–0.2 U/kg of regular insulin and 500 mg/kg of dextrose IV, calcium, or bicarbonate.
13. Treat any arrhythmias that develop using amiodarone, lidocaine, adenosine, procainamide, or any other drugs indicated according to the ACLS protocol. Dysrhythmias usually subside with the resolution of the hypermetabolic phase.
    a. Do not use calcium channel blockers (verapamil or diltiazem) to treat any of the associated arrhythmias as this may worsen the hyperkalemia.

### Post-operative

1. Alkalinize the urine and diurese. Monitor for acute renal failure.
2. Follow CK levels to track the severity of the rhabdomyolysis.
3. Follow all labs and vital signs closely. Beware of hypothermia, hyperkalemia, hypokalemia, and hypervolemic overshoot.
4. Watch for signs of DIC, including thrombocytopenia, hemolysis, and abnormal bleeding.
5. Elevated liver functions are often observed 12–36 hours post-MH crisis.
6. Follow CNS function serially after an MH crisis.
7. Continue dantrolene 1 mg/kg IV q 4–6 hours for up to 72 hours after an episode of MH.
8. Submit forms to the MH registry.
9. Continue to monitor the patient for up to 72 hours in the surgical ICU. Measurements should include urine output, arterial blood gases, pH, and serum electrolyte concentrations.
10. Recrudescence of MH occurs in 20% of patients after initial treatment. Mortality from MH is 6–10%.

## Masseter Muscle Rigidity (MMR)

### Sample Case

A 27-year-old male is scheduled for an elective cosmetic procedure. He has no significant medical or surgical history. After induction with IV propofol and succinylcholine, the resident notices that she is unable to open the patient's mouth. What are your concerns? Should you cancel the case?

### Clinical Issues

#### Definition of MMR

1. Rigidity of the jaw muscles after the administration of succinylcholine
2. MMR has a spectrum of severity from mildly increased jaw tension to "jaws of steel."
3. Patients who develop MMR after the administration of succinylcholine may have up to a 50% chance of developing MH.

4. If the MMR occurs with volatile anesthetics only, the correlation with MH is almost absolute.
5. The muscle rigidity does not decrease with a repeat dose of succinylcholine or the administration of a nondepolarizing muscle relaxant.

## Presentation

1. Jaw rigidity with flaccid limbs after the administration of succinylcholine
2. Isolated masseter spasm is usually a normal variant but can be a sign of MH.

## Differential Diagnosis

1. Myotonic syndrome/dystonia
2. Temporomandibular joint dysfunction
3. Underdosing of succinylcholine
4. Not allowing sufficient time for the succinylcholine to work prior to attempting intubation
5. Normal succinylcholine-induced increase in muscle tone
6. Inadequate analgesia
7. Opioid rigidity

8. Malignant hyperthermia

## KO Treatment Plan

### Mild Jaw Tension

1. The case may continue, but switch to a nontriggering anesthetic.
2. Make sure you have $ETCO_2$ and core temperature monitoring.
3. Observe for 12–24 hours for any signs of MH.
4. The patient must be alerted to the potential MH risk and need for further testing.

### "Jaws of Steel"

1. Delay the procedure unless it is an emergency.
2. This patient requires overnight observation.
3. Observe the patient for any signs of MH, including an increase in temperature, increased pulse rate, cola-colored urine, myoglobinuria, and increased CK levels.
4. The patient must be alerted to the potential MH risk and need for further testing.

## Bibliography

Barash PG, Cullen BF, Stoelting RK, et al. *Clinical Anesthesia*, 8th ed. Philadelphia: Lippincott Williams & Wilkins, 2017, pp. 622–3.

Duke J. *Anesthesia Pearls*. Philadelphia: Hanley & Belfus, 2003, pp. 151–4.

Malignant Hyperthermia Association of the United States. Home page. www.mhaus.org.

Rosenbaum HK, Rosenberg H. Malignant hyperthermia: diagnosis and management of acute crisis. In Jones SB, ed., *UpToDate*. 2021.

Stoelting RK, Dierdorf SF. *Anesthesia and Co-existing Disease*, 4th ed. Philadelphia: Churchill Livingstone, 2002, pp. 716–21.

# Anaphylaxis

## 81

Adrienne Gomez, Fouseena Pazheri, and Jessica A. Lovich-Sapola

## Sample Case

You are called to the MRI suite to see a 20-year-old female who is undergoing an MRI of her cervical spine with and without contrast dye. Anesthesia was called secondary to the patient becoming unresponsive and difficult to ventilate. The nurse reports a rash on the patient's arm. Vital signs include blood pressure 60/40 mm Hg and heart rate 110 beats/min. Auscultation of the lungs is significant for bilateral wheezing. What is the most likely cause? How would you treat this?

## Clinical Issues

### Definitions

1. Hypersensitivity response (allergy)

   a. Type I

      i. Anaphylactic or immediate-type hypersensitivity reactions

      ii. Physiologically active mediators are released from mast cells and basophils after antigen binding to IgE antibodies on the membranes of these cells.

      iii. Examples: anaphylaxis, extrinsic asthma, and allergic rhinitis

      iv. Anaphylaxis is a severe life-threatening systemic allergic reaction usually resulting from significant release of mast cell and/or basophil derived mediators into the circulation.

         (1) Such reactions are usually acute in onset and consist of allergens reacting with IgE antibodies bound to Fc receptors on mast cells and basophils, leading to activation of cells and potent mediator release.

         (2) Anaphylaxis requires prior exposure to the antigen.

   b. Type II

      i. Immune complex reactions

      ii. Antibody-dependent cell-mediated cytotoxic hypersensitivity or cytotoxic reactions

      iii. Mediated by either IgG or IgM antibodies directed against antigens on the surface of foreign cells

      iv. Examples: ABO-incompatible transfusion reactions, drug-immune hemolytic anemia, and heparin-induced thrombocytopenia

   c. Type III

      i. Results from circulating soluble antigens and antibodies that bind to form insoluble complexes that deposit in the microvasculature

      ii. Examples: classic serum sickness, immune complex vascular injury, and protamine-mediated pulmonary vasoconstriction

   d. Type IV

      i. Delayed hypersensitivity reactions

      ii. Interactions of sensitized lymphocytes with specific antigens

      iii. Manifest in 18–24 hours, peak at 40–80 hours, and disappear at 72–96 hours

      iv. This is a form of immunity important in tissue rejection, graft-versus-host reactions, and contact dermatitis.

## Diagnosis of Anaphylaxis

See Table 81.1.

### Non-IgE-Mediated Reactions

1. Nonimmunologic anaphylaxis, formerly known as anaphylactoid reactions, has an identical or a very similar clinical response but is not IgE-mediated.

2. Nonimmunologic anaphylaxis is the result of mediators released by mast cells and basophils in the absence of immunoglobulins.

3. Common medications associated with nonimmunologic reactions include:

   a. Most opioids: morphine, meperidine, codeine

   b. Radiographic contrast media

   c. Muscle relaxants: d-tubocurarine, atracurium, mivacurium

   d. Hyperosmotic agents: plasma expanders

## Incidence of Anaphylaxis

1. Between 1 in 3500 and 1 in 20,000 anesthetics

2. The mortality rate can be as high as 4%, with an additional 2% surviving with brain damage.

**Table 81.1** Diagnosis of anaphylaxis

| The diagnosis of anaphylaxis is made when one of the following 3 criteria is present: | |
| --- | --- |
| | 1 Acute onset of illness with involvement of:<br>• Skin and/or mucosa AND either:<br>• Respiratory symptoms and skin/mucosal involvement<br>OR<br>• Hemodynamic instability or evidence of end organ dysfunction |
| | 2 The presence of two or more occurring after exposure to a *possible* allergen:<br>• Gastrointestinal symptoms<br>• Respiratory symptoms<br>• Skin/mucosal involvement<br>• Hemodynamic instability or evidence of end organ dysfunction |
| | 3 Exposure to a *confirmed* allergen:<br>• Hemodynamic instability or evidence of end organ dysfunction |

Table adapted from information in Sampson HA, Munoz-Furlong A, Campbell RL, et al. Second symposium on the definition and management of anaphylaxis: summary report – Second National Institute of Allergy and Infectious Disease/ Food Allergy and Anaphylaxis Network symposium. *Food Allerg Dermatol Dis Anaphylaxis* 2006;117(2):391–7.

3. More than 90% of allergic reactions to intravenous (IV) mediations occur within 5 minutes of administration.

## Triggers of Anaphylaxis in Order of Approximate Frequency of Occurrence in the Peri-operative Period

1. Muscle relaxants, most notably succinylcholine, rocuronium, vecuronium, and atracurium, can cause up to 60–70% of anesthesia-related anaphylaxis.
   a. Cross-reactivity can occur with acetylcholine, choline, morphine, neostigmine, pentolinium, procaine, and promethazine.
   b. Pre-exposure to these drugs may sensitize a patient, resulting in anaphylaxis without prior anesthesia.

2. Latex is a common cause of anaphylaxis. Patients at high risk for anaphylaxis to latex include health care workers, children with spina bifida and genitourinary abnormalities, multiple prior surgeries, history of fruit allergies (including banana and avocado), and workers with occupational exposure to latex. These patients should receive medical treatment in a "latex-free" environment.

3. Antibiotics, particularly β-lactam antibiotics and vancomycin, can cause an anaphylactic reaction. Penicillin accounts for the greatest number of fatal anaphylactic drug reactions in the general population.

4. Induction agents or hypnotics such as propofol may cause a rare, but often life-threatening, reaction. An allergic reaction to propofol often presents with bronchospasm.

5. Opioid anaphylaxis is rare. Morphine more commonly evokes an anaphylactoid reaction secondary to histamine release from mast cells.

6. Volume expanders: including synthetic plasma protein solutions

7. Blood products: allergic reactions still occur in about 3% of properly cross-matched blood.

8. Protamine: increased risk in patients with a history of allergy to seafood (protamine is derived from salmon sperm) and patients with diabetes mellitus treated with protamine-containing insulin preparations. Men with vasectomies may develop circulating antibodies to spermatozoa, but increased risk is unlikely. Protamine can also cause a direct histamine response, especially if given too rapidly.

9. Methyl methacrylate (bone cement)

10. Radiographic contrast media evoke an allergic reaction in about 5% of patients. This reaction tends to be an anaphylactoid reaction and can be modified by pretreatment with corticosteroids and diphenhydramine.

11. Local anesthetics: local anesthetic-induced allergic reactions are rare. Ester-based local anesthetics are metabolized to a highly antigenic compound called para-aminobenzoic acid (PABA) and are more likely to evoke an allergic reaction than the amide-based local anesthetics. Esters and amides have very rare cross-reactivity and it is considered safe to choose a local anesthetic from the alternative group. A preservative-free solution should always be used.

## Clinical Signs and Symptoms

1. Signs and symptoms may be seen immediately in sensitized individuals. Anaphylaxis patterns include:
   a. Uniphasic
   b. Biphasic: recurrence of signs and symptoms of anaphylaxis after clinical resolution of the initial

reaction. Symptoms may occur up to 72 hours after initial presentation; however, most commonly occur within the first 8 hours.

c. Protracted anaphylaxis: reactions last for hours, days, or weeks in rare cases.

2. Signs and symptoms of anaphylaxis include:

a. Vasodilation

b. Feeling of impending doom

c. Cutaneous manifestations: burning, itching, and tingling

 i. Urticaria (hives)
 ii. Rash
 iii. Edema of the skin and face
 iv. Angioedema
 v. Erythema/flushing
 vi. Pruritus

d. Respiratory: dyspnea and chest discomfort

 i. Upper airway edema and obstruction
 ii. Lower airway obstruction
 iii. Bronchospasm
 iv. Pulmonary and laryngeal edema
 v. Wheezing
 vi. Coughing
 vii. Rhinitis symptoms, ocular symptoms (tearing, redness, pruritis)
 viii. Decreased pulmonary compliance
 ix. Acute respiratory failure
 x. Sneezing

e. Cardiovascular: dizziness, malaise, and retrosternal chest pain

 i. Hypotension secondary to hypovolemia
 ii. Tachycardia
 iii. Vasodilation at the levels of the capillary and postcapillary venule
 iv. Increased capillary permeability with up to 50% extravasation of intravascular fluid volume into extracellular fluid spaces
 v. Cardiovascular collapse with associated myocardial ischemia and cardiac dysrhythmias
 vi. Syncope
 vii. Dizziness
 viii. Disorientation
 ix. Diaphoresis
 x. Loss of consciousness
 xi. Cardiac arrest
 xii. Pulmonary hypertension

f. Gastrointestinal

 i. Nausea
 ii. Vomiting
 iii. Diarrhea

g. Miscellaneous

 i. Headache
 ii. Seizure

## Differential Diagnosis

1. Vasovagal reaction

a. Urticaria, flushing, angioedema, and pruritus are usually absent. Skin is usually cool and pale.
b. Bradycardia
c. Bronchospasm is absent.
d. Blood pressure is usually normal or increased.
e. Hypotension
f. Weakness
g. Nausea and vomiting
h. Diaphoresis

2. Acute anxiety

a. Panic attack
b. Hyperventilation syndrome

3. Myocardial dysfunction
4. Pulmonary embolism
5. Systemic mast cell disorder
6. Foreign-body aspiration
7. Acute poisoning
8. Hypoglycemia/hyperglycemia
9. Seizure disorder
10. Hereditary and medication-induced angioedema
11. Asthma
12. Urticaria pigmentosa
13. Basophilic leukemia
14. Shock (hemorrhagic, hypoglycemic, cardiogenic, or endotoxic)
15. Flushing syndromes

a. Niacin, nicotine, angiotensin-converting enzyme inhibitors (ACEIs), and alcohol
b. Postmenopausal

16. Carcinoid syndrome
17. "Red man" syndrome associated with vancomycin administration
18. Monosodium glutamate (MSG)
19. Sulfites
20. Pheochromocytomas
21. Capillary leak syndrome

## Treatment Goals

1. Correct arterial hypoxemia.
2. Inhibit further release of chemical vasoactive mediators.
3. Restore intravascular volume.

### Initial Therapy

1. Stop the administration of the antigen.

2. Airway maintenance

    a. 100% oxygen

3. Discontinue all anesthetic agents.
4. Intravascular volume expansion
5. Epinephrine (5–10 µg IV bolus; 0.1–1 mg IV with cardiovascular collapse)

### Secondary Therapy

1. Antihistamine (0.5–1 mg/kg diphenhydramine)
2. Catecholamine infusion
3. Bronchodilators
4. Corticosteroids (0.25–1 g hydrocortisone)
5. Sodium bicarbonate (0.5–1 mEq/kg with persistent hypotension or acidosis)
6. Refractory shock: vasopressin and additional monitoring

# KO Treatment Plan

## Pre-operative

Intravenous contrast material is the most frequently used agent that causes anaphylactoid reactions outside of the operating room. Pretreatment with diphenhydramine, H2-blockers, and corticosteroids (up to 1 g of methylprednisolone) has been reported to be useful in preventing or ameliorating anaphylactoid reactions to IV contrast material and perhaps narcotics.

Avoid all medications that may have a potential cross-reactivity. If the patient has a latex allergy, remove all latex from the operating room and suggest that the patient be scheduled as the first case of the day, when latex particles are at their lowest in the air.

## Intra-operative

1. Assess the patient's airway. Look and listen for signs of dysphonia, stridor, cough, wheezing, or shortness of breath.
2. Evaluate vital signs. Place standard ASA monitors. Monitor for hypotension or cardiac arrhythmias.
3. Assess the patient's state of consciousness.
4. Assess for diffuse or localized edema, pruritus, urticaria, and/or angioedema.
5. Stop the offending agent. Remove all latex from the environment. Discontinue all anesthetic drugs as soon as possible.
6. Call for help.
7. Ensure adequate oxygenation with 100% oxygen.
8. Secure the airway.
9. Administer intramuscular (IM) epinephrine (1:1000 = 1 mg/mL) 0.2–0.5 mL IM every 5 minutes (can be used for minor non-life-threatening symptoms such as a rash). IM dosing is the preferred route of initial administration. Pediatric dosing is 0.01 mg/kg to a maximum dose of 0.3 mg. The lateral thigh (vastus lateralis muscle) is the preferred location for medication administration. This technique should not be used for patients under general

anesthesia. IV epinephrine is commonly used in the operating room while the patient is monitored and IV access is readily available. The sample patient requires aggressive treatment because she is hemodynamically unstable.

10. Administration of IV epinephrine is indicated when the patient develops life-threatening symptoms such as cardiac arrest or profound hypotension that fails to respond to IV volume replacement and epinephrine IM. Administer epinephrine boluses 5–10 µg IV for hypotension, 100–500 µg IV for cardiovascular collapse, and 1–3 mg IV for cardiac arrest, followed by an infusion of 1–4 µg/min up to a maximum dose of 10 µg/min. If the patient is in cardiac arrest, follow ACLS protocol and consider atropine and transcutaneous pacing. Prolonged resuscitation is encouraged because efforts are more likely to be successful in a patient with anaphylaxis.
11. Fluid resuscitation: initiate immediately in patients who present with signs of hypovolemia and/or poor organ perfusion, including orthostasis, hypotension, and suboptimal response to IM epinephrine. Administer 1–2 L of crystalloid (normal saline) within the first few minutes of treatment. Additional IV fluids may be needed until a clinical response is observed. Patients should also be continuously monitored for signs of volume overload.
12. If the patient's hypotension is refractory to volume replacement and epinephrine, consider a vasopressor infusion. Consider dopamine, norepinephrine, phenylephrine, or vasopressin to maintain perfusion pressure until the intravascular volume can be restored.
13. Treat cardiac arrythmias.
14. Antihistamines are a second-line therapy to epinephrine and should never be used alone in the treatment of anaphylaxis. Use H1- and H2-antagonists combined.

    a. H1-antagonist: diphenhydramine 25–100 mg IV for adults and 1 mg/kg for children (up to 50 mg)
    b. H2-antagonist: famotidine 20 mg IV in adults and 0.25 mg/kg in children to a maximum of 20 mg/dose

15. IV corticosteroids should be given every 6 hours to a dose equivalent to 1–2 mg/kg/day. No effect may be seen for up to 4–6 hours.
16. Bronchospasm resistant to epinephrine should be treated with inhaled β-agonist bronchodilators (e.g., nebulized albuterol).
17. Aminophylline should be considered in patients with persistent bronchospasm and hemodynamic instability as a second-line therapy after β-agonist bronchodilators.
18. Consider a glucagon infusion of 1–5 mg IV given over 5 minutes followed by an infusion of 5–15 µg/min titrated to a clinical response when a concomitant β-adrenergic blocking agent complicates the treatment. Continue aspiration precautions secondary to the glucagon's increased side effects of causing nausea and emesis.

19. Sodium bicarbonate 0.5–1 mEq/kg IV can be given for persistent hypotension or acidosis.
20. Send the following labs:

a. Serum tryptase: peaks 1–2 hours after the onset of symptoms and can persist for up to 6 hours. Ideal measurement is obtained between 1 and 2 hours after the initiation of symptoms. Serum tryptase can be used to differentiate between true anaphylaxis and nonimmunologic anaphylaxis. Elevated tryptase can help distinguish anaphylaxis from other peri-operative events, such as cardiogenic shock. However, not all anaphylactic reactions result in elevations in tryptase levels, thus a normal tryptase does not exclude anaphylaxis. Elevations in serum tryptase are most often detected in cases of anaphylaxis that involve hypotension.

b. Plasma histamine metabolites: levels begin to increase within 5–10 minutes and remain elevated for only 30–60 minutes.

c. Urine histamine metabolites: levels may remain elevated for up to 24 hours.

d. Plasma-free metanephrine and urinary vanillylmandelic acid can be drawn to rule out a pheochromocytoma.

e. Serum serotonin and urinary 5-hydroxyindoleacetic acid can be drawn to rule out carcinoid syndrome.

## Post-operative

All patients who have experienced an anaphylactic reaction require 24 hours of continued ICU-like observation due to the fact that another wave of pro-inflammatory cytokines can promote the recurrence of symptoms. Elective surgeries should be postponed up to 24–36 hours after the symptoms resolve. Delay the surgery until the patient is stable and adequately resuscitated. A truly emergent surgery should proceed with caution. The patient can be transferred to the ICU intubated or remain in the OR for resuscitation prior to resuming the emergent surgery. Be prepared to treat any recurring anaphylaxis.

Counseling and allergy skin testing can be done to determine the true cause of the allergic reaction. However, if the clinical history to a specific agent is strong, allergy testing may be unnecessary or even dangerous. An allergist may be helpful if the diagnosis is doubtful, symptoms recur or are difficult to control, the patient is a candidate for sensitization, the patient requires daily medications for prevention, or the patient requires intense education. The patient should also be encouraged to wear a medical alert bracelet and carry self-administrable epinephrine.

## Bibliography

Barash PG, Cullen BF, Stoelting RK, et al. *Clinical Anesthesia*, 8th ed. Philadelphia: Lippincott Williams & Wilkins, 2017, pp. 204–18.

Butterworth JF, Mackey DC, Wasnick JD. *Morgan & Mikhail's Clinical Anesthesiology*, 6th ed. New York: McGraw-Hill Education, 2018, pp. 1246–51.

Campbell R, Kelso J. (2021) Anaphylaxis: emergency treatment. In Walls RM, Randolph AG, eds., *UpToDate*. www.uptodate.com/contents/anaphylaxis-emergency-treatment (accessed October 15, 2021).

Chacko T, Ledford D. Peri-anesthetic anaphylaxis. *Immunol Allergy Clin North Am* 2007;**27**(2):213–30.

Goldman L, Ausiello D. *Cecil Textbook of Medicine*, 23rd ed. Philadelphia: Saunders, 2007, chapter 458.

Gropper MA. *Miller's Anesthesia*, 9th ed. Philadelphia: Elsevier, 2020, pp. 1036–8.

Lieberman P, Kemo S, Oppenheimer J, et al. The diagnosis and management of anaphylaxis: an updated practice parameter. *J Allergy Clin Immunol* 2005:**115**(3) Suppl. 2: s483–523.

Rakel RE. *Textbook of Family Medicine*, 7th ed. Philadelphia: Saunders, 2007, figure 26.1.

Stoelting RK, Dierdorf SF. *Anesthesia and Co-existing Disease*, 4th ed. Philadelphia: Churchill Livingstone, 2002, pp. 612–20.

# Patient Blood Management

Jennifer Eismon

## Sample Case

A 73-year-old female, following a motor vehicle collision, is scheduled for an urgent spine open reduction internal fixation (ORIF) due to a Chance fracture sustained while wearing a lap belt. Her medical history consists of congestive heart failure (ejection fraction is 35%), atrial fibrillation on warfarin (Coumadin) (current INR 3.1), iron deficiency anemia (hematocrit 27), and thrombocytopenia (platelets 78). She also takes aspirin 81 mg. How will you reverse the warfarin for surgery? How will you manage her anemia? Will you transfuse her prior to the surgery? What management strategies will you institute if blood loss is expected to be high? What if she refuses blood transfusion?

## Clinical Issues

### Definition of Patient Blood Management

1. Pre-operative, intra-operative, and post-operative strategy for blood and blood component administration with a goal of reducing administration
2. Utilizing drugs and techniques to minimize blood loss and need for transfusion
3. Improve the patient's outcome by reducing the risk of adverse outcomes associated with transfusions, bleeding, or anemia.
4. Transfusion risks increase with advancing age, small body size, female gender, and chronic renal, hepatic, and connective tissue diseases.

### Patient Evaluation

1. Review medical records and conduct an interview.
   a. Previous blood transfusions
   b. Drug-induced coagulopathy
   c. Presence of congenital coagulopathy and screening for bleeding disorders
   d. History of thrombotic events
   e. Risk factors for organ ischemia which may influence transfusion trigger
2. Review laboratory results
3. Order additional laboratory tests if necessary
4. Inform patient of risk of transfusion

## Pre-admission Testing

1. Diagnosis and treatment of anemia occurring in advance of an elective surgery, ideally up to 30 days
   a. Pre-operative anemia is an independent predictor of morbidity and mortality post-operatively, and a risk factor for blood transfusion.
   b. Prevalence of anemia increases with age greater than 50; 20% incidence at age greater than 85.
   c. World Health Organization defines anemia by age:
      i. 0.5–5 years: hemoglobin (Hgb) 11 g/dL
      ii. 5–12 years: Hgb 11.5 g/dL
      iii. 12–15 years, and nonpregnant women ≥15 years: Hgb 12 g/dL
      iv. Pregnant women: 11 g/dL
      v. Men ≥15 years: 13 g/dL
   d. If the patient is anemic, consider sending iron, $B_{12}$, folate, and serum creatinine lab tests.
   e. Consider correcting anemia with iron supplementation and possibly erythropoietin, which may need an expert to direct treatment.
2. Discontinuation of anticoagulants and antiplatelet medications
   a. Consult a specialist prior to discontinuation before elective surgery.
   b. In advance, if possible, discontinue nonaspirin antiplatelet therapy.
      i. Exception: patients with percutaneous coronary stents
   c. Consider the risk of thrombosis versus the risk of bleeding.
3. Autologous blood collection
   a. Collected prior to surgery no later than three days before
      i. However, there is a risk of increased anemia prior to surgery.
      ii. Cost, blood storage, and waste of blood (if not transfused) should be considerations.

b.  Reduces the number of allogenic transfusions

c.  Autologous donation is only suggested if there is adequate time for erythropoietin administration.

d.  Similar intra-operative strategies to consider are acute normovolemic hemodilution and cell salvage technology.

# Pre-procedural Preparation

1.  Blood management

    a.  Multimodal protocols

        i.   Aids practitioners to identify decision points during a procedure whereby certain interventions can be utilized

        ii.  Predetermined interventions to reduce blood loss and transfusion requirements

        iii. Transfusion protocols

        iv.  Point-of-care testing

             (1) Thromboelastography (TEG) and rotational thromboelastometry (ROTEM) guided protocols reduce transfusion when compared with standard laboratory testing.

    b.  Liberal versus restrictive transfusion criteria

        i.   Liberal transfusion is not recommended, excluding scenarios where massive transfusion is indicated.

        ii.  Restrictive transfusion is strongly recommended:

             (1) When Hgb is less than 7 g/dL in hospitalized, hemodynamically stable patients (critically ill patients included)

             (2) When Hgb is less than 8 g/dL in patients having orthopedic or cardiac surgery or those with cardiovascular disease

    c.  Consider potential and actual ongoing blood loss, intravascular volume status, signs of organ ischemia, and cardiopulmonary reserve.

    d.  Administer red blood cells (RBCs) unit-by-unit to assess the further need for transfusion and minimize unnecessary transfusion.

    e.  Avoid transfusion in patients who refuse.

    f.  Massive transfusion protocol

        i.   In cases of life-threatening hemorrhage after trauma or during a procedure, avoid the following:

             (1) Dilutional coagulopathy

             (2) Consumptive coagulopathy

             (3) Hypothermia contributes to platelet dysfunction, reduced coagulation factor activity, and fibrinolysis, which is why it is important to utilize body and fluid warming devices.

             (4) Acidosis initiated by hypoperfusion and $Na^+Cl^-$ administration leads to impairment of the coagulation process and increased fibrinogen degradation.

        ii.  Transfusion of blood products in a higher amount (1:1:1; RBC:FFP: platelets)

        iii. Optimizes delivery of blood product to severely bleeding patients

2.  Optimize coagulation

    a.  Reversal of anticoagulants should be reviewed with an expert consultant pre-procedurally when possible.

    b.  Administration of 4-factor prothrombin complex concentrates (PCC)

        i.   Risk of thromboembolic events is 0.003%

        ii.  Dose is determined by starting INR and weight of patient, starting dose 25 units/kg.

        iii. Indicated for urgent reversal of vitamin K antagonists

        iv.  Administer vitamin K concurrently.

        v.   Superior efficacy in decreasing time to correct INR and a benefit of lower risk for thrombotic events when compared with fresh frozen plasma (FFP)

    c.  Administration of FFP when INR >2 in absence of heparin

        i.   15–30 cc/kg to normalize INR

        ii.  Risk of hypervolemia and possible transfusion-related acute lung injury (TRALI)

        iii. For urgent reversal of warfarin therapy when PCC not available

        iv.  Patients with INR <1.7 are not at risk for bleeding and do not need plasma therapy for minor procedures.

    d.  Administration of vitamin K for nonurgent reversal

        i.   10 mg IV

    e.  Use of antifibrinolytics to prevent excessive blood loss

        i.   Epsilon-aminocaproic acid (EACA) before and during the procedure is effective at reducing total blood loss.

             (1) Cardiac surgery

             (2) Orthopedic surgery: when compared to placebo, EACA reduces blood loss and blood transfusion after total knee replacement.

             (3) Liver surgery

        ii.  Tranexamic acid (TXA) given before and during the procedure is effective at reducing total blood loss and volume of transfused products.

3.  Acute normovolemic hemodilution

a. Involves collecting 500–1500 mL of the patient's blood prior to incision, then administering crystalloid or colloid to replace volume

b. Reduces volume of allogenic blood transfused and number of patients transfused in major cardiac, orthopedic, thoracic, or liver surgery especially combined with intra-operative RBC recovery

c. Reduction in storage lesions

d. No standardized protocol

## Intra-operative and Post-operative Management of Blood Loss

1. Meticulous surgical technique and, when possible, minimally invasive surgery

2. Allogenic RBC transfusion

   a. Age of stored blood; the studies are equivocal on new versus older stored blood on hospital mortality, 30-day post-discharge mortality, infection, and length of stay.

      i. Storage of RBCs:

         (1) Impairs RBC deformability
         (2) Decreased ATP levels
         (3) Decreases 2,3-diphosphoglycerate levels
         (4) Decreases nitric oxide-hemoglobin
         (5) Promotes endothelial adherence
         (6) Increases aggregation (pro-thrombotic effects)
         (7) Increased $K^+$, free hemoglobin, iron from hemolysis
         (8) Decreased pH

   b. Leukocyte reduction reduces complications associated with allogenic blood transfusion.

3. Autologous blood cell salvage and reinfusion of recovered blood cells reduces the volume of allogenic blood transfusion and is considered a blood-sparing technique.

   a. Use is relatively contraindicated in cancer, obstetrics, and bowel contamination surgeries.

   b. Potential risks are: bacterial contamination, febrile reactions, DIC, and coagulopathy caused by dilution.

4. Intra-operative and post-operative monitoring

   a. Blood loss entails viewing the surgical field and assessing blood present and presence of microvascular bleeding, surgical sponges, clot size, suction canisters, and post-operative surgical drain output.

   b. Perfusion of vital organs

      i. Standard ASA monitors with physical examination and observation of clinical symptoms

      ii. Consider echocardiography, renal monitoring, cerebral monitoring, arterial blood gas, and mixed venous oxygen saturation.

   c. Monitor for anemia by measuring serial hemoglobin and hematocrit when clinically justified. Measure blood loss and monitor clinical signs.

      i. Note that two-thirds of patients contract hospital-acquired anemia due to phlebotomy-induced blood draw. Blood loss is an average of 41–65 mL/day.

   d. Coagulopathy

      i. Standard coagulation tests (INR, aPTT, fibrinogen concentration), platelet count, and, if necessary, platelet function

      ii. Viscoelastic assays (TEG, ROTEM)

         (1) Viscoelastic guided algorithms are shown to reduce blood transfusion requirements.

   e. Adverse effects of transfusion; if suspected, stop the transfusion, notify the hospital's blood bank, order appropriate diagnostic testing, and initiate supportive therapy.

      i. ABO incompatibility; monitor for hyperthermia, hemoglobinuria, microvascular bleeding.

      ii. TRALI is the leading cause of transfusion-related death.

         (1) Appears within 6 hours of administration
         (2) Caused by donor antibodies in plasma interacting with antigens on patients' granulocytes (mostly FFP and platelets, occasionally RBCs)
         (3) Must be distinguished from transfusion-associated circulatory overload
         (4) Incidence of TRALI recently declined due to the preferential use of male donor plasma.
         (5) Look for fever, respiratory distress, hypoxemia, and increased peak airway pressure.
         (6) Consider ordering a chest radiograph and arterial blood gas.

      iii. Bacterial contamination; mostly associated with platelets

      iv. Allergic reaction; look for urticarial and hypotension, caused by immunoglobulin E antibodies in the patient against donor plasma.

      v. Citrate toxicity; look for hypocalcemia and hypomagnesemia.

5. Treatment of excessive bleeding due to coagulopathy

a. Plasma-derived treatment of excessive bleeding can be hindered by the large volume and time required for thawing and transfusion.

  i. Transfusion of platelets is indicated by the platelet count or platelet function test.

  ii. Transfusion of FFP is indicated by coagulation tests.

  iii. Transfusion of cryoprecipitate

    (1) Indicated when fibrinogen levels are less than 80–100 mg/dL

      (a) European guidelines recommend transfusion when fibrinogen is less than 150–200 mg/dL, which reflects clinical data supporting early fibrinogen replacement and higher target levels after major trauma, intra-operative blood loss, and hemodilution.

    (2) For pregnancy, transfuse fibrinogen when less than 250 mg/dL.

      (a) Higher target reflects physiological changes that occur during term pregnancy (350–650 mg/dL)

    (3) Cryoprecipitate is the cold, insoluble precipitate left behind from slowly thawed FFP, and contains fibrinogen, FVIII, von Willebrand's, and FXIII.

    (4) Fibrinogen content varies in cryoprecipitate (0.3 g/unit).

b. Pharmacologic treatment of excessive bleeding can rapidly restore deficient factors without precipitating volume overload.

  i. Desmopressin

  ii. Antifibrinolytics

  iii. Topical hemostatic such as fibrin glue and thrombin gel

    (1) Beware of allergic reactions.

  iv. PCC

    (1) Freeze-dried (FLyP) human plasma-derived vitamin K dependent factors (FII, FVII, FIX, FX)

      (a) Some preparations have heparin.

      (b) Use caution in patients with heparin-induced thrombocytopenia.

    (2) Administration is followed by a normalization of INR and a reduction in bleeding.

    (3) Off-label use of PCC has been utilized in acquired, nonwarfarin-related coagulopathy in major trauma and surgery.

  v. Coagulation factor concentrates (FVIIa) use is considered when traditional options have been exhausted in the presence of excessive bleeding.

  vi. Treatment of hypofibrinogenemia with fibrinogen concentrate. Each vial has a standard fibrinogen content of 900–1300 mg.

    (1) Contraindications are previous anaphylactic reactions, thrombosis, and myocardial infarction.

## KO Treatment Plan

### Pre-operatively

1. The Chance fracture is an unstable lumbar fracture and has a high association with intra-abdominal injury. This is a high-velocity injury usually associated with a lap belt.
2. Volume overload due to her heart failure using FFP is a concern as her elevated INR from her warfarin needs reversing, PCC 25 units/kg with concurrent vitamin K administration is the better choice after a thorough history to assess the patient's thrombosis risk. This should be administered prior to surgery and, if there is time, check a repeat INR after administration.
3. The patient has been taking aspirin, and with her underlying thrombocytopenia a platelet transfusion may be warranted pre-operatively. A platelet function assay could lend further information to pursue giving platelets.
4. Get further laboratory information if not already obtained; baseline coagulation studies including fibrinogen.
5. Type and cross-match should be performed.
6. Cell salvage system should be available.
7. A fluid warming device should be available and room temperature should be adjusted accordingly.
8. Antifibrinolytic therapy should be available.
9. Preinduction arterial line
10. Place a central line, as the patient would be in a prone position for surgical repair, and hypotension and resuscitation are considerations for placement.
11. There is no time to treat underlying anemia with iron therapy as this case is urgent.
12. I would not pre-emptively transfuse packed red blood cells (PRBCs) unless she was hemodynamically unstable.
13. Disposition intensive care setting
14. If the patient is refusing blood transfusion after discussion of risks and benefits and with the knowledge that her surgery has the potential for high-volume blood loss due to her injuries, verify with the patient exactly what she will accept (e.g., albumin, cell saver, etc.). Start antifibrinolytic therapy, discuss the use of pharmacological treatment, and discuss with the surgeon about meticulous surgical technique and possibility for staging surgery if possible.

## Intra-operatively

1. The patient most likely would have a cervical collar present and a rapid-sequence intubation should be performed with in-line stabilization, assuming she does not have a difficult airway and awake fiber-optic is not needed.

2. Due to the patient's congestive heart failure, consider etomidate as the induction agent.

3. Vasopressors should be available to treat hypotension after induction.

4. Judicious use of fluids during the case is necessary as she has ejection fraction 35% and would not tolerate fluid resuscitation.

5. Serial arterial blood gas (ABG), complete blood count (CBC), and thromboelastometry to direct transfusion therapy during the case and when clinically indicated

6. Vigilant observation of current blood loss, blood on the field, and communication with the surgeon is necessary to direct transfusion.

7. Cell salvage blood administration to the patient when dictated

8. If massive transfusion protocol is instituted this patient would have high mortality from ongoing blood loss but also resuscitation as cardiogenic pulmonary edema most likely would occur. Consider concurrent furosemide administration to promote diuresis.

9. If the patient underwent massive transfusion, consider keeping her intubated and transport to the surgical ICU. Otherwise, consider extubation and recovery in the postanesthetic care unit.

## Post-operative

1. Optimize erythropoiesis.

    a. Manage nutritional and correctable anemia.

    b. Be aware of medication interactions.

2. Minimize blood loss.

    a. Monitor for and manage post-operative bleeding.

    b. Maintain normothermia.

    c. Autologous blood salvage

    d. Hemostasis and anticoagulant management

3. Manage anemia.

    a. Maximize oxygen delivery.

    b. Minimize oxygen consumption.

    c. Avoid and treat infections promptly.

    d. Continue to follow evidence-based transfusion strategies.

## Bibliography

American Society of Anesthesiologists Task Force on Perioperative Blood Transfusion and Adjuvant Therapies. Practice guidelines for perioperative blood transfusion and adjuvant therapies: an updated report by the American Society of Anesthesiologists Task Force on Perioperative Blood Transfusion and Adjuvant Therapies. *Anesthesiology* 2015;**122**:241–75.

Bennett S, Harbi M. Anaemia and blood transfusion: incorporating patient blood management. *Surgery (Oxford)* 2019;**37**:424–30.

Goodnough LT, Shander A. Patient blood management. *Anesthesiology* 2012;**116**:1367–76.

Gropper, M. *Miller's Anesthesia*, 9th edition. Philadelphia: Elsevier, 2020, pp. 1579–602.

Hohmuth B, Ozawa S, Ashton M, et al. Patient-centered blood management. *J Hosp Med* 2014;**9**:60–5.

Johansson PI, Ostrowski SR, Secher NH. Management of major blood loss: an update. *Acta Anaesthesiol Scand* 2010;**54**:1039–49.

Shander A, Javidroozi M. Blood conservative strategies and management of perioperative anemia. *Curr Opin Anaesth* 2015;**28**:356–68.

Shander A, Van Aken H, Spahn D. Patient blood management in Europe. *Br J Anaesth* 2012;**109**(1):55–68.

Tanaka KA, Esper S, Bollinger D. Perioperative factor concentrate therapy. *Br J Anaesth* 2013;**111**(S1):i35–i49.

Chapter

# 83

# Liver Transplant

Robert St. Jules and Erica Fagelman

## Sample Case

A 59-year-old, 173 cm (5'8"), 75 kg man is scheduled for orthotopic liver transplantation. The patient was diagnosed with alcoholic cirrhosis 12 years ago. His current MELD score is 24. He has associated portal hypertension, ascites requiring regular large-volume paracentesis, mild encephalopathy, and esophageal varices that required banding 2 years ago. He quit drinking alcohol 2 years ago. His past medical history is significant for hypertension and noninsulin-dependent type 2 diabetes mellitus. He is a current smoker with mild chronic obstructive pulmonary disease (COPD). His medications include propranolol, metformin, famotidine, lisinopril, furosemide, lactulose, rifaximin, and a multivitamin.

What is the Model for End-stage Liver Disease (MELD) risk score?

What physiological changes associated with cirrhotic liver disease do you expect? How will these changes affect your intra-operative plan?

What pre-operative testing will you require for this patient?

What is a transjugular intrahepatic portosystemic shunt (TIPS)?

What are hepatorenal and hepatopulmonary syndromes?

What intra-operative monitors and vascular access will you employ?

What concerns do you have regarding the pre-anhepatic phase? The anhepatic phase? The neo-hepatic phase?

What potential post-operative complications are you concerned about following successful liver transplantation?

## Pre-operative Management

### Classification of Liver Disease Severity

1. Modified Child–Pugh score
   a. Utilizes serum bilirubin, albumin, prothrombin time (PT/INR), presence of ascites, and encephalopathy
   b. Increasing score correlates with decreasing 1- and 2-year patient survival.

2. MELD
   a. Prognostic scoring system utilizing serum bilirubin, creatinine, and INR.
      i. Newer model also incorporates serum sodium (MELD-Na)
   b. Currently used by the United Network for Organ Sharing (UNOS) for allograft allocation (in addition to blood type stratification)
   c. Higher scores correlate with worse 3-month survival and thus are ranked higher on the transplant waiting list.
   d. Certain conditions apply exception points to increase MELD score and thus position on the waiting list.
      i. Hepatocellular carcinoma (HCC), hepatopulmonary syndrome (HPS), portopulmonary hypertension (PPH), cholangiocarcinoma, hepatic artery thrombosis

## Indications for Liver Transplant

1. Acute liver failure
   a. Drug-induced, viral, or acute hepatitis

2. End-stage liver disease (cirrhosis)
   a. Alcoholic
   b. Nonalcoholic steatohepatitis (NASH)
   c. Chronic hepatitis
   d. Cholestatic disease
      i. Primary biliary cholangitis (PBC)
      ii. Primary sclerosing cholangitis (PSC)

3. Metabolic disorders
   a. Alpha-1 antitrypsin deficiency
   b. Cystic fibrosis
   c. Glycogen storage diseases
   d. Hemochromatosis
   e. Wilson's disease
   f. Acute intermittent porphyria

4. Hepatic neoplasms (if transplantation is curative)

5. Other miscellaneous
   a. Budd–Chiari syndrome, amyloidosis

## Contraindications for Liver Transplant

1.  Significant cardiopulmonary disease unable to be corrected prior to transplant

    a.  Significant coronary artery disease
    b.  Significant hypoxemia
    c.  Moderate to severe pulmonary hypertension (mean pulmonary artery pressure (mPAP) >50 mm Hg is an absolute contraindication; mPAP of 35–50 mm Hg depends on each transplant institution's criteria)

2.  Malignancy outside the liver (including spread of HCC outside the liver)
3.  Aggressive intrahepatic malignancy (cholangiocarcinoma, hemangiosarcoma)
4.  Uncontrolled sepsis (active infection requires clearance of infective source prior to transplant)
5.  Acquired immunodeficiency syndrome (AIDS)
6.  Specific anatomic abnormalities that preclude successful transplantation
7.  Lack of adequate social support or medical nonadherence

    a.  Continued alcohol or illicit drug use

## Pathophysiology of End-Stage Liver Disease

1.  Cardiopulmonary changes

    a.  Decreased systemic vascular resistance (SVR) leading to a hyperdynamic state (cardiac index [CI] often >5–6 L/min/m$^2$)

        i.  Increased portosystemic shunting allows bypassing of liver detoxification leading to increased systemic inflammatory cytokine levels and exposure to gut bacteria fragments/byproducts.
        ii.  Increased systemic nitric oxide production
        iii.  Decreased endogenous arginine vasopressin levels
        iv.  Decreased renal perfusion leads to activation of renin–angiotensin (RAS) system.

            (1)  Causes volume retention, increased cardiac output (CO) partially offsets decreased SVR

    b.  Cirrhotic cardiomyopathy

        i.  Pathologic hyperdynamic state with diminished response to pharmacologic agents and physiologic stressors

            (1)  Can precipitate overt heart failure in the setting of volume overload or sudden increase in afterload

    c.  Coronary disease

        i.  Cirrhotic patients are no more at risk for coronary artery disease compared to noncirrhotic patients.

            (1)  Exception is in patients with NASH: often associated with diabetes and metabolic syndrome and increased incidence of coronary artery disease

    d.  Decreased intravascular volume

        i.  Patients are often volume overloaded but intravascularly dry secondary to transudative losses.

            (1)  Decreased albumin/protein levels lead to lower oncotic pressure and generalized edema.
            (2)  Further loss via ascites from increased portal pressures

                (a)  Serum-ascites albumin gradient can help differentiate transudative versus exudative ascites.

    e.  Restrictive pulmonary disease

        i.  Large-volume ascites restricts diaphragmatic excursion and reduces functional residual capacity (FRC) and lung compliance.
        ii.  Hepatic hydrothorax may further exacerbate this (usually on the right).

    f.  Portopulmonary hypertension (PPH)

        i.  Pulmonary arterial hypertension associated with portal hypertension
        ii.  Pulmonary artery (PA) pressures are often high due to volume overload; may require right heart catheterization to obtain the pulmonary capillary wedge pressure (PCWP) to diagnose elevated pulmonary vascular resistance (PVR).

            (1)  Prolonged hyperdynamic state in the setting of volume overload can increase PVR over time.

        iii.  Often responsive to pulmonary vasodilators pre-operatively; however, if elevated at time of the transplant may preclude transplantation if unable to decrease with inhaled nitric oxide (NO) due to the high peri-operative mortality with moderate–severe pulmonary hypertension.

            (1)  Goal is mPAP <35 mm Hg with treatment
            (2)  mPAP >50 mm Hg is an absolute contraindication to liver transplantation.

        iv.  May worsen in the immediate post-transplant period; up to two-thirds of patients will show improvement or normalization of pulmonary pressures within 6 months after transplant.

    g.  Hepatopulmonary syndrome (HPS)

        i.  Ventilation–perfusion mismatch secondary to: pulmonary capillary dilation (limits oxygen diffusion: more common) and newly created arteriovenous connections (shunting: less common)

  (1) Often presents as progressive dyspnea and hypoxemia

  (2) Platypnea/orthodeoxia: increased dyspnea and decreased arterial oxygen tension in an upright position (relative to supine)

  (3) Alveolar–arterial gradient ≥15 mm Hg (or ≥20 in patients ≥65 years) with evidence of shunting on contrast echocardiography in patients with portal hypertension is diagnostic.

    (a) Severity is determined by room air $PaO_2$ (mild ≥80 mm Hg; moderate 60–80 mm Hg; severe 50–60 mm Hg; and very severe <50 mm Hg).

  (4) Pulmonary function tests (PFTs) are not very helpful, and will often show normal flow patterns

  ii. Treatment is oxygen supplementation until liver transplantation (resolves in days to up to 1 year following transplant).

2. Coagulation disorders

  a. Impaired hemostasis (bleeding risk)

   i. Decreased synthesis of coagulation factors

    (1) Levels of Factor VIII and vWF unaffected (produced by endothelium)

   ii. Vitamin K deficiency

   iii. Increased levels of nitric oxide and prostacyclin

   iv. Thrombocytopenia and thrombocytopathia

    (1) Splenic sequestration, decreased thrombopoietin levels, uremia secondary to renal failure

  b. Enhanced coagulation (clotting risk)

   i. Decreased production of anticoagulation factors (protein C and S, antithrombin III, α2-macroglobulin, heparin cofactor II, and ADAMTS-13)

   ii. Factor VIII and vWF may be elevated.

  c. Fibrinolytic disorders

   i. Can be increased or decreased; hyperfibrinolysis is more common secondary to decreased hepatic clearance of plasminogen activator.

  d. Standard studies (PT/INR, aPTT) often poorly characterize the current coagulation status due to this rebalanced hemostasis.

   i. Viscoelastic testing (TEG, ROTEM) provides a better picture but still requires clinical correlation (*in vitro* vs. *in vivo*).

  e. Vitamin K supplementation several days prior to surgery can decrease INR and bleeding risk (avoid fresh frozen plasma [FFP] pre-operatively unless bleeding emergency).

   i. Other goals similar to standard surgical patients: platelets ≥50 k and fibrinogen ≥200 mg/dL

  f. Patients with portal vein thrombosis (PVT) may be on some form of anticoagulation.

   i. Enoxaparin for acute PVT

   ii. Direct-acting oral anticoagulants may be used for secondary prevention.

3. Portal hypertension

  a. Diagnosed via hepatic venous pressure gradient (HVPG ≥6 mm Hg)

   i. Becomes clinically significant when HVPG ≥10 and at ≥12 there is increased risk of variceal bleeding and ascites formation

  b. Leads to formation of portosystemic shunts and ascites

   i. Esophageal/gastric varices

    (1) β-blockers are often utilized to minimize bleeding risk.

    (2) May require endoscopic therapy for banding.

    (3) TIPS procedure can decrease portal pressures for refractory varices/ascites (see below).

   ii. Other shunts include intra-abdominal varices, caput medusa, and hemorrhoids.

  c. Splenomegaly causes sequestration of up to 90% of the circulating platelet mass (functional thrombocytopenia).

  d. TIPS

   i. Iatrogenic shunt created to decrease portal pressures and minimize the complications associated with portal hypertension (refractory ascites, spontaneous bacterial peritonitis, or variceal bleeding)

   ii. Can worsen hepatic encephalopathy

   iii. Congestive heart failure (CHF), severe tricuspid regurgitation, and right ventricular dysfunction (with or without pulmonary hypertension) are contraindications as TIPS can significantly increase preload to the right heart.

4. Renal dysfunction

  a. Electrolyte disturbances

   i. Hyponatremia is the most common electrolyte disturbance.

(1) High circulating levels of antidiuretic hormone (ADH) can lead to free water retention.

(2) Correct acutely only if <120 mEq/L or with development of neurologic symptoms.

(3) Transplantation may need to be postponed for sodium levels <120 mEq/L as intra-operative overcorrection is more likely, increasing the risk for osmotic demyelination syndrome.

    ii. Potassium

(1) Hypokalemia may precipitate hepatic encephalopathy and should be corrected if <3.0 mEq/L.

(2) Hyperkalemia may be present in the setting of acute or chronic renal failure and should be corrected, especially prior to liver transplantation as packed red blood cells (PRBC) administration will worsen this.

b. Hepatorenal syndrome (HRS)

    i. Splanchnic arterial vasodilation and decreased intravascular volume can lead to hypoperfusion of the kidney, causing renal insufficiency.

(1) Type 1: more serious; 50% reduction in creatinine clearance in <2 weeks

(2) Type 2: less serious; progressive decline in kidney function, characterized by diuretic resistant ascites

    ii. If decreased function does not improve with fluid challenge (often 1.5 L), one must rule out other causes, including acute tubular necrosis or urinary obstruction.

    iii. Renal tubular function is preserved with hyperosmolar urine and urine sodium excretion <10 mEq/L; histology is often normal.

    iv. Both types carry a poor prognosis; treatment is supportive with the goal of improving hepatic function (correlates with improved renal function).

(1) Albumin, midodrine, and octreotide may improve kidney function.

(2) May require initiation of renal replacement therapy prior to liver transplant

(3) Up to 75% of HRS patients experience return to normal kidney function following liver transplant.

5. Neurologic

a. Hepatic encephalopathy (HE): altered mental status ranging from confusion to coma

    i. Secondary to increased shunting of intestinal nitrogenous waste normally filtered by liver

(ammonia is the most commonly described neurotoxin leading to HE).

    ii. Can be precipitated by hypoxia, hyponatremia, hypokalemia, hypovolemia, hypoglycemia, and alkalemia

    iii. Treated with lactulose and rifaximin to minimize systemic circulation of intestinal bacteria byproducts

b. Wernicke's encephalopathy: associated with chronic alcohol abuse; treated with vitamin B and thiamine

c. Cerebral edema: more commonly seen in acute liver failure; may require intra-operative intracranial pressure (ICP) monitoring (pupilometer, optic nerve sheath diameters, intraventricular catheter)

6. Hypoalbuminemia

a. Causes transudative fluid shifts, as mentioned previously

b. Can exaggerate the clinical effect of protein-bound drugs due to the increased unbound fraction

7. Hepatocellular carcinoma

a. Intrahepatic tumor associated with cirrhosis (also in chronic hepatitis B infection, even in the absence of cirrhosis)

    i. Diagnosed with elevated alpha-fetoprotein (AFP) level and radiographic evidence

b. Early treatment includes directed chemotherapy/radiotherapy (RFA, Y90).

    i. Multiple courses of treatment may complicate the dissection phase of transplant surgery.

c. Presence often precludes intra-operative use of cell salvage

d. Metastasis outside of the liver capsule precludes liver transplantation

## Pre-operative Testing

1. Laboratory testing

a. Complete blood count and comprehensive metabolic panel

    i. Hematocrit, renal function, and sodium and potassium levels are of importance immediately prior to transplant.

b. Basic coagulation testing (PT/INR, aPTT, fibrinogen) are useful in determining the extent of liver dysfunction, but often misrepresent actual coagulation status.

c. Type and cross-match

    i. Typically, 10 units of PRBC and 10 units of FFP are adequate; consider ordering more to start if there is concern for significant blood loss beyond the standard transplant.

  ii. Cryoprecipitate and platelets can be ordered intra-operatively in the presence of coagulopathic bleeding, with correlating viscoelastic testing.

2. Imaging

 a. Head CT: often obtained in acute/fulminant liver failure with mental status changes or in chronic liver failure with unexplained encephalopathy

  i. Presence of cerebral edema may require intra-operative ICP monitoring.

 b. Chest/abdomen/pelvis: often part of standard pre-transplant evaluation

  i. May provide evidence of underlying pulmonary disease

  ii. Complex abdominal anatomy may complicate the transplant, requiring a different surgical technique or may worsen intra-operative hemodynamics/blood loss.

   (1) Large portal vein thrombus, cavernous malformation of portal system, prior bowel/hepatic surgeries, anatomical variants

3. Cardiac testing

 a. Electrocardiogram

  i. Prior malignant arrhythmia, significant conduction defects, or high conduction blockade may necessitate placement of a pacemaker/defibrillator prior to transplant.

 b. Transthoracic echocardiogram

  i. Presence of elevated right ventricular systolic pressure (RVSP) or concerns for pulmonary hypertension should be further evaluated with a right heart catheterization.

  ii. Significant valvular stenosis may preclude transplantation until corrected.

   (1) Balloon valvuloplasty can be utilized as a bridge to liver transplant with a definitive valvular repair/replacement following a successful transplant.

  iii. Diminished function may be masked by comorbid cirrhotic cardiomyopathy.

  iv. Decreased right ventricular function or the presence of CHF may require venovenous bypass or piggyback technique (may not tolerate conventional caval replacement).

  v. Contrast-enhanced echocardiograms can further characterize intra- versus extracardiac shunts in patients with suspected HPS.

 c. Noninvasive stress testing

  i. No definitive guidelines on which patients to test. The algorithm is transplant institution-specific (often any patient age >40, some test any adult patient).

  ii. Dobutamine/adenosine stress testing may poorly characterize the presence of coronary artery disease (CAD) in patients on β-blockers for varices.

  iii. Dynamic left ventricular (LV) outflow obstruction is commonly seen (already hyperdynamic due to liver disease, exposure to chronotropic agents can worsen diastolic filling and lead to decreased LV volume).

 d. Cardiac catheterization

  i. Left heart catheterization is typically reserved for patients with a positive stress test, symptoms of active ischemia, or (in certain transplant institutions) if patients meet certain criteria (advanced age, presence of diabetes/hypertension, smoking, and/or significant atherosclerotic disease).

  ii. Significant coronary artery stenoses should be revascularized prior to transplant.

  iii. Right heart catheterization should be performed on any patient with concern for pulmonary hypertension with follow-up testing to evaluate efficacy of any treatments initiated.

4. Pulmonary testing

 a. PFTs: not standard in liver transplant evaluation; may be performed in patients with comorbid pulmonary disease (COPD, HPS)

 b. Pulse oximetry/arterial blood gas on room air can characterize the severity of HPS.

 c. Patients with recurrent hepatic hydrothorax may require pre-operative thoracentesis to improve respiratory function.

5. Endoscopy

 a. Esophagogastroduodenoscopy (EGD) and colonoscopy are performed to evaluate for the presence and severity of varices and to rule out colorectal cancer prior to any patient being placed on the transplant list.

 b. Recent (<1 month) treatment of varices or significant gastrointestinal bleeding may preclude intra-operative use of transesophageal echocardiogram (TEE) for pre-operative screening and intra-operatively.

6. Timing of surgery

 a. Deceased donor transplants are emergency surgeries; the case should not be delayed as increased organ ischemia times are correlated with worse outcomes.

i. If the patient presents poorly optimized for liver transplantation (uncontrolled pulmonary hypertension [pHTN], new or worsening CAD/CHF, active infection, severe hyponatremia), the case should be canceled and the organ should be allocated to a new recipient.

ii. Induction should occur only after the surgical team approves the allocated graft (may require visualization and/or biopsy upon harvest).

iii. ABO verification (between patient and incoming graft) must also occur before patient induction.

iv. Ensure availability of blood products prior to surgical incision.

b. Living donor transplants can be delayed for further optimization of donor/recipient if required as both cases often start simultaneously.

## Intra-operative Management

### Induction

1. Should always be considered a full stomach (decreased gastric emptying, presence of ascites)

   a. Consider H2-blocker and nonparticulate antacid.

   b. Nasogastric tubes should be placed with caution (or completely avoided) in patients with coagulopathy.

   c. Often these patients require only a working peripheral IV (PIV) for induction.

      i. Consider a pre-induction arterial line for patients with significant cardiopulmonary disease or adrenal insufficiency.

   d. Reverse Trendelenburg position can optimize ventilation and minimize the risk of passive regurgitation after induction

   e. Rapid-sequence intubation (double-dose nondepolarizing agent should be used if the patient's potassium is elevated, instead of succinylcholine).

2. Medications

   a. Induction with propofol is usually well tolerated; consider etomidate in patients with significant cardiovascular disease or concern for hemodynamic instability.

      i. All of these patients should be expected to have significant hypotension following induction (low SVR, relative hypovolemia).

      ii. Even with adequate preoxygenation, the decreased FRC (secondary to ascites) and increased CO will decrease time you have until hypoxia develops following induction.

   b. Maintenance of anesthesia with a combination of volatile anesthetic and IV opiate (usually fentanyl with a goal of <20 µg/kg total)

      i. Epidurals are contraindicated secondary to the significant coagulopathy associated with the anhepatic phase.

      ii. Avoid nitrous (long case; significant vascular manipulation leading to air entrainment/emboli).

      iii. Total IV anesthesia with propofol is a better choice in cases with increased ICP.

      iv. Benzodiazepines can minimize risk of intra-operative awareness if anesthetic reduction is required in an effort to decrease the effects on CO/SVR.

   c. Neuromuscular blockade can be maintained with any agent as hepatic clearance will improve following successful graft reperfusion.

      i. Consider cisatracurium with concomitant renal failure.

   d. Vasoactive agents should be drawn up and readily available prior to induction.

      i. Commonly vasopressin, norepinephrine, epinephrine

3. Monitors/vascular access

   a. Standard ASA monitors with five-lead ECG

   b. Defibrillator with pads placed on patient prior to induction

   c. Arterial line

      i. Often radial (axillary if unable to obtain radial)

      ii. Second catheter in femoral or opposite radial is utilized as backup in some institutions

   d. Reliable large-bore PIV (e.g., rapid infusion catheter [RIC] 7 Fr or 8.5 Fr)

      i. Should be connected to a rapid transfusion device (e.g., Belmont)

      ii. If unable to obtain peripherally, a large-bore (7 Fr sheath) central line can be utilized (if utilizing introducer lumen for pulmonary artery catheter [PAC], will require separate central venous catheter [CVC] for rapid transfusion).

      iii. If venovenous bypass (VVB) is planned, a second large-bore catheter should be available (either RIC or CVC is viable for VVB venous return).

   e. CVC with PAC through introducer port

      i. Central access should be via upper body (femoral is inadequate as inferior vena cava is often clamped during transplant).

      ii. PACs are common but dependent on each institution's practice.

(1) Allow real-time monitoring of CO, central venous oxygenation, PVR, and core temperature.

(2) In patients with known or suspected pHTN, a PAC should be placed pre-incision to rule out moderate–severe pHTN that may preclude transplantation.

(3) Complications include: PA dissection/rupture, arrhythmia, right bundle branch block, knotting/entrapment of catheter, air or thromboembolism, valve infection/rupture, and pulmonary infarction.

  iii. Central venous pressure (CVP) monitored via PAC; if no PAC, can transduce off side-port

  iv. Temporary dialysis catheter placement may be required if intra-operative and/or post-operative continuous venovenous hemofiltration (CVVH) is required.

f. TEE

  i. Similar to PACs; placement of TEE is common but institution-dependent.

  ii. Allows real-time monitoring of cardiac function, hemodynamics, and for development/progression of intracardiac thrombus or clinically significant emboli

  iii. Relative contraindications: very large varices, active GI bleeding, or recent variceal ligation

g. Gastric tube: improves surgical exposure but is associated with an increased risk of GI bleed

h. Neuromonitoring

  i. BIS monitor can assist in monitoring for intra-operative awareness (anesthesia is often decreased around the anhepatic period to minimize the effect on hemodynamics)

  ii. Cerebral oximetry: not commonly used but can be considered if concern for cerebral deoxygenation (significant carotid stenosis)

  iii. ICP monitoring should be continued if in place pre-operatively.

i. Foley catheter: monitoring of urine output and core temperature

j. Temperature management

  i. Combination of fluid/blood warmers and forced-air warming should be utilized.

4. Fluid/blood management

a. Combination of albumin and an isotonic buffered crystalloid (e.g., Plasma-Lyte)

b. Transfusion goal of hematocrit (HCT) is 25–30% (keep a slight buffer in case of sudden hemorrhage)

c. FFP is typically administered in a 1:1 ratio with PRBC administration to minimize the risk of dilutional coagulopathy.

d. Cell salvage should be utilized unless contraindicated (HCC, infection) and FFP administered with each "unit" of transfused salvage blood.

5. Antibiotics are often selected by an infectious disease team that specializes in transplant patients and should be administered as required peri-operatively.

## Pre-anhepatic

1. Surgical phase encompassing surgical incision until removal of the native liver

a. Management is influenced by the surgical technique utilized.

  i. Total caval occlusion (conventional caval replacement technique) will require aggressive fluid management prior to caval clamping to tolerate the significant decrease in venous return and accompanying hemodynamic instability.

(1) Existing collaterals (extrahepatic portosystemic shunts) provide variable flow around vascular clamps to maintain some venous return.

(2) In fulminant liver failure, collateral circulation has not yet developed, so conventional caval replacement is often not tolerated (requires VVB).

  ii. Piggyback and VVB techniques minimize the aforementioned hemodynamic effects, allowing more judicious fluid management.

(1) Piggyback technique requires appropriate anatomy to create anastomoses; native hepatic veins are reconstructed to allow donor suprahepatic vena cava to be anastomosed to the native vena cava (the donor infrahepatic vena cava is sewn or stapled closed).

(2) VVB utilizes a femoral or iliac vein cannula ± a portal vein cannula as the drainage lines; the venous return cannula is passed to the anesthesiology team and connected to a high-flow line (RIC or large vascular sheath, e.g., introducer or dialysis line).

(a) It is vital to ensure the appropriate inflow/outflow limbs of the circuit are connected to their appropriate positions.

(b) Complications include: air embolism, thromboembolism, hypothermia, vascular injury, and/or significant lymphedema.

b. Intermittent compression of native vessels with manipulation of the liver is common, leading to acute hemodynamic changes requiring constant surveillance and appropriate treatment.

2. Serial blood gases

a. Increases in potassium should be aggressively managed.

    i. Insulin (10 units) administered with dextrose bolus as needed
    ii. Furosemide if kidneys functioning
    iii. β-adrenergic agonists (e.g., albuterol)
    iv. Alkalosis (e.g., hyperventilation, sodium bicarbonate)
    v. Intra-operative CVVH (should be continued if on pre-operatively)
    vi. Washing of PRBCs if time allows

b. Baseline sodium should be checked

    i. Hyponatremia: avoid increases more than 0.5 mEq/h (risk of central pontine myelinolysis)
    ii. Increased ICP: typically target Na$^+$ at 145–150 mEq/L

c. Standard intra-operative glucose target of 80–180 mg/dL

d. Hypocalcemia from citrate toxicity should be corrected.

3. Viscoelastic testing

a. Baseline testing prior to incision allows establishment of baseline coagulation status and early identification of potential coagulopathy.

    i. Administration of platelets/cryoprecipitate should only occur with evidence of clinical bleeding following incision (transfusion is associated with risk of thrombosis and worse outcomes).

b. Consider repeating viscoelastic testing if new or significantly worsened coagulopathy occurs (also can rule in/out fibrinolysis).

4. Ascites drainage

a. Amount varies depending on reaccumulation rates and most recent large-volume paracentesis (LVP)

b. Sudden loss of intraperitoneal volume/pressure will lead to increased venous capacitance and decreased venous return.

c. Replace drained ascites in at least a 1:2 ratio (bottles of 5% albumin: liters of ascites).

5. Surgical dissection may be complicated by several factors leading to significant blood loss during this phase.

a. In combination with intermittent vascular compression

b. Acute hypotension is common.

6. Goals during this phase are ensuring adequate intravascular volume status (particularly important with caval replacement), management of electrolytes as above, and transfusion as required to keep up with surgical loses.

a. Fluid status can be a difficult compromise: adequate volume expansion is required to tolerate caval manipulation/clamping; however, increased CVP and liver swelling/congestion will worsen surgical bleeding and may compromise new graft function after reperfusion.

    i. Utilizing vasopressor infusions (particularly during the anhepatic phase) will allow less volume administration and help minimize risk of bleeding and new graft dysfunction.

## Anhepatic

1. Surgical phase encompassing removal of the native liver until reperfusion of the new liver

a. Begins with clamping of the portal vein followed by caval clamping

    i. Supra- and infrahepatic clamps are placed in the caval replacement and VVB.
    ii. A single-side clamp is placed in the piggyback technique (effect on venous return is variable depending on the amount of inferior cava clamped).

b. Hemodynamics following caval clamping should be monitored for a brief period before the surgical team transects and removes the native liver as this marks the point of no return.

    i. If caval clamping is not tolerated, the clamp should be removed and volume status improved or VVB utilized.

c. Vascular anastomoses are then completed with the new liver (caval, portal, ± hepatic artery).

d. This period from the new organ leaving its ice bath until reperfusion is the warm ischemia time, often 30–60 minutes.

    i. Prolonged warm ischemia times are correlated with diminished graft function and worse outcomes.

2. Progressive coagulopathy and metabolic acidosis during this phase

a. Aggressive management of fluid status, hematocrit, titration of vasopressors, and correction of hyperkalemia and hypocalcemia is vital in preparation for the significant hemodynamic insult presented by reperfusion of the new liver.

b. Citrate is normally metabolized by the liver; continued PRBC administration will worsen citrate toxicity and hypocalcemia.

c. No gluconeogenesis during this time

3. Vasopressors should be titrated during this phase while minimizing further fluid administration (except as required by significant hemorrhage or hypovolemia, as seen on monitors and TEE).

   a. Roughly 50% reduction in venous return associated with caval clamping will be returned on reperfusion; if further volume expansion occurs while the caval clamp is on, volume overload and associated venous congestion can cause acute heart failure and/or graft dysfunction following reperfusion.

   b. VVB will often flow ~1 L/min to minimize disruption of venous return.

     i. Utilization of VVB varies by institution and surgical team; it provides less benefit with short bypass runs, more benefit in patients with absent or poor collateral circulation (fulminant liver failure) or with significant cardiopulmonary disease that cannot tolerate caval clamping (e.g., heart failure, moderate–severe pHTN).

## Reperfusion

1. Reperfusion of the new liver with vascular clamp removal is often associated with significant hemodynamic instability, including severe hypotension, bradycardia, malignant arrhythmias, and even cardiac arrest.

   a. Cold, acidotic, hyperkalemic blood returning to the heart is likely the major etiology (cytokines and microemboli are also a factor).

   b. Sudden volume shifts associated with total caval occlusion may cause rapid distention of the right heart, leading to reduced contractility, bradycardia, or arrhythmias.

     i. This may lead to acute right heart failure, particularly in the setting of acute increase in PVR (thrombotic or air emboli, worsening of pHTN).

   c. Lidocaine and calcium chloride administration just prior to reperfusion may reduce the incidence of significant arrhythmias.

   d. Anticholinergic agents and/or epinephrine for severe bradycardia

   e. Acute hyperkalemia (peaked T waves, widening of QRS) should be aggressively treated to prevent progression to malignant arrhythmia or cardiac arrest.

   f. TEE should be monitored for overall cardiac function and the possibility of intracardiac thrombus or significant emboli.

   g. Post-reperfusion syndrome: definition/classification constantly changing, the main aspect is severe hypotension in the immediate post-reperfusion period.

     i. Treatment includes vasoactive agents such as vasopressin, norepinephrine, and epinephrine, as well as calcium chloride and sodium bicarbonate as required.

     ii. The initial phase often resolves after 3–5 minutes.

     iii. Overall hemodynamic instability can be seen for up to 4 hours following reperfusion.

## Neo-hepatic

1. Surgical phase that follows reperfusion of the new liver

   a. If the hepatic artery anastomosis was not performed prior to reperfusion, it will occur immediately following.

   b. Cholecystectomy and biliary duct anastomosis are the final steps prior to assurance of surgical hemostasis and abdominal closure.

2. Immunosuppression is often initiated following opening of the hepatic artery.

   a. Bolus dose of methylprednisolone is typical

   b. Discuss with surgical team

3. The new liver's function is monitored through clearance of lactic acid with improvement in acidosis, improved coagulation, and production of bile.

4. Hypothermia (from anastomoses of the previously cold organ and prolonged open abdomen) should be corrected to minimize coagulopathy and cardiovascular instability.

5. Repeat viscoelastic testing should be performed 30–60 minutes following reperfusion to diagnose and treat prolonged coagulopathy or fibrinolysis.

   a. Platelet/cryoprecipitate should be ordered only as dictated by clinical bleeding if there is evidence of decreased clot formation on the viscoelastic test.

   b. Antifibrinolytic agents should be administered with caution as intracardiac thrombus can be disastrous.

6. Transfusion should continue as required to a targeted HCT of 25–30%.

7. Vasopressor infusions should be minimized as tolerated to targeted mean arterial pressure (MAP) >65 mm Hg (unless a higher goal is required for cardiac or cerebral protection).

8. If the abdomen is unable to be closed (significant edema, large graft size), patients will remain intubated and paralyzed until a definitive abdominal closure can occur, often several days later.

## Post-operative Management
### ICU Course

1. Patients are often brought to the surgical ICU intubated and on mechanical ventilation until the new graft's function is adequately ensured with serial labs and assessment of vessel patency via ultrasonography, at which

time they can be extubated (often as early as a few hours following surgery).

   a. Earlier extubation is beneficial: positive-pressure ventilation can worsen splanchnic blood flow and increases CVP, which can worsen hepatic congestion.

     i. Early extubation also minimizes the risk of ventilator-associated pneumonia and ventilator-associated pulmonary injury.

   b. Indications for prolonged intubation: ongoing transfusion requirements, volume overload, airway or pulmonary edema, significant acidosis/alkalosis, persistent encephalopathy, or persistent hypoxemia secondary to HPS.

2. Early extubation in the operating room is possible if standard criteria are met (including monitoring and adequate reversal of neuromuscular blockade) and the surgical team is satisfied with the graft function.

   a. In some institutions, this may even allow bypassing of the surgical ICU.

3. Vasopressors should be utilized as required for the MAP goal, but often volume resuscitation is required (albumin allows less total volume administration).

   a. Increased CVP may worsen hepatic congestion and may compromise graft function.

   b. As new liver function improves, CO and SVR should begin to normalize.

4. A chest X-ray will confirm placement of the endotracheal tube, gastric tubes, and vascular devices, and assess lung parenchyma.

5. Normothermia should be maintained.

6. CVVH is often continued if utilized intra-operatively.

7. Post-operative analgesia is usually managed with intermittent opioid boluses or patient-controlled analgesia.

8. Patients with PPH should continue their pulmonary vasodilator therapies and wean as tolerated.

## Complications

1. Elevated liver function tests within the first 24 hours are common secondary to reperfusion injury; if not improving after 24 hours, it may require a return to the OR for exploration or possibly emergent relisting (status 1A).

   a. Possible causes include primary graft nonfunction, acute cellular rejection, or hepatic artery thrombosis.

2. Delayed graft function may contribute to prolonged coagulopathy requiring continued blood product administration (utilize viscoelastic testing to guide treatment).

   a. Significant bleeding may require a return to the OR for exploration and surgical control of ongoing bleeds.

3. Renal impairment is common in the immediate post-operative period; treatment is supportive, with avoidance of nephrotoxic agents and renal replacement therapy as needed.

4. Hyperglycemia is common secondary to peri-operative steroid administration and improving function of the new liver; this may require insulin infusion.

5. Hypertension may be seen secondary to immunosuppressive agents.

6. Arrhythmias including new atrial fibrillation may be seen secondary to electrolyte disturbances or peri-operative fluid shifts.

   a. Avoid amiodarone if possible due to potential hepatotoxicity.

7. Significant intra-operative transfusion requirements can lead to transfusion-associated circulatory overload (TACO)/transfusion-related acute lung injury, or acute respiratory distress syndrome (ARDS), requiring prolonged mechanical ventilation and possible tracheostomy.

8. Post-transplant or stress-induced cardiomyopathy may require continued supportive treatment (inotropes, vasopressors) in the days to weeks following transplant.

9. Cardiac tamponade is a rare complication associated with high vascular anastomoses that violates the cavoatrial junction.

10. Ischemic cholangiopathy is a more indolent complication that may present over the following weeks to months after transplant; may require retransplantation if unable to be corrected by other surgical or noninvasive intervention.

## Bibliography

Adelmann D, Kronish K, Ramsay MA. Anesthesia for liver transplantation. *Anesthesiol Clin* 2017;**35**(3):491–508.

Keegan MT, Kramer DJ. Perioperative care of the liver transplant patient. *Crit Care Clin* 2016;**32**(3):453–73.

Butterworth JF, Mackey DC, Wasnick JD, *Morgan & Mikhail's Clinical Anesthesiology*, 7th ed. New York: McGraw Hill, 2022, pp. 737–56.

Miller RD, Fleisher LA, Johns RA, et al. *Miller's Anesthesia*, 9th ed. New York: Churchill Livingstone; 2020, pp. 1960–92.

# Renal Transplant

John L. Parker and Jessica A. Lovich-Sapola

## Sample Case

A 47-year-old male is scheduled for a cadaveric kidney transplant. He is due for hemodialysis today. His last hemodialysis was 2 days ago. An EKG, chest X-ray, and labs are sent. He is complaining of chest pressure and tightness. He last ate 8 hours ago. What are your primary anesthetic concerns? Does it matter when his last dialysis was? His potassium ($K^+$) is 6.1 mEq/L. Does this change your anesthetic? The EKG and chest X-ray show left ventricular hypertrophy. Does that affect your management? Do you consider the patient to be NPO since he last ate 8 hours ago? Assuming you proceed with the surgery, what monitors will you use? Would you use general or regional anesthetic? What is your plan for the maintenance of anesthesia?

## Clinical Issues

### Increased Anesthetic Risks

1. End-stage renal disease (ESRD) can cause multisystem organ dysfunction.
2. Patients have a less predictable response to the anesthetic drugs and techniques.
3. They are at higher risk for cardiac and other peri-operative complications secondary to their underlying disease.
4. Cardiovascular complications are the leading cause of death after renal transplantation.

### Organ Matching and Allocation

1. Cadaveric and living donors
2. Initial testing is for ABO compatibility.
3. The second line of testing determines the HLA (human leukocyte antigen) profile of the recipient.
4. The final test is a cross-match that is performed by mixing the recipient blood with the donor blood cells to determine the presence of preformed reactive antibodies against the donor antigens.
5. In 2014, the United States began using the Kidney Donor Risk Index (KDRI) for kidney donors to provide grafts to patients with the maximum predicted posttransplant survival benefit.
   a. KDRI factors in age, height, weight, ethnicity, history of hypertension, history of diabetes, cause of death (if applicable), serum creatinine, hepatitis C status, and donation after circulatory death (DCD) status.

## Indication

1. ESRD caused by diabetes mellitus (most common)
2. ESRD caused by hypertension
3. ESRD caused by glomerular disease
4. Polycystic kidney disease
5. Familial or congenital diseases of the kidney
6. Tubulointerstitial disease

## Pathophysiology of ESRD

1. Once urine output falls below 400 mL/day, the patient becomes oliguric. This results in abnormalities in $Na^+$, $K^+$, $Ca^{2+}$, $Mg^{2+}$, phosphate levels, and uremia.
2. The resulting hypervolemia from oliguria leads to hypertension that further damages the kidneys, creating a positive feedback loop worsening the patient's hypertension.
3. The accumulation of uremic toxins and metabolic acids contributes to the poor myocardial performance.
4. Renal failure accelerates the progression of atherosclerosis.
5. Dilated cardiomyopathy and concentric hypertrophy develop in response to increased intravascular volume and afterload. Congestive heart failure results from the kidney's inability to excrete excess daily fluid intake.
6. The resulting cardiovascular diseases include acute myocardial infarction, cardiac arrythmias, pericardial disease, and cardiomyopathy. These diseases account for approximately 50% of the deaths of patients on dialysis. After transplantation, however, the cardiovascular risk diminishes from tenfold to twofold when compared to the general population.
7. Diabetes mellitus (DM) accounts for 35% of ESRD cases. Patients with DM and ESRD have a higher cardiovascular risk than patients with uremia alone.
8. Because chronic uremia causes delayed gastric emptying, all patients presenting for a kidney transplant should be considered to have a full stomach. Rapid-sequence induction should be considered.
9. Normochromic, normocytic anemia can occur secondary to the decreased erythropoiesis and retained toxins.
10. Qualitative platelet defect and coagulopathies are common.
11. Central nervous system disturbances may occur, including myoclonus, seizure, stupor, and coma.

## Exclusion Criteria for Renal Transplants

1. Severe heart, lung, or liver disease
2. Most malignancies
3. Active or untreatable infections such as tuberculosis

# KO Treatment Plan

## Pre-operative

1. Regarding the sample case, chest pain has a 65% sensitivity/specificity for coronary artery disease.
2. This patient requires a complete cardiac workup.
3. Kidney transplants are not emergent.
4. Well-tolerated, prolonged cold preservation of the cadaveric kidney provides enough time (up to 36 hours) for an adequate pre-operative exam.
5. The patient also should be dialyzed to allow normalization of electrolyte imbalances and volume status before surgery.
6. For heart failure, optimize medications and maintain intravascular volume.

## General Considerations for Evaluation during the Waiting List Period

1. Order pre-operative pulmonary function tests.
2. Screen the patient for any existing solid tumors or infections, including a dental evaluation, colonoscopy, prostate-specific Ag, mammography, Pap test, and viral serologies.
   a. Exclusion criteria include: severe heart, lung, or liver disease; most malignancies; active or untreatable infections, e.g., tuberculosis.
3. The patient should have good control of any diabetes, hypertension, or dyslipidemia.
4. Psychiatric evaluation

## Considerations in the Immediate Pre-operative Period

1. Estimate volume status by comparing the patient's current weight and his "dry weight."
   a. Consider using point-of-care-ultrasound to assess intravascular volume.
2. Order a basic metabolic panel.
   a. Potassium levels greater than 6.0 mEq/L require a delay in surgery and correction of the level with hemodialysis.
3. Pre-operative cardiac evaluation is extremely important.
   a. Pre-operative EKG/echocardiogram may be enough for a young patient with newly diagnosed ESRD unrelated to DM.
   b. Stress echocardiogram or cardiac catheterization may be indicated for a patient with long-standing ESRD associated with DM.

4. β-blockers are continued while angiotensin-converting enzyme (ACE)/angiotensin receptor blockers (ARBs) are held.
5. Evaluate the coagulation status with a prothrombin time (PT), INR, partial thromboplastin time (PTT), fibrinogen, and platelet count.
6. Order a hematocrit level.
7. Type and screen the patient for blood products.
8. Verify immunosuppressant pre-induction orders with the nephrologist/surgeon prior to induction.

## Intra-operative

1. Apply standard ASA monitors.
2. Renal transplants are usually done under general anesthesia but have been successfully done using neuraxial anesthesia. Regional anesthesia is often contraindicated, given concerns over uremic platelet dysfunction and residual heparin from the pre-operative dialysis.
3. Goals for induction and intubation should include careful control of heart rate and blood pressure to minimize the possibility of myocardial ischemia. This can be achieved by blunting the response to direct laryngoscopy with opioids such as fentanyl or remifentanil, or using a short-acting β-blocker such as esmolol.
4. Pretreat with a nonparticulate antacid.
5. Rapid-sequence induction should be performed secondary to a presumed full stomach unless the patient has a known difficult airway.
   a. Succinylcholine is not contraindicated in patients with ESRD, assuming that they have been recently dialyzed and their potassium level has been corrected.
   b. The increase in serum potassium with a bolus of succinylcholine is about 0.5 mEq/L for patients with or without ESRD.
6. General endotracheal anesthesia provides stable hemodynamics, muscle relaxation, and a predictable depth of anesthesia. Volatile anesthetics plus opioids or total IV anesthesia with opioids and propofol are both appropriate. Desflurane, isoflurane, and sevoflurane are all acceptable choices of volatile anesthetics.
7. Atracurium and cisatracurium are the preferred muscle relaxants secondary to their spontaneous Hoffman degradation and plasma cholinesterase metabolism. Pancuronium, gallamine, and curare are not recommended because they depend on the kidney for elimination and therefore have a prolonged duration of action in ESRD patients. Patients with ESRD also have been shown to have an increased sensitivity and prolonged duration of action with vecuronium; therefore, it is often not recommended.
8. Arterial line monitoring is common, especially for patients with more advanced comorbid conditions. Central venous pressure (CVP) is rarely used as it poorly predicts hemodynamics and fluid responsiveness; used primarily for administering vasoactive substances, if at all.

To optimize cardiac output and renal blood flow during the case, hemodynamic goals should be:

a. Systolic blood pressure (SBP) >90 mm Hg
b. Mean systemic pressure >60 mm Hg
c. CVP, if used, >10 mm Hg

9. Severe comorbid conditions such as symptomatic coronary artery disease or congestive heart failure should be monitored for the development of ischemia with a pulmonary artery catheter or transesophageal echocardiography.

10. Intravascular fluid balance should be maintained with balanced salt solutions such as Lactated Ringer's or Plasma-Lyte, which are preferred to hyperchloremic solutions such as normal saline (NS). NS has been paradoxically shown to increase $K^+$ more than potassium-containing crystalloids by producing hyperchloremic acidosis.

a. Colloids may also be used, depending on the institution.
b. Hydroxyethyl starch solutions should be avoided due to their nephrotoxicity.
c. Adequate hydration reduces acute tubular necrosis.

11. Always monitor the hemodialysis shunt or fistula during positioning and intra-operatively for the presence of a thrill, and document the patency. Avoid blood pressure cuffs and tourniquets over the shunt or fistula.
12. Antibiotics should be given prior to surgical incision.
13. Hypotension may occur with unclamping of the iliac vessels and reperfusion of the graft. Every effort should be made to avoid hypotension secondary to the renal graft function being so dependent on adequate perfusion.

a. Vasoconstrictors with strong α-adrenergic effects, such as phenylephrine, should be drugs of last resort.
b. The typical goal is to maintain the SBP greater than 90 mm Hg and the mean systemic pressures greater than 60 mm Hg.

14. Once the anastomosis of the kidney is begun by the surgeon, a diuresis should be initiated with mannitol and furosemide. Heparin and verapamil should be available in the operating room. The anesthesiologist may also be asked to give the first dose of the immunosuppressant. The kidney graft is not good at concentrating the urine and reabsorbing sodium initially; therefore, you should pay special attention to the patient's electrolytes.
15. Monitoring the urine output is very important. Immediate urine output is seen in over 90% of living donor kidney transplants and between 40% and 70% of cadaveric transplants. Near the end of the procedure, a decrease in urine output strongly suggests mechanical impingement of the graft, vessel, or ureter.

a. Intra-operative ultrasound can be used to examine the flow in the arterial and venous anastomoses.
b. Intra-operative urine output is frequently enhanced intra-operatively by infusions of mannitol, loop diuretics, and occasionally dopamine, but these measures have not been well studied.

16. Diabetic patients should have frequent blood glucose checks in an effort to maintain their blood glucose in a range from 80 to 110 mg/dL.
17. If the patient is cytomegalovirus (CMV) negative and is receiving a CMV-negative kidney, then they should receive CMV-negative blood.

## Post-operative

1. Pain control

a. Post-operative pain is usually mild to moderate.
b. Post-operative pain control can be managed with fentanyl, sufentanil, alfentanil, and remifentanil.
c. Caution should be used when administering morphine, meperidine, or oxycodone because they or one of their active metabolites is dependent on renal excretion and therefore may accumulate.
d. Patient-controlled analgesia is usually a good choice for post-operative pain management.
e. Nonsteroidal anti-inflammatory agents (NSAIDs) are contraindicated because of the resulting vasoconstriction and decreased blood flow to the kidneys.
f. Tramadol can be used as an alternative in these patients.

2. The plan should be for full reversal of the anesthetic and extubation if possible.
3. Monitor urine output closely. Re-exploration should not be delayed if kinking of the vascular attachments or obstruction of the ureter is suspected.
4. Common post-operative complications

a. Ureteral obstruction
b. Ureteral fistula
c. Vascular thrombosis
d. Lymphocele
e. Wound complications
f. Bowel perforation
g. Femoral neuropathy

## Bibliography

Barash PG, Cullen BF, Stoelting RK, et al. *Clinical Anesthesia*, 8th ed. Philadelphia: Lippincott Williams & Wilkins, 2017, pp. 1461–7.

Gropper MA. *Miller's Anesthesia*, 9th ed. Philadelphia: Elsevier, 2020, pp. 1962–9.

# Management of the Post-cardiac Transplant Patient

Quratulain Samoon and Jessica A. Lovich-Sapola

## Sample Case

A 57-year-old female is scheduled for an urgent appendectomy. She is on vacation. She reports that 3 years ago she had a cardiac transplant in her home state. She reports feeling well now, and that she is seen regularly for all of her required follow-up appointments. What further information would you like? What testing or labs would you like? How does her cardiac transplant affect your anesthetic?

## Clinical Issues

1. Cardiac denervation effects: loss of cardiac neural input and output

   a. The cardiac denervation happens during the donor heart removal.

   b. Leads to chronically increased sympathetic stimulation to the renin–angiotensin–aldosterone system

   c. Eliminates vagal-mediated parasympathetic influences

   d. Direct autonomic influences are absent.

   e. Cardiac impulse formation and conduction are normal.

   f. Sympathetic fibers are also interrupted, but the response to catecholamines is normal or even enhanced secondary to increased receptor density.

   g. Preload-dependent cardiac output

      i. The denervated heart depends on its Frank–Starling mechanism during stress, which shifts toward contractility. During stress or hypovolemia, it is unable to increase its heart rate in comparison to a native heart. It depends on venous return/preload. The systolic function of a transplanted heart remains normal, but it may have impaired diastolic relaxation and compliance.

      ii. Lack of efferent feedback might be the reason why transplant recipients are unable to experience angina pectoris during myocardial ischemia.

   h. Super-sensitivity to catecholamines affects inotrope and chronotrope response.

      i. Loss of baroreceptor reflexes in response to tracheal intubation, pain, or vasodilation

      ii. Lower cardiac index but preserved left ventricular ejection fraction

      iii. Lower oxygen consumption at rest and during exercise

      iv. Increased risk of arrythmias, especially atrial flutter and fibrillations; 76% of the recipients develop atrial premature beats.

      v. β-effects of epinephrine and norepinephrine are exaggerated. Isoproterenol is the main chronotropic treatment.

   i. Absence of parasympathetic innervation

      i. Higher resting heart rate with decreased heart rate variability. Resting heart rate is higher than normal: 90–110 beats/minute.

      ii. Valsalva maneuver and carotid sinus massage have no effect on the heart rate.

      iii. No effect of atropine in bradycardia

   j. No effect on cardiac atrial natriuretic peptide production and intrinsic nerve supply

   k. Results in:

      i. Increased resting heart rate (90–120 beats/min)

      ii. Less variation in heart rate throughout the day

      iii. Blunted heart rate response to exercise because the response is dependent on an increase in circulating catecholamines

      iv. Absence of angina

      v. No response of the heart rate to carotid massage

      vi. Low to normal cardiac output

2. Possible reinnervation over time

   a. The extent of reinnervation and regeneration is variable and unpredictable. The sympathetic reinnervation happens earlier than the parasympathetic, which may lead to an abnormal response during stress.

3. Coronary autoregulation is preserved.

4. Atria recipients remain innervated without any conduction across the suture line.

   a. Most EKGs demonstrate two P waves, which represent the recipient and donor's SA nodes. (This should not be confused with a complete heart block on an EKG.)

b.   AV-paced rhythm

5.   Incidence of atrial fibrillation/flutter is as high as 25%.

6.   Incidence of venous thromboembolism is as high as 8.5%.

# Pharmacology Considerations after Heart Transplant

1.   Indirect-acting agents

    a.   Ephedrine

    b.   Post-cardiac transplant effects: transplanted heart cannot respond

2.   Direct-acting sympathomimetic: works in a transplanted heart

    a.   Phenylephrine

    b.   Epinephrine and norepinephrine

        i.   β-effects when compared to α-effects are exaggerated for epinephrine and norepinephrine in heart transplant recipients

        ii.   Exaggerated sensitivity due to increased β-receptor density

        iii.   Used for refractory cardiogenic shock

    c.   Dobutamine

    d.   Isoproterenol

3.   Parasympathomimetic

    a.   Neostigmine

        i.   Risk of bradycardia and cardiac arrest despite the use of antimuscarinic agent

        ii.   Post-cardiac transplant effects: no effect on denervated heart

4.   Parasympatholytic

    a.   Atropine

    b.   Mechanism of action: blocks acetylcholine at parasympathetic sites

    c.   Post-cardiac transplant effects: not effective, no heart rate response

5.   β-blockers

    a.   Mechanism of action: inhibition of β-adrenergic receptors

    b.   Post-cardiac transplant effect: use with caution secondary to the reliance on circulating catecholamines and existing blunted heart rate during exercise.

6.   Digoxin

    a.   Mechanism of action: direct suppression of the AV node, enhanced vagal tone, positive ionotropic effect

    b.   Post-cardiac transplant effects: ionotropic effect is intact, but its action that relies on AV node

conduction is ineffective; ineffective to treat atrial fibrillation or supraventricular tachycardia.

7.   Adenosine

    a.   Mechanism of action: slows conduction time through AV node

    b.   Post-cardiac transplant effects: exaggerated sensitivity

# Hypertension is Common after Cardiac Transplant

1.   Related to multiple factors

    a.   Cardiac denervation

    b.   Immunosuppressive drug use

    c.   Ventricular vascular uncoupling

2.   Treatment of hypertension after a heart transplant

    a.   First-line therapy

        i.   Dihydropyridine calcium channel blockers

        ii.   Angiotensin-converting enzyme (ACE) inhibitors or angiotensin receptor blockers

        iii.   Diuretic

    b.   Second-line therapy

        i.   Diltiazem

        ii.   β-blockers

# Selected Drug–Drug Interactions

1.   Cardiac transplant patients are commonly on immunosuppressant therapy and therefore may be taking cyclosporin, tacrolimus, mycophenolate, azathioprine, antilymphocyte globulin, monoclonal antibodies, and corticosteroids for graft rejection and to improve overall graft survival.

    a.   About 40% of heart transplant recipients develop at least one episode of acute rejection.

2.   Chronic immunosuppressant agents have adverse effects such as:

    a.   Lowering seizure threshold (epilepsy)

    b.   Diabetes

    c.   Hypertension

    d.   Renal dysfunction

    e.   Bone marrow suppression

    f.   Lymphoproliferative disorders

    g.   Gastrointestinal bleeding and peptic ulcer

    h.   Coagulopathy

    i.   Electrolyte abnormalities: hyperkalemia and hypomagnesemia

# Antimicrobial Prophylaxis

1.   Transplant patients are at high risk for infections, especially if they are on immunosuppressants. However,

the antibiotic prophylaxis for surgical site prophylaxis is no different from the general population.

a. Prophylaxis antibiotics should be given an hour prior to incision. The timing ultimately depends on the hospital protocol. General guidelines are as follows:

   i. Cardiothoracic surgery – recommended antibiotics are:

      (1) First: cefazolin
      (2) Second: general antibiotics
      (3) In case of beta-lactam allergy, alternatives such as vancomycin and clindamycin can be considered.

   ii. Vascular surgery: cephalosporins
   iii. Colorectal surgeries: cefoxitin or cefotetan and metronidazole
   iv. Hip or knee arthroplasty: cefazoline or cefuroxime

## KO Treatment Plan

### Pre-operative

1. Focus on cardiac function and any symptoms of heart failure.

   a. EKG
   b. Transthoracic echocardiogram

2. It is very important to ensure the patient is fully optimized pre-operatively. A detailed history and physical exam should be done to assess the graft's performance based on the patient's daily activity level and exercise tolerance.

   a. Heart transplant recipients may have ongoing rejection with cardiac dysfunction or ischemia without any symptoms.
   b. Look for signs or symptoms of unintentional weight gain, fever, dyspnea, edema, shortness of breath, palpitations, or lightheadedness.
   c. Any form of transplant rejection should be ruled out pre-operatively.
   d. The ISHLT 2016 registry reported hypertension, hyperlipidemia, renal dysfunction, diabetes, and cardiac allograft vasculopathy as the most common morbidities.
   e. The risk of graft rejection is greatest during the first year.
   f. Renal dysfunction, malignancy, and cardiac allograft vasculopathy are the main causes of death after 1 year post-heart transplant.

3. Review pertinent investigations.

   a. Pertinent laboratory tests to rule out bone marrow suppression, renal or liver dysfunction, and coagulopathy (complete blood count, complete metabolic panel, liver function panel, PTT, INR, and PT).

b. Assess cardiac function and rhythm. Rule out signs of rejection, failure, or dysfunction.

   i. EKG: assess transplanted heart function and rhythm.
   ii. Pacemaker: an up-to-date pacemaker interrogation is required.
   iii. Echocardiogram: heart function and any graft vasculopathy
   iv. Cardiac catheterization: coronary artery disease

4. The dose of immunosuppressant should be continued peri-operatively to reduce the risk of rejection. If the patient is on oral cyclosporine, a dose of it should be given 4–7 hours prior to the surgery.

5. Add antimicrobial, DVT, and stress ulcer prophylaxis.

6. Peri-operative glucose levels should also be checked.

### Intra-operative

1. Standard ASA monitoring

   a. EKG

      i. Monitor for ischemia
      ii. Will often have two sets of P waves: recipient and donor SA node
      iii. The recipient's SA node will not affect cardiac function.

2. Heart transplant patients have a high incidence of post-operative wound infections. Sterile aseptic techniques should be followed. Remember that transplant patients are immunocompromised and may not show typical signs and symptoms of infection such as fever or leukocytosis.

3. Invasive hemodynamic monitors

   a. Arterial line placement is useful for closer monitoring of hemodynamic status and to avoid fluid shifts that can compromise loading conditions of the heart.
   b. Central venous pressure catheters or pulmonary artery catheters are not routinely required unless patients have decreased cardiac function or signs of cardiac failure.

4. General anesthesia is preferred over regional anesthetics because the denervated heart does not compensate for hemodynamic changes that occur with a regional anesthetic.

5. The goal of induction in a patient with a transplanted heart is to maintain hemodynamic stability and avoid vasodilation or an acute decrease in preload.

   a. Slow induction and titration of anesthetic agents is desirable as these patients do not have an adequate sympathetic response to hypotension. They rely on the Frank–Starling mechanism to increase their stroke volume.
   b. Consider inducing with etomidate to maintain hemodynamic stability.

c. Propofol may decrease preload, causing bradycardia, lowering systematic vascular resistance, and reducing cardiac output.

d. Fentanyl is safe for short-term use.

6. Acute appendicitis patients should be considered full stomach and require rapid-sequence intubation. Overall, the decision to use a neuromuscular blockade should be based on the type of surgery and intubating conditions.

   a. Gingival hyperplasia is present at times in patients taking cyclosporine, which may lead to bleeding and aspiration during airway management.

   b. An orogastric/nasogastric tube should be placed to decompress the stomach.

7. Avoid hypotension, hypertension, and arrythmias.

   a. Transplanted heart patients are at higher risk of developing atrial flutter or fibrillation.

   b. The transplanted heart is a preload-dependent heart. Maintain normovolemia.

   c. Try to maintain the patient's baseline heart and blood pressure. Transplanted hearts respond to direct-acting agents.

      i. Treat hypotension with direct-acting vasopressors like phenylephrine or norepinephrine. Remember, a transplanted heart will not respond to indirect vasopressors (ephedrine), parasympathomimetic (neostigmine), or parasympatholytic agents (atropine).

      ii. Have epinephrine and isoproterenol available to manage bradycardia or hypotensive emergencies.

8. Maintenance anesthesia can be safely implemented with inhalational or IV anesthetics.

9. Standard extubation criteria should be followed.

## Post-operative

1. Following surgery, close monitoring of blood pressure, heart rate, and rhythm should be continued.

2. Pay close attention to preload status and renal function.

3. Resume the patient's baseline medications, especially immunosuppressants and antihypertensive agents.

   a. Immunosuppressants like cyclosporin or tacrolimus require blood-level monitoring.

4. Early post-operative removal of CVP/arterial lines and urinary catheter

## Bibliography

Atallah B, Bader F, El-Lababidi, et al. Pharmacology considerations after heart transplant: what general cardiologists should know. *Healio News.* November 8, 2017.

Awad M, Czer LS, Hou M, et al. Early denervation and later reinnervation of the heart following cardiac transplantation: a review. *J Am Heart Assoc.* 2016;**5**(11): e004070.

Barash PG, Cullen BF, Stoelting RK, et al. *Clinical Anesthesia,* 8th ed. Philadelphia: Lippincott Williams & Wilkins, 2017, p. 350.

Brusich, KT, Acan I. Anesthetic considerations in transplant recipients for nontransplant surgery. 2018. www.Intechopen.com.

Butterworth JF, Mackey DC, Wasnick JD. *Morgan & Mikhail's Clinical Anesthesiology,* 6th ed. New York: McGraw-Hill Education, 2018, pp. 432–4.

Choudhury M. Post-cardiac transplant recipient: implications for anaesthesia.*Indian J Anaesth* 2017;**61**(9):768–74.

**Chapter**

# 86

# Delayed Emergence, Change in Mental Status, Delirium, and Agitation

Andrew Yurkonis and Jessica A. Lovich-Sapola

## Sample Case

A 67-year-old patient is in the post-anesthesia care unit (PACU) following a surgical repair of his left femur. He was found unconscious in the snow at a ski resort. He was awake prior to the induction of anesthesia. He denied any medical or surgical history. His toxicology screen was still pending. You are called to the PACU to see the patient because he is unarousable. What is your differential diagnosis? How will you treat this?

## Clinical Issues

### Definition

1. Delirium:
   a. Acute neuropsychiatric disorder
   b. Fluctuating disturbances in attention, awareness, and cognition
   c. Subtypes
      i. Hyperactive
      ii. Hypoactive
      iii. Mixed

### Risk Factors for Delayed Emergence, Delirium, and Agitation

1. Patient factors
   a. Age greater than 65 years
   b. History of dementia
   c. Pre-existing cognitive or psychiatric disorders
   d. Renal/hepatic impairment
   e. Current infection
   f. Intoxication
   g. Severe illness
   h. Hearing or vision impairment
   i. History of falls
   j. Malnutrition
   k. Pain
   l. Pre-operative anemia
   m. Obstructive sleep apnea

2. Surgical factors
   a. Increased incidence with prolonged procedures
   b. Hip fractures (up to 53.3% incidence)
   c. Total knee replacements
   d. Cataracts
   e. Cardiac surgery (especially after cardiopulmonary bypass)

3. Anesthesia factors
   a. Prolonged anesthesia
   b. Long-acting medications
   c. Absolute or relative overdose
   d. Polypharmacy

## Prognosis

1. 90% of patients regain consciousness within 15 minutes of admission to the PACU, but this could take up to 60–90 minutes after prolonged procedures.
2. The majority of patients recover with close observation and monitoring if life-threatening conditions are rapidly diagnosed and treated.
3. Post-operative delirium may take up to 5 days to present.
4. Once delirium occurs, interventions have little effect on severity or duration, which emphasizes the importance of primary prevention.
   a. Believed to be preventable in 30–40% of cases

5. Long-term effects
   a. Cognitive decline
   b. Decreased functional independence
   c. Increased risk of dementia
   d. Caregiver burden
   e. Increased health care costs
   f. Increased morbidity and mortality

## Differential Diagnosis

1. Hypoxia and hypercarbia
   a. Check an arterial blood gas (ABG), end-tidal $CO_2$, and pulse oximetry.
   b. Rule out $CO_2$ narcosis.

2. Hypoperfusion
   a. Hypotension
   b. Shock

3. Hypothermia

a. Less than 33 °C can produce profound unconsciousness.

b. Core temperature below 30 °C can cause fixed pupillary dilation, areflexia, and coma.

4. Residual medications and polypharmacy

   a. Pre-medications

      i. Benzodiazepines

   b. Induction drugs

      i. Ketamine

      ii. Droperidol

   c. Muscle relaxants (depolarizing and nondepolarizing)

   d. Volatile anesthetics

   e. Opioids

   f. Anticholinergics resulting in central anticholinergic syndrome

   g. Steroids (psychosis)

   h. Tricyclic antidepressants

   i. Antihistamines

5. Electrolyte abnormalities

   a. Diabetic ketoacidosis

   b. Hyperglycemia and hypoglycemia

   c. Hyponatremia

   d. Hypermagnesemia

   e. Hypercalcemia

   f. Acidosis/alkalosis

   g. Hypercalcemia

6. Adverse neurologic outcome

   a. Cerebral vascular accident (CVA)/cerebral edema/transient ischemic attack (TIA)

   b. Hepatic/renal encephalopathy

   c. Seizures and postictal state

   d. Anoxia

   e. Infection

   f. Increased intracranial pressure

7. Infections

   a. Meningitis

   b. Sepsis

   c. Pneumonia

   d. Urinary tract infections

8. Substance abuse

   a. Alcohol intoxication or withdrawal

   b. Cocaine

   c. Opioid intoxication or withdrawal

   d. Over-the-counter sleep aids

9. Endocrine abnormalities

   a. Addison's disease

   b. Cushing's disease

   c. Hypothyroid, hyperthyroid

10. Hepatic abnormalities

    a. Hepatic encephalopathy

    b. Delayed drug clearance

11. Renal/GU abnormalities

    a. Delayed drug clearance

    b. Urinary tract obstruction

    c. Uremia

12. Pain and anxiety

## Preventive Measures

1. Glasses and hearing aids immediately available in the PACU

2. Cognitive stimulation

   a. Orienting the patient to time and location

   b. Music therapy

3. Simple communication

4. Delirium screening tools

5. Prevent infection

6. Avoid physical restraints

7. Nutritional assistance

8. Early mobilization

9. Anesthetic management (variable benefit)

   a. Melatonin 5 mg given pre-operatively

   b. Bispectral Index (BIS)-guidance

   c. Dexmedetomidine infusion of 0.2–0.4 µg/kg/h during the surgery

   d. Antipsychotics: post-operative haloperidol 2.5 mg daily for 3 consecutive days

   e. Post-operative pain control

## KO Treatment Plan

Diagnose and treat the most likely cause. The differential diagnosis and treatment plan are essentially the same for delayed emergence, change in mental status, delirium, and agitation. If during the exam you are presented with any of these conditions, follow the step-wise approach listed below. Always start with the conditions that are most likely for your sample case.

## Primary Concerns in this Sample Case

1. Hypothermia
2. Undiscovered head injury
3. Unknown history of dementia
4. Possible intoxication

### Diagnostic Approach and Management

1. ABCs and vital signs: maintain patent airway, assess breathing and circulation

   a. Oxygen saturation

i. 100% $O_2$

ii. Jaw thrust

iii. Airway adjuncts: nasal pharyngeal airway, oropharyngeal airway

iv. Bag mask ventilation if needed

b. Pulse: rate/rhythm

i. Administer glycopyrrolate, atropine, metoprolol as needed.

c. Temperature

i. Apply a warming blanket if hypothermic.

d. Blood pressure

i. Maintain within 20% of baseline.

ii. Administer pressors, IV fluid, and blood as necessary.

e. Respiratory rate and end-tidal $CO_2$

i. If respiratory rate low: possible narcotic overdose

ii. If respiratory rate high: possible compensation for acidosis

f. Character of spontaneous ventilations

i. Cheyne–Stokes: oscillating periods of tachypnea and apnea associated with heart failure, head trauma, hemorrhage, meningitis, infarction

ii. Kussmaul: rapid and deep respirations associated with acidosis

2. Assess Glasgow Coma Scale and perform a neurologic exam.

3. Review all medications given for prolonged duration of action. Ensure no residual medications are in the IV lines.

4. Review the pre-operative level of consciousness and medical history.

5. Check the results of the toxicology screen.

6. Pharmacologic reversal agents if suspected overdose

a. Naloxone for suspected narcotic overdose

i. Pure opioid receptor antagonist

ii. Give 0.04 mg IV in increments every 2 minutes up to 0.2 mg.

iii. Has been found, in high doses, to reverse the effects of alcohol, barbiturates, and benzodiazepines

iv. No effect on volatile anesthetics

v. May partially antagonize ketamine and nitrous oxide

vi. May be useful in the treatment of post-anesthetic apnea in infants, even when no opioids have been given

b. Flumazenil

i. Benzodiazepine antagonist

ii. Give 0.2 mg IV per minute to a total of 1 mg.

c. Physostigmine

i. 1.25 mg IV can reverse the effects of some sedatives and inhaled anesthetics.

ii. Treats central anticholinergic syndrome

7. Prolonged muscle relaxant effect

a. Check TwitchView Train of Four

b. Administer neostigmine and glycopyrrolate or sugammadex as needed.

8. Check ABG, electrolytes, and blood glucose.

a. Rule out $CO_2$ narcosis and treat with hyperventilation if present.

b. Rule out hyponatremia.

c. If hypoglycemia is presumed, treat immediately with 50% dextrose IV, even before verifying the glucose value.

9. Review intra-operative records for labile blood pressures, irregular heart rhythm (atrial fibrillation/atrial flutter). Review patient history for CVAs, carotid stenosis/plaques, and atrial fibrillation.

10. Head CT scan and neurology consult if the condition is persistent and other etiologies are ruled out.

a. CT scan can determine elevated ICP and acute intracranial hemorrhage.

b. Consider a grand mal seizure, delirium tremens, and cerebral anoxia.

# Bibliography

Barash PG, Cullen BF, Stoelting RK, et al. *Clinical Anesthesia*, 8th ed. Philadelphia: Lippincott Williams & Wilkins, 2017, pp. 1557–8.

Fleisher LA, Rosenbaum SH. *Complications in Anesthesia*, 3rd ed. Philadelphia: Elsevier, 2018, pp. 535–538.

Ford MD, Delaney KA, Ling LJ, et al. *Clinical Toxicology*, 1st ed. Philadelphia: WB Saunders Company, 2001, chapter 56.

Gropper, M. *Miller's Anesthesia*, 9th edition. Philadelphia: Elsevier, 2020, pp. 2604–6.

Janssen TL, Alberts AR, Hooft L, et al. Prevention of postoperative delirium in elderly patients planned for elective surgery: systematic review and metanalysis. *Clin Interv Aging* 2019;14:1095–117.

McGee, MD. *Evidenced Based Physical Diagnosis*, 5th ed. Philadelphia: Elsevier, 2022, pp. 143–53.

# Post-tonsillectomy Hemorrhage

Dylan Elder

## Sample Case

A 9-year-old boy presents 6 days after an adenoidectomy and tonsillectomy for recurrent adenotonsillitis. He appears pale and lethargic. He is dizzy when upright, and lies on the bed throughout the entire exam. Mom states he woke up at 2:00 a.m. vomiting blood. He has a basin into which he is spitting blood-tinged saliva. Vital signs are heart rate (HR) 120, respiratory rate (RR) 26, and blood pressure (BP) 75/46 mm Hg. What are your concerns? How will you evaluate the patient's volume status? How will you induce general anesthesia in this patient?

## Clinical Issues

### Risk and Incidence of Post-tonsillectomy Hemorrhage

1. Post-tonsillectomy hemorrhage rates vary depending on the surgical method and study cohort, but are typically quoted to range between 1% and 6%.
2. Hemorrhages are categorized into two phases:
   a. Primary: occurs within 24 hours of surgery and is the most common time to present.
   b. Secondary: occurs after 24 hours, most commonly between post-operative days 5 and 10, when the fibrin clot sloughs off.

3. Risk factors for primary and secondary hemorrhage
   a. Age greater than 15
   b. Chronic recurrent infections as the indication for tonsillectomy
   c. Less than 5 years' experience of the surgeon
   d. Bleeding diathesis
   e. Peri-operative hypertension
   f. High intra-operative blood loss

### Patient Volume Status (Table 87.1)

1. The extent of blood loss and dehydration may be difficult to determine. Bleeding may be minor, with rapid resolution, or be life-threatening.
2. Light bleeding may precede more severe bleeding.
3. Typically, stabilization of bleeding may occur at bedside with silver nitrate, use of epinephrine-soaked

**Table 87.1** General principles for pediatric volume status

| | |
|---|---|
| The patient is sitting up and talking without dizziness. | 1. Mild to moderate hypovolemia<br>2. There is time to evaluate the volume status and obtain laboratory values. |
| The patient is lying down, pale, and hypotensive. | 1. May be on the verge of hypovolemic shock, with the development of lactic acidosis<br>2. Begin immediate volume resuscitation without delay for lab values.<br>3. Check hemoglobin and hematocrit after the resuscitation has begun. |
| The patient is tachycardic and hypertensive. | 1. Outpouring of catecholamines in the pediatric patient results from hemorrhage, hypovolemia, fear, or excitement<br>2. Peripheral vasoconstriction delays the clinical onset of severe hypotension in the awake patient. |

Adapted from Verghese ST, Hannallah RS. Pediatric otolaryngologic emergencies. *Anesthesiol Clin North Am* 2001;19(2):237–56.

pledgets, or even bedside electrocautery in the appropriate patient.
4. However, often hemostasis may need to be achieved in the operating room with adequate airway and anesthetic management.

## Intravenous Access

1. Good IV access must be established pre-operatively.
2. In an extremely agitated and hypovolemic child with acute vasoconstriction, it may be difficult to obtain an IV line. In this case, intraosseous infusion may be necessary.
3. Labs such as hemoglobin, platelet count, and coagulation studies, as well as a type and cross, should be obtained with the initial IV placement.

## Full Stomach Precautions

1. A patient who presents with a bleeding tonsil is considered a full stomach, due to the likelihood of swallowed blood.
2. Precautions in this case include:
   a. Two well-functioning suction devices with large-bore suction tubes
   b. Extra laryngoscope handles and blades
   c. Several cuffed endotracheal tubes with lubricated stylets in place

## KO Treatment Plan

### Pre-operative

1. Review the prior anesthetic record of the initial surgery to rule out any anesthetic issues.
2. Note any co-existing medical conditions, including loose teeth and the use of medications that could further exacerbate any bleeding.
3. Determine the child's volume status by performing a history and physical exam.
4. Anesthesia-induced vasodilation may lead to severe hypotension.
5. Initiate vigorous volume resuscitation with normal saline or lactated Ringer's solution immediately.
6. Blood is rarely used as the primary solution for volume replacement in these children.

### Intra-operative

1. Pre-medication is controversial; however, it may be indicated if the patient's condition permits. Sedation may be achieved with IV midazolam, ketamine, or dexmedetomidine.

2. After application of the standard ASA monitors, preoxygenate the child in a lateral, head-down position to allow the blood to drain out of the mouth.
3. After preoxygenating the patient, turn the child supine. Do not induce unless the surgeon is present and available to intercede. Either a classic (apneic) or controlled (gentle bag mask ventilation) rapid-sequence induction (RSI) is indicated.
   a. Controlled RSI is generally favored, as this leads to less hypoxemia and arterial hypertension during induction of anesthesia and tracheal intubation, with better direct laryngoscopic views.
   b. Bag mask ventilation does not increase pulmonary complications in this setting.
4. Intubate using a cuffed endotracheal tube to help prevent the blood from entering the trachea around the tube.
5. Decompress the stomach using a large-bore orogastric tube.
6. Do not extubate the patient until they are fully awake, with a normal gag and cough reflex, in order to avoid aspiration.

### Post-operative

1. After extubation, patient management is guided by the child's clinical condition before and immediately after surgery.
2. A child with a minor bleed may even be sent home immediately following surgery, though most cases that come to the operating room are monitored for 12–24 hours.
3. Patients who have come to the operating room hypotensive after a severe bleed may need to stay in the ICU in order to adequately manage their hemodynamics.

## Bibliography

Gropper MA. *Miller's Anesthesia*, 9th ed. Philadelphia: Elsevier, 2020, pp. 2223–4.

Heidemann CH, Wallen M, Aakesson M, et al. Post-tonsillectomy hemorrhage: assessment of risk factors with special attention to introduction of coblation technique. *Eu Arch Otorhinolaryngol* 2009;266:1011–15.

Kemper ME, Buehler PK, Schmitz A, et al. Classical versus controlled rapid sequence induction and intubation in children with bleeding tonsils (a retrospective audit). *Acta Anaesthesiologica Scandinavica* 2019;64:41–47.

Motoyama EK, Davis PJ. *Smith's Anesthesia for Infants and Children*, 7th ed. Philadelphia: Mosby Elsevier, 2006, pp. 798–9.

National Prospective Tonsillectomy Audit. Tonsillectomy technique as a risk factor for postoperative hemorrhage. *Lancet* 2004;364:697–702.

Verghese ST, Hannallah RS. Pediatric otolaryngologic emergencies. *Anesthesiol Clin North Am* 2001;19(2):237–56.

Wall JJ, Tay KY. Postoperative tonsillectomy hemorrhage. *Emerg Med Clin North Am* 2018;36(2):415–26.

# Neck Hematoma after Carotid Surgery

Garietta Falls and Jessica A. Lovich-Sapola

## Sample Case

You are called to evaluate a patient on the floor who underwent a carotid endarterectomy earlier in the day. She is 68 years old, with a history of coronary artery disease, hypertension, and chronic obstructive pulmonary disease. Upon entering the room, you notice that she has significant neck swelling over the incision site. She also seems anxious and is unable to speak in full sentences. You apply a face mask/Ambu bag and have difficulty ventilating. What do you do next? Do you attempt to intubate, or do you open the wound?

## Clinical Issues

### Neck Hematoma after Carotid Endarterectomy (Fig. 88.1)

1.  This is a rare occurrence.

    a.  The North American Symptomatic Carotid Endarterectomy Trial (NASCET) found an incidence of 5.5% of neck hematomas following the procedure.

    b.  Other more recent studies have documented incidences of 2–4%.

2.  Risk factors for development of hematoma include:

    a.  Pre-operative use of antiplatelet medications

    b.  Aggressive heparinization during the surgical procedure (goal activated clotting time generally 200–300 seconds) with failure to reverse with protamine

    c.  Use of anticoagulation after surgery

    d.  Post-operative hypertension

3.  A vast majority of the time, venous bleeding and/or capillary oozing are responsible for the hematoma. However, there can be significant arterial bleeding from the anastomosis of the carotid artery or due to iatrogenic injury of another smaller artery in the surgical field.

4.  Approximately 50% of neck hematomas require emergent re-operation.

    a.  Development of a significant hematoma can occur within minutes or hours.

    b.  One study found the average time between completion of carotid endarterectomy and neck exploration to be 6 hours.

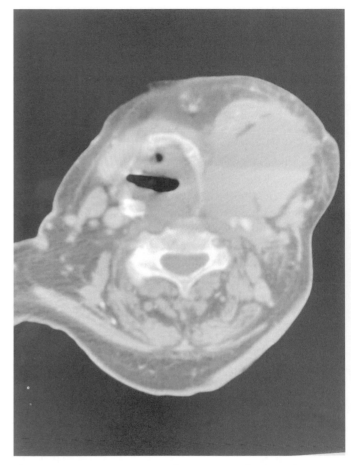

**Figure 88.1** Representation image from a computed tomography angiography of the neck showing a large post-operative hematoma displacing the trachea. Photo credit: Garietta Falls, MD.

## Possible Contributing Factors to Post-Carotid Respiratory Insufficiency

1.  Mass effect from large hematoma may cause significant tracheal deviation.

2.  Edema of recently traumatized tissues

3.  Deficient carotid body function leading to a loss in the ventilatory drive to increase respiration when the patient encounters a drop in $PaO_2$

4.  Nerve injury to the vagus or one of the laryngeal branches

    a.  Injury to the recurrent laryngeal nerve would result in paralysis of the ipsilateral vocal cord.

i. Changes in voice

ii. Hoarseness

iii. Breathy voice

iv. Difficulty breathing and shortness of breath

b. A recurrent laryngeal nerve, on either side, is generally within the thoracic outlet and distal to the surgical field.

c. A nonrecurrent laryngeal nerve (NRLN) is a rare anatomical variation.

   i. Iatrogenic injury can lead to vocal cord paralysis.

   ii. It occurs on the right in fewer than 1% of patients and is even more rare on the left.

   iii. The nerve in this case will cross from the vagus behind the common carotid artery, which could lead to injury during clamping of the vessel.

## KO Treatment Plan

## Post-operative

1. A small hematoma can initially by treated with external digital compression for 5–10 minutes and reversal of any residual heparin with protamine.

2. Rapidly expanding hematomas require prompt bedside evaluation and return to the OR secondary to the associated tracheal compression and loss of a secure airway.

   a. Call the surgical team. Bag mask ventilate the patient.

   b. Immediate evacuation at the bedside may be necessary if the airway is compromised. You may have to do it yourself. Use local anesthetic in the incision (if readily available) and use a #11 scalpel or suture-removal scissors to cut the skin and subcutaneous sutures. Evacuate the hematoma and apply pressure to any visible areas of bleeding.

   c. Consider alternatives to direct laryngoscopy because intubation can be difficult before re-exploration; GlideScope, laryngeal mask airway, or fiber-optic tracheal intubation.

   d. Aggressive post-operative blood pressure control

   e. Return to the operating room for surgical exploration if you have not done so already.

   f. Correct any associated coagulopathies.

3. Closely monitor the patient in an ICU setting post-operatively.

**TKO:** Remember that during the oral board exam you could have a very similar scenario with a post-thyroidectomy patient.

## Bibliography

Baracchini, C, Gruppo M, Mazzalai F, et al. Predictors of neck bleeding after eversion carotid endarterectomy. *J Vasc Surg* 2011;**54**:69–705.

Barash PG, Cullen BF, Stoclting RK. *Clinical Anesthesia*, 5th ed. Philadelphia: Lippincott Williams & Wilkins, 2006, pp. 953–4.

Miller RD, Fleisher LA, Johns RA, et al. *Anesthesia*, 6th ed. New York: Churchill Livingstone, 2005, p. 2105.

North American Symptomatic Carotid Endarterectomy Trial Collaborators. Beneficial effect of carotid endarterectomy in symptomatic patients with high grade carotid stenosis. *New Engl J Med* 1991;**325**:445–53.

Roussopoulou A, Lazaris A, Tsivgoulis G, et al. Risk of perioperative neck haematoma in TIA and non-disabling stroke patients with symptomatic carotid artery stenosis undergoing endarterectomy within 14 days from cerebrovascular event. *J Neurol Sci* 2019;**409**:116590.

Tomonori T, Morita A. Neck haematoma after carotid endarterectomy: risks, rescue, and prevention. *Br J Neurosurg* 2019;**33**:156–160.

Welling RE, Ramadas HS, Gansmuller KJ. Cervical wound hematoma after carotid endarterectomy. *Ann Vasc Surg* 1989;**3**:229–31.

**Chapter**

**89**

# Post-operative Nausea and Vomiting

Kara M. Barnett and Jessica A. Lovich-Sapola

## Sample Case

A 50-year-old female complains of persistent nausea and vomiting 5 hours after the drainage of a subhepatic abscess under general anesthesia. How will you proceed? What is your workup plan? What is your treatment plan?

## Clinical Issues

### Differential Diagnosis of the Causes of Nausea

1. Anesthetic medications: narcotics/volatile anesthetics/opioids/etomidate
2. Hypoxia
3. Hypotension
4. Pain
5. Anxiety
6. Infection
7. Chemotherapy
8. Gastrointestinal obstruction
9. Movement
10. Vagal response
11. Pregnancy
12. Increased intracranial pressure (ICP)

### Increased Risk of Post-operative Nausea and Vomiting

1. Patient-related factors
   a. History of motion sickness or post-operative nausea and vomiting
   b. Nonsmokers
   c. Female gender
   d. Younger age (≥3 years old, <50 years increases risk of post-discharge nausea and vomiting)
   e. Dehydration/hypovolemia
   f. Hypotension
   g. Hypercarbia
   h. Infection
   i. Menstrual cycle (conflicting evidence)
2. Anesthesia-related factors
   a. Opioids (dose-dependent)
   b. Volatile anesthetics
   c. Nitrous oxide (duration-dependent)
   d. Inadequate hydration

   e. Duration of anesthesia
   f. Gastric distension
   g. Neostigmine (conflicting evidence)

3. Surgery-related factors
   a. Operative procedure
      i. Laparoscopic surgery
      ii. Ear, nose, and throat surgery, including strabismus surgery
      iii. Bariatric surgery
      iv. Gynecological surgery
      v. Cholecystectomy
      vi. Major breast surgery
   b. Increased length of surgery time
   c. Blood in the gastrointestinal tract
   d. Premature ambulation
   e. Pain

4. Scoring system to identify patients at risk: use multimodal prophylaxis in those with one or more risk factors.
   a. Apfel simplified risk score for PONV
      i. One point each: female gender, nonsmoker, history of PONV and/or motion sickness, post-operative opioids
      ii. Risk of PONV based on number of points: 0, 1, 2, 3, 4 reflects risk of PONV of 10%, 20%, 40%, 60%, 80%, respectively
   b. Koivuranta score
      i. Four Apfel risk factors plus length of surgery >60 minutes
   c. Eberhart simplified risk score for post-operative vomiting (POV) in children
      i. One point each: surgery ≥30 minutes, age ≥3 years, strabismus surgery, history of POV or family history of PONV
      ii. Risk of POV based on number of points: 0, 1, 2, 3, 4 reflects risk of pediatric POV of 9%, 10%, 30%, 55%, 70%, respectively
   d. Post-discharge nausea and vomiting (PDNV) in adults

i. One point each: female gender, history of PONV, age <50, opioids in the post-anesthesia care unit (PACU), nausea in the PACU

ii. Risk of PDNV based on number of points: 0, 1, 2, 3, 4, 5 reflects risk of PDNV of 10%, 20%, 30%, 50%, 60%, 80%, respectively.

## KO Treatment Plan

## Pre-operative Treatment and Prevention

1. The best way to treat post-operative nausea and vomiting is to prevent it in the first place.

2. Medications

   a. 5-HT3 receptor antagonists

      i. Ondansetron (4–8 mg IV), granisetron (0.35–3 mg IV), palonosetron (0.075 mg IV) at the end of surgery

      ii. As prophylaxis or treatment of PONV

      iii. Lack sedative, dysphoric, and extrapyramidal side effects

      iv. May prolong QT interval

   b. NK1 receptor antagonists

      i. Aprepitant (40 mg PO), fosaprepitant (150 mg IV) given in pre-operative area for high-risk patients

      ii. May last 48 hours (half-life is 40 hours)

      iii. Recommend patients on hormonal birth control use a second method of contraception for 30 days after receiving a dose of aprepitant or fosaprepitant.

   c. Corticosteroids

      i. Dexamethasone (4–10 mg IV), methylprednisolone (40 mg IV) at induction because of its slow onset

      ii. May reduce analgesic requirements

      iii. Low dose for PONV may mildly increase blood glucose, but is not shown to increase the rate of wound infection or cancer recurrence.

   d. Dopamine antagonists

      i. Side effects may include QT prolongation, sedation, and extrapyramidal side effects.

      ii. Black box warning: severe tissue damage or gangrene if intra-arterial or subcutaneous injection; recommended to be administered intramuscularly.

      iii. Amisulpride (5 mg IV prophylaxis, 10 mg IV rescue treatment)

         (1) Lower dose used for PONV unlikely to cause QT prolongation

      iv. Droperidol (0.625 mg IV) at the end of surgery

         (1) Black box warning for QT interval prolongation and sudden cardiac death for doses >25 mg

      v. Haloperidol (0.5–2 mg IV/IM) at the end of surgery

         (1) Not FDA approved for PONV

      vi. Metoclopramide (10–50 mg IV)

         (1) Reduces gastric volume without an effect on acidity

         (2) Less effective at lower doses, higher doses associated with akathisia

      vii. Prochlorperazine (5–10 mg IV)

      viii. Perphenazine (5 mg IV)

      ix. Promethazine (6.25–50 mg IV/IM)

   e. Antihistamines

      i. Side effect of sedation limits their use

      ii. Dimenhydrinate (1 mg/kg IV)

      iii. Diphenhydramine (25–50 mg IV)

   f. Anticholinergics

      i. Transdermal scopolamine (1 mg/72 hours), place several hours prior to the surgery and remove 24 hours after surgery

         (1) Side effects include dry mouth, somnolence, mydriasis, vision disturbances, dizziness, and confusion.

   g. Gabapentinoids

      i. Gabapentin (600–800 mg PO)

         (1) Black box warning due to risk of respiratory depression when used with other central nervous system depressants such as opioids

   h. Benzodiazepines

      i. Midazolam (2 mg IV), lorazepam

   i. Ephedrine (0.5 mg/kg IM)

3. Nonpharmacologic prophylaxis

   a. Acupuncture

      i. Pericardium 6 acupuncture point stimulation: effective whether before or after anesthesia induction

      ii. Nerve stimulator over the median nerve may be effective for early PONV

      iii. Other acupuncture points are being studied.

   b. Hydration

      i. Supplemental crystalloids 10–30 mL/kg may be effective.

      ii. Colloids over crystalloids may be more effective in surgeries lasting more than 3 hours, otherwise there was no difference between two types of fluids.

# Bibliography

Fleisher LA, Rosenbaum SH. *Complications in Anesthesia*, 3rd ed. Amsterdam: Elsevier Health Sciences, 2017. pp. 588–600.

Gan TJ, Kumar BG, Belani KG, et al. Fourth consensus guidelines for the management of postoperative nausea and vomiting. *Anesth Analg* 2020;**131**(5):411–48.

Gropper MA, *Miller's Anesthesia*, 9th ed. New York: Churchill Livingstone, 2020, pp. 403–18, 2273–6.

# Awareness under Anesthesia

Kaitlyn Jakubec, Jessica A. Lovich-Sapola, and Donald M. Voltz

## Sample Case

A 46-year-old female with temporal-mandibular joint (TMJ) disease presents for a TMJ arthroplasty. This patient is a 155 cm, 62 kg woman with no known allergies or medical problems. She conveys to you that when she underwent a tubal ligation 7 years ago she remembers waking up during the surgery. As she describes her previous anesthetic misadventure, her anxiety level increases. What do you make of the previous anesthetic history in this patient? What would you tell this patient to alleviate her fears for this surgery? What are your anesthetic plan and management options for a patient with a prior episode of anesthetic awareness? What patients are at the highest risk of experiencing awareness under anesthesia?

## Clinical Issues

### Definitions

1. Awareness under anesthesia

   a. Awareness under anesthesia occurs when a patient is targeted for general anesthesia but at some point, during this plan, the patient emerges from a plane of surgical anesthesia into one where cortical activity is restored.

   b. This can occur during a period of:

      i. Decreased anesthetic delivery: hemodynamic compromise not allowing for adequate level of anesthesia

      ii. Increase in surgical stimulation for the given level of anesthetic agents: transition from surgical prep to surgical incision without adequate time for anesthetic deepening

      iii. Error in the delivery of anesthetic agents: error in delivery of anesthetic such as vaporizer under-filled or malfunctioning

   c. Awareness under anesthesia is a period when patients become aware of their surroundings when they should be amnestic of the events that occur during general anesthesia.

   d. This awareness may or may not be remembered by a patient after the surgical procedure is completed.

   e. An example of awareness under anesthesia is a patient purposefully reaching for the endotracheal tube immediately after intubation when an inadequate amount of anesthetic medication was delivered or not

enough time had passed prior to laryngoscopy. In this situation, a patient demonstrated purposeful movement that resulted from an inadequate level of anesthesia for the given level of stimulation. This episode is not likely to be remembered after the procedure is completed; however, it may be.

   f. Patients with awareness appear to be responding appropriately to stimulation or commands. However, they do not remember the circumstances following their anesthetic.

2. Intra-operative recall

   a. Intra-operative recall occurs when patients are able to remember specific events during the course of general anesthesia when they should have been completely amnestic.

   b. All patients with intra-operative recall also had awareness under anesthesia.

**TKO:** Remember, you may have awareness under anesthesia without recall!

## Memory Types

1. Explicit memory

   a. Conscious recollection of information or experiences by a patient

   b. This has also been called "direct memory"; it is tested by asking someone to recall what he or she remembers about a specific event.

   c. In the context of intra-operative recall, a patient with explicit memory of an event would be able to describe specific events that took place, such as the surgeon splitting the sternum during cardiac surgery or parts of a conversation that took place between operating room personnel.

2. Implicit memory

   a. The cortical processing of a sensory stimulation without resulting conscious recollection of that stimulus

   b. During the course of a surgical procedure under general anesthesia, patients can have subconscious processing of auditory or other sensory stimuli that they are later unable to consciously recall.

   c. In tests when patients were given paired words during various times under general anesthesia, the patients were able to provide the correct word when one of the pair was given to them.

d. It has been suggested that implicit memory of intra-operative events occurs more frequently than explicit recall; however, these types of studies are difficult to perform as well as interpret.

## Incidence

1. The actual incidence of both intra-operative recall and awareness under anesthesia is unclear due to the difficulty in studying these phenomena as well as not having an objective means of measuring a patient's level of consciousness.
2. Despite research difficulties, this is a defined complication of anesthesiology with a suggested rate of awareness being of 0.02–1.0%.
3. These suggested rates are for true explicit recall. The incidence of awareness under anesthesia (implicit memories) has been suggested to be higher.
4. 20% of all reported awareness with recall occurs at the end of the anesthetic.

## Legal Implications

1. ASA closed claims analysis reports 2% of cases were related to awareness, while British claims related to awareness were 12% of all cases brought against anesthesiologists.
2. In some of these cases cues to a light anesthetic were absent. Hemodynamic cues such as hypertension (15% of cases where awareness was reported) or tachycardia (7% of cases where awareness was reported) were not uncovered during retrospective analysis of the cases.

## Stages of Awareness

Transition from an awake state to one of adequate surgical anesthesia is a continuum that varies among patients and is influenced by the amount of surgical stimulation as well as the patient's physiological state. To obtain a better understanding of the progression from awake to amnestic states, Griffith and Jones define five perceptual stages that occur in general anesthesia.

1. Conscious perception of stimuli with explicit memory of the events
2. Conscious perception of stimuli without explicit memory of the events
3. Dreaming
4. Subconscious perception of stimuli with implicit memory of the events
5. No perception of stimuli and no memory of the events

## Risk Factors for Awareness under Anesthesia and Intra-operative Recall

1. Cardiac surgery
2. Emergency cesarean section
3. Trauma
4. Emergency surgery in patients with minimal physiologic reserve
5. Surgery in which neuromuscular blocking agents are used
6. Equipment failures
7. Patients with higher-than-normal anesthetic requirements: previous drug use and the development of tolerance

## Prevention

1. Delivery of anesthetics by well- and continuously trained individuals
2. Vigilance of medications delivered and the patient's response to them
3. Repeated checking of the medication delivery systems: infusion pumps, vaporizers
4. Avoidance of neuromuscular blocking agents and use of neuromuscular function monitoring (train of four) if required for the procedure
5. Continual monitoring and trending of anesthetic delivery and patient's physiologic variables
6. In situations when anesthesia may be light (cardiac, cesarean sections), inform the patient about the risk and ensure the patient that you will do everything possible to prevent awareness during these periods.
7. Avoidance of negative auditory stimuli in the OR (loud sounds, negative language, or language meant to reorient the patient) by limiting conversation or providing the patient with earplugs or noise-canceling headphones

**TKO:** Depth-of-anesthesia/bispectral index monitors (BIS) are not completely reliable for all individuals and all cases. In the future, the reliability of these monitors may improve.

## Treatment

1. Intra-operative awareness with recall is very disconcerting to the patients who experience it.
2. The feeling of helplessness and an inability to move or communicate this to their anesthesiology provider results in a high incidence of post-traumatic stress disorder (PTSD).
3. Review of these cases post-operatively often does not reliably uncover when or why the patient might have been aware.
4. In most cases of awareness, the classic signs of hypertension or tachycardia are absent.
5. In light of this, it is important to take every case seriously and initiate steps to help these patients.
6. Directly address a patient's fears and concerns in a sympathetic manner as well as arrange for these patients to be seen by a psychiatrist who has expertise in the area of PTSD treatment.

# KO Treatment Plan

## Pre-operative

1. A discussion of the patient's experience might be helpful in gaining additional information about her prior episode of anesthesia awareness and recall.

2. Reassure the patient that you will closely monitor her clinical condition and ensure that all steps are being taken to prevent awareness from occurring this time.

3. You might consider modifying your anesthetic plan from the previous one.

4. A review of her current medications as well as an investigation into what was administered during the previous case when awareness occurred could factor into the formulation of the new anesthetic plan.

5. Supplementing a volatile anesthetic with a propofol infusion with midazolam might lead to a more memory-suppressant anesthetic.

6. Currently, the ASA Practice Guidelines do not recommend the routine use of intra-operative depth-of-anesthesia (BIS) monitors for all cases of general anesthesia.

   a. The ASA does support the use of these monitors. However, the ASA also recommends multimodality monitoring such as heart rate, blood pressure, and expired volatile anesthetics.

   b. Diligent follow-up and intervention in cases of suspected or confirmed intra-operative recall and/or awareness

7. Vigilant clinical signs monitoring with the addition of depth-of-anesthesia monitoring will provide data for intra-operative clinical management of this patient.

8. Following the anesthetic, it is important to speak with the patient to ensure that no recollection occurred during this case, and provide support since her earlier experience might require further intervention, even if no recall or awareness occurred during this procedure.

# Bibliography

Bischoff P, Rundshagen I. Awareness under general anesthesia. *Dtsch Arztebl Int* 2011;**108**(1–2): 1–7.

Cascella M, Bimonte S, Amruthraj NJ. Awareness during emergence from anesthesia: features and future research directions. *World J Clin Cases*. 2020;**8**(2):245–54.

Griffith D, Jones JB. Awareness and memory in anaesthetized patients. *Br J Anaesth* 1990;**65**:603–7.

Sebel PS. Awareness and memory during general anesthesia. ASA Annual Meeting Refresher Course Lectures, 2007.

Tasbihgou SR, Vogels MF, Absalom AR. Accidental awareness during general anaesthesia: a narrative review. *Anaesthesia* 2018;**73**:112–22.

Wang M, Messina AG, Russell IF. The topography of awareness: a classification of intra-operative cognitive states. *Anaesthesia* 2012;**67**:1197–201.

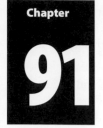

# Peripheral Nerve Blocks

Lori Ann Oliver and Jodi-Ann Oliver

## Sample Case

A 35-year-old 110 kg, 180 cm male presents for a right total knee replacement. A heavy smoker at two packs per day for 30 years, his past medical history also shows chronic bronchitis and type 2 diabetes, initially managed with oral antiglycemics such as metformin. He is now insulin-dependent and hypertensive. His medications include NPH with Novolog, lisinopril-HCTZ and fluticasone/salmeterol (Advair) Diskus and montelukast (Singulair) daily with albuterol as a rescue inhaler. HR 90, BP 160/75, RR 20, temperature 36 °C. EKG shows normal sinus rhythm, with a heart rate of 75 beats/min with nonspecific ST–T wave changes in V3–V5 and Hgb 14 g/dL.

1. What are the different options for post-operative pain management in this patient in terms of regional anesthesia? Which peripheral nerve blocks would you use and why?
2. What are the advantages and disadvantages of a peripheral nerve block placement compared to a neuro-axial block such as an epidural? Is catheter placement superior to single shot? Why or why not?
3. What are the different techniques used to perform peripheral nerve blocks and how does the use of ultrasonography aid in the placement of these blocks?
4. Do the patient's medical problems influence your choice of regional anesthetic technique? Any concerns? What if the patient is on any anticoagulants? How would this affect your management or decision?
5. What is local anesthetic toxicity and how does it present based on the type of local anesthetic used (e.g., lidocaine versus ropivacaine)?

**TKO:** Peripheral nerve blocks (PNBs) can be used either as the sole anesthetic, as an adjuvant to general anesthesia or sedation, and/or for post-operative pain relief. When implemented properly, they are a valuable tool in any anesthesiologist's armamentarium.

## Clinical Considerations

### Benefits of PNBs

1. Some studies have concluded the following:

    a. A PNB can provide superior post-operative analgesia when compared with parenteral opioids (usually intravenous (IV) morphine) and intra-articular opioids in joint operations.

    b. A PNB can contribute to faster post-operative recovery for inpatients and outpatients.

    c. A PNB can facilitate rehabilitation by providing pain control and increased passive joint mobility.

        i. There is also some evidence that this can decrease days of hospitalization and therefore reduce medical costs.

    d. The side effects of opioids may be avoided: nausea/vomiting, itching, respiratory depression, ileus, and constipation.

    e. The need for airway manipulation may be avoided (i.e., asthma).

        i. In the case of a difficult airway there is concern that although a PNB can obviate the need for a secure airway, failure or complications of a PNB can result in having to obtain an airway in an emergency situation with a difficult airway candidate.

    f. Other possible benefits

        i. Increased patient satisfaction
        ii. Reduced post-anesthesia care unit (PACU) care
        iii. Increased mental alertness and responsiveness and decreased post-operative delirium, especially in elderly patients
        iv. Faster ambulation
        v. Improved pain control, especially for patients with pre-existing chronic pain conditions and opioid tolerance

### General Contraindications for a PNB

1. Patient refusal
2. Proven allergy to local anesthetics

    a. Ester allergies are usually due to metabolism into para-aminobenzoic acid.

        i. Many people have skin irritation from this paraben, which is also found in some skin products such as sunscreens, lotions, and lip balms.

    b. Amide allergies are usually due to preservatives or antibacterial additives.

3. Systemic and local infection
4. Active bleeding in an anticoagulated patient

   a. Noncompressible vasculature may be a concern near nerve sites in the anticoagulated patient.

   b. There are guidelines for neuraxial regional techniques in the anticoagulated patient that can be extrapolated but generally are too strict to be applied to most PNB techniques, except for the placement of deep PNBs such as lumbar plexus and paravertebral nerve blocks.

5. Pre-existing peripheral/central nerve injury

   a. There is no evidence that a PNB will worsen a pre-existing neuropathy; however, the post-operative neurological assessment and follow-up may be complicated by a PNB, and in some cases may outweigh the benefits of the block.

6. Need for functional nerve assessment

   a. This may be the difference between doing the PNB pre-operatively versus post-operatively.

## Complications of a PNB

1. Peripheral nerve injury

   a. Most common mechanisms: needle trauma or intraneural injection

      i. Do not inject under pressure or if the patient experiences increased pain upon injection.

      ii. The etiology (surgical versus PNB) nerve injury is usually clinically indistinguishable.

         (1) Document any previous numbness or nerve injury prior to the PNB.

         (2) Attempt a PNB at a site higher than the surgical site. For example, popliteal sciatic nerve blocks are commonly placed for surgeries below the knee, such as ankle surgery.

      iii. Most peripheral nerve injuries will resolve without further incident, usually within 3 months.

         (1) However, some will require longer than 3 months to resolve while nerve regeneration takes place.

      iv. Consider a neurology consult with motor injuries and persistent sensory injuries that are unexplainable in relation to the operative technique or a pre-existing condition.

      v. Patient reassurance should also be part of the management. Be an active participant in patient follow-up.

2. Vascular puncture: hematoma
3. Local anesthetic toxicity

   a. Can occur either by intravascular injection or slow systemic absorption (delayed 5–30 minutes) in highly vascular sites

   b. The symptoms of local anesthetic toxicity are usually gradual and on a continuum.

      i. Signs of metallic taste, tinnitus, and circumoral paresthesia often appear first.

      ii. Followed by dizziness, lightheadedness, and anxiety

      iii. Neurological symptoms – seizure, agitation, and loss of consciousness – may appear next.

      iv. Cardiac arrest

   c. Always use standard monitors (EKG, blood pressure, and pulse oximetry) and have the appropriate resuscitation equipment nearby (oxygen, suction, bag mask, and intubation equipment) when placing a PNB.

   d. Inject the local anesthetic slowly with frequent aspiration.

   e. The patient receiving a PNB should always have functioning IV access.

   f. The patient should remain monitored for at least 20–30 minutes post-block to monitor for complications.

**TKO:** The presentation of local anesthetic systemic toxicity (LAST) versus intravascular injection will vary based on the type of local anesthetics used. If lidocaine is used, CNS symptoms will be present. However, if bupivacaine or ropivacaine is used in the event of intravascular injection, cardiac symptoms such as severe bradycardia followed by cardiac arrest might be the only presenting symptomology.

## LAST Management

1. Call for help.
2. Support ventilation
3. Life support

   a. CPR/ACLS

   b. Alert the facility of the possible need for cardiopulmonary bypass.

   c. Lipid emulsion: bolus 1.5 mL/kg then infuse 0.25 mL/kg/min

      (1) Cardiovascular instability: repeat bolus of 1.5 mL/kg

      (2) Hypotension: double infusion 0.5 mL/kg/min

      (3) Cardiovascular stability: continue infusion and monitor for 12 hours

4. Stop the seizure.

   a. Midazolam

**TKO:** For oral boards, use ABC and CPR prior to administering intralipid for resuscitation for LAST.

## PNB Techniques

1. Lumbar plexus block

   a. Indications: operations involving the femoral neck/shaft, anterior thigh, and knee

   b. Shortcomings: very vascular area

      i. Systemic absorption of local anesthetic from rich vascular beds can occur. Minimize this toxicity with slow injections and frequent aspirations.

      ii. Hematomas can occur, and large retroperitoneal hematomas have been reported.

   c. Complications specific to the lumbar plexus block

      i. Retroperitoneal hematomas

      ii. Epidural spread after accidental dural sheath injection: avoid injecting when you still have a muscle twitch while using a nerve stimulator at a voltage less than 0.2 mA.

      iii. Local anesthetic toxicity even without directly injecting into vessel

      iv. Note that weakness of the hip flexors may occur and should be considered with outpatients.

2. Femoral nerve block

   a. Indications: operations involving the knee

      i. Studies have shown that continuous femoral blocks used after major knee operations reduce IV morphine consumption and are comparable to epidural analgesia for pain control post-operatively.

   b. Shortcomings

      i. Need for proximal sciatic and possibly obturator (medial thigh) to completely cover the knee for some procedures

      ii. Can contribute to quadriceps weakness, which may contribute to falls

      iii. Is relatively contraindicated in ilioinguinal surgery and femoral vascular graft surgery

   c. Complications specific to the femoral nerve block

      i. Accidental puncture/injection of peritoneal space

3. Adductor canal block

   a. The same indications as femoral nerve block

      i. The saphenous nerve is a sensory branch of the femoral nerve and runs distally with the femoral artery and vein and at approximately the junction of the proximal two-thirds and distal one-third of the thigh. The saphenous nerves enter into the adductor canal with the femoral vessels. This nerve can be blocked.

      ii. Studies have shown the adductor canal nerve block is as efficacious as a femoral nerve block, but is motor sparing to the quadriceps.

      iii. The ultrasound probe is placed at the level of the mid-thigh with the goal to observe the femoral artery underneath the sartorius muscle. Place the needle tip medial to the artery in the adductor canal underneath the sartorius muscle and aspirate and inject local anesthetic.

   b. Shortcomings

      i. The same as femoral nerve block

      ii. Higher failure rate when compared to a femoral nerve block for knee surgery

   c. Complications specific to adductor canal nerve block

      i. The same as femoral nerve block

4. Sciatic nerve block

   a. Indications: operation on the sole of the foot and below the knee

   b. Shortcomings

      i. Will likely require blockade of the lumbar plexus, femoral, or saphenous nerves for supplementation

      ii. A proximal approach will cover tourniquet pain but contribute to hamstring weakness and can potentially block the parasympathetic nerves that control bladder emptying.

   c. Complications specific to the sciatic block: none; see general complication list.

**TKO:** For knee surgery such as total knee replacement, articular branches of the sciatic nerve can be blocked either at the antero-medial aspect of the knee or at the popliteal fossa to provide improved analgesia without involving the foot and ankle. This block is called the IPACK (infiltration between popliteal artery and capsule of the knee).

## Case Variation

The patient is now scheduled for a right total shoulder replacement instead of his right knee. How would the patient's medical history influence your choice of regional anesthetic? What are your concerns?

1. Interscalene brachial plexus block

   a. Indications: operations involving the shoulder, upper arm, and lower arm

   b. Shortcomings

      i. Can spare C8 and T1 nerve distribution (ulnar nerve) 15–30% of the time due to lack of local anesthetic spread to the lower nerve roots

      ii. Can be detrimental in patients with chronic obstructive pulmonary disease (COPD) (see below)

c. Complications specific to the interscalene block

    i. Pneumothorax

    ii. Spinal or epidural block: injection into the intervertebral foramina or dural sleeve

       (1) When using a nerve stimulator, avoid injecting when you still have a muscle twitch at a voltage less than 0.2 mA.

    iii. Vertebral artery injection/injury

    iv. Hoarseness: the most common side effect of this block

       (1) Occurs mostly with a right-sided injection

       (2) Incidence is 10–20%.

    v. Phrenic nerve paralysis and therefore diaphragmatic paralysis

       (1) The incidence is 100% due to the position of the nerve running anterior to the anterior scalene muscle.

       (2) Consider another technique on patients with severe pulmonary COPD and those dependent on the use of their accessory respiratory muscles.

       (3) Avoid bilateral interscalene blockade in patients with respiratory compromise.

    vi. Cervical plexus blockade can occur with the injection of large volumes of local anesthetic.

    vii. Horner's syndrome: local anesthetic spread to the sympathetic chain

       (1) Symptoms include:

          (a) Miosis: small pupil

          (b) Ptosis: drooping of upper eyelid

          (c) Anisocoria: unequal pupil size

          (d) Nasal stuffiness

             (i) Reassure the patient that the symptoms will resolve with the resolution of the block.

          (e) Anhidrosis: no sweating on the affected side

    viii. Intraneural injection of the C6 nerve root

2. Supraclavicular brachial plexus block

  a. Indications: operations involving the upper and lower arm but not the shoulder

    i. Most reliable upper extremity block because:

       (1) The three trunks are in close proximity to each other and to the skin.

       (2) The nerves are in one contiguous sheath at this level.

    ii. Rapid onset

  b. Shortcomings: should not be attempted bilaterally due to the possibility of bilateral pneumothoracies or phrenic nerve blocks.

  c. Complications specific to the supraclavicular block

    i. Pneumothorax: the incidence is not as high as previously recorded and can be prevented with good technique.

    ii. Phrenic nerve block with resulting diaphragmatic paralysis

       (1) 50% of the time

3. Infraclavicular brachial plexus block

  a. Indications: operations involving the upper arm and lower arm but not the shoulder

    i. A bilateral block can be attempted because there is little risk of phrenic nerve blockade. However, pneumothorax is still a small risk.

    ii. It is ideal for continuous infusions because there is a lower chance of catheter dislodgement due to less inherent movement in this area compared to the interscalene and supraclavicular

  b. Shortcomings: multiple injections are required.

    i. The musculocutaneous nerve may have already branched off and may require a separate injection.

    ii. As the brachial plexus moves peripherally, individual nerves may form separate compartments within the original brachial plexus sheath. A single injection may not reach all of the nerves due to fascial septation within the sheath.

  c. Complications specific to the infraclavicular block

    i. Pneumothorax

4. Axillary brachial plexus block

  a. Indications: operations of forearm, wrist, and hand

  b. Shortcomings

    i. The patient may need a separate block for the musculocutaneous nerve, which usually branches off the brachial plexus proximal to the axilla.

       (1) A separate injection of 5–10 mL of local anesthetic into the coracobrachialis muscle may be necessary to achieve anesthesia/analgesia of the lateral forearm.

    ii. The patient may need a separate injection to cover the inter-costobrachial and medial brachial cutaneous nerves if tourniquet pain is suspected.

       (1) This can be accomplished with a subcutaneous ring around the mid-upper arm.

    iii. The arm must be abducted to successfully perform the block.

(1) May be difficult and painful

    iv. This block will usually require more than one injection to provide analgesia/anesthesia to the radial, median, and ulnar nerves due to their position around the axillary artery and due to fascial septations that form around each nerve.

    v. Consider avoiding this specific block with the presence of axillary lymphadenopathy.

  c. Complications specific to the axillary block: none – see the general complication list.

## KO Treatment Plan

1. Identify the proper patient and the correct operation. Choose the technique that exemplifies the most benefits over the risks.
2. Consider surgical time, positioning, and the addition of sedation or general anesthesia when choosing a pre-operative technique.
3. Consider the need for post-operative nerve assessments, ambulation, and anticoagulation.

## Case Discussion

In this patient, a complete history and physical including an airway exam are needed before deciding if a PNB is right for him. If the patient proves to be a difficult airway, do not use the PNB as a way to avoid it. Remember, it is better to handle a difficult airway electively rather than emergently. Also, consider the patient's body habitus and the skill level of the regionalist. Consider the strength of the non-operative leg since the operative leg will be further weakened by the block and the patient may be more prone to falling.

## Case Variation

You are then told that the case will proceed under epidural anesthesia and that the patient forgot to mention that he was started on low molecular weight heparin 1–2 weeks ago prior to the surgery due to a strong family history of deep venous thrombus. How does this recent change in the patient's medication list and family affect our current plan? What are your concerns regarding anticoagulation and neuraxial placement?

## Complications

1. Increased risk of bleeding
2. Hematoma formation
  a. Vertebral canal hematoma
    i. Can result in permanent neurologic injury in patients who receive neuraxial blocks such as epidural and/or spinal anesthesia
    ii. This complication has to be recognized and managed by MRI imaging with surgical

intervention (resection of vertebral segment) within 8 hours of the hematoma.

## Guidelines for PNB Placement in Patients on Anticoagulation

1. Current guidelines on placement of PNBs in this patient population are based on recommendations by different societies in anesthesiology, such as the American Society of Regional Anesthesia (ASRA):
  a. No firm evidence for most recommendations
  b. ASRA 2021 guidelines include 32 cases of patients who had severe hemorrhagic complications following PNB placement.
  c. ASRA provides guidelines for time intervals when nerve blocks can be placed and/or removed in the case of catheter placement after discontinuing anticoagulation.
  d. Recommendations are based on:
    i. Type of anticoagulation (antiplatelet, heparin and derivatives, thrombolytics, anti-Xa inhibitors, warfarin)
    ii. Frequency of dosing
    iii. Type of block placement (single-shot versus catheter)
    iv. Location of block placement (deep versus superficial)
2. Complications associated with block placement in patients on anticoagulation:
  a. Hematoma formation

**TKO:** Central blockade such as epidurals and spinals are associated with the highest neurological complication (VCH) in patients on anticoagulation. Treat deeper PNBs such as paravertebral, lumbar plexus, and proximal sciatic (gluteal, sub-gluteal, para-sacral) nerve blocks as neuraxial blockade and use the neuraxial guidelines for block placement and/or catheter removal. Clinical judgment and risk–benefit analysis should be used when deciding whether it is appropriate to place nerve blocks in this patient population when deciding whether to discontinue anticoagulation for placement of nerve block (peripheral or neuraxial). For example, for a more superficial or compressible block, such as the brachial plexus or a femoral nerve block, it is safer to proceed with block placement compared to placement of a lumbar plexus nerve block.

**TKO:** The ASRA guidelines and ASRA Pain Medicine phone app are excellent resources for the most up-to-date guidelines for all anticoagulation medications.

1. How long to hold the mediation before the procedure
2. When to restart the medication after the procedure
3. How long to hold the medication before catheter removal
4. When to restart the medication after catheter removal

## Bibliography

Barash PG, Cullen BF, Stoelting RK, et al. *Clinical Anesthesia*, 8th ed. Philadelphia: Lippincott Williams & Wilkins, 2017, pp. 1583–98.

Finucane, BT. *Complications of Regional Anesthesia*. New York: Springer, 2007, pp. 39–52, 74–86.

Gitman M, Fettiplace M, Weinberg G. Local anesthetic toxicity. www.nysora.com (accessed August 4, 2022).

Hadzic A. *Textbook of Regional Anesthesia and Acute Pain Management*. New York: McGraw-Hill Professional, 2006, pp. 144–65, 403–543.

Mulroy MF. Regional anesthesia: when to say yes, when to say no. ASA Annual Meeting Refresher Course Lectures, 2007, p. 507.

Second Consensus Conference on Neuraxial Anesthesia and Anticoagulation. Regional anesthesia in the anticoagulated patient: defining the risks. 2002.

# Chapter 92

# Complex Regional Pain Syndrome Types I and II

Winston Singleton and Brendan J. Astley

## Sample Case

A 21-year-old female softball pitcher had a surgical ulnar nerve transposition/release for pain in her pitching arm three months ago. Now she still complains of severe pain daily. She can barely bend her elbow and has decreased function of her hand. She notes increased sensitivity to cold temperatures and generalized swelling, which is more pronounced on the ulnar side of her hand. She is in your office for pain management. What are your concerns? What is her diagnosis? How will you confirm the diagnosis? How will you treat the patient's pain?

## Clinical Issues

### Definition

Complex regional pain syndrome (CRPS) is a chronic progressive disease characterized by severe pain, swelling, and changes in the skin because of dysfunction of the central and peripheral nervous system. Historically, many terms that reference these symptoms have been used to depict this condition. Previously, the two subtypes of CRPS have been referred to as reflex sympathetic dystrophy and causalgia. Because these terms have lost their clinical utility, in 1994 the International Association for the Study of Pain (IASP) developed the term *complex regional pain syndrome* to emphasize the following clinical characteristics:

1. *Complex:* multiple and varied clinical features
2. *Regional:* majority of cases involve a region of the body, usually an extremity
3. *Pain:* cardinal feature, often out of proportion to original insult and essential to the diagnosis

   a. Type I: also known as reflex sympathetic dystrophy (RSD), Sudeck's atrophy, and shoulder and hand syndrome; does not have demonstrable nerve lesions.

   b. Type II: also known as causalgia; has evidence of obvious nerve damage.

## Typical Features of CRPS

### CRPS Types I and II

Features of both types that can be shared include:

1. Decreased function of the extremity
2. Pain out of proportion to known injury
3. Pain that is now chronic in nature
4. Skin changes such as mottling and cyanosis

5. Increased sweating of the affected limb during the acute phase
6. Allodynia: a painful sensation caused by non-noxious stimulation
7. Hyper-analgesia: an exaggerated painful response that is caused by a sensation that is usually noxious
8. Edema
9. Shiny skin at the affected site
10. Hair loss at the affected site
11. Temperature sensitivity: cold intolerance

### Type I

1. Caused by an unknown or minor limb injury
2. The pain is present in a nondermatomal distribution pattern.

### Type II

1. The pain presents after a known or major peripheral nerve injury.
2. The pain may or may not present with a dermatomal distribution.

In either type, the pain can spread into new dermatomes, especially if caused by sympathetic nervous system activation. Also, rarely (2% of cases) the pain and physical exam findings may include other extremities, usually in a mirror image fashion, which would suggest a more central origin for the pathology.

3. There are three stages of the disease:

   a. Stage 1 (0–3 months):

      i. Severe, burning pain at the site of the injury
      ii. Muscle spasm
      iii. Joint stiffness, restricted mobility, and decreased range of motion
      iv. Nail growth
      v. Puffy swelling
      vi. Redness and warmth
      vii. Hyperhidrosis
      viii. Radiographs are usually normal.
      ix. Positive bone scan
      x. Aggressive treatment at stage 1 yields the best outcome.

   b. Stage 2 (3–6 months from symptom onset):

i. Intense pain

ii. Skin atrophy with hard edema

iii. Diminished hair growth

iv. Nails become cracked, brittle, grooved, and spotty.

v. Osteoporosis develops quickly.

vi. Joints thicken.

vii. Muscles atrophy.

c. Stage 3 (6–12 months from symptom onset):

i. Irreversible changes occur in the skin, muscles, and bones.

ii. The pain becomes unyielding and may involve the entire limb.

iii. There is marked muscle atrophy with advanced contractions.

## Incidence

1. CRPS type I has an incidence of 1–2% after a fracture.
2. 2:1 to 4:1 female to male ratio
3. The mean age of presentation is 37–50 years old.

## Mechanism for CRPS Pain

1. The pathophysiology of this disease is still unclear.
2. The pain usually starts acutely within hours to days.
3. Most pain researchers believe CRPS is developed and maintained by abnormalities in the peripheral and central nervous systems.
4. The peripheral component is evidenced by:

a. Peripheral sensitization of primary nociceptive afferent neurons associated with sympathetic efferent coupling

b. Upregulation of ion channels and adrenergic receptors

c. Increased concentrations of neuropeptides

5. The central component is explained by spinal cord changes in the dorsal horn containing wide dynamic range (WDR) neurons.

a. Mechanisms of central sensitization resulting in increased perception of pain could include spontaneous firing of the WDR neuron as well as amplification of ascending signals or insufficient descending inhibitory signal.

b. Multiple neurotransmitters, receptors, and cytokines have been implicated.

i. Glutamate

ii. Magnesium

iii. Glycine

iv. Substance P

v. GABA

vi. NK (neurokinin)

vii. 5HT (serotonin)

viii. $\alpha_2$ receptors

ix. $\mu$-receptors

x. Prostaglandin

6. Newer imaging techniques – positron emission tomography (PET) and functional magnetic resonance imaging (MRI) – have confirmed a central reorganization of somatosensory sensations that improve with the treatment of the pain.

a. This means that actual areas of the brain have been "rewired" due to the chronic nature of this pain.

b. Therefore, there is an actual pathologic anatomy that may be the cause of, or result of, the chronic pain.

7. Vascular blood flow changes can occur after a major nerve injury.

a. This impaired blood flow can lead to dystrophic changes.

i. Skin and nail changes

ii. Impaired blood flow causing mottling

b. May be associated with hyperactive sympathetic discharge and impaired sympathetic function

8. Inflammatory cells such as macrophages and mast cells are implicated in inflammatory changes associated with CRPS, but whether their role is primary or secondary remains controversial.

a. Localized neurogenic inflammation may cause sweating, edema, and vasodilatation.

b. This inflammatory response is usually only seen in the acute phase, less than 6 months post-injury.

9. In CRPS, after the inflammation subsides from the initial event, it is thought that the nociceptors in the affected limb are still sending signals centrally. This causes the central nervous system to become hyperexcitable.

10. A genetic predisposition exists.

a. Certain women have a specific human leukocyte antigen (HLA) profile found on chromosome 6 and/or angiotensin-converting enzyme (ACE) gene deletion on chromosome 17.

## Tests to Help Confirm the Diagnosis

1. There is no single test used to diagnose CRPS.
2. Most physicians agree that the patient's clinical history is the most important factor in making the correct diagnosis. Physicians can use the "Budapest criteria" to aid in diagnosis. All of the following statements must be met.

a. Continuing pain, which is disproportionate to any inciting event

b. Must report at least one symptom in three or more of the following categories

c. Must display at least one sign at the time of evaluation in two or more of the following categories

d. There is no other diagnosis that better explains the signs and symptoms.

e. Categories

    i. Sensory: hyperalgesia (to pinprick), allodynia (to light touch, temperature sensation, deep somatic pressure, joint movement)

    ii. Vasomotor: temperature asymmetry, skin color changes, skin color asymmetry

    iii. Sudomotor/edema: evidence of edema, sweating changes, sweating asymmetry

    iv. Motor/trophic: decreased range of motion, motor dysfunction (weakness, tremor, dystonia), trophic changes (hair, nail, skin)

3. Response to sympathetic blockade

a. Previously, a reduced pain response to a sympathetic blockade was considered mandatory for the diagnosis of CRPS.

b. This is no longer the case because a sympathetic pain block may or may not alleviate the pain, even if the pain is sympathetically maintained.

c. The sympathetic block can help differentiate between sympathetically maintained pain (SMP) and sympathetically independent pain (SIP), but it does not definitively diagnose CRPS.

4. Sudomotor testing: sweat testing

a. During any stage of CRPS, the patient may have abnormalities in sweat gland function.

b. Sweating may be excessive or reduced.

c. Special tests can be used to measure resting sweat output, thermoregulatory sweating, and quantitative sudomotor axon reflex testing.

d. These tests are helpful if positive, but not if they are negative.

e. These tests are difficult to do and are currently available in only a few parts of the United States.

5. Three-phase bone scan

a. Osteopenia is common within one year from the beginning of the syndrome.

b. A three-phase bone scan can help confirm the diagnosis of CRPS-associated osteopenia.

c. It is not particularly useful because it is usually positive in only 50% of CRPS cases.

6. Skin temperature measurements at rest may be only slightly different in the affected limbs.

a. With whole-body cooling or warming, the differences dramatically increase the sensitivity and specificity for CRPS.

b. The variation in temperature between the extremities is due to vascular constriction and dilation caused by sympathetic nervous system dysfunction.

c. Infrared thermography is a diagnostic imaging procedure that records the body surface temperature by detecting heat emitted from the surface of the skin. It can detect very small differences in temperature.

7. Nerve conduction testing and electromyography (EMG)

a. Half of all CRPS patients will show an abnormality.

b. Not very useful, and rarely used for diagnosis of CRPS

8. Plain X-rays and MRI

a. More useful in later stages, and not as a screening tool

b. X-ray may show demineralization of bone.

c. MRI can show soft tissue changes and swelling.

9. Post-traumatic neuralgia (PTN) may mimic CRPS I and II.

a. In PTN, the pain is felt only in the area innervated by the injured nerve.

b. It usually presents with a less complex picture overall.

c. The patient may complain of burning pain.

d. There may be some cold sensitivity.

e. Sympathetic nerve blocks may relieve this pain but less often than in CRPS.

## KO Treatment Plan

The patient in the sample case likely has CRPS. Her diagnosis can be made by a thorough clinical examination. Treatment and physical therapy should begin immediately.

## Treatment

1. Physical therapy and occupational therapy are vitally important to maintain function in a given extremity. Physical therapy should be instituted as early as possible. Most patients require some medications/treatments to tolerate the physical therapy. Take advantage of the window of opportunity that exists after a block is performed. During this relatively pain-free period, intensive physical therapy should occur to improve function of the affected limb.

2. Nonsteroidal anti-inflammatory medications (NSAIDs)

a. These can be used to control low levels of pain and as an adjuvant therapy.

3. Opioids

a. Most experts would agree that these should be prescribed in the early phase of the disease.

b. Studies are lacking as to long-term benefits.

c. Opioids are considered as third-line drugs due to their potential adverse effects.

4. Steroids: high dose

a. May be helpful in the acute phase of the disease (<13 weeks)

5. Selective serotonin reuptake inhibitors (SSRIs) and tricyclic antidepressants (TCAs) may be helpful in CRPS, but studies are lacking.

6. Lidocaine IV does decrease the pain in CRPS.

a. IV lidocaine 2 mg/kg with 0.5 mg/kg of ketamine, given in a Bier block to the affected extremity, has been reported to give resolution of symptoms in CRPS.

b. Lidocaine PO (mexiletine) does not appear to be effective.

    i. It was previously thought that the membrane-stabilizing effects might be advantageous to people with CRPS.

    ii. This, however, has not been proven.

c. There have been reports of Lidoderm patches (5%) giving good pain relief with CRPS.

7. Anticonvulsant medications

a. Some experimental evidence has shown gabapentin to reduce pain associated with CRPS.

    i. A typical starting dose would be 300 mg at night, slowly increasing over the course of 1 week to three times daily dosing.

    ii. Titration of the medication should continue in a similar fashion to minimize side effects and optimize analgesic properties.

    iii. Daily maximum dosing should not exceed 3600 mg/day.

    iv. Decreased dosing is necessary for patients with renal impairment.

b. Pregabalin is effective in treating neuropathies, such as peripheral diabetic neuropathy and postherpetic neuralgia; unproven in CRPS.

    i. Doses used are 150–600 mg/day either two or three times daily dosing.

c. Carbamazepine is approved for trigeminal neuralgia. May be used as a second-line agent for CRPS.

    i. Doses used are 100–1000 mg/day, 2–4 times daily dosing.

8. Clonidine patches are also effective when smaller areas of pain are present.

a. The improvement of the pain is believed to be due to a reduction of the sympathetic nervous system activity.

b. A typical starting dose should be a patch of 0.1 mg/day applied weekly.

c. The patch should be applied to the affected area.

d. Caution should be taken when using clonidine as it may cause hypotension; also, if used for a prolonged period of time and abruptly stopped, it may lead to rebound hypertension.

e. The dose may be increased as tolerated if it is effective in relieving pain in a given small area and the patient's blood pressure can tolerate it.

9. Ketamine

a. The only potent N-methyl-D-aspartate (NMDA)-blocking drug currently available for clinical use

b. Ketamine IV 10–90 mg/h can be given over several treatment days.

c. Some studies show promising results.

    i. In one randomized placebo-controlled trial, IV ketamine given 0.35 mg/kg/h, up to 25 mg/h, over 4 hours for 10 days resulted in significant reductions in pain.

    ii. A Cochrane Review found evidence to support a course of IV ketamine for treating CRPS-related pain.

10. Bone-targeting drugs

a. Bisphosphonates: high-dose alendronate, IV pamidronate

    i. Mechanism of action for treating CRPS is unclear.

b. Calcitonin

    i. Mechanism of action for treating CRPS is unclear as well as unproven.

11. Sympathetic blocks

a. Stellate ganglion (upper extremity) block

    i. Should be performed in a series of 3–6 injections

    ii. Should give immediate pain relief

    iii. Physical therapy should be planned in conjunction with the improved pain control.

    iv. This block can be repeated weekly, or delayed longer if pain does not return.

    v. The block should result in good pain relief and the patient should have improved function in the extremity. If not, the block series should be discontinued.

    vi. The usual dose is 15 cc of bupivacaine 0.5%. This should give definite results and longer-lasting pain relief.

    vii. Horner's syndrome (miosis, enophthalmos, ptosis, and anhidrosis) is often seen as a side effect of the successful block.

    viii. Omnipaque is injected before the bupivacaine to ensure that the needle is in the proper position. Also, the omnipaque is injected with the bupivacaine to ensure that the medication travels inferiorly toward the T1 level, where the stellate ganglion lies.

    ix. The stellate ganglion block is typically performed at the C6 level due to the increased risk of vertebral artery puncture and pneumothorax at lower levels. The bupivacaine is injected caudally in the direction of the stellate ganglion.

b. Lumbar sympathetic (lower extremity) block

i. Effective at reducing pain compared with saline control injections up to 24 hours after the injection.

ii. Treatment goals are similar to those with the stellate ganglion block.

iii. Bupivacaine 0.5% about 20 cc with omnipaque would be a typical choice for injection.

iv. The omnipaque would be injected before the bupivacaine to make sure the needle is in the proper position. The omnipaque would also be injected and mixed with the bupivacaine to watch its spread, ensuring that the injection is not intravascular.

12. Other blocks that may be helpful depending on the site of pain include:

a. Celiac plexus block

i. Bupivacaine 0.5%, 15 cc per side can be used to determine if the cause of the pain can be relieved with this block.

ii. Usually used for pancreatic pain

(1) Palliative treatment, in cases such as terminal pancreatic cancer, can be performed and would include neurolytic block after the local anesthetic block has confirmed that the pain has been relieved with this block.

(2) Neurolytic agents, including phenol and alcohol

(a) Alcohol is painful on injection.
(b) Phenol is painless on injection.
(c) Alcohol and phenol have about the same efficacy.
(d) Neurolytic blocks are reserved for patients at the end of life as the pain can return in weeks to months.

b. Splanchnic nerve block

i. Again, one may use bupivacaine for the injections with the goal of reducing the pain acutely.

ii. If more permanent pain relief is desired based on the clinical situation, then alcohol or phenol may be used with a local anesthetic.

c. Hypogastric plexus and ganglion impar blocks

i. May be performed with a local anesthetic such as bupivacaine or with neurolytic agents

13. Transcutaneous electrical nerve stimulation (TENS)

a. This is a small battery-operated unit; electrodes are placed by the patient over the affected area.

b. The electrical current stimulation is mild; however, it can stop pain impulses from being transmitted to the central nervous system.

c. The TENS unit can also cause endorphins to be released centrally, which will modify the patient's perception of pain.

d. The unit is controlled by the patient; stimulation can be increased or decreased as desired.

14. Spinal cord stimulator (SCS)

a. The SCS leads are implanted dorsally in the epidural space.

b. The electrical impulses generate a tingling sensation that helps prevent painful impulses from being perceived by the patient.

c. Typically, a six-lead electrode is implanted for a trial period of 1 week.

d. The permanent implant surgery is performed in the operating room under sedation and the electrode is initially adjusted intra-operatively with the patient confirming that the electrical stimulation is covering the areas of pain.

e. Once the electrode wire is secured in place, the wires are attached to an external generator and the patient is taken to the recovery area for further adjustments of the stimulator.

f. A systematic review of the clinical and cost-effectiveness literature found that SCS appears to be an efficacious and cost-effective treatment for CRPS.

15. Intrathecal drug pumps

a. Implanted devices that deliver pain medications directly into intrathecal space

b. Medications typically used are baclofen, opioids, local anesthetics, and clonidine.

c. Delivery of medications in this way can decrease side effects and increase effectiveness.

d. CRPS can lead to dystonia, which is often refractory to standard treatment. Intrathecal baclofen has been shown to be effective in some patients with dystonia.

16. Psychiatric treatment

a. Psychiatry should be involved with these chronic pain patients at the beginning of their treatment.

b. Often these patients are frustrated and depressed.

c. The depression may set in early if their limb function does not improve with therapy.

d. They will also need to be involved before an SCS can be placed.

17. Surgical sympathectomy does not have good results for the vast majority of patients and therefore is not usually recommended.

# Prognosis

1. Follow-up studies show that the majority (62%) of patients are limited in daily activities at 5 years.

2. The majority (60%) of patients with CRPS II, even with intensive therapy, are still in pain at 1 year.

3.  Patients with CRPS I are much more likely to have a resolution of their symptoms at 1 year (74%) compared to patients with CRPS II.

4.  Some degree of functional dysfunction is likely to be present in the affected extremity for at least 13 months after the CRPS is diagnosed.

## Bibliography

Benzon HT, Raja SN, Molloy RE, et al. *Essentials of Pain Medicine and Regional Anesthesia*, 4nd ed. Philadelphia: Elsevier, 2018, pp. 223–232, e2.

Harden RN, Bruehl S, Stanton-Hicks M, Wilson PR. Proposed new diagnostic criteria for complex regional pain syndrome. *Pain Med* 2007;**8**(4):326–31.

Harden RN, Oaklander AL, Burton AW, et al. Complex regional pain syndrome: practical diagnostic and treatment guidelines, 4th edition. *Pain Med* 2013;**14**(2):180–229.

Waldman SD. *Pain Management*, Vol. **1**. Philadelphia: Saunders Elsevier, 2007, pp. 283–303.

# Opioid Addiction

Winston Singleton and Brendan J. Astley

## Sample Case

A 47-year-old female presents for a total knee arthroplasty. Her medical history is positive for hypertension, rheumatoid arthritis, and a previous history of opioid use disorder. Her current medications include hydrochlorothiazide (HCTZ), lisinopril, and buprenorphine hydrochloride (Subutex). The patient states that if possible she would like to avoid narcotics. What is your anesthetic plan? What is Subutex? How will it affect your anesthetic medications? Is it possible to completely avoid narcotics in the peri-operative period?

## Clinical Issues

### Definition of Opioid Addiction

As defined by the World Health Organization, "a state, psychic and sometimes also physical, resulting from the interactions between a living organism and a drug, that includes a compulsion to take the drug on a continuous or periodic basis in order to avoid the discomfort of its absence. Tolerance may or may not be present."

1. Opioid addiction is on the rise again
2. Most commonly abused opiates
   a. Heroin
   b. Fentanyl
   c. Morphine
   d. Oxycontin
   e. Vicodin

### Definition of Tolerance

1. A condition in which the typical effect of a drug is diminished due to previous drug exposure
2. The previous exposure has caused a change in the way a person deals with the drug either physically, mentally, or both.

### Opioid Receptor Types

1. Mu ($\mu_1$, $\mu_2$, $\mu_3$): analgesia, respiratory depression, euphoria, sedation, and gastrointestinal dysmotility
2. Kappa ($\kappa_1$, $\kappa_2$, $\kappa_3$): analgesia, dysphoria, diuresis, and psychotomimetic effects including hallucinations and delusions
   a. This is believed to be very important in spinal analgesia.

3. Delta ($\delta_1$, $\delta_2$): analgesia and other unknown effects
   a. Activation causes analgesia with minimal respiratory suppression.

## Properties of the μ, κ, and δ Receptors

1. These receptors are located in the central nervous system and the peripheral nervous system.
2. The analgesic components of these receptors are the primary target of drug therapy, with the μ receptor being the most important target.
3. Approximately 82% of patients on opioid therapy report opioid-related side effects.
   a. Constipation
   b. Nausea and vomiting
   c. Sedation
   d. Pruritis
   e. Respiratory depression
   f. Muscle rigidity
   g. Antitussive effect (this is usually a positive side effect).

## Appropriate Usage of Opioids

1. Opioids may be used for acute or chronic pain.
2. Opioids are very safe and effective pain killers with minimal short- or long-term side effects and tolerance profiles.
3. Opioids may be used in all patients, from pediatric to the elderly.
4. Opioids can be used in former addicts, although alternative techniques to alleviate pain should be tried first.

   a. See alternative techniques below.
   b. If opioids are chosen for former addicts, then great caution and close follow-up care are needed in this population.

      i. Effective communication with the rehabilitation physician and the patient's psychiatrist should be implemented.
      ii. The treatment plan should be coordinated with these officials and the pain management services.

   c. Opioids should not be avoided solely due to "former addict" status.

## Algorithm for Determining the Appropriate Opioid Usage for a Patient

1. Consider all the potential consequences if a patient has any of the expected side effects. Our primary goal is to do no harm. How will you treat any of the associated side effects? Develop a plan.
2. Does the patient have any previous opioid usage?
   a. Use the patient's daily opioid dose as the baseline of opioid needs.
   b. Start the acute pain regimen on top of that baseline dose.
   c. Know the signs of withdrawal.
3. Decide on the appropriate starting dose as mentioned above based on the patient's needs and previous opioid daily dosage.
4. Use a pain scale scoring system to assess the adequacy of pain control.
5. Monitor for over-sedation.
   a. Patients with a history of opioid usage are usually more sedated with higher pain scores post-operatively.
6. Use multiple techniques in addition to opioids.
   a. Regional/neuraxial blocks
   b. Anticonvulsants
   c. Sodium channel blockers
   d. NMDA receptor antagonists
   e. Nonsteroidal anti-inflammatory drugs (NSAIDs)
7. Prepare for daily routine events that typically cause increased pain (e.g., dressing changes).
   a. Compensate for these times with an appropriate breakthrough dose of a short-acting medication.
8. Be prepared to treat side effects, such as nausea and vomiting, and respiratory depression.
9. Patients with chronic opioid dependence should be monitored for compliance with therapy by using random urine toxicology screens.
10. Always believe the patient is in pain, but always be vigilant for any signs of complications, addiction, or manipulation.

## Signs of Addiction/Diversion

The signs of addiction should be watched for in every patient. Often, as physicians we are prescribing powerful medications that, in the hands of the wrong person, can do great harm – not only to the patient but also to others who may obtain access to the drug inappropriately, and to the community at large.

1. Multiple physicians are prescribing these patients pain medications.
2. The patients frequently report losing their prescriptions.
3. Requests for early refills

4. Unable to provide a urine toxicology screen when requested
5. The patient is requiring escalating doses of medication.
6. The patient inappropriately focuses on the narcotics during office visits.
7. The patient is not interested in a nonnarcotic means of pain relief, such as interventional methods, NSAIDs, and psychiatric treatment.
8. Diversion: borrowing/selling opioid medications from/to others.

## Signs of Substance Abuse and Dependance in an Anesthesia Provider

1. Signing out increasing quantities of narcotics
2. Volunteering for cases that require high doses of narcotics
3. Arriving early and staying late, taking extra calls, giving extra breaks
4. Refusing lunch or breaks; preferring to work alone
5. Additional bathroom breaks
6. Difficult to locate during breaks secondary to naps
7. Wearing long sleeve shirts to hide needle marks
8. Sloppy charting
9. Frequent job changes
10. Pinpoint pupils
11. Weight loss
12. Sweating
13. Tremors
14. Coma and death

## Behavioral Changes that are Signs of Substance Abuse and Dependance in an Anesthesia Provider

1. Mood swings and emotional lability
2. Social withdrawal
3. Increased impulsivity
4. Drug paraphernalia found
5. Decreased sex drive
6. Increased domestic issues

## Withdrawal and the Medications Used for Its Treatment

Withdrawal can be a frightening experience for a patient coming off opioids. However, this experience is usually not life-threatening.

## Signs and Symptoms of Withdrawal

### Physiological Symptoms
1. Increased lacrimation
2. Rhinorrhea
3. Sneezing
4. Nausea

5. Vomiting
6. Abdominal cramps
7. Diarrhea
8. Fever
9. Chills
10. Tremor
11. Tachycardia
12. Aches and pains, often in the joints
13. Elevated pain sensitivity
14. Elevated blood pressure
15. Piloerection
16. Pupillary dilation
17. Sweating
18. Dysphoria

**Cognitive Symptoms**

1. Suicidal ideation
2. Depression
3. Adrenal exhaustion
4. Adrenal fatigue
5. Spontaneous orgasm
6. Prolonged insomnia leading up to delirium
7. Auditory hallucinations
8. Visual hallucinations
9. Enhanced olfactory sense
10. Decreased sexual drive
11. Agitation
12. Panic disorder
13. Anxiety/irritability
14. Paranoia
15. Delusion
16. Opioid cravings

**TKO:** Only a physician licensed in drug rehabilitation may prescribe medications for the sole purpose of detoxification from opioids. For the oral boards it may be important to recognize these drugs and some of their general properties in case they are included in a given case.

# Commonly Prescribed Withdrawal Medications

## Agonists

1. Methadone

   a. Trade name: Dolophine

   b. Pharmacokinetics

      i. Oral peak concentration is 1–7.5 hours.
      ii. Elimination half-life is 7–59 hours.
      iii. These times are shorter for pregnant patients.
      iv. Variable bioavailability with resultant different duration of action and dosing regimens

   c. Used for drug detoxification, opioid abuse, neuropathic pain, and somatic pain

   d. The usual maintenance dose for abuse is 80–120 mg/ day orally (PO).

   e. The usual dose for pain treatment in an opioid-naïve patient can range from 2.5 to 10 mg PO every 3–6 hours as needed.

   f. Renal and hepatic impairment may increase the accumulation of methadone and therefore dosing should be adjusted.

   g. Black box warning: can cause QT prolongation and serious arrhythmias (Torsades de Pointes) in doses higher than 200 mg/day.

   h. Contraindications

      i. Respiratory depression
      ii. Bronchial asthma
      iii. Hypercarbia
      iv. Paralytic ileus

   i. Precautions

      i. Large daily doses
      ii. QT prolongation
      iii. Abuse
      iv. Electrolyte abnormalities may augment Torsades de Pointes.

         (1) Hypomagnesemia
         (2) Hypokalemia

## Agonist/Antagonist

1. Buprenorphine

   a. Buprenorphine is a semi-synthetic opiate with partial agonist and antagonist properties. Buprenorphine hydrochloride was first marketed in the 1980s as an analgesic. Today it is available in sublingual, buccal, transdermal, and IV formulations.

   b. Buprenorphine itself is a mixed agonist/antagonist. It blocks the activity of other opiates and induces withdrawal in opiate-dependent individuals who are currently physically dependent on another opiate. Therefore, users must wait until they are in withdrawal before beginning treatment with buprenorphine.

   c. Elimination half-life: intravenous (IV) 1.2–7.2 hours and sublingual 37 hours

   d. Used for opioid dependence and pain control

   e. This is a schedule III drug that is a partial μ-opioid receptor agonist and κ-opioid receptor antagonist.

      i. Since this drug is a partial μ-opioid receptor agonist, it makes reversing the overdose with naloxone difficult.

2. In 2002, the Food and Drug Administration (FDA) approved Suboxone and Subutex as high-dose sublingual pill preparations of buprenorphine for the treatment of opioid addiction.

   a. Subutex has a greater attraction to the opiate receptors than other drugs such as heroin and methadone, and it binds more tightly to these receptors.

i. This drug is used most commonly in drug treatment programs to discourage further opioid abuse because it has a "ceiling effect," meaning that only a certain, reduced level of pain control can be achieved and therefore gives a reduced feeling of reward for the patient taking this drug.

ii. This ceiling effect not only limits its maximal analgesic effect, but it also limits its associated amount of respiratory depression.

iii. The dependence dose is 12–16 mg/day.

iv. Precautions include:

(1) Compromised pulmonary function

(2) Head injury or increased intracranial pressure (ICP)

(3) Acute alcohol abuse

(4) Addison's disease

(a) Opioid receptor actions at the level of the hypothalamus can affect hormone secretion on the hypothalamic–pituitary axis and cause further adrenal–cortical insufficiency, leading to hypotension.

(5) Delirium tremens

(6) Infant risk with breastfeeding

(a) Decreased maternal milk production

(b) Buprenorphine is passed into the breast milk.

(7) Severe dysfunction of the hepatic, renal, or pulmonary systems. Ingestion of high doses of buprenorphine can result in severe hepatitis and acute renal failure.

(8) Severe opioid withdrawal may result with high doses.

v. Side effects

(1) Nausea and vomiting

(2) Dizziness and vertigo

(3) Sedation

(4) Arrhythmias

(5) An increase or decrease in blood pressure

(6) Dyspnea

(7) Respiratory depression

vi. Naloxone may not reverse the respiratory depression caused by buprenorphine.

b. Suboxone

i. Combination of buprenorphine and naloxone in a 4:1 ratio

ii. This combination is effective in reducing the misuse of this drug because, if crushed and injected (IV), the naloxone will precipitate withdrawal.

iii. If taken as directed (sublingual), then very little to no naloxone will be absorbed.

## Antagonists

1. Naltrexone

a. Medication approved to treat both alcohol and opioid use disorder

b. Blocks the euphoria and sedative effects

c. Binds and blocks opioid receptors

d. Reduces cravings for opioids

e. No abuse potential

f. Should not start until off opioids for 7–10 days

g. Side effects

i. Tissue reaction at the injection site

ii. Liver damage or hepatitis

iii. Serious allergic reaction

iv. Pneumonia

v. Depression

## Alternative Analgesics

Although implied, the following is specifically for chronic opioid users or those that have a previous abuse history. These patients have a more complicated background of pain and may require several extra therapies to get them through the peri-operative period successfully.

1. Regional anesthesia

a. Especially useful in orthopedics and vascular procedures

b. Regional anesthesia is easy to deliver to the upper and lower extremities, and usually has good results.

c. May be contraindicated in a patient with impending neurological complications: compartment syndrome.

2. Neuraxial anesthesia

a. A spinal or epidural may be an option depending on the site of surgery.

b. The epidural may have the added advantage of being used in the post-operative period for pain relief.

c. Bupivacaine is commonly used for spinal anesthesia.

i. Longer duration of action compared with lidocaine

ii. Less likely to cause transient neurologic syndrome when compared to lidocaine

(1) Patients with transient neurologic syndrome typically have complaints of pain and a burning sensation in the lower extremities and buttock.

(2) The pain may last for several hours to days after the procedure has been completed.

(3) Occasionally the pain may last for years.

(4) Transient neurologic syndrome has been associated with:

(a) Higher concentrations of local anesthetics (e.g., lidocaine 5%)

(b) Prone and lithotomy positions

d. Opioids and clonidine are effective in combination with bupivacaine or independently.

e. Lidocaine or bupivacaine can be used for epidural anesthesia.

   i. A combination of the two may be advantageous as lidocaine will have quicker onset of anesthesia and bupivacaine will have a longer duration of action.

3. NSAIDs and acetaminophen (Tylenol)

a. These give highly effective pain relief for the majority of pain that people experience on a day-to-day basis; however, these should be used in combination with other techniques for peri-operative care.

4. Muscle relaxants

a. These may be good additions in certain situations that involve muscle spasticity as the cause of pain.

b. Methocarbamol (Robaxin), carisoprodol (Soma), baclofen, metaxalone (Skelaxin), and diazepam (Valium) are examples of medications that cause central muscle relaxation.

5. Anxiety

a. This can be the main source of pain problems.

b. Often this can stem from social issues or a personality disorder.

c. Psychiatry can help resolve some of these issues over time, and in the acute peri-operative period benzodiazepine supplementation may be advantageous.

6. Neuropathic pain

a. Pain that is initiated or caused by a primary lesion or dysfunction in the nervous system

b. This may be considered if there is a burning component, numbness, or "electric shock" feeling to a patient's pain.

c. Medications that are useful supplements for this pain include gabapentin (Neurontin) and pregabalin (Lyrica).

7. Sleep

a. It is very important for all of us to sleep well; however, for a patient in pain (chronically or acutely) this can be a major source of concern and sleeping poorly may accentuate the patient's pain.

b. Lack of sleep should be treated aggressively.

c. A good pharmacological choice for the chronic pain patient would be amitriptyline. This medication can help relieve neuropathic pain, is not addictive, and is a sleep aid.

d. Other selective serotonin reuptake inhibitors (SSRIs)/antidepressants that have sedative properties may also be useful (e.g., trazadone).

e. Care should be taken to stay away from substances that have addictive potential, especially in patients with histories of addiction or who are at high risk for addiction.

## Opioid-Free Anesthesia

1. Dexmedetomidine
2. IV Tylenol
3. IV ketorolac
4. Ketamine
5. IV lidocaine
6. Gabapentin/pregabalin
7. Magnesium
8. Regional block and neuraxial block

## KO Treatment Plan

### Pre-operative

1. Obtain a detailed history concerning previous drug use/abuse, length of use, treatment medications, and the length of the treatment.

2. Focus on a nonnarcotic method of caring for the patient, if feasible.

3. Emphasize that if narcotics are used, it will only be in the peri-operative period and not for chronic therapy.

4. Be aware that some chronic users have decreased pain thresholds and increased opioid tolerance. Therefore, doses that would be effective normally may not be effective in this population.

5. If the patient is currently on an agonist/antagonist such as buprenorphine (Subutex), then she may experience a ceiling effect with narcotics peri-operatively. However, care should be taken when giving narcotics because side effects such as over-sedation and respiratory depression are still possibilities. Ideally, if opioids will be required in the peri-operative period, agonist/antagonists should be discontinued 1–2 weeks before any surgery and supplemented with another opioid agonist such as methadone. Therapy can be restarted after the surgery.

6. Choose a regional anesthetic for intra-operative and/or post-operative pain relief, if possible.

### Intra-operative and Post-operative

#### Sample Case: Plan to Provide an Opioid-Free Anesthetic

1. PO Tylenol pre-operatively
2. Spinal with bupivacaine
3. Adductor block with bupivacaine or ropivacaine
4. IV propofol and ketamine infusion for sedation
5. Consider dexmedetomidine infusion or boluses as needed.
6. IV ketorolac if approved by the surgeon at the end of the case
7. Close monitoring of the respiratory rate if ventilation is not controlled may be valuable as this should give you an idea of the patient's anesthetic requirements and pain

tolerance. Titrate the opioids to a goal respiratory rate of about 10 respirations per minute.

8. Monitoring for cardiac dysrhythmias is important with patients on high-dose methadone (>200 mg/day). This is especially important if other agents or conditions are present that could cause cardiac issues.

    a. Tricyclic antidepressants, secondary to the potential for an associated QT prolongation

    b. Electrolyte deficiencies, particularly calcium, potassium, and magnesium, because of their associated Torsades de Pointes or QT prolongation

    c. Lasix can lead to a further decrease in potassium concentrations, which can lead to dysrhythmias, and/ or decreased magnesium, which can also lead to Torsades de Pointes.

    d. Amiodarone and procainamide can also cause QT prolongation and worsen a patient's condition acutely.

    e. Hypothyroidism can also cause QT prolongation.

9. Titrate short- to medium-acting medications such as fentanyl until intra-operative pain is under control. There is still a risk of over-sedation in patients who are not opioid-naïve.

10. Consider using a low-dose propofol/ketamine infusion during the case, such as propofol/ketamine in a 4:1 concentration. Opioids can often be avoided entirely in this scenario.

    a. Ketamine helps with pain control by N-methyl-D-aspartic acid antagonism, instead of activation at the opioid receptors.

    b. Ketamine will help attenuate the decrease in blood pressure caused by propofol.

    c. Propofol will be useful as an anesthetic agent and as an antiemetic.

11. Consider using dexmedetomidine during the case as an adjunct for opioid sparing.

    a. Dexmedetomidine is an $\alpha_2$ receptor agonist with analgesic properties mediated through stimulation of the $\alpha_{2C}$ and $\alpha_{2A}$ receptor in the dorsal horn of the spinal cord.

    b. Pain transmission is suppressed by reducing the release of pronociceptive transmitters, such as substance P and glutamate, and hyperpolarization of interneurons.

12. Titrate in longer-acting agents at the end of the case for continued pain coverage in the post-anesthesia care unit (PACU) and afterward.

13. Consider an early regional block during the immediate post-operative period unless there are contraindications.

14. Keep in mind that, especially in this population, it is better to prevent severe pain than it is to treat it after the patient is very uncomfortable. Be proactive.

# Bibliography

Barash PG, Cullen BF, Stoelting RK, et al. *Clinical Anesthesia*, 8th ed. Philadelphia: Lippincott Williams & Wilkins, 2017 pp. 82–4.

Benzon HT, Raja SN, Molloy RE, et al. *Essentials of Pain Medicine and Regional Anesthesia*, 4nd ed. Philadelphia: Elsevier, 2018.

Gropper MA, Miller RD, Eriksson LI, et al. *Miller's Anesthesia*, 9th ed. New York: Churchill Livingstone, 2020, pp. 638–679.

Thomson Micromedex Healthcare Series. www.micromedex.dk

Waldman SD. *Pain Management*, **Vol. 1**. Philadelphia: Saunders Elsevier, 2007, pp. 939–61, 997–1001.

# Peri-operative Temperature Regulation

## 94

Rushi Gottimukkala, Alma Hoxha, and Jessica A. Lovich-Sapola

## Temperature Regulation

1. Thermoregulatory centers in the hypothalamus play an integral role in maintaining core body temperature within a very narrow range. Anesthetics interfere with these pathways.
2. Without intervention, core body temperature typically decreases 1–2 °C during the first hour of general anesthesia. This is followed by a more gradual decrease over the next 3–4 hours before reaching a steady state.
3. Typical clinical doses of all general anesthetics reduce the threshold for vasoconstriction to 33–35 °C.
4. General anesthetics increase threshold for sweating and active vasodilatation by 1 °C.
   a. Anesthesia profoundly alters the thermoregulatory system, markedly reducing cold-response thresholds while slightly increasing warm-response thresholds.
   b. This results in an approximately 4 °C range of core temperatures not triggering thermoregulatory deficiency intra-operatively. This inter-threshold range normally spans only a few tenths of a degree in the unanesthetized state.

## Temperature Monitoring and Thermal Management Guidelines

1. Core temperature should be monitored during general anesthesia exceeding 20–30 minutes.
2. Core temperature should be monitored during neuraxial anesthesia when changes in temperature are intended, anticipated, or suspected.
   a. Mechanism for hypothermia under neuraxial anesthesia
      i. Spinal and epidural anesthesia lead to an internal redistribution of heat from the core to the peripheral compartment.
      ii. Inhibition of both the afferent and efferent limbs of central thermoregulatory pathways
      iii. Loss of thermoregulatory vasoconstriction below the level of the spinal block
         (1) There is increased heat loss from body surfaces.
      iv. Altered thermoregulation under spinal anesthesia is characterized by a decrease in

vasoconstriction and shivering threshold and a slight increase in the sweating threshold.
3. Unless hypothermia is specifically indicated (e.g., for protection against cerebral ischemia), effort should be made to maintain a normothermic intra-operative core temperature.
   a. Normal body temperature is 36.7 °C to 37.0 °C ± 0.2–0.4 °C.
4. Temperature should always be monitored in any surgical patient who:
   a. Is receiving blood products
   b. Has a pre-existing fever
   c. Has an overt infection
   d. Has autonomic instability
5. Continuous monitoring of temperature is recommended; however, 15-minute intervals are acceptable for most patients.

## Temperature Monitoring Sites

1. Core
   a. Pulmonary artery
   b. Distal esophagus
   c. Tympanic membrane
   d. Nasopharynx
2. Intermediate
   a. Mouth
   b. Axilla
   c. Bladder
   d. Rectum
   e. Forehead skin surface: 1–2 °C less than the core temperature

## Hyperthermia

### Sample Case

A 63-year-old male with three vessel disease is brought to the operating room for a coronary artery bypass graft (CABG) surgery. The patient has a history of hypertension, gastroesophageal reflux diseases, diabetes mellitus, and hyperlipemia. He weighs 113 kg and is 169 cm tall. His pre-operative blood pressure is 130/66 mm Hg, heart rate is 72, oxygen saturation is 98%, respiratory rate is 18, and temperature is 36.7 °C. The patient has no prior surgical history. He is induced with etomidate and succinylcholine and intubated with a #8 endotracheal tube. The surgeon plans to perform this as an off-pump CABG. Anesthesia is maintained with isoflurane, fentanyl, and a vecuronium drip. During the procedure, your resident notes the patient to have an incremental increase in his temperature up to 38.3 °C. Is this a concern for you? What are the potential causes of this increase in temperature? What would you do?

## Clinical Issues

**TKO:** Hypothermia is by far the most common peri-anesthetic thermal perturbation. However, hyperthermia is more dangerous than a comparable degree of hypothermia.

### Definitions

1. Hyperthermia: core body temperature exceeds normal values (>37.5 °C).

    a. The body produces or absorbs more heat than it can dissipate.

    b. The body temperature is raised without the consent of the body's heat control centers.

    c. Body temperatures greater than 40 °C can be life-threatening.

    d. At 41 °C, brain death begins to occur.

    e. At about 45 °C, death is imminent.

    f. Internal temperatures above 50 °C cause muscle rigidity and death.

2. Passive intra-operative hyperthermia

    a. Excessive patient heating

    b. Most common in infants and children

    c. Frequently seen when effective active warming is used without adequate body temperature monitoring

3. Malignant hyperthermia (MH)

    a. Results secondary to an enormous increase in metabolic heat produced by both internal organs and skeletal muscle in response to a volatile anesthetic or succinylcholine

    b. Central thermoregulation presumably remains intact during an acute crisis. (Please see Chapter 80 on MH for further information.)

4. Fever

    a. Regulated increase in the core temperature targeted by the thermoregulatory system

    b. Fever results when endogenous pyrogens increase the thermoregulatory target temperature ("set point").

    c. The anterior hypothalamus sets the body's core temperature higher.

    d. Fever is relatively rare during general anesthesia.

        i. Volatile anesthetics and opioids inhibit the expression of fever.

### Differential Diagnosis of Hyperthermia

1. Iatrogenic

    a. Increased room temperature

    b. Warming devices

    c. Airway humidifiers and warmers

    d. Excessive rewarming after cardiopulmonary bypass

2. Infectious

    a. Pre-operative fever associated with upper respiratory tract infection or condition related to surgical indication

    b. Sepsis

    c. Bacteremia or sepsis associated with surgical manipulation (i.e., oral surgery)

    d. Infusion of blood components with infectious contamination

3. Pulmonary

    a. Aspiration pneumonia

    b. Atelectasis

    c. Deep venous thrombosis or pulmonary embolus

4. Metabolic

    a. Pheochromocytoma

    b. Thyrotoxicosis or thyroid storm

    c. Adrenal insufficiency

5. Central nervous system

    a. Status epilepticus

    b. Hypothalamic pathology

    c. Parkinson's disease

6. Drug-induced

    a. Malignant hyperthermia

    b. Neuroleptic malignant syndrome

    c. Anticholinergic effect

    d. Cocaine

    e. Tricyclic antidepressants

    f. Antibiotic-induced drug fever

    g. Monoamine oxidase inhibitors interacting with opioids, especially meperidine

7. Miscellaneous

    a. Monitoring error

    b. Connective tissue disease

    c. Hematoma

    d. Transfusion reactions

### Signs and Symptoms of Hyperthermia

1. Skin

    a. Perspiration

        i. Evaporative cooling

        ii. When the body is no longer capable of sweating secondary to dehydration or the sweat does not evaporate due to high relative air humidity, the patient's core temperature will rise rapidly.

   b. The skin initially becomes red as the blood vessels dilate in an attempt to increase heat dissipation, which reduces vascular resistance and blood pressure.

   c. Once the patient's blood pressure begins to drop, cutaneous blood vessels will begin to contract and the skin may start to look pale and bluish (this is a bad sign).

2. Cardiac

   a. Blood pressure may drop significantly from dehydration or vasodilation.

      i. Syncope or dizziness can be seen in an awake patient.

   b. Increased heart rate and cardiac output

   c. Increased metabolic rate and therefore increased oxygen consumption

      i. Myocardial ischemia occurs if the cardiac demand exceeds the oxygen delivery.

   d. Decreased intravascular volume and preload due to the hyperthermia-associated perspiration and vasodilation

3. Respiratory

   a. Increased respiratory rate

   b. If the cellular demand exceeds the oxygen delivery, acidosis occurs.

   c. Rightward shift of the oxyhemoglobin dissociation curve

4. Neurologic

   a. If awake, hyperthermic patients may become confused and hostile.

      i. Headache

      ii. Appear intoxicated

      iii. Seizure

      iv. Temporary blindness

      v. Unconsciousness

   b. Cerebral blood flow increases by 5–7% for each degree Celsius increase in body temperature.

   c. Reduces the latency of the somatosensory evoked potentials

5. Electrolytes

   a. Loss of electrolytes and free water secondary to perspiration and the associated nausea and vomiting

### Treatment of Hyperthermia

1. Treatment of hyperthermia depends on the etiology of the elevated temperature, with the critical distinction between fever and other causes of hyperthermia.

2. Review the patient's history and examine the patient for clues to the possible causes of hyperthermia.

   a. Medications

   b. Surgical procedure

   c. Peri-operative complications

   d. Iatrogenic

3. First line of treatment: treat the underlying cause.

   a. Passive cooling

      i. Remove any external warming devices: heating blankets, pads, fluid warmers, etc.

      ii. Lower the room temperature.

      iii. Remove excess blankets, clothing, or surgical drapes.

   b. Stop any blood transfusions if a reaction is occurring.

   c. Stop volatile anesthetic and change to a total IV anesthetic if the patient has signs of hypermetabolism and you are concerned about MH.

   d. Urine culture

   e. Chest X-ray

4. Second line of treatment: administration of antipyretic medications (this step is not always possible during the surgical procedure).

   a. Acetaminophen

   b. Aspirin

   c. Nonsteroidal anti-inflammatory drugs (NSAIDs)

5. Third line of treatment: active cooling should be considered when temperature exceeds 39 °C or the patient is believed to be hemodynamically unstable secondary to temperature perturbation.

   a. Turn off warming devices and blow cool air over the patient.

   b. Cooled IV fluids

   c. Ice packs on the torso, head, neck, and groin

   d. A fan can be used to aid evaporation.

   e. Flush cool water into the nasogastric tube and Foley catheter.

   f. In desperate situations, use of cardiopulmonary bypass provides rapid cooling.

   g. A hyperthermia vest can be placed if available.

## KO Treatment Plan

### Pre-operative

1. Careful pre-operative history and physical examination

   a. History of MH

   b. Known sepsis

   c. Pheochromocytoma

   d. Thyroid dysfunction

2. What is the patient's pre-operative temperature?

3. The sample patient does not have an elevated pre-operative temperature, and he has no history of any diseases associated with hyperthermia.

### Intra-operative

1. Iatrogenic hyperthermia is prevented by monitoring the patient's core temperature after the establishment of a baseline temperature and using a blanket cooling or warming device as necessary.

2. If hyperthermia occurs, review recent intra-operative events.

    a. Blood transfusion
    b. MH: triggering agents – volatile anesthetics and succinylcholine
    c. Where is the site of the surgery?
    d. Recent medications given

3. Differential diagnosis for the sample patient

**TKO:** On the oral board exam you should be able to list this differential quickly and efficiently, and in the order of most to least likely. The oral board examiners want to know that you have a complete differential in your mind, but they also really want to know what you think is going on, and that you have a plan to treat it quickly. See differential diagnosis above.

4. Diagnosis

    a. Review the patient's medical history.
    b. Verify the temperature reading and check all other vital signs.

        i. Look for signs of hypermetabolism.

            (1) Tachycardia
            (2) Acidosis
            (3) Hypercarbia
            (4) Hypoxemia

        ii. Look especially for changes in end-tidal $CO_2$.

            (1) Potential clue to MH or a pulmonary embolism

    c. Review all of the pre-operative and intra-operative medications that the patient has received.
    d. Send an arterial blood gas immediately.
    e. Chest X-ray
    f. Culture any possible infected areas.

        i. Blood
        ii. Urine
        iii. Sputum
        iv. Wound

            (1) This will not give you an immediate answer, but it can be used for diagnosis if other possibilities are ruled out.

### Post-operative

1. Although some mild hyperthermia or fever may be beneficial with an infection, the potential physiologic effects on the heart and brain can be detrimental, especially in the elderly.

2. Hyperthermia should be treated aggressively in at-risk patients.

# Hypothermia

## Sample Case

A 67-year-old male is brought to the operating room for an emergency surgery to repair his perforated esophagus. The patient was found lying in bed by his family members. He was cold and diaphoretic. His chest X-ray showed capsules in his stomach. The patient has a history of hypertension, hypothyroidism, gastroesophageal reflux disease, and depression. Vital signs: blood pressure 96/55 mm Hg, heart rate 61, respiratory rate 20, and temperature 33.8 °C. What do you think about the patient's body temperature? Is this a concern for you? How will the patient's hypothermia affect your anesthetic? Does it affect the muscle relaxant reversal? What are the effects of hypothermia on cardiovascular function? What are the effects of hypothermia on coagulation? What physiologic effects are you concerned about in a hypothermic patient?

## Clinical Issues

### Definition

1. Hypothermia:

    a. Defined as a core body temperature less than 36 °C
    d. The thermoregulatory system in an awake patient usually maintains a core body temperature within 0.2 °C of normal (37 °C).
    c. Usually caused by prolonged exposure to low temperatures

2. Mild hypothermia:

    a. About 1–2 °C below normal
    b. Triples the incidence of a morbid cardiac outcome
    c. Triples the incidence of wound infections
    d. Directly impairs immune function

        i. Impairs resistance to some bacteria *in vitro*

    e. Prolongs drug metabolism
    f. Prolongs hospitalization by 20%
    g. Significantly increases surgical blood loss and the need for allogenic transfusion

        i. Impairment of platelet aggregation secondary to decreased release of thromboxane A3
        ii. Impairment of coagulation secondary to decreased enzymatic activity of coagulation factors

**TKO:** Hypothermia during anesthesia by far is the most common peri-operative thermal disturbance. Hypothermia results from a combination of anesthetic-impaired thermoregulation and exposure to the cold operating room environment.

## Clinical Hypothermia

1. Mild: 32–35 °C
2. Moderate: 26–31 °C
3. Deep: 20–25 °C
4. Profound: 14–19 °C

## Incidence

1. More common than hyperthermia
2. Less dangerous than hyperthermia
3. The core temperature usually decreases by 0.5–1.5 °C in the first 30 minutes after the induction of anesthesia.

   a. Internal redistribution of heat

## General Causes of Hypothermia

1. Decreased heat production
2. Decreased metabolic rate
3. Increased heat loss
4. Heat transfer

   a. Radiation
   b. Convection
   c. Conduction
   d. Evaporation

## Mechanisms of Heat Loss

1. Radiation loss

   a. Largest component of heat loss
   b. Occurs in the form of infrared electromagnetic waves

2. Convection loss

   a. Secondary to "wind chill"
   b. Transfer of heat between the body and the air
   c. Heat rises from the skin, which creates a convection current.

3. Conduction loss

   a. Due to direct skin contact
   b. Exchange of heat between objects in direct contact
   c. Conductors pull heat away from the body.

      i. Water
      ii. Metals

4. Evaporative loss

   a. Usually less significant
   b. Important with premature babies
   c. Conversion of water from a liquid to a gas requires energy in the form of heat that is taken from the body.

## Differential Diagnosis of Hypothermia

1. Environmental

   a. Wind chill
   b. Cold water immersion

2. Impaired thermoregulation

   a. Extremes of age: neonates, elderly
   b. Prolonged immobilization
   c. Drugs

      i. Alcohol intoxication
      ii. Central nervous system depressants
      iii. Drug overdose

3. Medical conditions

   a. Hypothyroidism
   b. Large body surface area burns
   c. Malnutrition
   d. Hypoglycemia
   e. Hypothalamic stroke or tumor
   f. Unconsciousness

4. Iatrogenic causes of hypothermia

   a. Prolonged anesthesia and surgery without proper monitoring and regulation
   b. Prolonged cardiopulmonary resuscitation
   c. Blood or blood product transfusions (especially if the blood products are given rapidly and not warmed properly)
   d. Large-volume fluid resuscitation (especially without a proper warming device)

## Physiological Consequences of Hypothermia

1. Initial homeostatic responses in an effort to maintain normothermia: increased sympathetic nervous system activation, tachycardia, hypertension, increased cardiac output, increased oxygen consumption, hyperventilation, shivering
2. Increasing duration and degree of hypothermia leads to exhaustion of homeostatic responses and progressive decreases in metabolism, organ function with eventual respiratory and cardiovascular collapse.

## Organ Function during Hypothermia

1. Metabolism

   a. Abnormal response to drug administration

      i. Drug responses are often exaggerated. Decreased metabolic enzymatic activity leads to prolonged action of drugs to varying degrees.
      ii. The minimum alveolar concentration (MAC) for a volatile anesthetic decreases by 5–7% per degree Celsius fall in body temperature.

   b. Hyperglycemia secondary to decreased insulin secretion, decreased glucose metabolism

2. Brain

   a. Cerebral blood flow decreases in proportion to the metabolic rate during hypothermia because of an autoregulatory increase in cerebrovascular resistance.

   b. Cerebral function is well maintained until the patient's core temperature falls below 33 °C.

3. Heart

   a. Initial increase in heart rate, stroke volume, cardiac output, and blood pressure (MAP) secondary to sympathetic stimulation

      i. If the sympathetic response is blunted by anesthesia or other medications, there is a proportional decrease in cardiac output, heart rate, and MAP, with little change in stroke volume, and an increase in peripheral vascular resistance.

      ii. Decrease in the heart rate, cardiac output, and blood pressure with extremes of hypothermia

   b. As hypothermia progresses, SA node pacing becomes erratic and ventricular irritability increases.

4. Kidney

   a. Renal blood flow decreases as renal vascular resistance increases.

   b. Inhibition of tubular reabsorption maintains normal urinary volume.

   c. As the temperature decreases, reabsorption of sodium and potassium is progressively inhibited and an antidiuretic hormone-mediated "cold diuresis" results.

5. Respiratory

   a. Increase in oxygen consumption with an associated increase in respiratory rate with the initial fall in temperature

   b. Ultimately, hypothermia leads to respiratory depression.

   c. There is a 6% fall in oxygen consumption per degree Celsius fall in body temperature as hypothermia progresses.

   d. Respiratory strength is decreased at temperatures less than 33 °C, but ventilatory $CO_2$ response is minimally affected.

   e. Increased physiologic and respiratory dead space

6. Liver

   a. Hepatic blood flow and function decrease.

      i. Significantly inhibits the metabolism of some drugs

         (1) Propranolol

         (2) Verapamil

         (3) Prolongs elimination of nondepolarized muscle relaxants

7. Tissues

   a. The tolerance to tissue hypoxemia is increased during hypothermia.

8. Blood

   a. Rise in hematocrit

   b. Increase in viscosity

   c. Leukopenia

   d. Thrombocytopenia

## Treatment of Hypothermia

1. Surface rewarming

   a. Warmed blankets

   b. Forced-air heating blankets

2. Heated inspired gases

3. Fluid warmer

4. Increase the operating room temperature.

5. Warm body cavity lavage: bladder, stomach, chest, and abdominal cavity

6. An arterial line should be placed for continuous pressure monitoring and frequent blood gas determinations.

7. A pulmonary artery catheter may be helpful to follow cardiac output, but there is a risk of cardiac arrhythmia due to its placement.

8. Bladder catheterization

   a. Monitoring urine output reflects the adequacy of intravascular volume and organ perfusion.

9. Continuous core temperature monitoring

10. Warm the patient slowly.

**TKO:** Patients are not dead until they are warm and dead!

# KO Treatment Plan

## Pre-operative

The management and prevention of hypothermia are inseparable and include the following:

1. Pre-operative skin warming

2. Adjusted ambient temperature in the operating room

3. Intra-operative temperature monitoring

4. Heated and humidified anesthesia circuits

5. Forced-air warming blankets and other devices

6. Warmed IV fluids and blood products

7. Prevention and treatment of post-operative shivering

   a. Meperidine: 25 mg IV (treatment)

   b. Clonidine: 0.15 mg IV (treatment)

   c. Tramadol: 1 mg/kg IV (treatment and prophylaxis)

   d. Ondansetron: 8 mg IV (prophylaxis)

8. Anticipation and treatment of rewarming vasodilatation

## Intra-operative

1. Treatment of intra-operative hypothermia

   a. Preventing redistribution hypothermia

      i. Active pre-warming for as little as 30 minutes helps prevents redistribution hypothermia.

b. Airway heating and humidification

  i. Even though airway heating and humidification are effective in infants/children, cutaneous warming still remains more effective and transfers more than 10 times as much heat as airway heating.

c. IV fluids

  i. One unit of blood or 1 L of crystalloid solution administered at room temperature will decrease the mean body temperature by approximately 0.25 °C.

  ii. Fluid warmers minimize this loss and should be used when large amounts of IV fluid or boluses are administered.

d. Cutaneous warming

  i. Room temperature 23 °C for adults and 26 °C for children is needed to maintain normothermia.

  ii. Operating room temperature influences the rate at which heat is lost by radiation and convection from the skin and by evaporation from within surgical incisions.

  iii. The easiest way of decreasing cutaneous heat loss is to apply passive insulation to the skin surface.

    (1) Insulators are readily available in most operating rooms. Cotton blankets, surgical drapes, plastic sheeting, and reflective composites are examples.

    (2) A single layer of each reduces heat loss approximately 30%, with no clinical difference noted among the insulation types.

  iv. Cutaneous heat loss is roughly proportional to the surface area throughout the body.

    (1) 90% of metabolic heat is lost through the skin surface.

    (2) Only cutaneous warming will transfer sufficient heat to prevent hypothermia.

  v. For intra-operative use, forced-air cutaneous heating devices should be used.

2. Predisposition of hypothermia during general and regional anesthesia

a. Heat loss is common in all patients during general anesthesia because anesthetics alter thermoregulation, prevent shivering, and produce peripheral vasodilation.

  i. Volatile anesthetics impair the thermoregulatory center in the hypothalamus and also have direct vasodilatory properties.

  ii. Opioids reduce the vasoconstrictive mechanism of heat conservation.

  iii. Barbiturates cause peripheral vasodilation.

  iv. Muscle relaxants reduce muscle tone and prevent shivering thermogenesis.

b. Regional anesthesia also may produce sympathetic blockade, muscle relaxation, and sensory blockade of thermal receptors, thus inhibiting compensatory responses.

3. Attention should be paid to the effect of hypothermia on the patient's cardiac physiology.

a. Vasoconstriction causes hypoperfusion and hypoxia.

b. Shivering increases oxygen consumption by up to 300%.

  i. Also results in increased myocardial oxygen consumption

c. As hypothermia worsens, the heart rate, cardiac output, and oxygen consumption decrease.

d. Later symptoms include ventricular arrhythmias and myocardial depression.

4. Hypothermia leads to decreased platelet function. In addition, visceral sequestration of platelets results in thrombocytopenia.

5. Drug effects are prolonged by decreased hepatic blood flow, metabolism, renal blood flow, and clearance.

a. Protein binding increases as body temperature decreases.

b. The MAC of inhalation agents is decreased about 5–7% per degree Celsius fall in core temperature.

c. Hypothermia may prolong the duration of neuromuscular blocking agents because of decreased metabolism.

## Post-operative

1. Hypothermia delays discharge from the post-anesthesia care unit (PACU) and may prolong the need for mechanical ventilation.

a. Delayed emergence from volatile anesthetics (decreased MAC) and prolonged neuromuscular blockade

2. Shivering (see the pre-operative section for treatment).

# Bibliography

Atlee JL. *Complications in Anesthesia*, 2nd ed. Philadelphia: Saunders Elsevier Health Sciences, 2006, pp. 419–25

Ben-David B, Solomon E, Levin H. Spinal anesthesia, hypothermia, and sedation: a case of resedation with forced-air warming. *Anesth Analg* 1997;**85**:1357–8.

Butterworth JF, Mackey DC, Wasnick JD. *Morgan & Mikhail's Clinical Anesthesiology*, 6th ed. New York: McGraw-Hill Education, 2018, pp. 1213–21.

Faust RJ, Cucchiara RF. *Anesthesiology Review*, 3rd ed. Philadelphia: Churchill Livingston, 2001, pp. 91–2.

Gropper MA. *Miller's Anesthesia*, 9th ed. Philadelphia: Elsevier, 2020, pp. 2341–7.

Malignant Hyperthermia Association of the United States. Homepage. www.mhaus.org.

Wong KC. Physiology and pharmacology of hypothermia. *West J Med* 1983;**138**(2):227–32.

# Chapter 95

# Myasthenia Gravis

Ryan J. Gunselman and Jessica A. Lovich-Sapola

## Sample Case

A 45-year-old male is scheduled for a resection of a tumor in his colon. He has a history of myasthenia gravis (MG). He takes pyridostigmine 360 mg/day. What are your anesthetic concerns with this patient? How would you assess the adequacy of his therapy? How would you manage his pre-operative medications? Should he have pulmonary function tests (PFTs) pre-operatively? Would a spinal/epidural be a good choice for this case? Will the patient need or not need muscle relaxant during this case? Would succinylcholine be a good choice? If you used a nondepolarizing muscle relaxant (NDMR), would you reverse it at the end of the case?

## Clinical Issues

### Definition of Myasthenia Gravis

1. Autoimmune disease in which nicotinic acetylcholine receptors (nAChRs) are attacked by IgG antibodies
2. Functionally, MG will decrease the available number of nAChRs, causing muscle weakness and fatigue.
3. It is the most common disorder of neuromuscular transmission.

### Incidence

1. 0.25–2 per 100,000
2. Peak of onset
   a. Females: second and third decades of life
   b. Males: sixth to eighth decades of life

### Classification

1. Seropositive: antibodies to nAChRs found: 80% of MG patients
2. Seronegative: no antibodies to nAChRs: 20% of MG patients
   a. 70% of seronegative patients have antibodies against muscle-specific tyrosine kinase, an enzyme mediating the arrangement of nAChRs.

### Anatomical Origin

1. Thymus
   a. Hyperplasia found with production of antibodies to nAChRs

b. Thymectomy does not cure MG: the patient also has production of antibodies from lymphocytes that develop in other locations.

### Clinical Signs

1. Two major types of symptoms
   a. Ocular
      i. Weakness of the eyelids and extra-ocular muscles: ptosis and diplopia
   b. Generalized (bulbar)
      i. Weakness of the face, limbs, and respiratory muscles in addition to the ocular muscles
         (1) Weakness with chewing
         (2) Expressionless look
         (3) Head drop
         (4) Respiratory insufficiency
      ii. The most common complaint is fluctuating weakness in the muscles.
   c. Symptoms usually are worse later in the day or after exercise and are often transient early in the disease process.
   d. 50% of patients present with ocular symptoms.

### Differential Diagnosis

1. Generalized fatigue
2. Graves' disease
3. Amyotrophic lateral sclerosis (ALS)
4. Lambert–Eaton myasthenic syndrome
5. Congenital myasthenic syndrome
6. Penicillamine-induced myasthenia
7. Botulism
8. Statin medication side effects

### Diagnostic Testing

1. Primarily based on the patient's clinical symptoms
2. Tensilon test
   a. Can be used as a screening test at the bedside in patients with suspected MG
   b. A small dose of a fast-onset acetylcholinesterase inhibitor will increase the Ach in the neuromuscular

junction and should improve muscle contractile force in patients with MG.

    i.   Classically, a 10 mg dose of edrophonium is used.

3. Ice pack test

    a.   Used in patients when the muscarinic effects of edrophonium may be deleterious (i.e., patients with heart block, bradycardia, etc.)

    b.   In patients with ptosis, cooling the eyelid often improves neuromuscular transmission.

4. Serologic testing for AChR antibodies
5. Electrophysiologic testing

    a.   Repetitive nerve stimulation (RNS)

    b.   EMG studies

## Treatment

1. Usually starts with the use of anticholinesterase therapy
2. Steroids and other immunosuppressants
3. Plasmapheresis
4. IV immunoglobulin
5. Thymectomy

## Anesthetic Implications

1. Muscle relaxants

    a.   Patients with MG who are not receiving anticholinesterase treatment

        i.   Depolarizing muscle relaxants

           (1)   Due to an overall decrease in nAChRs, patients with MG are more resistant to succinylcholine.

           (2)   ED95 of succinylcholine in a patient with MG is 2.6 times that of a patient without MG.

        ii.   NDMRs

           (1)   MG patients are typically more sensitive to NDMRs.

           (2)   Avoid long-acting agents (i.e., pancuronium).

           (3)   Sensitivity, however, will vary.

    b.   Patients receiving treatment for MG with anticholinesterase therapy

        i.   Depolarizing muscle relaxants

           (1)   These MG patients tend to be more sensitive to succinylcholine.

           (2)   Therapy may increase the duration of action of succinylcholine.

        ii.   NDMR

           (1)   These MG patients tend to be more resistant to NDMRs.

           (2)   Therapy may decrease sensitivity to NDMRs compared to an MG patient who is not receiving anticholinesterase treatment.

           (3)   Remember that since these patients are prone to respiratory insufficiency, the smallest dose of NDMR that provides relaxation should be used despite the associated resistance.

    c.   Reversal of NDMRs

        i.   May result in a cholinergic crisis due to an excess of Ach in the MG patient treated with anticholinesterase therapy

        ii.   May be ineffective in patients who are receiving anticholinesterase treatment because much of the anticholinesterase inhibition already exists

        iii.   Many clinicians will avoid neuromuscular blockade completely, if possible.

        iv.   If muscle relaxation is necessary, it is now recommended that rocuronium with sugammadex reversal be utilized.

           (1)   If rocuronium/sugammadex is unavailable and relaxation is needed, clinicians can consider atracurium and cisatracurium for the MG patient because the patient's metabolism can obviate the need for reversal.

        v.   Train-of-four monitoring can be used to assess the degree of blockade.

2. Inhaled anesthetics

    a.   In normal patients, volatile agents provide some degree of muscle relaxation; in MG patients this may be more pronounced.

3. Regional anesthesia

    a.   Epidural/spinal anesthesia may be used, but at lower doses.

        i.   Caution must be used in patients with respiratory insufficiency. Avoid anesthetic spread to midthoracic or higher levels.

        ii.   Regional techniques, however, will allow the practitioner to avoid the use of muscle relaxants, which will decrease the likelihood of post-operative mechanical ventilation.

    b.   Local anesthetics potentiate the neuromuscular blockade; limited amounts should be used if possible.

    c.   If a brachial plexus block is being utilized, consider risk of phrenic nerve paresis.

4. Post-operative need for mechanical ventilation

    a.   All possible anesthetics can increase the likelihood of mechanical ventilation post-operatively.

    b.   The most important predictor is a proper pre-operative history and testing (see below).

# KO Treatment Plan

## Pre-operative

1. Detailed history and physical exam
2. MG-specific pre-operative assessment should include the following

   a. Detailed history of duration, severity, progression, and treatment of the disease (this may require consultation/discussion with the patient's neurologist).

   b. Depending on the presence of bulbar symptoms, PFT may be needed.

      i. Inability to clear secretions
      ii. Patients are at increased risk of aspiration due to the inability to protect their airway.
      iii. If a thymoma is present, flow-volume testing may also be indicated.

   c. In-depth discussion with the patient about the possible need for controlled ventilation post-operatively

      i. Predictors for post-operative mechanical ventilation may include, but are not limited to
         (1) MG for greater than 6 years
         (2) Chronic pulmonary disease
         (3) Daily pyridostigmine requirement 750 mg or higher with bulbar symptoms
         (4) Vital capacity less than 40 mL/kg
         (5) Pre-operative bulbar symptoms
         (6) History of myasthenic crisis
         (7) Intra-operative blood loss >1 L
         (8) Serum Ach receptor antibody >100 nmol/mL
         (9) Pronounced decremental response on low-frequency repetitive nerve stimulation

   d. MG medications

      i. Patients should continue pyridostigmine therapy pre-operatively, keeping in mind the effects on neuro-muscular blocking drugs.
      ii. Recent changes in pyridostigmine dose can help assess the status/severity of MG.
      iii. Patients on glucocorticoids should take their normal daily dose. Stress dose is not recommended unless the patient is on 5 mg or more of daily prednisone for more than 3 weeks within 6 months of surgery or if the patient appears Cushingoid.
      iv. If the severity of the patient's symptoms has increased during the pre-operative period, plasmapheresis may be needed before the patient undergoes surgery.

   e. Discuss the need for muscle relaxation with the surgeon.

   f. Often, the most sensitive indicator of the adequacy of the patient's therapy will be the patient's subjective history of his or her symptoms.

## Intra-operative

1. Anesthetic technique is largely dependent on the type of surgical procedure.

   a. If possible, avoidance of neuromuscular blockade is preferred (i.e., spinal/epidural, general anesthesia without muscle relaxation).

   b. For this particular case, a general anesthetic utilizing rocuronium and sugammadex could be used. In addition, barring any coagulopathy or other contraindication, one could choose to use a combined spinal–epidural (provided the surgical technique is not laparoscopic/robotic).

      i. With this technique, the neuraxial blockade can be extended if the procedure is prolonged.
      ii. Avoids the need for mechanical ventilation

2. If muscle relaxation is utilized, one should use rocuronium and sugammadex reversal; remember to use very small doses of NDMRs.

   a. Succinylcholine can be used safely in most cases.

3. Narcotics should be used judiciously to avoid respiratory depression in patients with underlying respiratory insufficiency.

   a. A remifentanil infusion may be a good option since it is short-acting.

   b. Utilize a multimodal approach to analgesia (consider utilizing ketamine, dexmedetomidine, etc.).

4. Patients should be extubated at the completion of the case only if stringent criteria are met.

   a. Patient should be awake, alert, and following commands.
   b. Sustained head lift greater than 5 seconds
   c. Vital capacity greater than 15 mL/kg
   d. Respiratory rate less than 20
   e. Oxygenation should be adequate: $PaO_2/FiO_2 = 200$ mm Hg or greater
   f. Maximum negative inspiratory pressure greater than 20 cm $H_2O$

5. If there is any concern that the patient may fail extubation, the patient should be kept on mechanical ventilation in the immediate post-operative period.

## Post-operative

1. If the patient is maintained on mechanical ventilation post-operatively, weaning should be gradual and performed in an intensive care setting.
2. The patient should continue anticholinesterase therapy through the peri-operative period.

3. Post-operative pain management with narcotics should be carefully monitored following extubation to minimize any respiratory depression.
4. Supplemental oxygen as needed
5. A neurologist should be contacted if there are any additional concerns.

## Bibliography

Abel M, Eisenkraft J. Anesthetic implications of myasthenia gravis. *Mount Sinai J Med* 2002;**69**:31–37.

Barash PG, Cullen BF, Stoelting RK, et al. *Clinical Anesthesia*, 8th ed. Philadelphia:

Lippincott Williams & Wilkins, 2017, pp. 1065–8.

Bird SJ. Clinical manifestations of myasthenia gravis. In Shefner, JM, ed., *UpToDate*. www.uptodate.com/contents/clinical-manifestations-of-myasthenia-gravis.

Gropper MA. *Miller's Anesthesia*, 9th ed. Philadelphia: Elsevier, 2020, pp. 1113–40.

Kveraga R, Pawlowski, J. Anesthesia for the patient with myasthenia gravis. In Jones BJ, Shefner JM, eds., *UpToDate*. www.uptodate.com/contents/anesthesia-for-the-patient-with-myasthenia-gravis.

# Obesity

Serle Levin, Jeffrey A. Brown, and Jessica A. Lovich-Sapola

## Sample Case

A 48-year-old, 223 kg female is scheduled for a gastric bypass surgery. Her medical history is significant for osteoarthritis, hypertension, type II diabetes mellitus, and gastroesophageal reflux disease. She uses a continuous positive airway pressure (CPAP) machine at home. What are your concerns? How would you approach this patient? Are there any tests you would like to have before surgery? How would you induce anesthesia in this patient? What would you use for maintenance of anesthesia?

## Clinical Issues

Currently more than two-thirds of adults in the United States are considered overweight or obese. Obesity is second only to smoking as the most common cause of preventable deaths. These patients represent a challenge from a medical standpoint as well as an increased risk of a difficult airway. The wise anesthesiologist will know how to manage these patients effectively.

## Definitions

1. Overweight: body mass index (BMI) $\geq$25 kg/m$^2$
2. Obesity: BMI $\geq$30 kg/m$^2$
3. Extreme ("morbid") obesity: BMI $\geq$40 kg/m$^2$
4. Super obesity: BMI $\geq$50 kg/m$^2$
5. Super-super obesity: $\geq$60 kg/m$^2$

## Physiologic Effects of Obesity

1. Cardiovascular
   a. Due to their often-sedentary nature, obese patients may not complain of angina or dyspnea with exertion.
   b. Careful history taking may prompt further testing such as EKG, echocardiography, or cardiac stress testing.
   c. Cardiac output is increased 0.1 L for every 10 kg of extra body fat.
      i. Increased stroke volume
   d. Cardiac hypertrophy
      i. Biventricular heart failure
   e. Chronic hypoxemia may lead to pulmonary hypertension and later cor pulmonale.

   f. Increased absolute blood volume
   g. Fatty infiltrate of the cardiac conduction system
      i. Increased risk of arrhythmias
   h. Acceleration of atherosclerosis
      i. Increased risk of coronary artery disease and hypertension

2. Respiratory
   a. Fat in the thorax and abdomen leads to decreased chest wall and lung compliance.
   b. Decreased vital capacity (VC) and total lung capacity
   c. Obese patients have decreased functional residual capacity (FRC) secondary to the decreased expiratory reserve volume, resulting in rapid hypoxemia during induction of general anesthesia.
      i. FRC may fall below closing capacity which may cause ventilation–perfusion mismatch.
   d. Increased oxygen consumption and carbon dioxide production at rest
   e. Patients should be kept in a semi-recumbent state as long as possible prior to induction.
   f. Ventilation with 100% oxygen is mandatory.
      i. At least four VC breaths should be sufficient for denitrogenation.
   g. Obese patients may suffer from obstructive sleep apnea (OSA).
      i. Overnight polysomnogram
         (1) Apnea–hypopnea index (AHI)
            (a) Mild: AHI 5–14
            (b) Moderate: AHI 15–30
            (c) Severe: AHI >30
      ii. The STOP-Bang questionnaire:
         (1) Easy, concise screening tool for OSA
         (2) Consists of eight questions

**S: Snoring:** Do you snore loud enough to be heard through closed doors?
**T: Tired:** Do you often feel tired or sleepy during the daytime?
**O: Observed:** Has anyone ever observed you stop breathing during sleep?
**P: Pressure:** Do you have or are you being treated for high blood pressure?

**B: BMI:** BMI more than 35 kg/m$^2$?
**A: Age:** Age over 50?
**N: Neck circumference:** >40 cm$^2$?
**G: Gender:** Male?

If patients answer "yes" to three or more of these questions, they are considered at high risk for OSA.

    h.   Patients who use CPAP at home should bring their machines with them to the hospital on the morning of surgery.

3.   Airway

    a.   Neck circumference alone is an independent predictor of a difficult airway.

        i.   Neck circumference greater than 60 cm represents a 35% chance of difficulty with intubation.

        ii.   These patients may often require an awake fiber-optic intubation or video laryngoscope.

    b.   Many authors now recommend "ramping" patients' shoulders and neck so that the external auditory meatus is in line with the sternal notch prior to induction to aid in visualization of the vocal cords, especially in the setting of direct laryngoscopy.

4.   Gastrointestinal

    a.   Gastric volume is increased, even in a fasted obese patient.

    b.   Delayed gastric emptying

        i.   Gastric emptying is faster with fat emulsions, but because of the larger gastric volume the residual volume is greater.

    c.   Increased gastric acidity

        i.   The pH of the gastric juice is reduced, predisposing the patient to aspiration pneumonitis should aspiration occur.

        ii.   Increased incidence of severe pneumonitis if aspiration occurs

        iii.   Patients should be pre-medicated with H2-blockers and metoclopramide prior to surgery.

    d.   A fasting obese surgical patient with no diabetes or gastroesophageal reflux is unlikely to have increased gastric volume or pH.

        i.   These patients are able to follow routine fasting guidelines.

    e.   Increased risk of nonalcoholic fatty liver disease and nonalcoholic steatohepatitis (NASH)

5.   Endocrine

    a.   Impaired glucose tolerance

        i.   Obese patients have a much higher incidence of type II diabetes mellitus than nonobese patients.

    b.   They may require exogenous insulin to oppose the catabolic response to surgery and maintain normal glucose levels during the peri-operative period.

    c.   25% of all morbidly obese patients have subclinical hypothyroidism.

    d.   Metabolic syndrome (syndrome X)

        i.   Insulin resistance syndrome

        ii.   Cluster of metabolic abnormalities associated with an increased risk of diabetes and cardiovascular events

6.   Musculoskeletal

    a.   Increased risk of osteoarthritis

7.   Renal

    a.   increased incidence of glomerular hyperfiltration

8.   Pharmacology: IV drug dosing in obesity

    a.   Dosed at lean body weight (LBW)

        i.   Propofol (induction dose)

        ii.   Rocuronium, vecuronium, atracurium, cisatracurium

        iii.   fentanyl, sufentanil, remifentanil

    b.   Dosed at total body weight (TBW)

        i.   Propofol (infusion)

        ii.   Succinylcholine

        iii.   Dexmedetomidine

        iv.   Neostigmine

        v.   Sugammadex

9.   Mechanics

    a.   Difficult IV access

    b.   Longer needles for IVs and regional techniques

    c.   Noninvasive blood pressure can be inaccurate because the cuff does not match the arm's shape.

        i.   Consider placement of an arterial line.

# TKO

1.   Have a high index of suspicion for OSA.
2.   An awake fiber-optic or video laryngoscopic intubation should be considered in many obese patients.
3.   Neck circumference is an independent indicator of a difficult airway.
4.   Pulmonary embolism is the major cause of 30-day mortality in bariatric surgery patients.

    a.   Measures to prevent deep vein thrombosis must be taken.

5.   Drugs with a short duration of action should be used during maintenance of anesthesia.

a. If long-acting narcotics must be used, then the obese patient may require hospitalization overnight with continuous oxygen saturation monitoring.

# KO Treatment Plan

## Bariatric Surgery

1. Bariatric surgery is the most effective treatment for morbid obesity.
2. BMI >40 kg/m$^2$ or <35 kg/m$^2$ if they have obesity-related comorbidities

## Pre-operative

1. Complete history and physical
2. Determine the severity of her OSA.

   a. This will help you decide if she should stay overnight with continuous pulse oximetry monitoring and help determine your anesthetic plan.

3. A pre-operative EKG should be obtained if deemed necessary after a careful history.

   a. Chest pain
   b. Shortness of breath
   c. Orthopnea
   d. Poor functional capacity

4. Chest X-ray: heart size and pulmonary vasculature (evidence of pulmonary hypertension)
5. Pre-operative blood glucose should be checked and treated.
6. Evaluate her airway.
7. The patient in the above sample case is at an increased risk for aspiration pneumonia, secondary to her diabetes and gastroesophageal reflux disease; she should be pre-medicated with intravenous (IV) metoclopramide and ranitidine the morning of surgery.
8. Avoid pre-medication with any respiratory depressant medications.

## Intra-operative

1. I would intubate the patient via an awake fiber-optic intubation.

   a. Risk for rapid desaturation

      i. Pre-medication

         (1) Glycopyrrolate 0.2 mg IV
         (2) Conservative doses of sedation while monitored in the operating room

            (a) 1–2 mg IV midazolam
            (b) 50 μg of IV fentanyl

         (3) Adequate topicalization either via nebulized lidocaine 2–4% for 10 minutes or having the patient gargle with 5 mL of 2% viscous lidocaine

         (4) The patient should have the standard ASA monitors applied prior to any sedation or topicalization.
         (5) Supplemental oxygen should be given during the intubation.

**TKO:** The patient may not be cooperative or may refuse an awake fiber-optic intubation. In this situation, a rapid-sequence induction with intubation with a video laryngoscope and a solid understanding of the difficult airway algorithm may be required. Make sure the patient is properly positioned prior to the induction of anesthesia.

2. Once the patient is successfully intubated, I would induce with propofol 1–2 mg/kg because of its rapid onset and short duration of action.
3. If paralysis is required (it is not always needed) full reversal and demonstration of return of muscular strength (i.e., with 5 second head lift) is mandatory prior to extubation.

   a. Consider using sugammadex

4. Pharmacological considerations

   a. I would use a remifentanil infusion and sevoflurane/desflurane for maintenance anesthesia because their effects are short-lived.

      i. There is very little, if any, residual respiratory depression from these agents.
      ii. Metabolism of remifentanil is via nonspecific plasma esterase.

   b. Desflurane is a very insoluble agent, which is ideal for a patient with a large amount of adipose tissue.

      i. A downside is the associated risk of bronchospasm

5. Enhanced recovery after surgery (ERAS) protocols

   a. Pre-operative carbohydrate drink
   b. Extensive antiemetic therapy
   c. Multimodal and regional pain management techniques

      i. Limited opioids, adjuvant medications: ketamine, lidocaine, magnesium
      ii. TAP blocks

   d. Goal-directed fluid therapy
   e. Glucose management

6. Hemodynamic management

   a. Blood pressure management with alterations in table position

7. Ventilation management

   a. Intra-operative use of PEEP
   b. Anticipate elevated airway pressures, atelectasis
   c. Recruitment maneuvers to ensure lung expansion prior to extubation

## Post-operative

1. Respiratory failure is the biggest post-operative concern. Consider post-operative CPAP, BiPAP, or noninvasive positive-pressure ventilation (NIPPV).

2. Extubation criteria are the same as for nonobese patients.

   a. I would be much stricter in following the established criteria:

      i. VC greater than 15 cc/kg
      ii. Respiratory rate 10–20 breaths/min
      iii. Reasonable arterial blood gas results
      iv. Negative inspiratory force greater than 20 cm $H_2O$

3. I would extubate the patient and apply her CPAP.

4. Elevated head of the bed, incentive spirometry, continuous pulse oximetry post-operatively

5. She should be monitored overnight with continuous oxygen saturation monitoring, secondary to her OSA.

6. Other common post-operative concerns include:

   a. Wound infection
   b. Deep venous thrombosis
   c. Pulmonary embolism
   d. Anastomotic/gastric leak

      i. Bleeding

   e. Small bowel obstruction
   f. Sepsis

## Bibliography

Barash PG, Cullen BF, Stoelting RK, et al. *Clinical Anesthesia*, 8th ed. Philadelphia: Lippincott Williams & Wilkins, 2017, pp. 1277–93.

Butterworth JF, Mackey DC, Wasnick JD. *Morgan & Mikhail's Clinical Anesthesiology*, 6th ed. New York: McGraw-Hill Education, 2018, pp. 767–9.

Chung F, Yegneswaran B, Liao P, et al. STOP Questionnaire: a tool to screen for obstructive sleep apnea. *Anesthesiology* 2008;**108**:812–21.

Gounden R, Blackman M. Clinical pharmacology: dosing in the obese patient. *Clin Pharmacol* 2006;**24**(7):399–400.

Groper MA. *Miller's Anesthesia*, 9th ed. Philadelphia: Elsevier, 2020, pp. 1911–28.

Stenberg E, Dos Reis Falcão LF, O'Kane M, et al. Guidelines for perioperative care in bariatric surgery: Enhanced Recovery After Surgery (ERAS) Society Recommendations: a 2021 update. *World J Surg* 2022. doi:10.1007/s00268-021-06394-9.

Vikram M, Hashmi J, Singh R, et al. Comparative evaluation of gastric pH and volume in morbidly obese and lean patients undergoing elective surgery and effects of aspiration prophylaxis. *J Clin Anesth* 2015;**27**(5):396–400.

# Sickle Cell Anemia

Ali G. Ali, Sheila Chiu, and Jessica A. Lovich-Sapola

## Sample Case

An 11-year-old male with sickle cell disease is scheduled for a repair of his ankle fracture. What are the anesthetic implications of sickle cell disease? How would you anesthetize this child? Would you use regional or general anesthesia? Can the surgeon use a tourniquet?

## Clinical Issues

### Definition

1.  Sickle cell disease is a hereditary hemoglobin disorder that stems from structural deformation and irreversible sickling of red blood cells due to polymerization of hemoglobin.
2.  The most common forms of the disease include sickle cell anemia (SS disease), sickle hemoglobin C disease (SC disease), sickle β-thalassemia, and sickle cell trait (SA disease).
3.  The pathologic hallmark of this disease is a vaso-occlusive crisis that arises when erythrocytes with irreversibly sickled hemoglobin aggregate in the blood vessels, impeding blood flow and oxygen to tissues, which can lead to venous thrombosis, organ infarction, and severe pain.

### Pathophysiology of Sickle Cell Anemia

1.  Normal adult hemoglobin (Hb A) is a protein with two α-globin and two β-globin chains.
2.  Sickle hemoglobin (Hb S) has two normal α-globin chains and two sickle β-globin chains.
3.  Genetic mutation in the β-globin gene where the neutral amino acid (valine) substitutes for an acidic amino acid (glutamic acid) at the sixth position
4.  When hemoglobin S deoxygenates, a gel polymer of hemoglobin forms, resulting in sickling of the red blood cell molecule.
5.  Physiologic conditions that affect the rate of deoxygenation determine the extent of gel formation.
6.  Low arterial oxygen tension, acidosis, and vascular stasis are powerful stimuli of sickle cell formation.

    a.  Sickling occurs at a $PaO_2$ <50 mm Hg and is most pronounced at a $PaO_2$ <20 mm Hg.

7.  Polymerized sickle hemoglobin is relatively insoluble, rigid, and unstable.

8.  Sickling and adhesion of red cells in the blood vessels cause a decrease in oxygen delivery to the tissues and a subsequent ischemia and destruction of end organs.
9.  Splenic sequestration (acute and painful enlargement of the spleen) can occur in children less than 6 years old.
10. Hemolysis can occur, resulting in a hemolytic crisis.
11. Bone marrow exhaustion can occur, leading to an aplastic crisis and severe anemia.

### Sickle Cell Anemia (Hb SS)

1.  Incidence is 0.3% among African Americans
2.  Homozygous genotype
3.  70–98% of hemoglobin is S and the remainder is hemoglobin F (fetal).

### Sickle Cell Trait (Hb AS)

1.  Present in 8–10% of African Americans
2.  Heterozygous genotype showing via incomplete dominance
3.  One β-globin gene codes for sickle hemoglobin and the other for hemoglobin A.
4.  10–40% hemoglobin S
5.  Hemoglobin A (α2β2) and fetal hemoglobin F (α2γ2) can prevent polymer formation and are responsible for the minimal clinical symptoms in sickle cell trait.
6.  Asymptomatic and not clinically significant unless the $PaO_2$ is <20 mm Hg when Hb AS begins to sickle

### Sickle Hemoglobin C Disease

1.  One β-globin gene codes for sickle globin and the other for hemoglobin C (where lysine replaces glutamic acid in the sixth position of the β-globin chain)
2.  Hemoglobin C can likewise form polymers with Hb S, resulting in SC disease.

### Sickle β-Thalassemia

1.  One β-globin gene has a sickle cell mutation and the other has a thalassemia mutation.
2.  The synthesis of the β-globin chain can be completely or partially suppressed.

## Triggers of Sickle Cell Crisis

1. Low oxygen saturation/desaturated hemoglobin S
2. Acidosis
3. Hypothermia/hyperthermia
4. Infection
5. Emotional stress
6. Physical exertion
7. Alcohol consumption
8. Dehydration
9. Surgery

## Clinical Signs and Presentation (Percentage Equals the Incidence per Lifetime)

1. Neurological
   a. Pain crisis: >70% of patients
   b. Stroke: 20% of patients
   c. Proliferative retinopathy, peripheral neuropathy, and chronic pain syndrome are rare.
   d. Major cause of morbidity and mortality
2. Cardiovascular
   a. Myocardial infarction
3. Pulmonary
   a. Acute chest syndrome (ACS)
      i. Occurs in 40% of patients
      ii. Pneumonia-like complication
      iii. Clinically presents as chest pain, fever >38.5 °C, tachypnea, wheezing, or cough.
      iv. ACS diagnosis is based on a new pulmonary infiltrate involving at least one lung segment.
   b. Airway hyper-reactivity: 35% of children
   c. Restrictive lung disease: 10–15% of patients
   d. Major cause of morbidity and mortality
4. Genitourinary
   a. Chronic renal insufficiency: 5–20%
   b. Urinary tract infection
   c. Priapism: 10–40% men
   d. Obstetric complications
      i. Higher number of vaso-occlusive events
5. Gastrointestinal
   a. Cholelithiasis: 70% adults
   b. Liver disease: 10%
      i. Viral hepatitis from transfusion (up to 10% of adults)
      ii. Liver failure (<2% patients)
6. Hematological
   a. Hemolytic anemia
   b. Acute aplastic anemia
   c. Splenic enlargement/fibrosis
7. Orthopedic
   a. Osteonecrosis: 50% adults
   b. Osteomyelitis
   c. Dactylitis
8. Vascular
   a. Ischemic leg ulcer: 20%
9. Immunologic
   a. Increased susceptibility to infection
   b. Increased incidence of transfusion erythrocyte alloimmunization and therefore hemolytic transfusion reaction

## Peri-operative Complications

1. Sickle cell patients have a high incidence of peri-operative problems, including pain crisis, ACS, transfusion reactions, and other nonspecific complications such as fever, infection, bleeding, thrombosis, embolism, and even death.
2. Peri-operative management should include stratifying risks for complications.
   a. High surgical risk, longer duration of general anesthesia, increased age, recent/active crisis, frequent hospitalizations, abnormal chest X-ray, pregnancy, pre-existing infections, and organ failures increase risk.
   b. Since sickling cannot be reversed, the best type of management is prevention of sickling.

# KO Treatment Plan

## Pre-operative

1. Obtain a detailed history and physical examination
   a. Sickle cell trait or anemia or other variant hemoglobinopathy
   b. Previous transfusions and related complications
   c. Recent or active sickle cell crisis and/or hospitalization
      i. Patients in current active sickling crisis should NOT undergo surgery except for emergencies, and only after an exchange transfusion.
   d. Presence of any chronic organ dysfunction
   e. Surgical history (e.g., splenectomy) that predisposes the patient to infections by encapsulated organisms
2. Labs and other tests
   a. Hematocrit (Hct) and the percentage of hemoglobin S (via electrophoresis) to determine whether simple or exchange transfusions (apheresis used to remove a person's red blood cells or platelets and replace them

with a transfused blood product) are needed prior to the procedure.

   i. A patient with sickle cell disease should have a hemoglobin S ratio less than 40% prior to any elective surgery.

b. Blood urea nitrogen (BUN), creatinine for baseline kidney function

c. Urinalysis to detect hematuria, proteinuria, and the presence of an infection

d. Pulse oximetry as a noninvasive measure of oxygenation

e. Chest X-ray

   i. For patients with recent upper or lower respiratory tract symptoms or asthma exacerbation

   ii. To detect the presence of pulmonary fibrosis, calcified spleen, and calcified marrow

f. Type and screen for antibodies

   i. Leukocyte-reduced/filtered, sickle hemoglobin (Hb S) negative and phenotype/antigen-matched red cells are preferred to minimize alloimmunization and transfusion reactions.

g. Pre-operative transfusion guidelines

   i. Intravenous (IV) fluids with no transfusion (even with a Hct <30%)

      (1) Local anesthetic

      (2) Minor and brief procedure

      (3) General anesthetic less than 60 minutes

      (4) No pulmonary compromise

   ii. Simple transfusion

      (1) Goal is to correct anemia; associated with improved mortality

      (2) Hct <30% with a goal of 30–35%

      (3) Higher-risk patients

      (4) Nontonsillectomy, nonlaparotomy, nonthoracotomy procedures

   iii. Repeated simple transfusion

      (1) Elective procedures of the airway, open thoracotomy or general anesthetic >90 minutes

      (2) Goal for Hb S is less than 30%.

   iv. Exchange transfusion

      (1) Goal is to decrease Hb S concentration.

      (2) Any Hct

         (a) Urgent procedures of the airway, open laparotomy, thoracotomy, or anesthesia >90 minutes

         (b) Elective noncardiac procedures with a goal of reducing the concentration of

Hb S to less than 30%. Hb S levels <5% are desirable for cardiac surgery involving cardiopulmonary bypass.

      (c) Patients with a history of severe ACS and/or chronic pulmonary disease

h. Other tests such as pulmonary and liver function tests, arterial blood gas, EKG, neurological imaging if indicated for a specific organ disease process

3. Avoid pre-operative sedative medications that may affect ventilation if patients have a pulmonary component to their sickle cell disease.

a. Remember that these patients may have an increased tolerance for sedatives due to their prior treatment of pain crisis.

## Intra-operative

1. Maintain normothermia with convection thermoregulation devices and fluid warmers.

a. Hypothermia depresses sickling but promotes peripheral vasoconstriction and vascular stasis.

b. Hyperthermia can promote hemoglobin S gel formation and sickling.

c. Your goal is to maintain normothermia.

2. Circulatory stasis and acute hypovolemia can be avoided with adequate hydration and anticipation of intra-operative volume loss.

a. IV fluids up to 1–1.5 × maintenance fluids especially if the kidneys are unable to concentrate urine

b. Must use fluids with caution if cardiac function is compromised to avoid pulmonary edema.

3. Correct acidemia and hypoxia.

4. Avoid areas of pressure stasis that promote sickling.

5. While no single anesthetic technique is considered more favorable in reducing sickle cell-associated complications, I would choose:

a. Preoxygenation to minimize hypoxia

b. Induction with fentanyl for pre-emptive analgesia and propofol for rapid onset of sedation (in the presence of IV access)

c. Inhalation induction with sevoflurane if no pre-operative IV access

   i. Inhaled, halogenated anesthetics accelerate precipitation of hemoglobin S *in vitro* but no known clinical significance has been shown.

d. Maintenance with isoflurane

   i. Potential neuroprotective and cardioprotective effects of isoflurane, especially in the event of ischemic episodes during anesthesia

e. Muscle relaxation

i. There is no contraindication for using a depolarizing or nondepolarizing muscle relaxant in sickle cell anemia patients.
ii. One study by Dulvadestin et al. showed that the onset time for atracurium is delayed in sickle cell anemia patients, but not the duration of the neuromuscular blockade.

f. Choice of anesthetic technique can be general or regional anesthesia as long as perfusion and oxygenation are maintained during the surgery.

i. General anesthesia may be preferred for a young and anxious child; however, regional analgesia (e.g., epidural anesthesia) has been used safely in the pediatric population.
ii. Regional anesthesia may lead to compensatory vasoconstriction and decreased oxygen delivery to nonblocked areas, resulting in red cells in nonblocked areas more vulnerable to sickling. However, it is not a contraindication.

6. The use of an extremity tourniquet is controversial. It is not contraindicated, but avoid use if possible.

a. There is no definitive study to prove the safety or danger of the use of a tourniquet in a sickle cell patient; however, the incidence of peri-operative complications is increased with their use.
b. The anesthesiologist and surgeon must weigh the benefits of tourniquet use and the risks associated with induced vaso-occlusive and vascular stasis effects of the tourniquet.

## Post-operative

1. Early mobilization to prevent venous stasis
2. Pulmonary toilet such as frequent suctioning and incentive spirometry to prevent hypoxia and atelectasis
3. Early effective analgesia using a variety of techniques such as opioids, nonnarcotic analgesics, and epidural analgesia
4. Supplemental oxygen in the presence of hypoxia

a. Avoid the routine use of supplemental oxygen, which can suppress erythropoiesis.

5. Prompt recognition and treatments for possible complications such as pain crisis or ACS

## Bibliography

Dulvadestin P, Gilton A, Hernigou P, Marty J. The onset time of atracurium is prolonged in patients with sickle cell disease. *Anesth Analg* 2008;**107**(1):113–16.

Firth PG, Head CA. Sickle cell disease and anesthesia. *Anesthesiology* 2004;**101**:766–85.

Gropper MA. *Miller's Anesthesia*, 9th ed. Philadelphia: Elsevier, 2020, pp. 1051–2.

Hines RL, Marschall K. *Stoelting's Anesthesia and Coexisting Disease*, 7th ed. Philadelphia: Elsevier, 2018, pp. 483–4.

Humes HD. *Kelley's Textbook of Internal Medicine*, 4th ed. Philadelphia:

Lippincott Williams & Wilkins, 2000, pp. 1788–94.

New England Pediatric Sickle Cell Consortium. Blood transfusion for pediatric patients with sickle cell disease. 2003.

**Chapter**

**98**

# Stress Dose Steroids

Michael Dale Bassett and Jessica A. Lovich-Sapola

## Sample Case

A 65-year-old male is admitted to the emergency department and found to have an acute appendicitis. His past medical history is significant for rheumatoid arthritis. The patient has taken prednisone 10 mg/day for several years. After an uneventful appendectomy, the patient becomes hypotensive with a blood pressure of 76/40 mm Hg in the post-anesthesia care unit. The patient received a 2 L normal saline IV bolus without improvement. Would you recommend that the patient receive stress dose steroids in this situation?

## Clinical Issue

### Normal Physiology

1. Glucocorticoids (including cortisol) are produced in the zona fasciculata of the cortex of the adrenal gland.
2. Glucocorticoid production is regulated by adrenocorticotropic hormone (ACTH) secreted from the anterior pituitary under the influence of corticotropin-releasing hormone (CRH) from the hypothalamus.
3. ACTH and CRH are controlled by negative feedback through cortisol.
4. Normal daily production of cortisol when not stressed is 8–10 mg/day.
5. Acute physical or psychological stress activate the hypothalamic–pituitary–adrenal (HPA) axis, resulting in increased levels of CRH, ACTH, and ultimately cortisol.

### Actions of Cortisol

1. Stimulation of gluconeogenesis

    a. Increases protein catabolism
    b. Increases lipolysis
    c. Decreases insulin sensitivity of adipose tissue

2. Anti-inflammatory effects

    a. Induces the synthesis of lipocortin (an inhibitor of phospholipase $A_2$)
    b. Inhibits production of interleukin-2 (IL-2)
    c. Inhibits release of histamine and serotonin from mast cells and platelets

3. Calcium homeostasis

    a. Stimulates osteoclasts; inhibits osteoblasts
    b. Reduces intestinal calcium absorption
    c. Stimulates parathyroid hormone release
    d. Increases urinary calcium excretion
    e. Decreases reabsorption of phosphate

4. Suppresses immune response by inhibition of IL-2 and T-lymphocytes
5. Maintains vascular response to catecholamines by upregulating $\alpha_1$ adrenergic receptors on arterioles
6. Increases cardiac output
7. Causes loss of collagen and connective tissue

### Effect of Surgery

1. Surgery is a potent activator of the HPA axis.
2. The degree of activation depends on the type of surgery, anesthetic agents used during the procedure, age of the patient, medication usage, and concurrent illness.
3. Deep general or regional anesthesia delays the usual intra-operative glucocorticoid surge to the post-operative period.
4. Cortisol release enhances survival by improving: cardiac output, the body's responsiveness to catecholamines, work capacity of skeletal muscles, and the ability to mobilize energy sources.
5. Plasma ACTH and cortisol

    a. Increase at time of incision
    b. Increase during surgery
    c. Greatest increase occurs during reversal of anesthesia, extubation, and in the immediate post-operative period, primarily due to pain

6. Cortisol levels are measured at:

    a. 50 mg/day during minor procedures
    b. 75–100 mg/day during major procedures
    c. Can reach 200–500 mg/day with severe stress
    d. Output rarely exceeds 150 mg/day even in response to major surgery.
    e. Rare to be greater than 200 mg/day 24 hours after surgery

### Chronic Glucocorticoid Therapy

1. Suppresses the HPA axis
2. Impairs wound healing

3.  Increases friability of skin, superficial blood vessels, and other tissues
4.  Increases risk of fractures, infections, gastrointestinal hemorrhage, and ulcers

## Acute Adrenal Insufficiency Crisis

1.  Chronic glucocorticoid therapy, including inhaled and topical steroids as well as intra-articular and spinal glucocorticoid injections, exert negative feedback on the HPA axis by suppressing CRH and ACTH release and can cause a secondary adrenal insufficiency.
2.  The adrenal gland atrophies and can no longer secrete cortisol.
3.  These patients cannot increase their cortisol levels during a stressful event and can suffer from an acute adrenal insufficiency crisis.
4.  Acute adrenal insufficiency rarely occurs, but it can be life threatening.
5.  Adrenal insufficiency crisis
    a.  Fatigue
    b.  Nausea and vomiting
    c.  Fever
    d.  Abdominal pain
    e.  Anorexia
    f.  Hyponatremia
    g.  Hypoglycemia
    h.  Confusion
    i.  Hypotension
    j.  Shock
    k.  Coma
6.  Peri-operative adrenal crisis for the anesthesiologist requires a high index of suspicion as most of the signs and symptoms are nonspecific and can be absent in the anesthetized patient.
7.  After cessation of steroid therapy, recovery of the HPA axis is variable and depends upon a variety of factors, but it can take 12 months or longer.

## Criteria Regarding HPA Axis Suppression

1.  Low risk: The following patients can be considered to be at low risk for a suppressed HPA axis, and therefore do not require stress dose steroids in the peri-operative period.
    a.  Patients receiving morning doses of prednisone (or its glucocorticoid equivalent) 5 mg/day or less for any length of time
    b.  Patients treated with alternate-day glucocorticoid therapy at physiologic doses (less than 10 mg prednisone every other day)
    c.  Patients on any dose of glucocorticoid for less than 3 weeks
2.  Intermediate risk: these patients have considerable variability in their HPA axis suppression. They should either undergo pre-operative evaluation of their HPA axis

if time permits or be considered high risk and treated empirically with stress dose steroids.
    a.  Any patient taking 5–20 mg/day of prednisone (or its glucocorticoid equivalent) for more than 3 weeks within the previous year
    b.  Patients taking less than the equivalent of 5 mg of prednisone daily in the evening
3.  High risk: the following patients should be considered to be at increased risk for suppression of their HPA axis and therefore require stress dose steroids in the peri-operative period.
    a.  Any patient who has received more than 20 mg/day of prednisone (or its glucocorticoid equivalent) for more than 3 weeks within the previous year
    b.  Any patient who has clinical Cushing's syndrome

## HPA Axis Evaluation

1.  In patients whose HPA axis status is uncertain, one can test for responsiveness of the adrenal gland to stress; however, investigation for adrenal suppression is rarely done pre-operatively. In addition, emergent cases will not permit the time for the testing to occur.
2.  Measurement of morning serum cortisol levels
    a.  If the morning cortisol is <5 µg/dL, the patient likely has a suppressed HPA axis.
    b.  If the morning cortisol is >10 µg/dL, the patient likely does not have significant suppression of their HPA axis.
    c.  If the morning cortisol is 5–10 µg/dL, further evaluation is necessary.
3.  Measurement of cortisol levels during insulin-induced hypoglycemia
    a.  Most sensitive test of response to stress
    b.  Not commonly used due to it being difficult to perform and risky; it is likely more dangerous to perform than just administering glucocorticoids.
4.  1 µg ACTH (cosyntropin) stimulation test
    a.  Cosyntropin 1 µg is given intravenously.
    b.  Plasma cortisol is measured before and 30 minutes after cosyntropin administration.
    c.  Adrenal function is considered normal if plasma cortisol level is at least 18 µg/dL at 30 minutes.
    d.  ACTH levels obtained with the 1 µg test are equivalent to ACTH levels after stressful situations, such as surgery or hypoglycemia.
5.  250 µg cosyntropin stimulation test
    a.  Cosyntropin 250 µg is given intravenously or intramuscularly.
    b.  The plasma cortisol is measured before and 30–60 minutes following the cosyntropin administration.

c. Adrenal function is considered normal if the plasma cortisol level is at least 18 µg/dL before or 30–60 minutes following administration. All patients should see an increase in plasma cortisol of at least 9 µg/dL above baseline unless they have adrenal insufficiency.

d. Limitations to this test are that the dose of cosyntropin is much higher than that often observed in the body in response to most stressful situations. This explains why patients with a partially suppressed HPA axis fail to respond to the 1 µg test but respond normally to the 250 µg cosyntropin test.

6. In each of these stimulation tests, cross reaction between exogenous glucocorticoids and the test can occur.

a. Can lead to falsely elevated cortisol values

b. Glucocorticoids should be stopped 24 hours prior to testing.

c. Dexamethasone does not affect these tests.

## KO Treatment Plan

### Peri-operative Management

1. Patients who are considered to not have functional suppression of their HPA axis by the criteria outlined above should continue on their usual dose of glucocorticoids peri-operatively if still taking them. If they are no longer on glucocorticoids, they do not require any additional steroid prior to surgery.

2. Patients who are considered to have HPA axis suppression by the defined criteria or through testing should be treated based on the surgery being performed.

3. The literature shows variation in dosing guidelines; however, the supplementation guidelines all maintain the need for additional glucocorticoid coverage tailored to the patient's need and anticipated surgical stress.

a. Minor procedures or surgery under local anesthesia: take the usual morning steroid dose. No extra supplementation is necessary.

    i. EGD/colonoscopy
    ii. Dental work

    iii. Inguinal hernia repair
    iv. Laparoscopic appendectomy

b. Moderate surgical stress: take the usual morning steroid dose. Give hydrocortisone 50 mg IV on induction and 25 mg IV every 8 hours for 24 hours. Resume the usual dose thereafter.

    i. Exploratory laparotomy
    ii. Total joint replacement
    iii. Lower limb revascularization

c. Major surgical stress: take the usual morning steroid dose. Give 100 mg hydrocortisone IV before induction of anesthesia and 50 mg IV every 8 hours for 24 hours. Taper the dose over 2–3 days to maintenance level. It may be advisable to consult an endocrinologist post-operatively to assist in management.

    i. Cardiothoracic surgery
    ii. Whipple procedure
    iii. Liver resection
    iv. Severe trauma

4. For patients that fall into the intermediate category regarding their HPA axis, they can be treated with glucocorticoids or, if time permits, can be tested for responsiveness of the adrenal gland to stress.

5. It is unusual to have laboratory data regarding HPA axis suppression pre-operatively and the risk of providing glucocorticoid supplementation is low. Rather than delay surgery or test most patients, we assume that any patient that falls into the intermediate or high-risk category has suppression of their HPA axis and will require peri-operative stress dose steroids.

6. Etomidate should be avoided in patients with suspected suppression of their HPA axis.

7. An anti-nausea prophylactic dose of dexamethasone (8 mg IV) is roughly equivalent to 200 mg hydrocortisone and alone should suffice to prevent an acute adrenal insufficiency crisis in all but those undergoing a major surgical stress.

## Bibliography

Brown CJ, Buie WD. Perioperative stress dose steroids: do they make a difference? *J Am Coll Surg* 2001;**193** (6):678–86.

Draper R. Precautions for patients on steroids undergoing surgery. Egton Medical Information Systems (EMIS). 2011.

Hamrahian AH, Roman S, Milan S, et al. The management of the surgical patient taking glucocorticoids. In Nieman LK, Carty SE, eds., *UpToDate*. www.uptodate.com/con

tents/the-management-of-the-surgical-patient-taking-glucocorticoids

Jabbour SA. Steroids and the surgical patient. *Med Clin North Am* 2001;**85** (5):1311–17.

Jung C, Inder W. Management of adrenal insufficiency during the stress of medical illness and surgery. *Med J Aust* 2008;**188** (7):409–13.

Leach CI, Kaye AD. Preanesthetic assessment of the patient with Addison's Disease. *Anesthesiol News* 2014;**40**(6):16–19.

Liu MM, Reidy A, Saatee S, Collard CD. Perioperative steroid management, approaches based on current evidence. *Anesthesiology.* 2017:**127**(1):166–72.

Miller, RD. *Miller's Anesthesia*, 9th ed. ED. et al. Saunders: Philadelphia, 2019. pp 1010–1013

Reed, AP. *Clinical Cases in Anesthesia*, 4th ed. Elsevier: Philadelphia, 2014, pp. 137–140.

Wing E, Schiffman F. *Cecil Essentials of Medicine* 10th ed. Philadelphia: Saunders, 2021, pp. 645–656.

# Transfusion Therapy

## 99

Vera V. Borzova and Jessica A. Lovich-Sapola

## Sample Case

A 36-year-old G3P2 with pregnancy-induced hypertension was admitted to the hospital at 34 weeks' gestation with a chief complaint of severe abdominal pain and tenderness. On admission she was pale, with cold and clammy skin, heart rate of 140 and blood pressure of 87/46 mm Hg. Diagnosis of suspected placental abruption was confirmed by the ultrasound. The obstetrician on call decided to proceed with an emergent cesarean delivery. What are your anesthetic concerns? What laboratory tests would you like to obtain? What additional preparations would be required? What complications are you anticipating and how do you plan to address them?

## Clinical Issues

Transfusion of blood products remains one of the most common procedures. Recently, patient-centered blood management has emerged and aims at administering the right product for the right patient at the right dose and time. This approach effectively makes the universal transfusion threshold obsolete and instead offers evidence-based guidelines tailored to specific patient populations. Clinical trials over the last decade established safety and noninferiority of the restrictive transfusion practices (Hgb threshold <7–8 g/dL).

## Blood Products

1. Whole blood: renewed interest in lower-titer group O whole blood that contains functional platelets in an actively bleeding patient in a pre-hospital setting.
2. Red blood cells (RBC)
3. Platelets: apheresis from the single donor (93% of transfusions) or pooled random donor platelets.
4. Fresh frozen plasma (FFP): contains all of the coagulation factors, including labile factors V and VIII.
5. Cryoprecipitate: contains concentrated amounts of fibrinogen, Factor VIII: C, Factor VIII: von Willebrand factor (vWF), Factor XIII, and fibronectin.
6. Factor concentrates including prothrombin complex concentrate (PCC) for urgent reversal of the warfarin.
7. Synthetic factors: Factor VIIa and erythropoietin

## Indications for Transfusions of RBC

1. The goal is to increase oxygen-carrying capacity in the presence of impaired tissue oxygenation.

2. RBC are usually administered to keep hemoglobin above 6 g/dL, with the majority of the societies recommending hemoglobin >7 g/dL in asymptomatic ICU patients, above 8 g/dL in the presence of acute coronary syndrome, and 7–9 g/dL in patients with acute neurologic injuries as well as actively bleeding patients.
3. Do not use blood products to replace intravascular fluid volume. Anemia produces physiologic compensation mechanisms that maintain tissue oxygenation as long as intravascular volume is maintained (isovolemic anemia).
4. One unit of packed RBC increases Hb by 1 g/dL and hematocrit by 2–3% in a euvolemic patient.
5. Use ABO-compatible RBC.

## Indications for Transfusion of Platelets

1. Indicated for treatment of thrombocytopenia and/or platelet dysfunction.
   a. Nonbleeding noncoagulopathic patients transfused for platelets <10,000/μL
   b. Central line placement with threshold of 20,000/μL
   c. Spinal and epidural anesthesia with a threshold of 20,000–50,000/μL
   d. Flexible bronchoscopy or gastrointestinal (GI) endoscopy with threshold of 20,000–50,000/μL
   e. Bone marrow biopsy with threshold of 10,000–20,000/μL
   f. Major elective nonneuraxial surgery and liver biopsy with threshold of 50,000/μL
   g. Ophthalmologic or central nervous system surgery with a threshold of 100,000/μL
   h. Patients with massive transfusion with a threshold of 75,000–100,000/μL

2. One apheresis unit (single donor) increases the platelet count by 30,000–60,000/μL. It is advisable to check for expected response within 1 hour of transfusion to detect platelet refractoriness in the absence of ongoing consumption.
3. Platelets suspended in plasma should be ABO-compatible.

## Indications for Transfusion of FFP

1. Indications
   a. Bleeding due to deficiency of multiple coagulation factors

b. Urgent reversal of warfarin when 4-factor PCC is unavailable and time does not permit vitamin K administration

c. Massive transfusion with coagulopathic bleeding

d. Single coagulant factor deficiency when concentrate is unavailable

e. Heparin resistance secondary to antithrombin (AT) deficiency when AT concentrate is unavailable.

f. Liver dysfunction with clinical signs of bleeding

2. FFP should be given to achieve a minimum of 30% of plasma factor concentrations. Generally speaking, it is required when PT or aPTT >1.5 times the control, or INR >2.0. This usually requires administration of 10–20 mL/kg of FFP.

3. Use ABO-compatible FFP.

a. Group AB plasma is suitable for all blood types.

## Indications for the Transfusion of Cryoprecipitate

1. Indicated for bleeding associated with fibrinogen deficiencies

a. Congenital fibrinogen deficiency: normal level of fibrinogen is 200–400 mg/dL

b. Disseminated intravascular bleeding with fibrinogen <150 mg/dL

c. Hemorrhage or massive transfusion with fibrinogen <150–200 mg/dL

d. Recombinant or virus-inactivated Factor VIII: C, Factor VIII: vWF, and Factor XIII are preferred to cryoprecipitate. Cryoprecipitate can be used in the absence of the above factor concentrates.

2. ABO compatibility is not required but often performed when transfusing cryoprecipitate.

## Leading Causes of Transfusion-Relates Death

1. TACO: transfusion-associated circulatory overload
2. TRALI: transfusion-related acute lung injury
3. TAS: transfusion-associated sepsis
4. HTR: hemolytic transfusion reaction

## Complications of Blood Transfusions

1. Infectious

a. Bacterial contamination, especially of platelets stored at room temperature

b. Viral disease examples

i. Cytomegalovirus (CMV)

ii. Hepatitis B and C

iii. Human immunodeficiency virus (HIV)

iv. Human T-cell lymphotropic virus (HTLV)

v. West Nile virus

vi. Prion diseases with long incubation period, such as variant Creutzfeldt–Jakob (vCJD) disease

2. Non-infectious

a. Acute hemolytic transfusion reactions

i. Usually result from ABO incompatibility

ii. Results from immunologic destruction of transfused RBC coming in contact with pre-existing IgM or IgG antibodies of the recipient, leading to immediate intravascular hemolysis

iii. Signs are nonspecific under general anesthesia

(1) Fever

(2) Tachycardia

(3) Hypotension

(4) Disseminated intravascular coagulation (DIC) with diffuse bleeding

(5) Bronchospasm

(6) Urticaria

(7) Dark urine

iv. Diagnosis

(1) High index of suspicion

(2) Anemia

(3) Positive direct antiglobulin (Coombs) test

(4) Decreased serum haptoglobin

(5) Elevated plasma and urine hemoglobin

(6) Increased unconjugated bilirubin

(7) Laboratory markers of DIC, platelet counts

v. Treatment

(1) Immediately discontinue transfusion, notify blood bank, re-identify the patient, and recheck the blood.

(2) Supportive treatment

(a) Maintain cardiovascular function with fluids and pressors.

(b) Place a urinary bladder catheter and maintain adequate urine output to avoid acute renal failure (fluids, pressors, diuretics, and sodium bicarbonate to alkalinize the urine).

(c) Monitor and treat DIC.

b. Delayed hemolytic transfusion reaction

i. Anamnestic antibody response in the recipient to donor antigens; often Kell, Duffy, or Kidd.

ii. Causes extravascular hemolysis, which occurs in days/weeks.

iii. Symptoms are mild (fever, jaundice, elevated bilirubin, anemia).

iv. Positive direct Coombs test

v. Treatment: supportive

3. Febrile reactions to donor leukocytes

a. Tend to be mild and self-limited

b. Leukoreduction decreases frequency of febrile reactions.

c. Treatment with antipyretics

4. Allergic reactions

    a. Reaction to the proteins in the donor plasma

    b. Treatment is supportive (fluids, IV epinephrine, corticosteroids, H1- and H2-blockers)

    c. Consider anaphylactoid reaction in IgA-deficient patient with anti-IgA antibodies on exposure to IgA-containing products. Washing blood products to remove residual plasma or using IgA-deficient donors serves as a prevention.

5. Transfusion-related acute lung injury

    a. Acute onset of hypoxemia and noncardiogenic pulmonary edema as a result of activation of host leukocytes by donor antibodies

    b. Occurs within 6 hours of transfusion

    c. Treatment is supportive.

        i. Immediately stop transfusion.
        ii. Notify the blood bank to screen the donor unit for anti-leukocyte antibodies.
        iii. Rule out other causes of acute lung injury and pulmonary edema.
        iv. Institute measures to improve oxygenation. It may require mechanical ventilation with lung-protective strategies.

6. Transfusion-associated circulatory overload

    a. Acute respiratory distress within 6 hours of transfusion

    b. Hydrostatic pulmonary edema occurs as a result of an acute left heart failure due to excessive rate or volume of transfusion.

    c. Treatment: address fluid overload, use diuretics.

7. Transfusion-associated graft-versus-host disease (GVHD)

    a. Passenger donor lymphocytes engraft in the recipient and mount an immune response against the immunocompromised host.

    b. Pancytopenia, rash, fever, and liver/gastrointestinal dysfunction that develops in days to weeks and is often fatal.

    c. Irradiation of blood products prevents GVHD as leukoreduction alone is not enough.

8. Posttransfusion purpura

    a. Severe thrombocytopenia occurs due to antiplatelet antibodies destroying both transfused and recipient platelets.

    b. Intravenous immunoglobulin is the treatment of choice.

    c. Plasmapheresis is the second line of therapy.

9. Metabolic derangements usually in a context of massive transfusion

    a. Hypothermia leading to platelet and coagulation factor dysfunction, arrhythmias, hepatic dysfunction, decreased drug metabolism, and myocardial depression.

    b. Hyperkalemia leading to ventricular arrhythmias and cardiac arrest (peaked T waves, prolonged PR interval, widened QRS on ECG). Treatment: stop the transfusion, administer calcium, bicarbonate, insulin, and glucose.

    c. Citrate toxicity leads to chelation of calcium with clinical signs of hypocalcemia (muscle weakness, tetany, arrhythmias, myocardial dysfunction, and coagulopathy). Treatment with calcium chloride or gluconate

    d. Leftward shift of the oxygen–Hb dissociation curve due to decrease in the 2,3-DPG of the stored RBC

    e. Acid–base disturbances: metabolic acidosis due to elevated lactate in the stored RBC followed by metabolic alkalosis as lactate and citrate in the transfused blood are converted to bicarbonate. Ongoing acidosis is most likely due to underlying tissue hypoxia.

10. Transfusion-related immunomodulation

    a. Systemic immunomodulation of the host by the transfused blood products. Pathophysiology is complex and multifactorial.

    b. Of note, despite theoretical concerns, age of the stored blood was not showed to be associated with the increased risk of complications in the diverse groups of populations observed in several studies.

**TKO:** Complications of massive blood transfusion: transfusion of more than the patient's own blood volume.

1. Hypothermia
2. Volume overload
3. Dilutional coagulopathy: decrease in fibrinogen, Factors II, V, and VIII, and platelets.
4. Leftward shift of the oxygen–Hb dissociation curve due to a decrease in the 2,3-DPG of the stored RBC
5. Citrate intoxication can occur with a rate of transfusion of 1 unit of RBC every 5 minutes in an adult.

    a. Watch for signs of hypocalcemia from citrate chelation effects: hypotension, narrow pulse pressure, elevated central venous pressure (CVP), and prolonged QT interval on ECG.

6. Hyperkalemia is possible when large volumes of older stored blood are given rapidly.

    a. ECG shows peaked T waves, prolonged PR interval, and a widened QRS.

    b. If ECG changes are observed, stop the transfusion, administer calcium, bicarbonate, insulin, and glucose.

7. Acid–base disturbances

a. Metabolic acidosis with transfusion of stored blood occurs followed by metabolic alkalosis as the lactate and citrate in the transfused blood are being converted to bicarbonate in the liver.

## Compatibility Testing

1. ABO, Rhesus typing: most fatal hemolytic transfusion reactions result from ABO incompatibility.
2. Antibody screens identify recipient antibodies against donor RBC antigens. When the plasma screen is positive, the blood bank will proceed to identify the antibody. Use appropriate antigen-negative donor units for the transfusion.
3. Cross-match: Donor cells get mixed with recipient serum. It is performed in three phases:
   a. First phase: 1–5 minute duration; confirms ABO and Rh type
   b. Second phase: 30–45 minute duration; detects antibodies to different blood group systems
   c. Third phase: 60–90 minute duration; is performed only when the screening is positive. It detects antibodies in low titers and antibodies that do not agglutinate easily.

## Emergency Transfusion

1. When crossed-matched blood is unavailable, use type-specific, partially crossed-matched blood.
2. If type-specific, partially crossed-matched blood is unavailable, use type-specific, uncrossed-matched blood.
3. If type-specific blood is unavailable, use type O Rh-negative blood: the universal donor.
   a. Do not withhold Rh-positive blood from an exsanguinating Rh-negative patient if Rh-negative blood is unavailable. In other words, it is less than ideal but acceptable to give O-positive blood to an O negative recipient in an emergency situation.
4. If more than 10–12 units of O negative blood were administered to nongroup O patient, continue with O negative blood even if type-specific blood becomes available unless the blood bank confirms that anti-A or anti-B antibodies are present in the low titers only.
5. Anti-A and anti-B antibodies, when combined with group O RBC, can cause hemolysis of A, B, or AB RBC.
6. Of note, group AB is the universal donor plasma and avoids transfusing anti-A or anti-B antibodies against the patient's RBC.

## Intra-operative Blood Salvage

1. Intra-operative blood salvage (IOBS) was shown to reduce allogenic blood transfusion in major surgery (multilevel spine fusions and cardiac surgery).
2. It may be beneficial in patients with low pre-operative hemoglobin and in:

a. Patients unsuitable for pre-operative autologous blood donations or acute normovolemic hemodilution
b. Patients not willing to accept allogenic transfusion
c. Patients with multiple alloantibodies

3. Salvaged blood has better oxygen-carrying capacity and tissue oxygenation.
4. Typical hematocrit of salvaged blood is 60–70%.
5. The only absolute contraindications to IOBS are microbial contamination and gross contamination by cancer cells.

## KO Treatment Plan

### Pre-operative

1. Keep in mind that placental abruption can be associated with significant uterine atony, amniotic fluid embolism, and development of DIC. All of these can require massive transfusion and appropriate treatment.
2. There is minimal opportunity to optimize this hemodynamically unstable patient. If time permits, obtain or check:
   a. Blood type and cross-match blood
   b. Baseline coagulation studies (INR, PT, aPTT)
   c. Complete blood count
3. Communicate with the blood bank the possibility of massive blood loss and need for massive transfusion of blood products.
4. Obtain at least two large-bore IV lines.
5. Start supportive therapy with blood and crystalloids prior to induction.
6. Consider IOBS if available (peripartum hemorrhage and concern for amniotic fluid embolism are not absolute contraindications).

### Intra-operative

1. Rapid-sequence induction and intubation
2. Placement of arterial line
3. Insert a Foley catheter to monitor urine output and check for hemoglobinuria.
4. Continue volume resuscitation with crystalloids.
5. Continue or start blood transfusion.
   a. Can use O negative blood if type and screen are unavailable
   b. Switch to cross-matched blood as soon as possible.
6. Monitor the patient's vital signs, temperature, acid–base status, electrolytes, and hemoglobin/hematocrit.
   a. Keep in mind that hemoglobin/hematocrit are affected by the patient's fluid status and may not be an accurate indicator of the blood oxygen content in the presence of active bleeding.
7. Treat hypothermia aggressively.

423

8. In the presence of ongoing microvascular bleeding, consider dilutional coagulopathy or the development of DIC.

   a. Draw coagulation studies, thromboelastography (TEG,) rotational thromboelastometry (ROTEM), complete blood count (CBC), and send blood for fibrinogen and fibrin split products.

9. Consider correcting coagulopathy with platelets, FFP, and cryoprecipitate as needed. Activate massive transfusion protocol if available and was not activated previously.

10. Monitor the surgical site for bleeding. Keep open communication with the obstetrician. Discuss therapeutic options to control hemorrhage.

    a. Pharmacologics to increase uterine tone
    b. Bimanual compression of the uterus
    c. Intrauterine gauze packing
    d. Balloon tamponade
    e. Consider safety and suitability of arterial embolization that may require transfer of the unstable patient to the interventional radiology suite.
    f. Hysterectomy

11. In the presence of established DIC, surgical control alone (including hysterectomy) might not be enough. Consider the possibility of amniotic fluid embolism that can worsen DIC and lead to multi-organ failure.

## Post-operative

1. Anticipate the need for an ICU bed and continuing resuscitation.
2. Prepare to transport this critically ill, intubated patient.

## Bibliography

American Red Cross. *A Compendium of Transfusion Practice Guidelines*, 4th ed. 2021. https://www.redcross.org/content/dam/redcrossblood/hospital-page-documents/334401_compendium_v04jan2021_bookmarkedworking_rwv01.pdf.

American Society of Anesthesiologists Task Force on Perioperative Blood Management. Practice guidelines for perioperative blood management: an updated report by the American Society of Anesthesiologists Task Force on Perioperative Blood Management. *Anesthesiology* 2015;**122**:241–75

Barash PG, Cullen BF, Stoelting RK, et al. *Clinical Anesthesia*, 8th ed. Philadelphia: Lippincott Williams & Wilkins, 2017, pp. 419–54.

Dunn PF. *Clinical Anesthesia Procedures of the Massachusetts General Hospital*, 7th ed. Philadelphia: Lippincott Williams and Wilkins, 2006, pp. 603–20.

# Tourniquet Physiology

**Chapter 100**

Zaid H. Jumaily and Jessica A. Lovich-Sapola

## Sample Case

A 63-year-old female underwent surgery for a left total knee replacement, lasting 2 hours. After the tourniquet was released, her blood pressure rapidly fell to 70/40 mm Hg. How would you manage this drop in blood pressure? What if her oxygen saturation fell to 86%? How would you manage this drop in oxygenation?

## Clinical Issues

### Indication for Tourniquet

1. Applied to upper or lower extremities to decrease intra-operative bleeding and improve operative conditions
2. Emergent use to stop acute hemorrhage
3. Regional technique (Bier block)

### Relative Contraindications

1. Sickle cell disease

   a. Possible precipitation of sickle cell crisis secondary to the low concentration of oxygen in the ischemic limb.

   b. If a tourniquet is considered mandatory to decrease the blood loss and improve the operative visualization, maintenance of adequate hydration, warmth, and blood volume is critical.

2. Infection and thrombosis

   a. Potential systemic spread during the exsanguination step; a risk–benefit analysis should be conducted prior to applying a tourniquet.

### Physiologic Changes

1. Neurologic

   a. Somatosensory evoked potentials and nerve conduction are ablated within 30 minutes.

   b. Pain and hypertension can be seen at 45–60 minutes.

   c. Post-operative neurapraxia occurs at 2 hours.

   d. Nerve injury may occur at the skin level under the edge of the tourniquet. Direct pressure from the cuff is more damaging than the distal ischemia.

2. Muscle

   a. Cellular hypoxia occurs within 8 minutes.

   b. Cellular creatinine levels decline.

   c. Progressive cellular acidosis

   d. Endothelial capillary leak develops in 2 hours.

   e. The limb becomes progressively colder.

3. Systemic effects of tourniquet inflation

   a. Expansion of central venous blood volume

   b. Arterial and pulmonary artery pressure increases.

4. Systemic effects of tourniquet release

   a. Transient fall in core temperature by 0.7 °C occurs within 90 seconds of deflation.

   b. Transient metabolic acidosis

   c. Transient fall in central venous oxygen tension by about 20% within 30–60 seconds (a decrease in arterial oxygen saturation is unusual).

   d. Acid metabolites are released into the central circulation.

   e. Transient fall in pulmonary and systemic arterial pressures

   f. The fall in blood pressure can be significant and has resulted in cardiac arrest.

   g. 10–15% increase in heart rate

   h. 5–10% increase in serum potassium

   i. Transient increase in end-tidal carbon dioxide ($ETCO_2$)

   j. Increased oxygen consumption

5. Local effects of tourniquet inflation

   a. Mitochondrial partial pressure of oxygen decreases to zero within 8 minutes.

   b. Anaerobic metabolism begins.

   c. Tissue edema begins with inflation lasting longer than 60 minutes.

   d. Closure of the wound may be more difficult secondary to edema.

   e. Injury to the muscle beneath the tourniquet may delay rehabilitation.

6. Prolonged inflation

   a. Hypertension occurs after 45–60 minutes.

      i. Treat with deepened anesthesia.

      ii. The refractory treatment is antihypertensives such as IV hydralazine, nifedipine, or labetalol.

   b. Neurologic problems may occur if inflated greater than 2 hours.

425

c.   Deflate the cuff every 90–120 minutes to minimize the risk of neurapraxia.

## KO Treatment Plan

### Intra-operative

1.   A transient fall in blood pressure is common with the deflation of the tourniquet. Monitor closely and treat as needed.

2.   A persistent drop in blood pressure and pulse oximetry may be ominous.

   a.   Verify the patient's vital signs.
   b.   Check for a pulse.
   c.   Look at the cardiac rhythm and ETCO$_2$.
   d.   Consider a differential diagnosis that includes fat embolism, anaphylaxis, and cardiac arrest.
   e.   Treat accordingly.
   f.   ACLS if indicated

## Bibliography

Barash PG, Cullen BF, Stoelting RK, et al. *Clinical Anesthesia*, 8th ed. Philadelphia: Lippincott Williams & Wilkins, 2017, p. 1453.

Gropper MA. *Miller's Anesthesia*, 9th ed. Philadelphia: Elsevier, 2020, pp. 1048, 1312, 2094, 2377, 2768.

Kumar L, Railton C, Tawfic Q. Tourniquet application during anesthesia: "What we need to know?". *J Anesthesiol Clin Pharmacol* 2016;**32**(4):424–30.

Sharma JP, Salhotra R. Tourniquets in orthopedic surgery. *Indian J Orthopaed* 2012;**46**(4):377–383.

# Chapter 101

# Electroconvulsive Therapy

Wesley G. Dougall, Kelly P. Jones, and Jessica A. Lovich-Sapola

## Sample Case

A 57-year-old male with known hypertension and major depressive disorder refractory to medical management presents on the day of his electroconvulsive therapy (ECT) with an elevated blood pressure of 180/95 mm Hg. All other vitals are within normal limits. This is not his first treatment. Would you go ahead with the procedure?

## Clinical Issues

### Definition of ECT

1. A procedure in which a programmed electrical stimulus is passed through the brain, deliberately triggering a brief seizure
2. EEG seizure activity lasting 25–60 seconds is assumed to be optimal.
3. The current is administered to both hemispheres or only the nondominant hemisphere.
   a. Stimulation of only one hemisphere may be associated with reduced memory loss.
4. The stimulus produces a grand mal seizure: brief tonic phase followed by a more prolonged clonic phase.
5. A patient usually requires 6–12 treatments during a hospitalization and then continued treatments weekly or monthly.
6. Exact mechanism for therapeutic effect remains unknown despite decades of use

### Indications for ECT

1. Definitely effective for:
   a. Major depression refractory to antidepressant therapy
   b. Need exists for a rapid treatment response, such as in pregnancy
   c. Medical comorbidities prevent the use of antidepressant medication.
   d. Previous response to ECT
   e. Depression with psychotic features
   f. Catatonic stupor
   g. Severely suicidal
   h. Food refusal leading to nutritional compromise
   i. Bipolar disorder
   j. Schizophrenia
   k. Mania
   l. Atypical psychosis

2. May be effective in:
   a. Neuroleptic malignant syndrome
   b. Organic delusional disorder
   c. Organic mood disorder
   d. Obsessive-compulsive disorder
   e. Neuroleptic-induced Parkinsonism
   f. Neuroleptic-induced tardive dyskinesia
   g. Catatonia secondary to medical conditions

### Relative Contraindications for ECT

1. Unstable or severe cardiovascular disease
2. Space-occupying intracranial lesion or elevated intracranial pressure (ICP)
3. Recent cerebral hemorrhage or stroke
4. Bleeding or unstable intracerebral aneurysm
5. Severe pulmonary disease
6. ASA class 4 or 5

### Morbidity and Mortality

1. Approximately 4 deaths per 100,000 treatments

### Physiologic Effects of ECT

1. Cardiovascular
   a. Initiation of the electrical stimulus triggers a brief parasympathetic discharge that can lead to a 10–15 second period of bradycardia with or without hypotension, premature atrial or ventricular contractions, or asystole.
   b. This is then followed by sympathetic nervous system stimulation of several minutes in duration, with an associated catecholamine surge that produces tachycardia and hypertension. This can be countered with short-acting β-blockers and nitroglycerin.
   c. The postictal state may present with compensatory bradycardia that can be effectively treated with anticholinergics if needed.

2. Central nervous system
   a. Increased cerebral blood flow
   b. Increased cerebral oxygen consumption

---

c. Increased ICP

d. Possible increased blood–brain permeability

e. Memory loss is the most common long-term side effect of ECT.

f. Disorientation can last from minutes to hours and appears to be related to the treatment parameters.

g. Delirium occurs in approximately 10% of patients recovering from anesthesia.

   i. Several conditions have been identified that increase the risk for delirium post-ECT.

     (1) Stroke within 1 year

     (2) Parkinson's disease

     (3) Advanced age

h. Headache is also a common complaint after ECT.

   i. Ibuprofen has been shown to be effective in prophylaxis of post-ECT headache.

# KO Treatment Plan

## Pre-operative

A complete presurgical evaluation should be performed with special attention to the areas listed below.

1. Pre-existing medical conditions

  a. Cardiac disease: arrhythmia, ischemia, congestive heart failure

    i. 2014 American Heart Association and the American College of Cardiology practice guidelines consider ECT a low-risk procedure.

    ii. It is well tolerated even in at-risk patients because the duration of hemodynamic changes is brief.

  b. Neurologic disease: space-occupying lesion, stroke, dementia

  c. Osteoporosis or other causes of fragile bones

  d. Medications: one study showed 54% of patients with psychiatric illnesses use alternative medicine in addition to physician-prescribed pharmacotherapy.

  e. Labs: the American Psychiatric Association suggest no routine medical labs are required unless indicated by other medical conditions such as hypertension treated with diuretics.

  f. Ensure the patient is adequately fasted.

## Intra-operative

1. Induction agents
Many IV anesthetics have been used for ECT.

  a. Methohexital 0.75–1 mg/kg is the traditional drug for ECT and is considered the gold standard.

    i. Rapid onset and rapid recovery

    ii. Short duration of action

    iii. Minimal anticonvulsant side effects

    iv. Methohexital provides longer seizure duration when compared to propofol.

    v. Fewer side effects than etomidate

    vi. Faster wake-up than thiopental

    vii. US shortages of barbiturates may require use of alternative agents.

  b. Propofol 0.75–2.5 mg/kg

    i. Decreased seizure duration when compared to methohexital and possibly etomidate

    ii. Comparable EEG seizure duration, with shorter recovery, when compared to thiopental

    iii. No difference in outcome was demonstrated when compared to methohexital.

    iv. Lower blood pressure and heart rate response to ECT

  c. Etomidate 0.15–0.3 mg/kg

    i. May prolong seizure duration

    ii. Good choice for patients when seizure duration was deemed too short with other agents

    iii. It may also prolong recovery.

  d. Thiopental 2–3 mg/kg

    i. Produces tachycardia and hypertension more often than propofol

    ii. Avoids pain at the injection site

    iii. No advantage over methohexital

    iv. Prolonged recovery time when compared to methohexital

    v. Not currently available in the United States

  e. Ketamine 0.7–2.8 mg/kg

    i. May prolong or enhance ECT seizures

    ii. Should be used cautiously in patients with cardiovascular comorbidities in view of more pronounced blood pressure elevations

    iii. May result in higher rates of restlessness, disorientation, delirium, psychosis, and prolonged reorientation time after the procedure

2. Neuromuscular blocking agents
Used to decreased excessive seizure motor activity which could result in bony injuries such as fractures and dislocations

  a. Succinylcholine 0.3–0.5 mg/kg

    i. Most commonly used neuromuscular blocker for ECT

    ii. It has a short duration of action and low frequency of side effects.

    iii. *Uncommonly* associated with myalgias (only ~2% of patients)

b. Rocuronium 0.3 mg/kg

    i. Viable alternative to succinylcholine when used with sugammadex, 2–8 mg/kg, which allows for rapid, complete reversal to be achieved without additional safety concerns

3. Adjuvants

  a. Glycopyrrolate 0.2–0.4 mg

    i. Given pre-operatively as an antisialagogue

    ii. Decreases the bradycardia associated with ECT

  b. Caffeine is given 3–5 minutes before initiation of ECT in varied doses.

    i. Shown to increase seizure length

  c. β-blockers (e.g., esmolol 1 mg/kg) given just prior to induction

    i. Used to control tachycardia and hypertension post-stimulus (appears better than labetalol for this purpose)

    ii. Has been shown to decrease the seizure duration

    iii. There are reports of asystole after β-blocker treatment and ECT.

    iv. Routine treatment with β-blockers is not recommended because the hemodynamic changes are usually self-limited.

## Sample Case

I would proceed with this case if there are no signs of unstable cardiac disease. Hypertension alone is not a contraindication. As noted above, this is a low-risk procedure, and hemodynamic changes are usually short-lived and self-limited. I would avoid ketamine as an induction agent and have β-blockers available at the bedside. I would not pretreat with β-blockers because of the reported risk of prolonged bradycardia and asystole.

1. Pre-operative evaluation including review of all pertinent areas
2. Always review the patient's previous anesthetic ECT records. They are usually a good guide for current anesthetics.
3. IV access
4. Placement of standard ASA monitors

5. Placement of electroconvulsive leads
6. Glycopyrrolate 0.2–0.4 mg IV
7. Preoxygenate with 100% oxygen.
8. Placement of a second blood pressure cuff/tourniquet on the extremity without the IV to monitor seizure activity

  a. Seizure activity should also be monitored by an EEG.

9. Methohexital or induction agent of choice
10. Bite block placement and hyperventilate the patient by mask ventilation
11. Inflate the tourniquet on the arm without the IV.
12. Succinylcholine at the reduced dose noted above, or muscle relaxant of choice
13. Initiation of the ECT
14. Follow the length of seizure by following the arm with the tourniquet and the EEG.
15. Esmolol or labetalol as indicated for prolonged tachycardia or hypertension
16. Assist with ventilation via bag, valve mask until recovery of protective airway reflexes. (Give sugammadex for reversal if rocuronium is used.)
17. Transport to recovery for continued post-operative monitoring.

## Post-operative

There are three stages of recovery after surgery. Regardless of whether the ECT procedure is done as an outpatient or inpatient procedure, the patient should be monitored in accordance with standard monitoring guidelines and meet the discharge criteria set by your institution.

1. Early

  a. Time from emergence to recovery of protective airway responses and early motor activity

  b. This often occurs in the operating or procedure room of ambulatory centers.

2. Intermediate

  a. Time when the patient may be moved to a phase 2 recovery

  b. There is progression to ambulating, voiding, and oral intake.

3. Late

  a. Resumption of normal daily activity

  b. Usually occurs at home

## Bibliography

Abrams R. The mortality rate with ECT. *Convuls Ther* 1997;**13**(3):125–7.

Abrams R. *Electroconvulsive Therapy*, 2nd ed. New York: Oxford University Press, 1992.

American Psychiatric Association. Indications for electroconvulsive therapy. *Am J Psychiatry* 2000;**157**:1.

American Psychiatric Association. *The Practice of Electroconvulsive Therapy: Recommendations for Treatment, Training, and Privileging*, 2nd ed.

Washington, DC: American Psychiatric Association, 2001.

Daniel WF, Crovitz HF. Autobiographical amnesia with ECT: an analysis of the roles of stimulus wave form, electrode placement, stimulus energy, and seizure length. *Biol Psychiatry* 1983;**18**:121.

Decina P, Malitz S, Sackeim HA, et al. Cardiac arrest during ECT modified beta-adrenergic blockade. *Am J Psychiatry* 1984;**141**:298.

Fleisher LA, Fleischmann KE, Auerbach AA, et al. 2014 ACC/AHA guideline on perioperative cardiovascular evaluation and management of patients undergoing noncardiac surgery: a report of the American College of Cardiology/American Heart Association Task Force on Practice Guidelines. *Circulation* 2014;**130**:278–333.

Hines R, Jones S, *Stoelting's Anesthesia and Co-existing Disease*, 8th ed. Philadelphia: Elsevier, 2022, pp. 619–44.

Gelb AW, Maties O. Anesthesia for electroconvulsive therapy. In: Joshi GP, Jones S, eds., *UpToDate*. www.uptodate.com/contents/anesthesia-for-electroconvulsive-therapy (accessed October 20, 2021).

Gropper MA. *Miller's Anesthesia*, 9th ed. Philadelphia: Elsevier, 2020, pp. 832–64.

Knaudt PR, Conner KM, Weisler RH, Churchill LE, Davidson JR. Alternative therapy use by psychiatric outpatients. *J Nerv Ment Dis* 1999;**187**(11):692–5.

Larson G, Swartz C, Abrams R. Duration of ECT-induced tachycardia as a measure of seizure length. *Am J Psychiatry* 1984;**14**:1269.

Lihua P, Su M, Ke W, Ziemann-Gimmel P. Different regimens of intravenous sedatives or hypnotics for electroconvulsive therapy (ECT) in adult patients with depression. *Cochrane Database Syst Rev* 2014;**4**: CD009763.

Martin M, Figiel G, Mattingly G, et al. ECT-induced interictal delirium in patients with a history of CVA. *J Geriatr Pyschiatry Neurol* 1992;**5**:149.

Prabhakar H. *Essentials of Neuroanesthesia*. Philadelphia: Elsevier, 2017, pp. 805–11.

# Remote Anesthesia

Jocelyn Loy and Jessica A. Lovich-Sapola

## Sample Case

You are called by the neurologist to sedate a 6-month-old child for an MRI (magnetic resonance imaging) scan. What are your pre-operative concerns? What do you need to take with you to the MRI scanner? What safety concerns do you have for you and the patient? Can you use your usual monitors?

## Clinical Issues

2018 American Society of Anesthesiologists statement on non-operating room anesthetizing locations: guidelines for nonoperating room anesthetizing locations:

1. It is the responsibility of the anesthesiologist to ensure that the location meets the ASA guidelines for safety. The anesthesiologist must maintain the same high standard of anesthetic care provided in the operating suite.
2. Reliable piped oxygen source with a full backup E cylinder of oxygen
3. Suction source for the patient and the scavenging system
4. Waste gas scavenging system if inhalational agents are used
5. Adequate monitoring equipment that complies with the ASA standards
6. Anesthesia machine that has an equivalent function to the machines used in the operating rooms
7. Self-inflating hand resuscitator bag to deliver positive-pressure ventilation
8. Adequate anesthetic drugs and supplies
9. Sufficient safe electrical outlets with isolated electrical power or ground fault circuit interrupters
10. Adequate light and battery-powered backup
11. Sufficient space for imaging and anesthesia equipment, monitors, personnel, and patient
12. Emergency cart with defibrillator, emergency drugs, and emergency equipment
13. Means of reliable two-way communication to request immediate assistance from the OR in the event of an emergency
14. Compliance with safety and building codes
15. Adequately trained staff to support the anesthesia team
16. Adequate equipment for transport
17. Post-anesthesia care facilities

## Remote Monitoring

1. Qualified anesthesia personnel must be present for the entire case.
2. Continuous monitoring of the patient's oxygenation, ventilation, circulation, and temperature
3. Oxygen concentrations of inspired gas: low oxygen concentration alarm
4. Blood oxygenation: pulse oximetry
5. Ventilation: observation, end-tidal carbon dioxide ($ETCO_2$) detection, and disconnect alarm
6. Circulation: EKG, pulse oximetry, and arterial blood pressures every 5 minutes or continuous invasive blood pressures
7. Understand that the standards of anesthesia care and patient monitoring are the same regardless of the location.

## Remote Facilities and Equipment

1. Familiarize yourself with the physical layout of the location, anesthetic equipment, and anesthetic implications of the procedure being performed prior to the induction of anesthesia.
2. Verify the availability of assistance.
3. Check piped-in gases and gas tanks.
4. Check suction.
5. Check power outlets (i.e., grounding and electrical requirements).

## Remote Recovery Care

1. The patient must be medically stable before transport.
2. The patient must be accompanied to the recovery area by qualified anesthesia staff.
3. Provisions for oxygen delivery and monitoring on the transport cart are required.
4. Appropriate recovery facilities and staff must be provided.

## Radiology Suite

1. Includes ultrasound (US), computed tomographic scanning (CT), MRI, radiofrequency ablation (RFA), neurosurgical embolization and coiling, and nuclear medicine.
2. The rooms are often crowded, with bulky fixed imaging equipment with some type of energy hazard.

3. Patients are often required to hold still for long periods of time.
4. Unique hazard
   a. Radiation exposure
      i. Increases risk of leukemia and fetal abnormalities
      ii. Dosimeters are required to measure the level of radiation exposure a staff member receives. (A maximum exposure of 50 millisieverts (mSv) annually, a lifetime of 10 mSv × age, and monthly exposure of 0.5 mSv for pregnant women is allowed.)
      iii. Exposure can be limited by lead aprons, thyroid shields, leaded glass screens, protective goggles, and remote video monitoring.
   b. Iodinated contrast media
      i. Older ionized contrast media were hyperosmolar and toxic.
      ii. Newer nonionized contrast media have lower osmolality and improved side effect profiles.
      iii. Overall incidence of an adverse drug reaction from contrast media is about 3%.
      iv. The incidence of a severe reaction is 0.04%.
   c. High magnetic fields
   d. High-voltage equipment

## Reactions to Iodinated Contrast Media

1. Mild: nausea, vomiting, perception of warmth, fever, chills, facial flushing, headache, itchy rash, and mild urticaria
2. Moderate: edema, bronchospasm, hypotension, and seizures
3. Severe: vomiting, rigors, feeling faint, chest pain, severe urticaria, bronchospasm, dyspnea, arrhythmias, and renal failure
4. Life-threatening: glottic edema/bronchospasm, pulmonary edema, prolonged hypotension, loss of consciousness, arrhythmias, cardiac arrest, and seizures/ unconsciousness
5. Associated renal dysfunction due to contrast-induced nephropathy
   a. The contrast media is eliminated by the kidneys.
   b. Increased risk in patients with pre-existing renal dysfunction, especially if it is associated with diabetes, or patients on chronic nonsteroidal anti-inflammatory drugs
   c. Reduction in nephrotoxicity is associated with pre-procedure fluid hydration, careful urine output monitoring, and the use of low-osmolarity contrast media.
   d. Studies have shown benefits with the pre-procedure administration of acetylcysteine or sodium bicarbonate.

6. Pre-treatment: oral methylprednisolone and diphenhydramine may be considered for patients with a history of IV contrast reaction.
7. Treatment of a reaction: call for help, stop the injection of the causative agent, place the patient on oxygen, secure the airway, and give bronchodilators, fluids, epinephrine, corticosteroids, and antihistamines.

## CT

1. Two-dimensional, cross-sectional image
2. Each cross-section requires a few seconds of radiation exposure.
3. Patient immobility is required. Procedures are short and uncommonly require sedation.
4. It is often noisy, warm, and can induce claustrophobia.
5. CT can be used for diagnostic and therapeutic purposes.
6. The number one problem is inaccessibility of the patient.

## Indications for CT

1. Diagnostic purposes
2. Vascular malformations
3. Tumors
4. Invasive therapeutic procedures
5. CT-guided radiofrequency ablation
6. Head trauma
7. Acute stroke
8. Primary intracerebral hemorrhage
9. Meningioma
10. Aortic dissection screening

## MRI

1. Able to obtain images in any plane
2. Excellent soft tissue contrast
3. Does not produce ionizing radiation, is noninvasive, and does not produce biologically deleterious effects
4. MRI is often very time-consuming and any patient movement, including physiologic motion, can produce artifacts.
5. Obese patients may not fit in the MRI bore.
6. Hearing protection is mandatory (produces loud noises >90 dB).
7. Thermal injury has been reported at the site of MRI-unsafe EKG leads, areas where skin contacts the machine, from coiled or frayed MRI-safe monitor cables, and from looping of temperature probes and pulse oximeter cables.
8. The most significant risk in the MRI suite is the effect of the magnet on ferrous objects. The magnet is always "on."

## Indications for MRI

1. MRI can produce better resolution between gray and white matter.
2. Evaluation of blood flow and cerebrospinal fluid

3. Contraction and relaxation of organs
4. Images of tissue surrounded by bone because calcium does not emit an MRI signal
5. Evaluating the posterior fossa and parasellar regions of the brain
6. Diagnosis of multiple sclerosis, epilepsy, and brain tumors
7. Better than CT for small brain tumors
8. Arteriovenous and cardiac malformations
9. Multiple sclerosis
10. Syringomyelia
11. Congenital spinal cord abnormalities
12. Other indications: autism, hypotonia, metabolic/mitochondrial disorders, evaluation of obstructive sleep apnea, infectious processes.

## Contraindications for MRI

1. Shrapnel, vascular clips and shunts, wire spiral endotracheal tubes, cardiac pacemakers, automatic implantable cardioverter-defibrillators (AICDs), mechanical heart valves, recently placed sternal wire, implanted biological pumps, intraocular ferromagnetic foreign bodies, spinal cord or vagus nerve stimulators, programmable insulin pumps, VP shunts, coronary artery stents, and middle ear or cochlear implants

   a. In 2011, the US FDA approved the use of pacemakers and leads as MRI-conditional for certain patients, scans of certain parts of the body, and under certain scanning parameters. It is important to collaborate with the referring physician, radiologist, pacemaker specialist or cardiologist, and device manufacturer.

2. Tattoo ink with high concentrations of iron-oxide (permanent eyeliner) can cause burns in rare instances but is not an absolute contraindication.

3. Ferromagnetic items should never be allowed in the vicinity of the MRI magnet, including but not limited to: scissors, pens, keys, gas cylinders, anesthesia machines, anesthesia monitors, syringe pumps, stethoscopes, batteries, watches, pagers, phones, steel chairs, jewelry (including piercings and rings), and magnetic dental keepers.

4. Identification badges, credit cards, or any other swipe cards with magnetic strips will be demagnetized.

## MRI Zones

Zone 1: main entry to the facility, outside of MRI suite, freely accessible to the public

Zone 2: "meet and greet" area. Personnel and patient are screened. Emergency equipment is available. May be used for anesthetic induction and post-anesthesia care.

Zone 3: restricted area just outside of the MRI scanner suite. MRI-unsafe objects should already have been eliminated. Location of slave displays of patient monitors in zone 4. Breathing circuits from MRI-incompatible anesthesia

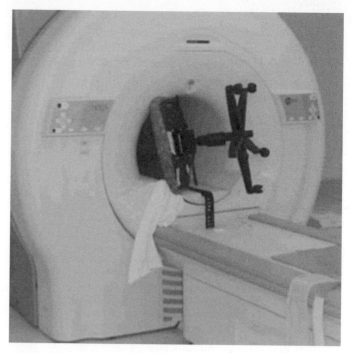

**Figure 102.1** Chair in the MRI scanner. Source: Courtesy of Moriel NessAiver, PhD, www.simplyphysics.com.

machine, infusion tubing, and cables of monitors in this area are passed through copper wave guides to get to zone 4.

Zone 4: MRI scanner magnet suite. Limited to screened individuals and MRI-safe or conditional objects. MRI-safe and conditional airway equipment and suction should be immediately available at all times.

### Equipment Categories in MRI Environment 4

MRI "safe": no ferromagnetic parts or radiofrequency interference

MRI "unsafe": have ferromagnetic parts or affected by radiofrequency interference (Fig. 102.1)

MRI "conditional": may be safe in certain locations of the suite depending on gauss lines, but cannot be identified as having no ferromagnetic parts

## Cerebral Coiling

1. This type of case should be treated like a cerebral artery aneurysm clipping in the operating room.
2. You should use all of the same IV access and monitors.
3. Place a pre-induction arterial line.
4. Always have two large-gauge IVs in place.

   a. For medication infusion
   b. For rapid fluid administration

5. General anesthesia with an endotracheal tube is usually required. The case can be long and the patient is required to hold still. Consider a muscle relaxant infusion to help ensure patient immobility during critical coiling events.

Check for adequate relaxation with a twitch monitor. Communication with the radiologist is important.

6. Have a fluid warmer and forced-air warmer available to warm the patient after the procedure. Mild hypothermia may be requested during the procedure.
7. Infusion pumps to deliver medications
8. Medications (including but not limited to)

    a. Nitroglycerine
    b. Nitroprusside
    c. Esmolol
    d. Labetalol
    e. Heparin
    f. Protamine
    g. Mannitol
    h. Phenytoin
    i. Dexamethasone

9. An activated clotting time (ACT) machine should be available because heparin is usually given during the procedure.
10. Stay in constant communication with the operating room in case of an emergency.
11. The patients are often transported directly to the ICU post-operatively.

## KO Treatment Plan

### MRI Road Trip; What to Bring

1. Anesthesia cart (pediatric or adult) fully stocked
2. Anesthesia machine/circuits (pediatric or adult)
3. Monitors for transport
4. ETCO$_2$ monitor
5. Temperature monitor
6. MRI-compatible monitoring equipment is usually available in the MRI suite. Remember that the usual anesthesia monitors are not safe in the MRI scanner.
7. Airway equipment: oral and nasal airways, nasal cannula, masks, laryngoscopes, laryngeal mask airways, and endotracheal tubes
8. Long, corrugated ventilation tubing: the anesthesia machine must often be placed a long distance from the patient (Fig. 102.2)
9. Self-inflating hand resuscitator bag
10. Syringe pump, preferably MRI-safe infusion pump, and at least three extension sets
11. Medications (including but not limited to)

    a. Propofol
    b. Remifentanil
    c. Ketamine
    d. Midazolam
    e. Fentanyl
    f. Dexmedetomidine
    g. Succinylcholine
    h. Nondepolarizing muscle relaxants

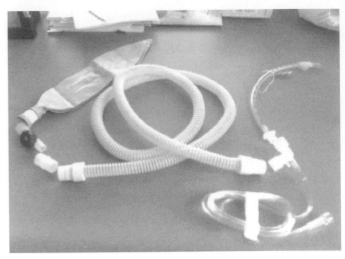

**Figure 102.2** Long-distance MRI ventilation set-up. Photo credit: J. Lovich-Sapola, MD.

    i. Ephedrine
    j. All other emergency drugs

12. IV tubing and IV fluids
13. Papers needed for charting if no electronic medical record keeping

### MRI Safety

1. Keep all ferromagnetic objects away from the MRI scanner.
2. Always wear ear protection secondary to the loud noises >90 dB.

### MRI Anesthetic

1. Initial workup

    a. Vital signs
    b. Pre-operative history
    c. Physical examination

2. Set up your equipment and familiarize yourself with physical layout and location.

    a. Verify the availability of assistance.
    b. Check gases, suction, and the MRI monitors.

3. The decision to deliver general anesthesia with a secured airway vs. deep IV sedation highly depends on the following:

    a. Special requirements for the procedure (breath holding)
    b. Pain tolerance or discomfort of patient lying flat in the thinly padded scanner bed
    c. Position of patient required for the procedure
    d. Child's comorbidities and NPO status
    e. Weight of the patient vs. the risk of airway compromise

f. Experience and comfort level/preference of the anesthesiologist with deep sedation techniques

g. Availability of support staff and equipment

h. Presence of any MRI-incompatible "devices" that need to be modified (e.g., Bivona tracheostomy tubes). Shiley tracheostomy tubes are considered MRI-safe by the US FDA.

4. If general anesthesia is planned, induce and secure the patient's airway in the induction room or holding area on an MRI-safe bed, and then transport the patient to the MRI suite with monitors, modified Mapleson anesthesia circuit connected to a full E cylinder oxygen tank or wall oxygen source, and MRI-safe infusion pump for total IV anesthesia (TIVA) or an MRI-compatible anesthesia machine if using volatile anesthetics.

5. For deep sedation with a spontaneously breathing patient, infusion of propofol or dexmedetomidine, nasal ETCO$_2$ cannula, and oxygen supplementation are commonly used.

6. Do not take anything metal into the MRI room!

7. Leave the MRI-unsafe monitors, anesthesia machine, oxygen cylinder, etc. outside of the MRI room.

8. Position the patient on the MRI table, provide supplemental oxygen, and use MRI-compatible monitors only.

9. ASA standard monitors are required.

a. EKG
b. Pulse oximetry
c. Noninvasive blood pressure
d. Capnography
e. Temperature if available

10. After the scan, it is safer to extubate the patient under general anesthesia outside of the MRI suite.

11. Transport the patient to the post-anesthesia care unit along with the ASA standard monitors.

# Bibliography

ASA Task Force on Anesthetic Care for MRI. Anesthesiology practice advisory on anesthetic care for magnetic resonance imaging: an updated report by the ASA Task Force on Anesthetic Care for MRI. *Anesthesiology* 2015;**122** (3):495–520.

Barash PG, Cullen BF, Stoelting RK. *Clinical Anesthesia*, 5th ed. Philadelphia: Lippincott Williams & Wilkins, 2006, pp 1331–42.

Campbell K, Torres L, Stayer S. Anesthesia and sedation outside the operating room. *Anesthesiol Clin* 2014;**32**:25–43.

Miller RD, Fleisher LA, Johns RA, et al. *Miller's Anesthesia*, 8th ed. New York: Churchill Livingstone, 2015, pp. 2646–7.

NIH Consensus Development Program. What are the clinical indications for MRI, and how does it compare to other diagnostic modalities? Outdated Consensus Development Reports. http://consensus.nih.gov.

**Chapter**

# 103

# Anesthetic Considerations of Cancer Chemotherapy

Neel Pandya and Matthew A. Joy

## Sample Case

A 48-year-old female with Hodgkin's lymphoma presents to the emergency department with severe abdominal pain. Plain films reveal free air under the diaphragm and she is suspected to have a perforated abdominal viscus. She is taken to the operating suite for an emergent exploratory laparotomy. What specific questions about this patient's history are important? How might this information affect the patient's pre-operative workup? What side effects and complications of chemotherapy might impact peri-operative care? What post-operative considerations must be made for cancer patients?

## Clinical Issues

A growing number of patients receive surgical procedures shortly after undergoing chemotherapy. It is important for the consultant physician anesthesiologist to have knowledge of the pharmacological implications of chemotherapeutic agents and how these might significantly change the plan for peri-operative care.

1. The most common toxicities to chemotherapeutic agents include:
   a. Cardiac
   b. Pulmonary
   c. Hematologic
   d. Bone marrow
   e. Gastrointestinal effects (ulceration and bleeding of the gastrointestinal tract)
   f. Coagulopathies
   g. Thrombocytopenia
   h. Anemia

## Chemotherapeutic Classes

### Alkylating Agents

1. *Mechanism of action*: a diverse set of drugs that interact and bind with different nucleic acids and proteins. They bind to the alkyl group in DNA and interfere with mitosis.
2. *Dose-limiting factor*: bone marrow suppression
3. Agent(s):
   a. Cyclophosphamide
      i. Side effect/toxicity
         (1) Inhibits pseudocholinesterase activity
         (2) Exerts ADH-like effect on the kidneys
         (3) Hemorrhagic cystitis
         (4) Inhibits CYP450 enzymes
         (5) Cardiac toxicity: congestive heart failure (CHF) second to hemorrhagic myocarditis (at doses of over 120 mg/kg over 2 days)
         (6) Pulmonary fibrosis
      ii. Anesthesia consideration
         (1) May prolong neuromuscular blockade when given with succinylcholine (may last up to 3–4 weeks from last dose)
         (2) Watch fluid management carefully when preventing hemorrhagic cystitis due to possibility of life-threatening hyponatremia.
   b. Chlorambucil
      i. Side effect/toxicity
         (1) Bone marrow suppression
   c. Busulfan
      i. Side effect/toxicity
         (1) Pulmonary fibrosis
         (2) Cardiac toxicity
         (3) Seizures (may occurs 24 hours after last dose)
      ii. Anesthesia consideration
         (1) Most sensitive indicator to assess for pulmonary damage: decrease in diffuse capacity for carbon monoxide (>10–15% from baseline)
   d. Cisplatin/carboplatin
      i. Side effect/toxicity
         (1) Dose-dependent peripheral neuropathy
         (2) Nephrotoxic (dose-limiting factor); a single dose of 2 mg/kg can produce toxicity in 25–30% of patients) (cisplatin).
         (3) Delayed pulmonary toxicity (carboplatin)
         (4) Cardiac toxicity
      ii. Anesthesia consideration
         (1) When considering regional anesthesia, a careful and detailed history and physical

436

exam should be done to assess for possible neuropathies.

(2) Nonsteroidal anti-inflammatory drug (NSAID) use may precipitate renal failure.

## Antimetabolites

1. *Mechanism of action*: structurally similar to metabolites used in DNA and RNA synthesis. They cause crosslinking and abnormal base pairing and therefore interfere with DNA production and halting tumor growth.
2. Agent(s):

   a. Methotrexate

      i. Side effect/toxicity

         (1) Life-threatening hepatic necrosis (also seen with 6-mercaptopurine and L-asparaginase)
         (2) CNS toxicity: encephalopathy
         (3) Acute nephrotoxicity

      ii. Anesthesia consideration

         (1) Check liver function tests (LFTs) and use an inhalation agent with minimal metabolism (i.e., desflurane).
         (2) NSAIDs decrease excretion of methotrexate.

   b. 5-Fluorouracil

      i. Side effect/toxicity

         (1) Cardiac toxicity: angina/myocardial infarction due to coronary spasm
         (2) Cerebellar ataxia

   c. Cytarabine

      i. Side effect/toxicity

         (1) Pulmonary toxicity

   d. Gemcitabine

      i. Side effect/toxicity

         (1) Thrombocytopenia

## Antitumor Antibiotics (Anthracyclines)

1. *Mechanism of action*: inhibit topoisomerase II and the intercalation between DNA/RNA base pairs.
2. Most likely class of chemotherapy drugs to cause cardiotoxicity and only class shown to cause delayed cardiotoxicity

   a. Delayed toxicity causing dysrhythmias is unrelated to dosing.

3. Agent(s):

   a. Bleomycin

      i. Side effect/toxicity

         (1) Pulmonary fibrosis is seen in 2–40% of patients (risk factors: total dose >450 mg, age >70, and renal failure).
         (2) Acute pericarditis

      ii. Anesthesia consideration

         (1) Check pulmonary function tests (PFTs), use lowest $FiO_2$ possible to maintain saturation at 90% or greater and use PEEP (recent bleomycin use and high $FiO_2$ can exacerbate existing damage), and employ careful fluid management.
         (2) Chest X-ray may show bilateral basal and peri-hilar infiltrates with fibrosis.
         (3) Most sensitive indicator to assess for pulmonary damage: decrease in diffuse capacity for carbon monoxide (>10–15% from baseline)

   b. Doxorubicin (adriamycin)/daunorubicin

      i. Side effect/toxicity

         (1) Cardiotoxic (dose-dependent)
         (2) Myelosuppression
         (3) Dose-dependent QTc prolongation (doxorubicin)
         (4) Risk of developing CHF in children is >9% if cumulative dose >500 mg/m$^2$.
         (5) General CHF risk: 7% at 550 mg/m$^2$, 15% at 600 mg/m$^2$, and 35% at 700 mg/m$^2$

      ii. Anesthesia consideration

         (1) Check the echocardiogram to evaluate left ventricular ejection fraction percentage (less than 45% can indicate drug-induced cardiac toxicity).
         (2) Empiric limiting dose is 550 mg/m$^2$.
         (3) Earliest sign of toxicity is tachycardia.

## Mitotic Inhibitors (Vinca Alkaloids)

1. *Mechanism of action*: inhibit a cell's ability to divide by blocking the formation of the microtubule complex in the cell cytoplasm.
2. Agent(s):

   a. Vinblastine

      i. Side effect/toxicity

         (1) Neurotoxicity: encephalopathy, peripheral nervous system neuropathic changes

   b. Vincristine

      i. Side effect/toxicity

         (1) Neurotoxicity (dose-limiting factor): encephalopathy, peripheral nervous system neuropathic changes
         (2) SIADH secretion

ii. Anesthesia consideration

(1) The earliest and most consistent asymptomatic sign of neurotoxicity is loss of Achilles tendon reflex and most consistent symptomatic sign is paresthesia in hands and feet.

**Mitotic Stabilizers**

1. *Mechanism of action*: binds and stabilizes the newly formed microtubule complex and prevents mitosis from progressing.
2. Agent(s):
   a. Docetaxel
      i. Side effect/toxicity
         (1) Inhibition of CYP450 enzymes
         (2) Bradycardia and arrhythmias
   b. Paclitaxel
      i. Side effect/toxicity
         (1) Neurotoxic: peripheral neuropathy, autonomic neuropathy
         (2) Nephrotoxic
         (3) Ventricular tachycardia (when given with cisplatin)

## Common Malignancies and Selected Chemotherapy Regimens

1. Malignancy
   a. Non-Hodgkin's lymphoma
      i. Common treatment regimen
         (1) CHOP: cyclophosphamide, vincristine, doxorubicin, and prednisone
      ii. R-CHOP: rituximab + CHOP
   b. Hodgkin's disease
      i. Common treatment regimen
         (1) ABVD: adriamycin, bleomycin, vinblastine, dacarbazine
   c. Breast cancer
      i. Common treatment regimen
         (1) AC: adriamycin, cyclophosphamide
         (2) FEC: 5-fluorouracil, epirubicin, cyclophosphamide
         (3) CMF: cyclophosphamide, methotrexate, 5-fluorouracil
   d. Lung cancer, nonsmall cell
      i. Common treatment regimen
         (1) Cisplatin or carboplatin

(a) Used in combination with gemcitabine or paclitaxel or docetaxel
   e. Lung cancer, small cell
      i. Common treatment regimen
         (1) Carboplatin or etoposide
   f. Esophageal
      i. Common treatment regimen
         (1) Cisplatin or 5-fluorouracil
   g. Ovarian
      i. Common treatment regimen
         (1) Gemcitabine

## Summary

## Common Complications Associated with Cancer Chemotherapy Agents

1. Cardiac toxicity: doxorubicin, busulfan, cisplatin, cyclophosphamide, daunorubicin, 5-fluorouracil
2. Pulmonary toxicity: methotrexate, bleomycin, busulfan, cyclophosphamide, cytarabine, carmustine
3. Renal toxicity: methotrexate, L-asparaginase, cisplatin, carboplatin, ifosfamide, mitomycin-C
4. Hepatic toxicity: actinomycin D, methotrexate, androgens, L-asparaginase, busulfan, cisplatin, azathioprine
5. CNS toxicity: methotrexate, cisplatin, interferon, hydroxyurea, procarbazine, vincristine
6. SIADH secretion: cyclophosphamide, vincristine

## Clinical Presentations of Chemotherapeutic Complications

1. Cardiac toxicity
   a. Chemotherapy agents may depress myocardial contractility, may cause dysrhythmias, CHF, or pericarditis.
   b. Patients may present with presyncope, syncope, chest pain, shortness of breath, nausea/vomiting, diaphoresis, or palpitations.
   c. Chemotherapy may also predispose patients to supraventricular tachycardia (SVT), complete heart block, prolonged QT syndrome, ventricular fibrillation, and ventricular tachycardia.
2. Pulmonary toxicity
   a. Pulmonary fibrosis
   b. Pneumonitis
   c. Patients may present with cough, dyspnea, or chest pain
3. Renal toxicity

a. Nephrotoxicity is a common complication of chemotherapy agents.

b. 30% of patients receiving cisplatin will develop nephrotoxicity.

c. This can lead to both accumulation and wasting of electrolytes, which can lead to peri-operative complications.

4. Hematologic toxicity

a. Bone marrow function in cancer patients may be disturbed by primary bone marrow disorders (e.g., leukemia), bony metastases (e.g., from breast cancer), as well as myelosuppressive chemotherapy.

b. The production of blood proteins and clotting factors may be impaired.

c. There may be dysfunctional coagulation in these patients.

5. Hepatic toxicity
6. Central nervous system toxicity
7. Tumor lysis syndrome
8. Chemotherapy-impaired wound healing

## KO Treatment Plan

### Pre-operative

1. Assess the effects of cancer and cancer therapies on the patient.
2. Obtain a full history and physical.

3. Routine clinical tests including a complete blood count and basic metabolic panel. If time permits, other relevant tests may include a hepatic function panel, PT/PTT/INR, arterial blood gas, chest X-ray, EKG, PFTs, and ECG.

4. Optimize the patient's physical status depending on the emergent vs. urgent vs. elective nature of the procedure.

### Intra-operative

1. All cancer patients receiving chemotherapy are treated with immune-suppression precautions, including careful aseptic techniques (i.e., meticulous sterile technique when placing invasive lines and monitors, cleaning IV ports with alcohol prior to injection).

2. For patients with severe pulmonary fibrosis or pneumonitis, lung protective strategies should be utilized (TV 6–8 cc/kg, PEEP to optimize oxygenation).

3. For patients who have received bleomycin, high $FiO_2$ should be avoided and colloid rather than crystalloid should be used for fluid replacement.

4. Invasive arterial blood pressure recordings and pulmonary artery catheterization may be necessary if significant myocardial impairment is present.

### Post-operative

1. Pain control
2. Address do not resuscitate (DNR) and do not intubate (DNI) requests.

## Bibliography

Allan N, Siller C, Breen A. Anesthetic implications for chemotherapy. *Contin Edu Anesth Crit Care Pain* 2012;**12**:52–6.

Bosek, V. Anesthetic implications of chemotherapy. *Curr Rev Clin Anesth* 2003;**23**:269–80.

De Souza, P. Cancer drug toxicities and anesthesia. 2007. https://perioperative .files.wordpress.com/2018/05/cancer-drug-toxicities.pdf (accessed January 14, 2023).

Foley J, Vose J, Armitage JA. *Current Therapy in Cancer*, 2nd ed. Philadelphia: Saunders, 1999, pp. 485–91.

Huttemann E, Sakka S. Anesthesia and anti-cancer chemotherapeutic drugs. *Curr Opin Anesthesiol* 2007;**18**:307–14.

Gehdoo RP. Anticancer chemotherapy and it's anaesthetic implications. *Indian J Anaesth* 2009;**53**(1):18–29.

Lefor AT. Perioperative management of the patient with cancer. *Chest* 1999;**115**:165S–171S.

Maracic L, Van Nostrand J, Beach D. Anesthetic implications for cancer chemotherapy. *AANA J Course* 2007;**75**:219–26.

Stephen P. Fischer preoperative evaluation of the cancer patient. *Anesth Clin North Am* 1998;**16**:533–46.

# Retrobulbar Block and Associated Complications

Marcos A. Izquierdo and Michael Prokopius

## Sample Case

A 76-year-old man presents to the ambulatory surgery center for cataract extraction. The surgeon informs you that the procedure will be performed under retrobulbar block. Vital signs at the beginning of the case are heart rate (HR) 76, respiratory rate (RR) 15, and blood pressure (BP) 156/76 mm Hg. Sedation is started with a remifentanil 40 µg bolus IV. Shortly after the block is performed, the patient is nonresponsive. What is your differential diagnosis? What are your next steps?

## Clinical Issues

### Anatomy

1.  The retrobulbar block is performed for akinesia and anesthesia of the eye.

    a.  Local anesthetic is injected behind the eye into the cone formed by the extraocular muscles

    b.  A 25-gauge needle penetrates the lower lid. The needle is advanced from the inferolateral border of the orbit approximately 15 mm along the wall of the orbit, turned superiorly, and 2–3 mL of local anesthetic is injected between the extraocular muscles and into the muscle cone.

    c.  Patients are often given a brief period of deep sedation during the block using remifentanil, etomidate, or propofol

    d.  Aspiration to avoid intravascular injection and then injection of local anesthetic

    e.  The successful block results in anesthesia, akinesia, and abolishment of the oculocephalic reflex (blocked eye does not move during head turning).

    f.  Retrobulbar block is avoided:

        i.   Patients with bleeding disorders or on anticoagulant therapy

        ii.  Severe myopia (elongated globe increases the risk of perforation)

        iii. Open-eye injury (injection of fluid behind the eye may case extrusion of the intraocular contents through the wound)

2.  Facial nerve block

    a.  Used to prevent blinking during the procedure.

    b.  Major complication is subcutaneous hemorrhage

## Complications of the Retrobulbar Block

1.  Retrobulbar hemorrhage (occurs in 1% of retrobulbar injections)

    a.  Arterial bleed: rapid orbital swelling, marked proptosis, inability to close the lid, and massive blood staining of the conjunctiva and lids

        (1) Compressive hematoma can threaten retinal perfusion, increase intraocular pressure, and lead to vision loss.

    b.  Venous bleed: spreads slowly and patients rarely have long-term visual complications

2.  Globe perforation

    a.  A potentially catastrophic ophthalmic complication

3.  Optic nerve injury

4.  Intravascular injection: small dose, therefore rarely symptoms

5.  Oculocardiac reflex

    a.  More common with topical anesthesia of the eye

    b.  More common in pediatric patients having strabismus surgery

6.  Trigeminal nerve block

7.  Respiratory arrest

8.  Acute neurogenic pulmonary edema

9.  Seizure

    a.  Secondary to a forceful injection into the ophthalmic artery causing retrograde flow to the brain

    b.  Local anesthetic toxicity

10. Postretrobulbar block apnea syndrome

    a.  Injection of local anesthetic into the optic nerve sheath with spread to the cerebrospinal fluid

    b.  High local anesthetic concentration in the central nervous system leads to mental status changes and possible unconsciousness.

    c.  Apnea results within 20–60 minutes.

    d.  Treatment

        i.  Supportive measures

        ii. Positive-pressure ventilation

11. Allergic reaction

## Differential Diagnosis

1. Over-sedation
   a. Elderly patients with comorbidities will be highly sensitive to sedatives.
   b. Continuously monitor end-tidal $CO_2$ ($ETCO_2$) and administer supplemental oxygen throughout the procedure.

2. Arrhythmias
   a. Bradycardia
   b. AV conduction blocks
   c. Asystole
   d. Secondary to the stimulation of the oculocardiac reflex

      i. Traction on the extraocular muscle or pressure on the globe causes bradycardia, atrioventricular block, ventricular ectopy, or asystole.
      ii. Pathway

         (1) Afferent of the reflex limb arises from the ophthalmic division of the trigeminal nerve and continues to the trigeminal ganglion and the sensory nucleus of the trigeminal nerve near the fourth ventricle
         (2) Afferent limb synapses with the motor nucleus of the vagus nerve
         (3) Efferent impulses travel to the heart via the vagus nerve
         (4) Leads to decreases in both heart rate and contractility of the heart

**Oculocardiac Reflex Pathway**

Orbital content → Ciliary ganglion → Ophthalmic division of the trigeminal nerve → Sensory nucleus of the trigeminal nerve → Motor nucleus of the vagus nerve → vagus nerve → Sinoatrial node

      iii. Assess the arrhythmia and check the blood pressure and mental status.
      iv. Instruct the surgeon to stop the manipulation.
      v. Avoid hypoxia and hypercapnia.
      vi. Consider treatment with an anticholinergic – atropine vs. glycopyrrolate.
      vii. If bradycardia is significant or persists, give epinephrine.

3. Intravascular injection
   a. Systemic toxicity is rare as the dose of local anesthetic used is very low.
   b. Intra-arterial injection can transiently increase brain levels, causing central nervous system excitation and seizures.

4. Intrathecal injection
   a. The optic nerve sheath is continuous with the subarachnoid space.
   b. A high spinal anesthetic can result in respiratory arrest, obtundation, and hemodynamic instability.

## KO Treatment Plan

Evaluate and intervene quickly in this situation. Regardless of the cause, the patient is not adequately ventilating. Airway, breathing, and circulation should be quickly addressed. The most likely cause of apnea in this patient is over-sedation, but as stated above there can be profound hemodynamic effects from the retrobulbar block. You will need to treat the patient while ruling out other less likely but significant problems.

## Pre-operative

1. Discuss the anesthetic plan with the surgeon.
   a. Topical anesthetic vs. regional block
   b. Level of sedation required
   c. Chance for extraocular muscle manipulation

2. Assess the need for general anesthesia.
   a. Inability to lie flat for prolonged periods
   b. Intractable cough
   c. Claustrophobia

3. Anticholinergic medications and emergency airway equipment should be readily available.
   a. Consider pretreatment with an anticholinergic in patients at higher risk for oculocardiac reflex.
   b. AV blocks
   c. Prone to vasovagal syncope
   d. Avoid anticholinergics and tachycardia in patients with underlying coronary artery disease.

4. Address the other comorbidities found in this elderly population.

## Intra-operative

1. Confirm apnea
   a. $ETCO_2$
   b. Pulse oximetry
   c. Observe respiratory effort.
   d. Listen to bilateral breath sounds.
   e. Mental status

2. Assess hemodynamics
   a. Blood pressure
   b. Heart rate
   c. Heart rhythm
   d. Carotid pulse

3. Treat
   a. Jaw thrust and chin lift

b. Stimulate the patient; instruct him to take a deep breath.

c. Bag mask ventilate

d. Consider the need for a laryngeal mask airway or endotracheal tube.

4. Communicate with the surgeon the need for airway manipulation.

5. Rule out seizure activity.

6. A high spinal will require a definitive airway with endotracheal intubation and supportive care.

## Bibliography

Butterworth JF, Mackey DC, Wasnick JD. *Morgan & Mikhail's Clinical*

*Anesthesiology*, 6th ed. New York: McGraw-Hill Education, 2018, p. 779.

Gropper MA. *Miller's Anesthesia*, 9th ed. Philadelphia: Elsevier, 2020, pp. 2194–209.

# Laser Safety

**105**

Aditya Reddy and Jessica A. Lovich-Sapola

## Sample Case

A 24-year-old male professional recording artist presents to an otolaryngologist with the complaint of hoarseness. On exam he was found to have vocal cord nodules and a laser laryngoscopy was scheduled. This patient has no significant medical history. His surgical history is significant for a tonsillectomy and adenoidectomy as a child under general anesthesia without any complications. What type of laser may be used? What safety precautions will be necessary in the operating room?

## Clinical Issues

Definition of laser: an acronym that stands for light amplification by stimulated emission of radiation.

## Indications for Laser Treatments

1. Vocal cord nodules and polyps
2. Malignant neoplasm: vocal cord cancers
3. Laryngoceles and benign cyst in the laryngoceles
4. Recurrent respiratory papillomatosis
5. Subglottic hemangioma
6. Laryngomalacia
7. Congenital and acquired anterior glottic webs
8. Subglottic and glottic stenosis
9. Condyloma acuminatum of external genitalia and urethra
10. Ureteral stricture or bladder neck contracture
11. Carcinoma of the penis, bladder, ureter, and renal pelvis
12. Laser resurfacing for facial cosmetic procedures (such as perioral and periorbital creases and wrinkles)
13. Laser ablation of endometriosis
14. Coagulation of small or superficial blood vessels

## Different Types of Medical Lasers and Their Specific Applications

1. Argon laser
   a. It is absorbed by hemoglobin.
   b. It has a modest tissue penetration of 0.05–2 mm.
   c. It provides the ability to penetrate skin or ocular structures and selectively coagulate vascular or pigmented regions.
   d. It is mainly used in ophthalmologic and dermatologic procedures.

2. Potassium–titanyl–phosphate (KPT) or yttrium–aluminum–garnet (YAG) laser
   a. Absorbed by hemoglobin
   b. Has a penetration similar to an argon laser

3. Neodymium-doped yttrium–aluminum–garnet (Nd-YAG) laser
   a. Very powerful
   b. Tissue penetration of 2–6 mm
   c. It can be used for tumor debulking – particularly the upper airway, trachea, and mainstem bronchi.

4. Carbon dioxide ($CO_2$) laser
   a. Very little tissue penetration
   b. Best precision
   c. Can be used for cutting
   d. It is absorbed by water; hence, minimal heat is dispersed to the surrounding tissues.
   e. It is primarily used for procedures in the oropharynx and around the vocal cords.

5. Helium–neon (He-Ne) laser
   a. Produces an intense red light
   b. Used for aiming $CO_2$ and Nd-YAG lasers
   c. It has very low power and will not cause any significant damage.

6. Ruby laser
   a. Primarily used for tattoo and nevi removal
   b. Absorbed well only by cells containing dark pigment

7. Direct diode laser
   a. Primarily used for hair removal
   b. Diodes emit infrared laser light at 800–810 nm.
   c. Longer wavelength than ruby laser but less than Nd-YAG

## Complications and Hazards of Laser Surgery

1. Vaporization of tissue by lasers can produce a plume of smoke and fine particulates that can be deposited in lungs.
   a. Viral DNA has been detected in smoke from condylomas and skin warts.
   b. Viable bacteria
   c. Environmental toxins

2. Perforation of larger blood vessels that are not coagulable by the laser
3. Laser-induced pneumothorax: after laryngeal procedures
4. Venous gas embolism: especially with Nd-YAG lasers during hysteroscopic surgery
5. Corneal injury: $CO_2$ lasers
6. Retinal injury: argon, KTP, Nd-YAG, diode, and ruby laser
7. Thermal injury to the skin
8. Surgical fires

## Anesthetic Technique/Management for Laser Surgery

1. The most effective way to prevent operating room personnel from exposure to the viral and chemical content of the laser plume is to use a smoke evacuation system, with the suction held close to the tissue being vaporized.

    a. In addition, operating room personnel should wear gloves and high-efficiency filter masks.

2. The operating room staff and the patient should have proper eye protection during laser surgery.

    a. Safety goggles or lenses specific for the laser in use
    b. Protective covers over the patient's eyes

3. One of the major caveats during laser surgery (laryngoscopy) is to supply a gas mixture with the lowest potential for combustion.

    a. Ideally the lowest inspired oxygen concentration required to safely oxygenate the patient should be used.
    b. The ideal mixture would be air and oxygen or helium and oxygen.

**TKO:** Remember, nitrous oxide ($N_2O$) is as combustible as oxygen.

4. Total intravenous anesthesia (TIVA) is preferred because volatile anesthetics can potentially decompose into toxic compounds when exposed to airway fires.

    a. Modern volatile anesthetics are nonflammable and nonexplosive.

5. Use a laser-resistant endotracheal tube.

    a. Traditional endotracheal tubes

        i. Polyvinyl chloride (PVC)

            (1) Inexpensive and nonreflective
            (2) Low melting point and highly combustible

        ii. Silicone rubber

            (1) Nonreflective
            (2) Combustible and turns into toxic ash with fire

        iii. Red rubber

            (1) Puncture resistant and nonreflective
            (2) Highly combustible

    b. Metal endotracheal tubes

        i. Combustion and kink resistant
        ii. Cumbersome, flammable cuff; transfers heat and reflects the laser
        iii. Types

            (1) Bivona Fome-Cuff

                (a) Aluminum spiral tube with a silicone polyurethane foam cuff in a silicone envelope
                (b) Recommended for use with $CO_2$ lasers
                (c) The foam part of the cuff is self-inflating and remains inflated if the envelope ruptures.
                (d) High incidence of sore throat

            (2) Xomed Laser-Shield

                (a) Silicone elastomer tube containing metallic powder
                (b) To be used with $CO_2$ lasers only
                (c) Risk of perforation and fragmentation into silica ash

            (3) Mallinckrodt Laser-Flex

                (a) Airtight stainless steel, spiral wound endotracheal tube
                (b) It has two separate PVC cuffs.

                    (i) The cuffs should be filled with colored saline.
                    (ii) Recommended for $CO_2$, KTP, and Nd-YAG lasers (not the original YAG laser)

    c. Wrapped endotracheal tubes

        i. Aluminum foil, copper foil, or a thinly metal-coated plastic tape
        ii. Disadvantages

            (1) No cuff protection
            (2) Adds thickness to the endotracheal tube
            (3) Not FDA-approved
            (4) Reflective
            (5) Rough edges may damage the mucosa.

6. Inflate the endotracheal tube cuff with water or saline (+ methylene blue to facilitate leak detection).

## Airway Fire Prevention

1. Avoid ignition sources near oxygen-enriched atmosphere.
2. Configure the drapes to minimize oxygen accumulation.

3. Allow sufficient time for flammable skin preps to dry.
4. Moisten sponges and gauze when used near the ignition source.

## Treatment Plan for Airway Fires

In case of an airway fire, the surgeon (usually the first person to recognize an airway fire) and anesthesiologist must act quickly, decisively, and in a coordinated fashion. The following steps must be taken:

1. Remove the source of the fire.
2. Stop ventilation by disconnecting the breathing circuit from the anesthesia machine and turning off the oxygen flowmeters.
3. Remove the object on fire (usually the endotracheal tube).
4. Sterile water or saline should be poured on the fire.
5. If the fire is not immediately extinguished with water, use a carbon dioxide fire extinguisher.

   a. Close the operating room doors.
   b. Activate the fire alarm.
   c. Turn off medical gas supply to the operating room.

6. Ventilation with 100% oxygen should be provided by mask.

   a. Stop all volatile anesthetics.
   b. Continue IV anesthetics.

7. Direct laryngoscopy and rigid bronchoscopy should be performed to examine the airway and remove any debris if present.
8. Reintubate if needed.
9. Evaluate the face and oropharynx.
10. Chest X-ray
11. Distal fiber-optic bronchoscopy as needed
12. Severe damage may require a low tracheostomy.
13. Consider steroids.

## Treatment of a Nonairway Fire

1. Stop the flow of all airway gases.
2. Remove the drapes and all burning and flammable materials.
3. Pour saline on the fire.
4. Extinguish the fire by other means if necessary if saline does not work.

   a. Carbon dioxide fire extinguisher

5. Activate the fire alarm.
6. Evacuate the patient.
7. Close the OR doors.
8. Turn off gas supply to the room.

## KO Treatment Plan

### Pre-operative

1. The $CO_2$ laser is widely used for vocal cord surgery since it can precisely vaporize superficial tissue.
2. The patient's eyes must be protected with moistened gauze and taped.
3. All of the operating room personnel must wear protective goggles.
4. The laser should always be placed in "standby" mode when not in use.

### Intra-operative

1. Induction of anesthesia should be performed in a standard manner.

   a. Standard ASA monitors
   b. IV propofol can be used as an induction agent because of its rapid onset and short duration of action.
   c. Rocuronium is a good choice for muscle relaxation since it is very important that the vocal cords must remain motionless during laser surgery.

2. A smaller-diameter, laser-safe endotracheal tube (Mallinckrodt Laser-Flex) should be placed to facilitate visualization of the larynx and vocal cords.
3. Place methylene blue-dyed normal saline in the endotracheal tube cuff(s).

   a. This will help the surgeon to identify if he or she has ruptured the cuff with the laser.

4. Use the lowest possible $FiO_2$ (<0.3–0.4) and avoid nitrous oxide.

   a. Both oxygen and nitrous oxide support combustion.

5. Maintenance of anesthesia

   a. TIVA

      i. Propofol and remifentanil infusion
      ii. Especially useful with jet ventilation and/or intermittent apnea techniques

   b. When the endotracheal tube is used for the entire case, then volatile anesthetic gases may be used in addition to the propofol and remifentanil infusions.

### Post-operative

1. Be vigilant for complications resulting from laser use.

   a. Eye trauma
   b. Airway compromise
   c. Esophageal perforation
   d. Pneumothorax/mediastinal air: may present as hypotension and cardiovascular collapse

## Bibliography

Apfelbaum JL, Practice advisory for the prevention and management of operating room fires: an updated report by the American Society of Anesthesiologists Task Force on Operating Room Fires. *Anesthesiology* 2013;**118**:271–90.

Barash PG, Cullen BF, Stoelting RK, et al. *Clinical Anesthesia*, 8th ed. Philadelphia: Lippincott Williams & Wilkins, 2017, pp. 131–3, 1367–8.

Butterworth JF, Mackey DC, Wasnick JD. *Morgan & Mikhail's Clinical Anesthesiology*, 6th ed. New York: McGraw-Hill Education, 2018, pp. 22–5.

Faust JR, Cucchiara RF, Rose SH, et al. *Faust's Anesthesiology Review*, 3rd ed. Philadelphia: Churchill Livingstone, 2002, pp. 250–1.

Groper MA. *Miller's Anesthesia*, 9th ed. Philadelphia: Elsevier, 2020, p. 2278.

Jaffe AR, Samuels IS. *Anesthesiologist's Manual of Surgical Procedures*, 3rd ed. Philadelphia: Lippincott Williams & Wilkins, 2004, pp. 150, 235–8, 434, 606–8, 685, 882, 962.

Reed PA, Yudkowitz SF. *Clinical Cases in Anesthesia*, 3rd ed. Philadelphia: Churchill Livingstone, 2005, pp. 265–8.

# Chapter 106

# Electrical Safety in the Operating Room

Kristen Oswald and Jessica A. Lovich-Sapola

## Sample Case

A broken equipment ground wire produces 0.1 milliamperes (mA) of leakage current. This current ultimately conducts through an indwelling right ventricular catheter of a patient undergoing coronary artery bypass graft surgery and causes ventricular fibrillation. Is this an example of microshock or macroshock? How could it have been prevented?

## Clinical Issues

### Principles of Electricity

Ohm's law: $E = I \times R$

**E** = electrical force (volts)

**I** = current (ampere)

**R** = resistance (ohms)

### Understanding Electrical Power Systems

1. Electrical utilities provide power to homes and hospitals that is grounded.
2. An isolation transformer converts the grounded power on the primary side from the main power source to an ungrounded power system on the secondary side of the transformer.
3. This ungrounded electrical service is called an isolated power system (IPS).

### The Line Isolation Monitor

1. The line isolation monitor (LIM) continuously monitors the integrity of the IPS to ensure that it is isolated from ground.
2. Leakage current degrades the integrity of isolation and can be from faulty electrical equipment or from several pieces of normal functioning equipment.
3. The LIM meter indicates in milliamperes (mA) the total amount of leakage current in the system.
4. The reading on the LIM is the amount of current that would flow in the event of a first fault. A second fault is required to create a dangerous situation (Fig. 106.1).
5. If the set limit of 2 mA (older systems) or 5 mA (newer systems) is exceeded, visual and audio alarms are triggered.

6. This alarm is not useful for leakage currents in the microshock range.

## Ground Fault Circuit Interrupter

1. This is a circuit breaker used to prevent electrical shock in a grounded power system.
2. A ground fault circuit interrupter (GFCI) monitors for changes in the equality of current flow within a grounded power system. It is able to detect very small current changes.
3. Imbalance of current flow may be created if an individual contacts faulty equipment. The GFCI will detect the change and will interrupt current flow to the faulty equipment and prevent a shock.
4. GFCI are rarely used in the operating room setting due to the risk of sudden interruption of power to life-saving equipment.
5. When in use in the operating room, only one outlet should be protected by each GFCI to prevent the potential interruption of electrical current flow to multiple pieces of equipment.
6. GFCI are commonly used in residential homes.

## Electrical Concepts and Considerations for the Operating Room

1. A conductor is any substance that permits the flow of electrons.
2. Direct current (DC) is characterized by electrons always flowing in the same direction.
3. Alternating current (AC) is characterized by electron flow that reverses direction at regular intervals or oscillates.
4. Impedance is the sum of forces that oppose electron flow in an AC circuit.

    a. The current flow is inversely proportional to the impedance.

    b. A short circuit occurs when there is zero impedance and a very high current flow.

5. Capacitance is the measure of a substance's ability to store charge.

    a. The capacitance of electrical equipment and AC wiring in the operating room contribute to the total amount of leakage current.

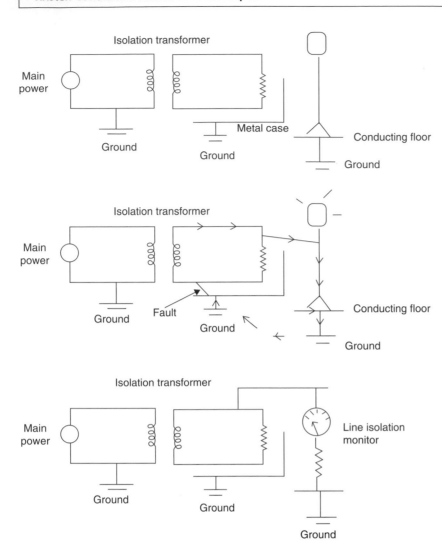

**Figure 106.1** (a) No electric shock occurs if an isolated power line is touched. (b) An electric shock does occur if a faulted secondary power line is touched. (c) A line isolation monitor can watch for a fault. Source: This figure was published in *Anesthesia*, 6th ed., RD Miller, LA Fleisher, RA Johns, et al., Page 3142, Copyright Elsevier (2005). Adapted with permission.

6. Current density is the amount of current that is applied per unit area of tissue.

   a. A smaller-caliber catheter has a higher current density and requires a lower amount of current to cause fibrillation.

7. Inductance refers to a property of AC circuits in which an opposing electromagnetic field is generated in the circuit.

## Electrical Shock

1. An electrical accident or shock occurs when an individual completes an electrical circuit by making two points of contact along the circuit, and a source causes current to flow through the individual.
2. Shock severity is determined by the amount of current and the duration of current flow (Table 106.1).
3. Macroshock is a large amount of current (≥1 mA) applied to the surface of the body.
4. Microshock is a small amount of current (0.05–0.1 mA) and is only a risk for an electrically susceptible patient.
5. Electrical susceptibility is defined by the presence of an external conduit with a direct connection to the heart.

   a. Intracavity or epicardial pacemaker wires
   b. Indwelling saline-filled catheters such as a central venous or pulmonary artery catheters

      i. Never touch an electrical device and a saline-filled central catheter and external pacing wires at the same time.
      ii. When handling central venous or pulmonary or pacing wires, insulate oneself by wearing rubber gloves.

6. Microshock may cause cardiac dysrhythmias including ventricular fibrillation.
7. National code requires less than 0.01 mA maximum permissible leakage through electrodes or catheters that directly contact the heart.

## Electrosurgery

1. An electrosurgery unit (ESU) works by generating very high-frequency currents from 500,000 to 1 million Hz.
2. Heat is created as tissue resists the passage of current flow and this produces the therapeutic cut or coagulation function.

**Table 106.1** Effects of 60 Hz AC current on an average human for 1 second duration of contact

| Current (milliamperes, mA) | Event | Shock level |
|---|---|---|
| 0.01 mA | Maximum recommended 60 Hz leakage current | Microshock |
| 0.1 mA | Ventricular fibrillation | Microshock |
| 1 mA | Threshold of perception | Macroshock |
| 5 mA | Maximum harmless current intensity | Macroshock |
| 10–20 mA | "Let go" value exceeded; sustained muscle contraction next | Macroshock |
| 50 mA | Pain, exhaustion, mechanical injury, possible fainting, cardiorespiratory functions continue | Macroshock |
| 100–300 mA | Ventricular fibrillation, respiratory center intact | Macroshock |
| >6000 mA | Sustained myocardial contraction followed by normal rhythm, transient respiratory center paralysis, burns when current density >100 mA/cm$^2$ | Macroshock |

Adapted from Barash PG, Cullen BF, Stoelting RK, et al. *Clinical Anesthesia*, 8th ed. Philadelphia: Lippincott Williams & Wilkins, 2017, pp. 333–4.

3. Current from the ESU is concentrated at the ESU tip, where it produces an effect on the tissue, then it passes through the patient to a dispersive electrode and ultimately returns to the ESU.

4. An improperly applied dispersive electrode or a compromised dispersive electrode cord can be sources of injury to the patient.

   a. Burns result when the surface area of the return site or alternate return site is less than the dispersive electrode pad due to the increase in current density.

5. Low-frequency (50–60 Hz) "stray current" from the ESU can cause ventricular fibrillation when used near the heart or when the patient has a central venous or pulmonary catheter present.

## Case Discussion

1. The sample case is an example of a microshock.

   a. A small current leak, such as 0.1 mA, can cause a microshock in a susceptible patient, such as this patient with a direct central access to the right ventricle via the catheter.

   b. This current is sufficient to cause ventricular fibrillation.

   c. Prompt recognition of the problem and early removal of the catheter causing the fibrillation can facilitate more effective resuscitation intra-operatively.

2. Prevention of current leakage pre-operatively is the key to avoiding this adverse event.

## KO Treatment Plan

### Pre-operative

1. Understand the structure, function, and safety features of the electrical power system of the operating room.

2. Inspect operating room equipment for signs of damage or compromise in structure. Ensure that electrical cords are intact and free from compression.

3. Confirm regular maintenance of operating room equipment.

### Intra-operative

1. If the LIM alarm sounds, each piece of electrical equipment should be unplugged one at a time, starting with the most recently plugged in, until the faulty piece of equipment is identified.

2. A vital piece of life-support equipment can continue to be used safely.

3. No other electrical equipment should be connected for the remainder of the case or until the faulty equipment has been removed from the operating room.

4. Make sure the dispersive electrode is placed properly on the patient if ESU is used.

   a. The dispersive electrode should be rechecked during long cases and should be replaced if necessary.

5. Emergency equipment should be immediately available in case of an electrical shock or fire.

## Bibliography

Barash PG, Cullen BF, Stoelting RK, et al. *Clinical Anesthesia*, 8th ed. Philadelphia: Lippincott Williams & Wilkins, 2017, pp. 109–37.

Butterworth JF, Mackey DC, Wasnick JD. *Morgan & Mikhail's Clinical Anesthesiology*, 6th ed. New York: McGraw-Hill Education, 2018, pp. 17–25.

Faust JR, Cucchiara RF, Rose SH, et al. *Faust's Anesthesiology Review*, 3rd ed.

Philadelphia: Churchill Livingstone, 2002, pp 247–9.

Hensley FA, Martin DE, Gravlee GP. *A Practical Approach to Cardiac Anesthesia*, 4th ed. Philadelphia: Lippincott Williams & Wilkins, 2008, pp. 138–40.

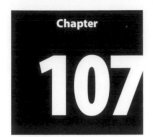

# Ethics

Maureen Harders and Jessica A. Lovich-Sapola

## Clinical Issues

### Definitions

1.  Informed consent
    a.  The cornerstone of the patient–physician relationship
    b.  It is a legal condition whereby a person gives consent based upon an appreciation and understanding of the facts, implications, and future consequences of an action.
    c.  The person must have adequate reasoning faculties and be in possession of all of the relevant facts at the time that consent is given.
    d.  The goal is to maximize the ability of the patient to make substantially autonomous informed decisions.
    e.  It is unreasonable to expect a patient with no prior medical training to be fully informed.
    f.  Autonomy: the ability to choose without controlling interferences by others and without personal limitations
    g.  Informed consent does not prevent legal liability when an adverse event occurs.

2.  Competence
    a.  Legal determination
    b.  Several elements are required to demonstrate competence
        i.   Understanding and appreciation of their medical situation and the consequences of their choices
        ii.  Demonstration of reasoning in their thoughts
        iii. Evidence of their awareness that they have a choice

3.  Capacity
    a.  Necessary skills to participate in medical decision-making

4.  Negligence
    a.  Conduct that is culpable because it falls short of what a reasonable person would do to protect another individual from a foreseeable risk of harm
    b.  May occur if the anesthesiologist provides a disclosure that is insufficient to allow a patient to make an informed decision and an injury subsequently occurs, even if the injury was foreseeable and in the absence of medical error

5.  Causation
    a.  The causal relationship between conduct and the result
    b.  Assesses whether the omitted information would have caused the patient to choose a different option.

6.  Disclosure
    a.  Exception to the obligation of full disclosure occurs with emergencies and situations of therapeutic privilege.

### Malpractice Suit

The patient must prove all four of the following:

1.  Duty: the anesthesiologist owed the patient a duty.
2.  Breach of duty: the anesthesiologist failed to fulfill his or her duty.
3.  Causation: a reasonably close causal relation exists between the anesthesiologist's actions and the resultant injury.
4.  Damages: the actual damage resulted because of the breach of the standard of care.

### Do Not Resuscitate Order

1.  A competent patient has the right to refuse life-sustaining medical treatment.
2.  All do not resuscitate (DNR) orders should be reevaluated and discussed with the patient or their surrogate pre-operatively in light of the surgical and anesthetic options. The discussion and decision reached should be well documented.
    a.  A DNR order is not automatically suspended in the peri-operative setting.
    b.  Determine the patient's goals regarding surgery and resuscitation.
    c.  Establish exactly what is meant by "resuscitation" in contrast to routine anesthetic care.
    d.  Educate the patient on the risks and benefits of resuscitation in the operating room.
    e.  Document the agreements reached.
        i.   Intubation
        ii.  Vasoactive medications
        iii. Chest compression
        iv.  Cardioversion

3. DNR orders may be modified to meet the individual patient's wishes.
    a. Full attempt at resuscitation
    b. Limited attempt at resuscitation regarding certain procedures
    c. Limited attempt at resuscitation regarding patient goals and values

## Organ Procurement

1. Brain death
    a. The irreversible end of all brain activity, including involuntary activity necessary to sustain life, due to total necrosis of the cerebral neurons following a loss of blood or oxygenation
    b. The patient has no clinical evidence of brain function upon physical examination.
        i. No response to pain
        ii. No cranial nerve reflexes: pupillary response, oculocephalic reflex, corneal reflex
        iii. No spontaneous respirations
    c. Before an official diagnosis of brain death can be made, conditions that mimic brain death must be ruled out.
        i. Barbiturate intoxication
        ii. Alcohol intoxication
        iii. Sedative overdose
        iv. Hypothermia
        v. Hypoglycemia
        vi. Coma
        vii. Chronic vegetative states
    d. Brain death is declared using neurologic criteria, prior to the patient's being taken to the operating room.
        i. Requires a neurologic exam by two independent physicians
        ii. The exam must show a complete absence of brain function.
        iii. The exam may include two isoelectric EEGs 24 hours apart, but this is not mandatory.
        iv. The patient must have a normal temperature and be free of any medications that can suppress brain activity.
        v. A radionuclide cerebral blood flow scan that shows the absence of intracranial blood flow can be used to confirm the diagnosis.
    e. The nonliving donor is kept on ventilator support until the organs have been surgically removed.

2. A more controversial topic is organ donation after cardiac death (DCD).
    a. Cardiac death
        i. Death declared on the basis of cardiopulmonary criteria
        ii. Irreversible cessation of circulatory and respiratory function
        iii. It is determined that the patient has no significant likelihood for survival after the withdrawal of life support.
    b. Examples
        i. Nonrecoverable and irreversible neurologic injury resulting in ventilator dependency but not fulfilling the brain death criteria
        ii. End-stage musculoskeletal disease, pulmonary disease, and high spinal cord injury
    c. Protocol
        i. A suitable candidate is selected.
        ii. Consent is obtained from the next of kin to withdraw care and retrieve the organs.
        iii. Life-sustaining measures are withdrawn under controlled circumstances in the ICU or operating room.
        iv. When the donor meets the criteria for cardiac death, a physician pronounces the patient as dead. This physician can in no way be associated with the organ procurement due to the obvious conflict of interest.
        v. The time from the onset of asystole to the declaration of death is usually 2–5 minutes.
        vi. The organs, kidneys, liver, pancreas, lungs, and in some rare cases the heart, are recovered.
        vii. If a patient does not die quickly enough to permit the recovery of organs, end-of-life care continues and any planned donation is canceled. This occurs in 20% of cases.
    d. This technique increases the number of organs available for donation.

## Refusal to Provide Care

1. Anesthesiologists may refuse to provide care when they ethically or morally disagree with the procedure, such as an elective abortion.
2. Anesthesiologists are obligated to make a reasonable effort to find a competent, willing replacement.
3. They may also refuse to provide care if they are not qualified to provide the needed care.
4. An anesthesiologist cannot refuse care based on gender, race, or disease status.

## Jehovah's Witness

1. Current doctrine
    a. Blood is sacred to God.
    b. Blood must not be eaten or transfused.

c. Blood that leaves the human body must be disposed of.

d. Therefore, the patient refuses blood products based on his or her religious beliefs.

2. Prohibited blood products
   a. Red blood cells: allogenic and autologous
   b. White blood cells
   c. Platelets
   d. Blood plasma

3. Usually accepted techniques
   a. Hemodilution therapy
   b. Intra-operative blood salvage
   c. Cardiopulmonary bypass
   d. Dialysis
   e. Epidural blood patch
   f. Plasmapheresis
   g. Blood labeling or tagging

4. Most accept synthetic colloid solutions, dextran, erythropoietin, and iron supplementation.

5. A court order can be obtained for a minor to receive blood products, even if the parents refuse.

## Emancipated Minor

1. A legal mechanism by which a child is freed from control by his or her parents/guardians, and the parents/guardians are free from any and all responsibility to the child

2. Patients less than 18 years old who have been given the global right to make their own health care decisions

3. Circumstances under which a person can become emancipated
   a. Marriage
   b. Having a child of his or her own
   c. Enlisted in the military
   d. Court order from a judge

4. Pregnancy does not necessarily qualify one as an emancipated minor.

## Sample Case 1

A 46-year-old male had an epidural placed for post-operative pain relief after a radical cystectomy. The epidural was discontinued earlier this morning. You are called to see the patient for progressive bilateral lower extremity motor and sensory loss. You immediately begin testing to rule out an epidural hematoma or abscess. The patient tells you that your colleague never warned him of these potential risks. What do you say?

## KO Treatment Plan

These are never easy situations. The best approach is to talk openly and honestly with the patient. Tell the patient that while you are not sure what was discussed earlier with your colleague, you plan on doing everything to diagnose the current situation and prevent further progression of his symptoms. Do not say anything bad about your fellow physician. In the event of an ethical dilemma that is beyond your scope of practice, consult the hospital ethics service. The ethics committee will act in an advisory role to resolve the ethical dilemma.

## Sample Case 2

Two weeks ago you were involved in a large trauma case during which 17 units of blood were given. The patient is currently doing well. She has been discharged to the rehabilitation site. The blood bank calls to notify you that one of the units of red blood cells that were given was crossed to a different patient. Do you tell the patient? If so, what do you tell the patient?

## KO Treatment Plan

It is your responsibility to notify the patient, despite the fact that no complications occurred. It would be appropriate to consult your legal department prior to the conversation and have a representative from the blood bank present to help answer any questions. It is never a good idea to lie or try to cover up information.

## Bibliography

American Society of Anesthesiologists. Ethical guidelines for the anesthesia care of patients with do-not-resuscitate orders or other directives that limit treatment.

Developed by: Committee on Ethics. Reaffirmed: October 17, 2018 (original approval October 17, 2001).

Barash PG, Cullen BF, Stoelting RK, et al. *Clinical Anesthesia*, 8th ed. Philadelphia:

Lippincott Williams & Wilkins, 2017, pp. 1662–3.

Gropper MA. *Miller's Anesthesia*, 9th ed. Philadelphia: Elsevier, 2020, pp. 231–47.

# Index